JAYPEE — The Health Sciences Publisher

emedicine360.com

Register

- Visit emedicine360.com
- Click "Sign Up"
- Fill in your user information
- Click "Create Account"

Activate Your Book

- Scratch off your 'Activation Code' on this page below
- Login into portal to redeem the 'Activation Code' for accessing the digital copy of the book
- Click the "Redeem" button present below the book cover image and title, from the portal
  (Note: You need to ensure that the book title on the portal matches with that of physical copy)
- Enter the 'Activation Code' into the "Discount Code - Enter your coupon code here" section
- Click "Redeem Code" and then Click on "Checkout" button
- You will be directed to the 'Checkout' page where you need to confirm billing address details
- Click "Continue" button
- Next on 'Payment Method' and 'Payment Information' sections, click "Continue" button
  (Note: You will not be charged anything here as you will get free access to digital copy of the book using the 'Activation Code')
- Click "Confirm" and click "Continue" button on the order completion/Thank you page
- The book will get added to your "My Library" page from where you can access the same

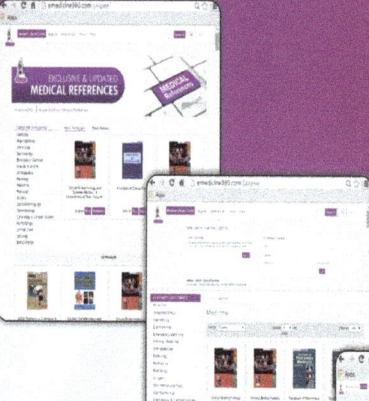

Scratch

Activation Code

For assistance
email: helpdesk@emedicine360.com

FAQs
on Vaccines and Immunization Practices

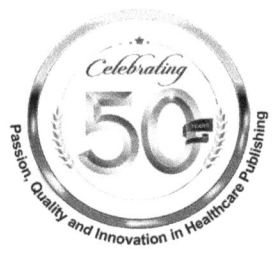

FAQs
on Vaccines and Immunization Practices

3rd Edition

Chief Editor

Vipin M Vashishtha
MD FIAP
Director and Consultant Pediatrician
Mangla Hospital and Research Center
Bijnor, Uttar Pradesh, India

Editor

Ajay Kalra
MD DCH MNAMS FIAP
Erstwhile Professor
Department of Pediatrics
SN Medical College
Agra, Uttar Pradesh, India

Foreword

Walter A Orenstein

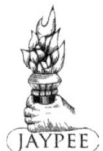

JAYPEE BROTHERS MEDICAL PUBLISHERS
The Health Sciences Publisher
New Delhi | London

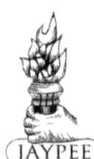 **Jaypee Brothers Medical Publishers (P) Ltd**

Headquarters

Jaypee Brothers Medical Publishers (P) Ltd
EMCA House, 23/23-B, Ansari Road
Daryaganj, New Delhi 110 002, India
Landline: +91-11-23272143, +91-11-23272703
+91-11-23282021, +91-11-23245672
Email: jaypee@jaypeebrothers.com

Corporate Office

Jaypee Brothers Medical Publishers (P) Ltd
4838/24, Ansari Road, Daryaganj
New Delhi 110 002, India
Phone: +91-11-43574357
Fax: +91-11-43574314
Email: jaypee@jaypeebrothers.com

Overseas Office

J.P. Medical Ltd
83, Victoria Street, London
SW1H 0HW (UK)
Phone: +44 20 3170 8910
Fax: +44 (0)20 3008 6180
Email: info@jpmedpub.com

Website: www.jaypeebrothers.com
Website: www.jaypeedigital.com

© 2021, Jaypee Brothers Medical Publishers

The views and opinions expressed in this book are solely those of the original contributor(s)/author(s) and do not necessarily represent those of editor(s) of the book.

All rights reserved. No part of this publication may be reproduced, stored or transmitted in any form or by any means, electronic, mechanical, photocopying, recording or otherwise, without the prior permission in writing of the publishers.

All brand names and product names used in this book are trade names, service marks, trademarks or registered trademarks of their respective owners. The publisher is not associated with any product or vendor mentioned in this book.

Medical knowledge and practice change constantly. This book is designed to provide accurate, authoritative information about the subject matter in question. However, readers are advised to check the most current information available on procedures included and check information from the manufacturer of each product to be administered, to verify the recommended dose, formula, method and duration of administration, adverse effects and contraindications. It is the responsibility of the practitioner to take all appropriate safety precautions. Neither the publisher nor the author(s)/editor(s) assume any liability for any injury and/or damage to persons or property arising from or related to use of material in this book.

This book is sold on the understanding that the publisher is not engaged in providing professional medical services. If such advice or services are required, the services of a competent medical professional should be sought.

Every effort has been made where necessary to contact holders of copyright to obtain permission to reproduce copyright material. If any have been inadvertently overlooked, the publisher will be pleased to make the necessary arrangements at the first opportunity. The **CD/DVD-ROM** (if any) provided in the sealed envelope with this book is complimentary and free of cost. **Not meant for sale.**

Inquiries for bulk sales may be solicited at: jaypee@jaypeebrothers.com

FAQs on Vaccines and Immunization Practices

First Edition: 2011
Second Edition: 2015
Third Edition: **2021**

ISBN: 978-93-90020-60-7

Contributors

A Parthasarathy
MD DCH DSc (Hon) FIAP
Senior Consultant Pediatrician
AP Child Care, Chennai
Former Distinguished Professor
Department of Pediatrics
The Tamil Nadu Dr MGR
Medical University
Retired Senior Clinical Professor
Department of Pediatrics
Madras Medical College, Chennai
Deputy Superintendent
Institute of Child Health and
Hospital for Children
Chennai, Tamil Nadu, India

Aashay A Shah MD (Ped)
Fellow, Pediatric Gastroenterology
Hepatology and Nutrition
Medanta—The Medicity
Gurugram, Haryana, India

Abhay K Shah
MBBS (Gold Medalist) MD (Gold Medalist)
DPed (UNI FIRST) FIAP
Senior Pediatrician and Infectious
Diseases Specialist, Ahmedabad
Director, Children Hospital and
Neonatal Center
Ahmedabad, Gujarat, India
Member ACVIP 2020-2021, 2018-19
Chairperson Infectious Diseases
Chapter of IAP 2015

Adarsh Bansal MPH PhD(c)
Project Officer
Department of Community
Medicine and School of
Public Health
Postgraduate Institute of
Medical Education and Research
Chandigarh, India

Ajay Kalra MD DCH MNAMS FIAP
Erstwhile Professor
Department of Pediatrics
SN Medical College
Agra, Uttar Pradesh, India

Arun Wadhwa MD (Ped)
Visiting Consultant
Rainbow Children's Hospital
New Delhi, India

Ashok K Banga MD (Ped)
Director and Consultant
Department of Pediatrics
Chirayu and Astha Hospitals
Gwalior, Madhya Pradesh, India

Ashok K Dutta MD (Ped)
Former Director Professor and Head
Department of Pediatrics
Lady Hardinge Medical College
New Delhi, India

Atul Kumar Agarwal MD FIAP
Consultant Pediatrician
Department of Pediatrics
Atul Latika Hospital
Bareilly, Uttar Pradesh, India

Baldev S Prajapati
MD DPed FIAP MNAMS
Professor and Head
Department of Pediatrics
GCS Medical College Hospital and
Research Center, Ahmedabad
Aakanksha Children Hospital and
Postgraduate Institute
Ahmedabad, Gujarat, India

Canna Jagdish Ghia MD
Therapy Lead
Department of Medical Affairs
Pfizer Vaccines
Mumbai, Maharashtra, India

Contributors

Chandra Mohan Kumar
MD PGDAP MAMS
Additional Professor
Department of Pediatrics
All India Institute of Medical Sciences
Patna, Bihar, India

Chandrakant Lahariya MBBS MD
MBA Diplomate of Nat Board PGDHHM
FICMCH FIPHA MNAMS
Senior Public Health Specialist and
National Professional Officer
Department of Health Systems
Design and Development
World Health Organization (WHO)
Country Office for India
New Delhi, India

CP Bansal MD (Ped)
Consultant Pediatrician and
Director, Department of Pediatrics
Shabda-Pratap Hospital
Gwalior, Madhya Pradesh, India

Dewesh Kumar MD DNB MPS
Assistant Professor
Department of Preventive and
Social Medicine, Rajendra Institute
of Medical Sciences
Ranchi, Jharkhand, India

Dhanya Dharmapalan MBBS MD
Consultant in
Pediatric Infectious Diseases
Apollo Hospitals
Navi Mumbai, Maharashtra, India

Digant D Shastri
MD (Ped) FIAP PGDHHM
Senior Consultant Pediatrician
Killol Children Hospital
Surat, Gujarat, India
Immediate Past President, Indian
Academy of Paediatrics
Member, Standing Committee
International Paediatric Association
2019-21

Managing Editor, Asia Pacific
Journal of Pediatrics and
Child Health

Dipti Agarwal MD (Ped) MAMS
Associate Professor
Department of Pediatrics
Dr Ram Manohar Lohia Institute
and Medical Sciences
Lucknow, Uttar Pradesh, India

Gautam Rambhad MD
India Vaccines Medical Lead
Department of Medical Affairs
Pfizer Vaccines
Mumbai, Maharashtra, India

Geeta MG MD (Ped)
Additional Professor
Department of Pediatrics
Medical College
PSG FRI FAIMER Fellow 2015
Calicut, Kerala, India

Harish K Pemde MD (Ped) FIAP
Director-Professor
Department of Pediatrics
Lady Hardinge Medical College and
Kalawati Saran Children's Hospital
New Delhi, India

Hitt Sharma MBBS MBA
Additional Director
Department of Clinical Research
and Pharmacovigilance
Serum Institute of India Pvt Ltd
Pune, Maharashtra, India

Jaydeep Choudhury
MBBS DNB (Ped) MNAMS FIAP
Professor
Department of Pediatrics
Institute of Child Health
Kolkata, West Bengal, India

Sachidanand Kamath MD (Ped)
Senior Consultant Pediatrician
Department of Pediatrics
Indira Gandhi Co-operative Hospital
Ernakulam, Kerala, India

M Surendranath MD DCH FACI
Head, Department of Pediatrics
Vijay Marie Hospital
Hyderabad, Telangana, India

Madhu Gupta MD PhD
Professor, Department of
Community Medicine and
School of Public Health
Postgraduate Institute of
Medical Education and Research
Chandigarh, India

Meeta Dhaval Vashi MBBS MD (PSM)
Surveillance Medical Officer
WHO
Mumbai, Maharashtra, India

Naveen Thacker MD FIAP
Director
Deep Children Hospital and
Research Center
Gandhidham, Gujarat, India

Neha Goel MD
Resident, Department of Pediatrics
Vardhaman Mahavir Medical
College and Safdarjung Hospital
New Delhi, India

Nigam P Narain
MD DCH PhD MRCP (UK) FRCPCH (UK)
FIAP FNNF
Retired Professor and Head
Department of Pediatrics
Patna Medical College
Patna, Bihar, India

Nupur Ganguly MBBS DCH DNB FIAP
Professor
Department of Pediatric Medicine
Institute of Child Health
Kolkata, West Bengal, India

Obeid Shafi
MD Diplomate of American
Board of Pediatrics
Specialist, Department of Pediatrics
Manipal Hospital, New Delhi, India

Omesh Kumar Bharti
MBBS DHM MAE (Epidemiology)
State Epidemiologist
State Institute of Health and
Family Welfare, Parimahal
Department of Health and
Family Welfare
Government of Himachal Pradesh
Shimla, Himachal Pradesh, India

Parang N Mehta MD (Ped)
Consultant Pediatrician
Department of Pediatrics
Mehta Childcare
Surat, Gujarat, India

Piyali Bhattacharya
DCH MD (Ped) FIAP FRCP (London)
Consultant Pediatrician
Department of Pediatrics
General Hospital
Sanjay Gandhi Postgraduate
Institute of Medical Sciences
Lucknow, Uttar Pradesh, India

Prem Pal Singh DCH
Senior Consultant Pediatrician
District Combined Hospital
Amroha, Uttar Pradesh, India

Premashish Mazumdar
DM (Neonatology) MD (Ped)
Consultant Pediatrician and
Neonatologist, Department of
Pediatrics and Neonatology
Global Rainbow Hospital
Agra, Uttar Pradesh, India

Pritesh Nagar MD
Pediatric Intensivist
Department of Pediatric and
Neonatal Intensive Care, Aditya Hospital
Hyderabad, Telangana, India

Priya Marwah MBBS DNB (Ped) MBA (Human Resource Management)
Clinical Program Director cum Bone Marrow Transplant Physician
Department of Bone Marrow Transplant
South East Asia Institute for Thalassemia, Jawahar Circle
Jaipur, Rajasthan, India

Puneet Kumar MBBS
Owner-Consultant
Kumar Child Clinic
New Delhi, India

Rakesh Bhatia MD (Ped)
Ex-Professor,
Department of Pediatrics
SN Medical College
Agra, Uttar Pradesh, India

Rashna Dass Hazarika MD (Ped)
Chief, Department of Pediatrics and Neonatology
Nemcare Superspecialty Hospital
Guwahati, Assam, India

Ravitanaya Sodani MD (Ped)
Assistant Professor
Department of Pediatrics
Lady Hardinge Medical College and Kalawati Saran Children's Hospital
New Delhi, India

Sangeeta Sharma MBBS MD
Professor and Head
Department of Pediatrics
National Institute of Tuberculosis and Respiratory Diseases
New Delhi, India

Sanjay Niranjan DCH MD
Ex Pool Officer
Department of Pediatrics
King George Medical University
Lucknow
Founder and Director
Neochild Clinic
Lucknow, Uttar Pradesh, India

Sanjay Srirampur MD DCh
Head, Department of Pediatrics
Aditya Hospital
Hyderabad, Telangana, India

Sanjay Verma MD
Professor (Pediatrics)
Infectious Disease Unit
Department of Pediatrics
Advanced Pediatric Center (APC)
Postgraduate Institute of Medical Education and Research
Chandigarh, India

Satish Kamtaprasad Tiwari
MD (Ped) LLB
Professor
Department of Pediatrics
PDM Medical College
Amravati, Maharashtra, India

Satish V Pandya
MD (Ped) PGDAP PGDGC
Consultant Pediatrician and Counselor
Department of Pediatrics
Varun Complete Healthcare
Vadodara, Gujarat, India

Srinivas G Kasi MBBS MD
Consultant Pediatrician
Kasi Clinic
Bengaluru, Karnataka, India

Shalabh Agarwal MD Pediatrics
Consultant Pediatrician
Department of Pediatrics
Surabhi (Mother & Child Care)
Moradabad, Uttar Pradesh, India

Shobha Sharma MD FIPNA FISPN
Professor
Department of Pediatrics
Vardhaman Mahavir Medical College and Safdarjung Hospital
New Delhi, India

Shweta Singh MD
Associate Professor
Department of Biochemistry
Hamdard Institute of Medical
Sciences and Research
New Delhi, India

Sudhir Kumar Choudhary MD FIAP
Consultant Pediatrician
Department of Pediatrics
Chiranjeev Children Hospital
Dehradun, Roorkee, Uttarakhand,
India

Sumit Mehndiratta
BBS DCH DNB (Ped) MNAMS FIMSA
Specialist Grade II
Department of Pediatrics
Vardhaman Mahavir Medical
College and Safdarjung Hospital
New Delhi, India

Unmesh A Upadhyaya MD (Ped)
Consultant Pediatrician and
Neonatologist
Department of Pediatrics
Vismay Childcare Hospital
Ahmedabad, Gujarat, India

Vijay N Yewale MD DCH
Consultant Pediatrician
Department of Pediatrics
Director
Dr Yewale Multispecialty Hospital
for Children, Navi Mumbai
Head, Institute of Child Health
Apollo Hospitals, Navi Mumbai
Navi Mumbai, Maharashtra, India

Vipin M Vashishtha MD FIAP
Director and Consultant
Pediatrician
Mangla Hospital and
Research Center
Bijnor, Uttar Pradesh, India

Vivek R Pardeshi
MBBS MD (PSM) DNB
Surveillance Medical Officer
WHO
Mumbai, Maharashtra, India

Yash Paul MBBS DCh
Consultant Pediatrician
Department of Pediatrics
Shah Hospital
Jaipur, Rajasthan, India

Foreword

Few measures in preventive medicine can compare with the impact of vaccines. Smallpox has been eradicated and polio is on the verge of eradication. Two of the three wild poliovirus serotypes have been certified as eradicated. Measles transmission has been terminated in large areas of the world. Most recommended vaccines are highly effective in preventing vaccine-preventable diseases in vaccine recipients. But nearly all vaccines have another special property, the induction of herd immunity or community protection. Most vaccine-preventable diseases are transmitted from person to person in a chain of transmission from infectious case to susceptible. When a transmitting case comes in contact with an immune person, transmission does not occur and the chain of transmission is broken. Since infectious cases do not have unlimited contacts, if the immunity levels are high enough in a community, the likelihood that such cases will meet a susceptible is very low. Thus, transmission can be terminated for many diseases in a given community before 100% vaccine coverage is achieved. Who are the people indirectly protected? They are children too young for vaccination, persons with compromised immunity who cannot make adequate immune responses to vaccines, persons with contraindications to vaccination, and persons who do not respond to vaccine for other reasons. All are protected indirectly by high levels of immunity in the population.

Prevention from vaccines is very attractive because generally with a few doses, long-term, even lifelong, protection can be achieved with many vaccines. In contrast, the lifestyle changes needed to prevent many chronic diseases require a lifetime of continued implementation.

During the last few decades, there has been a revolution in Vaccinology. Vaccines have been produced that prevent cancer. The Human Papillomavirus Vaccine (HPV) prevents approximately 70% of cervical cancers globally. And hepatitis B vaccine can prevent one of the major causes of liver cancer. Antibodies against polysaccharides are key to the defense against several bacteria that cause pneumonia, meningitis, and other serious clinical syndromes. However, young infants make poor immune responses against plain polysaccharides. By conjugating polysaccharides to protein carriers, excellent immune responses can be achieved even in very young infants. Conjugation technology is the basis for vaccines against Haemophilus influenzae type b (Hib), pneumococci, and meningococci. We can now prevent one of the most common causes of severe diarrhea and dehydration, leading to death, rotavirus. And other new technologies, including the use of recombinant DNA, messenger RNA, vaccine vectors, genetic reassortment and other techniques are being brought to bear to bring us new and better vaccines.

Efforts are underway to develop new vaccines against more infectious diseases as well as enhancing more widespread and better use of existing vaccines. No where is this more apparent than in the massive efforts to develop safe and effective vaccines to protect against SARS-CoV-2, the virus that causes COVID-19. Hopefully, some vaccines to mitigate the COVID-19 pandemic will be available for use in the coming year.

The most favorable benefits of vaccines are only achieved when they are used widely in populations for whom they are recommended. Vaccines do not save lives, vaccinations save lives. A vaccine dose that remains in the vial is 0% effective regardless of the results of clinical trials show. And this handbook provides a major resource to vaccine providers in using vaccines optimally. This book is devoted to answering practical questions on recommended vaccines, recommended schedules, indications, contra-indications, and precautions. It tries to answer questions regarding particular clinical situations, which may not be easily answered from reading existing recommendations. Use of the book, will help you minimize the risks of vaccine-preventable diseases in the populations you serve while maximizing the safe use of those vaccines.

Walter A Orenstein MD
Professor of Medicine
Pediatrics, Global Health and Epidemiology
Emory University and
Associate Director, Emory Vaccine Center
Former Deputy Director for Immunization Programs
Bill and Melinda Gates Foundation
Former Assistant Surgeon General
United States Public Health Service
Former Director, National Immunization Program
Centers for Disease Control and Prevention

Preface

The quest for vaccines is no longer limited to infectious diseases, but to anything which even remotely has some possible involvement of the immune system. That means more vaccines and greater research. And more the vaccines, more the questions which will need to be answered. Moreover, research and development of vaccines occurs exponentially, making it expedient for updates to be brought out more frequently than ever before.

This third edition continues to provide an avenue to answer many of the queries that arise in the mind of the inquisitive, especially keeping in view the advances that have taken place since the last edition. Earlier chapters have been intensively scrutinized and revised and new ones have been added on newer topics. Therefore, some esteemed authors have now joined us, both to revise the earlier chapters and to contribute to newer subjects. Our grateful thanks to these invaluable colleagues.

The year 2020 is an exceptional year. The whole world is in the grip of a deadly pandemic of Covid-19 caused by an SARS-CoV-2 virus. Vaccines against coronavirus have become the most anticipated product to rapidly end this scourge of mankind. An unprecedented number of vaccine candidates against Covid-19 are in the pipeline and some employing new platforms like mRNA, DNA, viral vector, antigen presenting cell vaccines, etc. has never been tested before. In the coming year or so billions of people around the globe are going to witness an unprecedented, massive immunization drive on a scale that has never been seen by mankind before. There is a sudden surge in the online searches regarding vaccines, immunity, correlate of protection, durability of immune responses, T cell immunity, neutralizing antibodies, etc. not only amongst health care professionals but in the general population as well. Hence, the publication of a new edition of this book is in sync with this heightened demand of updating knowledge about vaccines and immunization process.

We hope that this edition will also enjoy the same reputation that its predecessors did so fondly.

Vipin M Vashishtha
Ajay Kalra

Acknowledgments

We are especially thankful to Shri Jitendar P Vij (Group Chairman), Mr Ankit Vij (Managing Director), Mr MS Mani (Group President), Ms Chetna Malhotra Vohra (Associate Director—Content Strategy), Ms Pooja Bhandari (Production Head), and Ms Savleen Kaur (Development Editor) of M/s Jaypee Brothers Medical Publishers (P) Ltd, New Delhi, India, for giving the go-ahead at the very beginning and helping us in every way possible to bring out this book.

Contents

SECTION 1: GENERAL VACCINATION

1. **Vaccine Immunology: Basics and Beyond** — 3
   Yash Paul, Vipin M Vashishtha

2. **Elementary Epidemiology in Vaccination** — 28
   Vipin M Vashishtha, Yash Paul

3. **Vaccination Schedules** — 39
   Yash Paul, Satish V Pandya

4. **Practice of Vaccination** — 48
   Yash Paul, Satish V Pandya, Atul K Agarwal

5. **Vaccine-preventable Diseases Surveillance** — 62
   Meeta Dhaval Vashi

6. **Vaccination in Special Situations** — 75
   Abhay K Shah

7. **Adverse Events following Immunization, Vaccine Safety, and Misinformation against Vaccination** — 93
   Meeta Dhaval Vashi, Vivek R Pardeshi

8. **Cold Chain and Vaccine Storage** — 104
   Digant D Shastri

9. **Control and Eradication of Infectious Diseases** — 118
   Yash Paul, Priya Marwah

10. **Development and Licensing of Vaccine** — 124
    Gautam Rambhad, Canna Jagdish Ghia

11. **National Immunization Technical Advisory Group** — 145
    Madhu Gupta, Adarsh Bansal

12. **Medicolegal and Ethical Issues in Immunization** — 151
    Satish Kamtaprasad Tiwari, Yash Paul

13. **Vaccine Schedules including National Immunization Program** — 158
    Meeta Dhaval Vashi, Vivek R Pardeshi

14. **Vaccine Hesitancy** — 167
    Chandrakant Lahariya, Dewesh Kumar

SECTION 2: LICENSED VACCINES

15. **Bacillus Calmette-Guérin Vaccine** — 177
    Vipin M Vashishtha, A Parthasarathy, Hitt Sharma

16. **Polio Vaccines** — 199
Naveen Thacker, Prem Pal Singh, Vipin M Vashishtha

17. **Diphtheria, Tetanus and Pertussis Vaccines** — 224
Vipin M Vashishtha, Unmesh A Upadhyay

18. **Measles Vaccines** — 259
Baldev S Prajapati, Arun Wadhwa

19. **Measles, Mumps and Rubella Vaccines** — 266
Arun Wadhwa, Baldev S Prajapati, Sudhir Kumar Choudhary

20. **Hepatitis B Vaccines** — 281
Ajay Kalra, Sanjay Verma

21. **Hepatitis A Vaccines** — 302
Arun Wadhwa, Nigam P Narain

22. **Varicella Vaccines** — 312
Vijay N Yewale, Dhanya Dharmapalan

23. **Typhoid Vaccines** — 333
Chandra Mohan Kumar, Vipin M Vashishtha, Ajay Kalra

24. ***Haemophilus influenzae* Type B Vaccines** — 356
Jaydeep Choudhury

25. **Pneumococcal Diseases Vaccines** — 363
Shobha Sharma, Neha Goel

26. **Rabies Vaccines** — 389
Omesh Kumar Bharti, Jaydeep Choudhury, Vipin M Vashishtha

27. **Japanese Encephalitis Vaccines** — 405
Vipin M Vashishtha, Chandra Mohan Kumar

28. **Rotavirus Vaccines** — 434
Rakesh Bhatia

29. **Human Papillomavirus Vaccines** — 446
Jaydeep Choudhury, Srinivas G Kasi

30. **Influenza Vaccines** — 462
Sanjay Srirampur, Pritesh Nagar, Vipin M Vashishtha

31. **Meningococcal Vaccines** — 481
Parang N Mehta

32. **Cholera Vaccines** — 491
Nupur Ganguly

33. **Dengue Vaccines** — 498
Dipti Agarwal

34. **Malaria Vaccines** — 509
Abhay K Shah

35.	**Combination Vaccines** *Ashok K Dutta*	519
36.	**Yellow Fever Vaccines** *Chandra Mohan Kumar, Obeid Shafi, Shweta Singh*	525
37.	**Ebola Vaccines** *Arun Wadhwa*	532

SECTION 3: VACCINES IN THE PIPELINE

38.	**Respiratory Syncytial Virus Vaccines** *M Surendranath*	541
39.	**Newer Tuberculosis Vaccines** *Sangeeta Sharma*	549
40.	**Coronavirus Disease 2019 Vaccines** *Arun Wadhwa*	556
41.	**Human Immunodeficiency Virus Vaccines** *Dipti Agarwal*	568
42.	**Cytomegalovirus Vaccines** *Unmesh A Upadhyaya*	574
43.	**Enteroviral Vaccines (EV71)** *Piyali Bhattacharya*	582
44.	**Diarrheal Disease Vaccines other than Rotavirus** *Shalabh Agarwal*	588
45.	**Hepatitis E Vaccines** *Dipti Agarwal*	594
46.	**Hepatitis C Vaccines** *Abhay K Shah, Aashay A Shah*	599
47.	**Zika Virus Vaccines** *M Surendranath*	611
48.	**Chikungunya Vaccines** *Sachidanand Kamath, Geeta MG*	617

SECTION 4: NOVEL VACCINE STRATEGIES

49.	**Deoxyribonucleic Acid Vaccines** *Sumit Mehndiratta*	629
50.	**Chimeric Vaccines** *Puneet Kumar*	639

51.	**Therapeutic Vaccines**	647
	Ajay Kalra, Srinivas G Kasi, Premashish Mazumdar	
52.	**Newer Adjuvants Vaccines**	656
	Puneet Kumar, Sanjay Niranjan	

SECTION 5: VACCINATION OF SPECIAL GROUPS

53.	**Adolescent Immunization**	677
	CP Bansal, Ashok K Banga	
54.	**Vaccination Strategies for Travelers**	691
	Rashna Dass Hazarika	
55.	**Maternal Immunization**	700
	Harish K Pemde, Ravitanaya Sodani	
56.	**Vaccines for Healthcare Professionals**	711
	Rashna Dass Hazarika	

Annexure 1: National Immunization Schedule 2020 723

Annexure 2: Indian Academy of Pediatrics— Advisory Committee on Vaccines and Immunization Practices Recommended Immunization Schedule 2019 727

Index 735

SECTION 1

General Vaccination

1. **Vaccine Immunology: Basics and Beyond**
   Yash Paul, Vipin M Vashishtha

2. **Elementary Epidemiology in Vaccination**
   Vipin M Vashishtha, Yash Paul

3. **Vaccination Schedules**
   Yash Paul, Satish V Pandya

4. **Practice of Vaccination**
   Yash Paul, Satish V Pandya, Atul K Agarwal

5. **Vaccine-preventable Diseases Surveillance**
   Meeta Dhaval Vashi

6. **Vaccination in Special Situations**
   Abhaya K Shah

7. **Adverse Events following Immunization, Vaccine Safety and Misinformation against Vaccination**
   Meeta Dhaval Vashi, Vivek R Pardeshi

8. **Cold Chain and Vaccine Storage**
   Digant D Shastri

9. **Control and Eradication of Infectious Diseases**
   Yash Paul, Priya Marwah

10. **Development and Licensing of Vaccine**
    Gautam Rambhad, Canna Jagdish Ghia

11. **National Immunization Technical Advisory Group**
    Madhu Gupta, Adarsh Bansal

12. **Medicolegal and Ethical Issues in Immunization**
    Satish Kamtaprasad Tiwari, Yash Paul

13. **Vaccine Schedules including National Immunization Program**
    Meeta Dhaval Vashi, Vivek R Pardeshi

14. **Vaccine Hesitancy**
    Chndrakant Lahariya, Dewesh Kumar

CHAPTER 1

Vaccine Immunology: Basics and Beyond

Yash Paul, Vipin M Vashishtha

1. Are vaccination and immunization same?

Broadly speaking, both terms appear to be same and frequently used interchangeably. However, there is minor technical difference. "Vaccination" is a process of inoculating the vaccine/antigen into the body. The vaccine may or may not seroconvert to vaccine whereas the process of inducing immune response, which can be "humoral" or "cell mediated" in the vaccine is called "immunization". Vaccines can be administered through different routes, e.g., nasal mucosa, gut mucosa, or by injection which may be given intradermal, subcutaneous, or intramuscular. This process is called "vaccination" or "active immunization". In case immunoglobulins or antisera are administered, it is called "passive immunization".

Thus, administration of immunoglobulins or antisera is not vaccination, although it provides immunity or protection for a short period.

2. What are "humoral" and "cell-mediated immunity"?

Vaccines confer protection against diseases by inducing both antibodies and T cells. The former is called "humoral" response and the latter "cellular" response or "cell-mediated immunity (CMI)". Antibodies are of several different types [immunoglobulin G (IgG), immunoglobulin M (IgM), immunoglobulin A (IgA), immunoglobulin D (IgD), and immunoglobulin E (IgE)] and they differ in their structure, half-life, site of action, and mechanism of action. Humoral immunity is the principal defense mechanism against extracellular microbes and their toxins. B lymphocytes secrete antibodies that act by neutralization, complement activation, or by promoting opsonophagocytosis. CMI is the principal defense mechanism against intracellular microbes. The effectors of CMI, the T cells, are of two types. The helper T cells secrete proteins called cytokines that stimulate the proliferation and differentiation of T cells as well as other cells including B lymphocytes, macrophages, and natural killer (NK) cells. The cytotoxic T cells act by lysing infected cells.

3. What are innate and adaptive immunity?

Innate immunity comprises of the skin and mucosal barriers, phagocytes (neutrophils, monocytes, and macrophages), and the NK cells. It comes into play immediately on entry of the pathogen and is nonspecific. Adaptive immunity is provided by the B lymphocytes (humoral/antibody-mediated immunity) and T lymphocytes (cellular/CMI). The innate immune system triggers the development of adaptive immunity by presenting antigens to the B lymphocytes and T lymphocytes. Adaptive immunity takes time to evolve and is pathogen specific (**Fig. 1 and Table 1**).

4. What are "B" and "T" cells? What role do they play in regard to immunology of vaccines?

Immune system is almost nonexistent at birth; maternal antibodies transferred transplacentally provide some protection during early childhood. After birth, baby comes in contact with microbes which gradually activate immune system. B cells form the most important component of immune

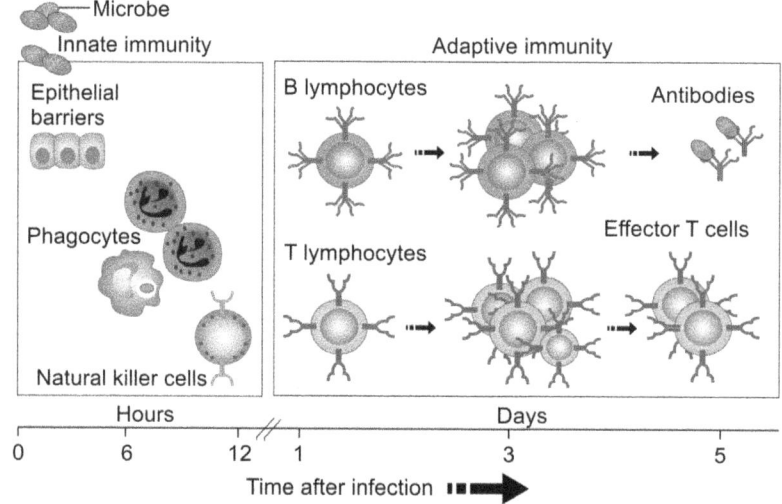

Fig. 1: Innate and adaptive immunity.

Source: Abbas AK, Lichtman AH, Pillai S. Introduction to the immune system. In: Basic Immunology. 6th edition, Elsevier, 2019.

TABLE 1: Comparison of innate and adaptive immunity.	
Nonspecific immunity (innate)	*Specific immunity (adaptive)*
Its response is antigen independent	Its response is antigen dependent
There is immediate response	There is a lag time between exposure and maximal response
It is not antigen specific	It is antigen specific
Exposure does not result in induction of memory cells	Exposure results in induction of memory cells
Some of its cellular components or their products may aid specific immunity	Some of its products may aid nonspecific immunity

system in the body. These are produced in liver in fetal life and mature in bone marrow in humans. In other species, these cells mature in an organ called "bursa of Fabricius", thus these lymphocytes are called B cells. On activation by an antigen contained in microorganisms and vaccines, the B cells proliferate and get converted to plasma cells, which, in turn, produce antibodies. For effective production of antibodies, B cells need help from T-helper cells. T lymphocytes are the cells that originate in the thymus, mature in the periphery, and become activated in the spleen/nodes if (1) their T-cell receptor (TCR) binds to an antigen presented by a major histocompatibility complex (MHC) molecule and (2) they receive additional costimulation signals driving them to acquire killing (mainly CD8$^+$ T cells) or supporting (mainly CD4$^+$ T cells) functions.

B cells have immunoglobulin surface receptor, which binds with the appropriate antigen present on the infective pathogen. The processed antigen stimulates the B cell to mature into antibody-secreting plasma cell and generates IgM. T helper 2 (Th2) cell leads to switch in the production from IgM to IgG and IgA or IgD. The B cells can directly respond to the antigen and process the antigen, but the T cells do not react with the antigen directly unless processed and presented by special cells called antigen-presenting cells (APCs).

5. What are antigen-presenting cells (APCs) and dendritic cells? What functions do they perform?

Antigen-presenting cells are the cells that capture antigens by endo- or phagocytosis, process them into small peptides, display them at their surface through MHC molecules, and provide costimulation signals that act synergistically to activate antigen-specific T cells. APCs include B cells, macrophages, and dendritic cells (DCs), although only DCs are capable of activating naïve T cells (**Fig. 2**).

Dendritic cells are major APC in the body in addition to the B cells and the macrophages. The major role of these cells is to identify dangers, which is done by the special receptors on the APC named Toll-like receptors (TLRs).

Vaccine antigens are taken up by immature DCs activated by the local inflammation, which provides the signals required for their migration to draining lymph nodes. During this migration, DCs mature and their surface expression of molecules changes. DCs sense "danger signals" through their TLRs and respond by a modulation of their surface or secreted molecules. Simultaneously, antigens are processed into small fragments and displayed at the cell surface in the grooves of MHC [MHC-human leukocyte antigen (HLA) in humans] molecules. As a rule, MHC class I molecules present peptides from antigens that are produced within infected cells, whereas phagocytosed antigens are displayed on MHC class II molecules. Thus, mature DCs reaching the T cell zone of lymph nodes display MHC-peptide complexes and high levels of costimulation molecules at their surface. CD4$^+$ T cells recognize antigenic peptides displayed by class II MHC molecules, whereas CD8$^+$ T cells bind to class I MHC peptide complexes.

SECTION 1 General Vaccination

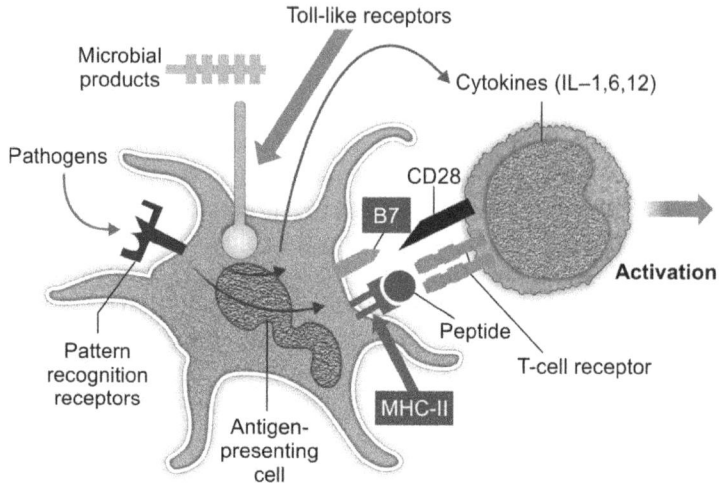

Fig. 2: Schematic presentation of a dendritic cell and its activation by pathogens.
Source: Siegrist CA. Vaccine immunology. Presentation delivered at 20th Advanced Course of Vaccinology, Annecy, France 2019. Available from: https://www.advac.org/images/files/members/files_presentations/2019/0900_SIEGRIST_ADVAC_2019_Immunology_slides_-_9h-11h30.pdf
(IL-1: interleukin-1; MHC: major histocompatibility complex)

Antigen-specific TCRs may only bind to specific MHC molecules (e.g., HLA-A2), which differ among individuals and populations. Consequently, T-cell responses are highly variable within a population.

6. What are adjuvants? How do they affect performance of a vaccine?

Adjuvants are agents which increase the stimulation of the immune system by enhancing antigen presentation (depot formulation, delivery systems) and/or by providing costimulation signals (immunomodulators). Aluminum salts are most often used in today's vaccines. Hence, the adjuvants improve the immunogenicity of vaccines. Many new generations of adjuvants are in fact analogs of TLRs, for example, CpG-ODN is used in new generation of Japanese encephalitis vaccines.

Most nonlive vaccines require their formulation with specific adjuvants to include danger signals and trigger a sufficient activation of the innate system. These adjuvants may be divided into two categories: (1) delivery systems that prolong the antigen deposit at site of injection, recruiting more DCs into the reaction and (2) immune modulators that provide additional differentiation and activation signals to monocytes and DCs. Although progress is being made, none of the adjuvants currently in use trigger the degree of innate immune activation that is elicited by live vaccines, whose immune potency far exceeds that of nonlive vaccines.

7. What are "germinal centers" and "marginal zone"?

Germinal centers (GCs) are dynamic structures that develop in spleen/nodes in response to an antigenic stimulation and dissolve after a few weeks.

GCs contain a monoclonal population of antigen-specific B cells that proliferate and differentiate through the support provided by follicular DCs and helper T cells. Immunoglobulin class switch recombination, affinity maturation, B-cell selection, and differentiation into plasma cells or memory B cells essentially occur in GCs.

"Marginal zone" is the area between the red pulp and the white pulp of the spleen. Its major role is to trap particulate antigens from the circulation and present it to lymphocytes.

8. What do the terms "epitope" and "paratope" mean?

An "epitope" refers to the specific target against which an individual antibody binds. When an antibody binds to a protein, it is not binding to the entire full-length protein. Instead, it is binding to a segment of that protein known as an "epitope". Hence, an epitope is a specific part of the antigen that elicits an immune response.

Binding between the antibody and the epitope occurs at the antigen-binding site, which is called a "paratope" and is located at the tip of the variable region on the antibody. This paratope is only capable of binding with one unique epitope.

9. What is the difference between "antibody affinity" and "avidity"?

The antibody affinity refers to the tendency of an antibody to bind to a specific epitope at the surface of an antigen, i.e., to the strength of the interaction. The avidity is the sum of the epitope-specific affinities for a given antigen. It directly relates its function.

10. What do the terms "CD4+ T cells" and "CD8+ T cells" stand for? What are the functions of these lymphocytes?

CD4+ T cells are those T lymphocytes that express the cluster of differentiation 4 (CD4) glycoprotein at their surface. CD4 is a glycoprotein expressed on the surface of T-helper cells, regulatory T cells, monocytes, macrophages, and DCs. It was discovered in the late 1970s and was originally known as Leu-3 and T4 (after the OKT4 monoclonal antibody that reacted with it) before being named CD4 in 1984. In humans, the CD4 protein is encoded by the *CD4* gene. CD4 is a coreceptor that assists the TCR to activate its T cell following an interaction with an APC. Using its portion that resides inside the T cell, CD4 amplifies the signal generated by the TCR by recruiting an enzyme, known as the tyrosine kinase Lck, which is essential for activating many molecules involved in the signaling cascade of an activated T cell. CD4 interacts directly with MHC class II molecules on the surface of the APC using its extracellular domain.

T cells expressing CD4 molecules (and not CD8) on their surface, therefore, are specific for antigens presented by MHC class II and not by MHC class I (they are MHC class II-restricted). The short cytoplasmic/intracellular tail (C) of CD4 contains a special sequence of amino acids that allow it to interact with the Lck molecule described above.

CD8+ cells are those T lymphocytes that express the CD8 glycoprotein at their surface. These cells recognize their targets by binding to antigen associated with MHC class I, which is present on the surface of nearly every cell of the body. Through IL-10, adenosine, and other molecules secreted by regulatory T cells, the CD8+ cells can be inactivated to an anergic state, which prevent autoimmune diseases such as experimental autoimmune encephalomyelitis. CD8+ cells are cytotoxic T lymphocytes (CTLs) and destroy virally infected cells and tumor cells and are also implicated in transplant rejection (**Fig. 3**).

CD8+ T cells do not prevent, but reduce, control, and clear intracellular pathogens by:

Directly killing infected cells (release of perforin, granzyme, etc.)
Indirectly killing infected cells through antimicrobial cytokine release.

CD4+ T cells do not prevent but participate to the reduction, control, and clearance of extra- and intracellular pathogens by:

Producing interferon-γ (IFN-γ), tumor necrosis factor-α/-β (TNF-α/-β), interleukin-2 (IL-2) and IL-3, and supporting activation and differentiation of B cells, CD8+ T cells, and macrophages [T helper 1 (Th1) cells].

Producing IL-4, IL-5, IL-13, IL-6 and IL-10, and supporting B-cell activation and differentiation (Th2 cells).

11. What are toll-like receptors (TLRs) and their role in vaccine immunogenicity?

Toll-like receptors are a family of 10 receptors (TLR1 to TLR10) present at the surface of many immune cells, which recognize pathogens through conserved microbial patterns and activate innate immunity when detecting danger. TLRs are a key driver of innate immune response. They can recognize an invading pathogen through structurally conserved molecules of that particular pathogen collectively referred to as pathogen-associated molecular patterns (PAMPs) that are different from the host molecules. They later activate a cascade of immune responses that clear the infection. Many TLRs are now employed as adjuvants in novel vaccine products.

12. What are the differences between live attenuated and inactivated vaccines?

Live vaccines are attenuated (modified) live organisms, which have immunogenicity, i.e., can generate antibodies, but have lost pathogenicity, i.e., capability to cause disease. Live vaccines can be viral as well as bacterial. The live vaccine particles (viruses or bacteria) replicate or multiply in the body after administration and stimulate the immune system. The older concept that single dose of live vaccines induces lifelong immunity perhaps does not hold true, we need many doses of oral polio vaccine (OPV) and booster doses are required for live vaccines such as measles vaccine, varicella, rubella, and live oral typhoid vaccines. Inactivated vaccines may consist of whole-inactivated organisms such as whole-cell pertussis, typhoid, rabies; inactivated polio vaccine, modified exotoxins called "toxoids" such as diphtheria toxoid or tetanus toxoid; subunits such as polysaccharide antigens of *Salmonella typhi*, *Haemophilus influenzae* type b (Hib), and surface proteins of hepatitis B virus.

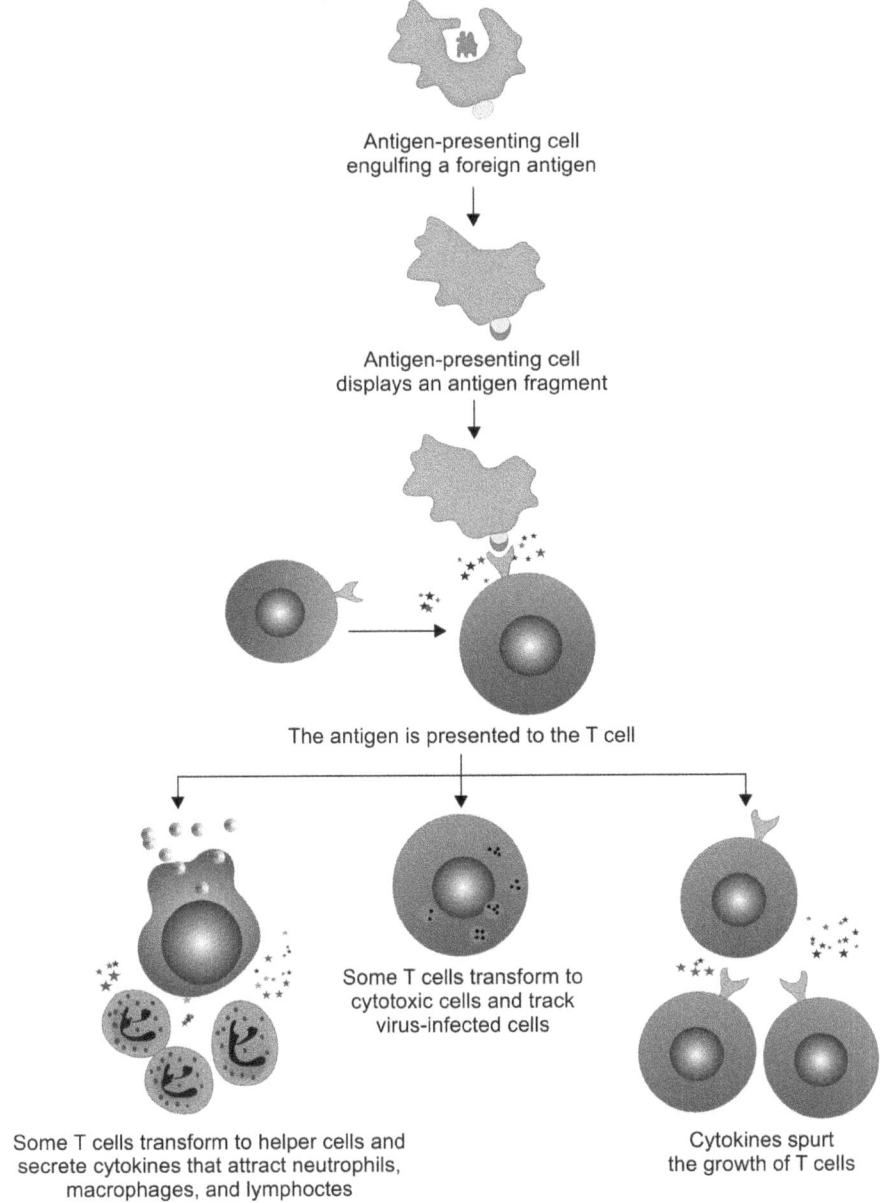

Fig. 3: T lymphocyte activation pathway.

Conjugation of the polysaccharide with a protein carrier significantly improves the immune response.

Live viral vaccines do efficiently trigger the activation of the innate immune system, presumably through pathogen-associated signals [such as viral ribonucleic acid (RNA)] allowing their recognition by pattern recognition receptors (PRRs)—TLRs. Following injection, viral particles rapidly disseminate throughout the vascular network and reach their target tissues. This pattern is very similar to that occurring after a natural infection, including the initial mucosal replication stage for vaccines administered through the nasal/oral routes. Following the administration of a live viral vaccine and its dissemination, DCs are activated at multiple sites, migrate toward the corresponding draining lymph nodes, and launch multiple foci of T- and B-cell activation. This provides a first explanation to the generally higher immunogenicity of live versus nonlive vaccines.

The strongest antibody responses are generally elicited by live vaccines that better activate innate reactions and thus better support the induction of adaptive immune effectors. Nonlive vaccines frequently require formulation in adjuvants, of which aluminum salts are particularly potent enhancers of antibody responses and thus included in a majority of currently available vaccines. This is likely to reflect their formation of a deposit from which antigen is slowly deabsorbed and released, extending the duration of B- and T-cell activation, as well as the preferential induction of IL-4 by aluminum-exposed macrophages.

Very few nonlive vaccines induce high and sustained antibody responses after a single vaccine dose, even in healthy young adults. Primary immunization schedules, therefore, usually include at least two vaccine doses, optimally repeated at a minimal interval of 3–4 weeks to generate successive waves of B cell and GC responses. These priming doses may occasionally be combined into a single "double" dose, such as for hepatitis A or B immunization. In any case, however, vaccine antibodies elicited by primary immunization with nonlive vaccines eventually wane.

13. What is the difference between T cell-dependent and T cell-independent immune response?

Certain antigens, primarily proteins, induce both B-cell and T-cell stimulation leading to what is called T cell-dependent immune response. Infants of 6 weeks of age onward are capable of T cell-dependent response. This type of response usually results in higher titers of IgG type and long lasting. It also shows booster effects with repeated exposures.

On the other hand, T cell-independent response being only B-cell mediated is not possible below 2 years of age. It is predominantly IgM type with low titers. The response is short lasting and repeated doses of vaccine do not lead to boosting effect. IgA is not produced and hence there is no local mucosal protection with this type of antigens, while in case of T cell-dependent response IgA antibodies are also produced which help in providing mucosal protection and eradication of the carrier state. Few examples of T cell-independent vaccines include bacterial polysaccharide (PS) vaccines such as *Streptococcus pneumoniae* (*S. pneumoniae*), *Neisseria meningitidis*, *Haemophilus influenzae* (*H. influenzae*), and *Salmonella typhi*.

14. What are conjugate vaccines?

As already mentioned in answer to above question, regarding the difference between T cell-dependent and T cell-independent immune response, in

T cell-independent immune response, being B-cell mediated, younger children do not respond to such vaccines. A T cell-independent antigen like PS can be made into T cell dependent by the technique of conjugation. Such conjugated vaccines can be administered to children <2 years of age also. This technique is used to produce conjugated Vi typhoid, Hib, and pneumococcal and meningococcal vaccines.

15. How do vaccines elicit their responses? Which are the main effectors of vaccine responses?

The nature of the vaccine exerts a direct influence on the type of immune effectors that are predominantly elicited and mediate protective efficacy (**Table 2**). Capsular PSs elicit B-cell responses in what is classically reported as a T-independent manner, although increasing evidence supports a role for $CD4^+$ T cells in such responses. The conjugation of bacterial PS to a protein carrier (e.g., glycoconjugate vaccines) provides foreign peptide antigens that are presented to the immune system and thus recruits antigen-specific $CD4^+$ T helper cells in what is referred to as T-dependent antibody responses. A hallmark of T-dependent responses, which are also elicited by toxoid, protein, inactivated, or live attenuated viral vaccines, is to induce both higher-affinity antibodies and immune memory. In addition, live attenuated vaccines usually generate $CD8^+$ cytotoxic T cells. The use of live vaccines/vectors or of specific novel delivery systems [e.g., deoxyribonucleic acid (DNA) vaccines] appears necessary for the induction of strong $CD8^+$ T-cell responses. Most current vaccines mediate their protective efficacy through the induction of vaccine antibodies, whereas Bacillus Calmette-Guérin (BCG)-induced T cells produce cytokines that contribute to macrophage activation and control of *Mycobacterium tuberculosis*. The induction of antigen-specific immune effectors (and/or of immune memory cells) by an immunization process does imply that these antibodies, cells, or cytokines represent surrogates or even correlates of vaccine efficacy. This requires the formal demonstration that vaccine-mediated protection is dependent—in a vaccinated individual—upon the presence of a given marker such as an antibody titer or a number of antigen-specific cells above a given threshold. Antigen-specific antibodies have been formally demonstrated as conferring vaccine-induced protection against many diseases.

Passive protection may result from the physiological transfer of maternal antibodies (e.g., tetanus) or the passive administration of immunoglobulins or vaccine-induced hyperimmune serum (e.g., measles, hepatitis, varicella, etc.). Such antibodies may neutralize toxins in the periphery at their site of production in an infected wound (tetanus) or throat (diphtheria). They may reduce binding or adhesion to susceptible cells/receptors and thus prevent viral replication (e.g., polio) or bacterial colonization (glycoconjugate vaccines against encapsulated bacteria) if present at sufficiently high titers on mucosal surfaces. The neutralization of pathogens at mucosal surfaces is mainly achieved by the transudation of vaccine-induced serum IgG antibodies. It requires serum IgG antibody concentrations to be of sufficient

TABLE 2: Correlates of vaccine-induced immunity.

Vaccines	Vaccine type	Serum IgG	Mucosal IgG	Mucosal IgA
EPI vaccines				
Diphtheria toxoid	Toxoid	++	(+)	
Pertussis, whole cell	Killed	++		
Pertussis, acellular	Protein	++		
Tetanus toxoid	Toxoid	++		
Measles	Live attenuated	++		
Polio Sabin	Live attenuated	++	++	++
Polio Salk	Killed	++	+	
Tuberculosis (BCG)	Live mycobacterial			
Non-EPI vaccines				
Hepatitis A	Killed	++	(+)	
Hepatitis B (HbsAg)	Protein	++		
Hib PS	PS	++	(+)	
Hib glycoconjugates	PS protein	++	++	
Influenza	Killed subunit	++	(+)	
Influenza intranasal	Live attenuated	++	+	+
Meningococcal PS	PS	++	(+)	
Meningococcal conjugate	PS protein	++	++	
Mumps	Live attenuated	++		
Pneumococcal PS	PS	++	(+)	
Pneumoccoccal conjugates	PS protein	++	++	
Rabies	Killed	++		
Rotavirus	VLPs	(+)	(+)	++
Rubella	Live attenuated	++		
Typhoid PS	PS	+	(+)	
Varicella	Live attenuated	++		
Yellow fever	Live attenuated	++		
Typhoid conjugate	–	–	–	

(BCG: Bacillus Calmette-Guèrin; EPI: Expanded Program on Immunization; Hib: *Haemophilus influenzae* type b; IgA: immunoglublulin A; IgG: immunoglobulin G; PS: polysaccharide; VLPs: virus-like particles)

Source: With permission from Siegrist CA. Vaccine immunology. In: Plotkin SA, Orenstein W, Offit P (Eds). Vaccines, 5th edition. Philadelphia: Saunders Elsevier; 2008. pp. 17-36.

affinity and abundance to result into "protective" antibody titers in saliva or mucosal secretions. As a rule, such responses are not elicited by PS bacterial vaccines but achieved by glycoconjugate vaccines, which therefore prevent nasopharyngeal colonization in addition to invasive diseases.

Under most circumstances, immunization does not elicit sufficiently high and sustained antibody titers on mucosal surfaces to prevent local infection. It is only after having infected mucosal surfaces that pathogens encounter vaccine-induced IgG serum antibodies that neutralize viruses, opsonize bacteria, activate the complement cascade, and limit their multiplication and spread, preventing tissue damage and thus clinical disease. That vaccines fail to induce sterilizing immunity is, thus, not an obstacle to successful disease control, although it represents a significant challenge for the development of specific vaccines such as against human immunodeficiency virus-1 (HIV-1). Current vaccines mostly mediate protection through the induction of highly specific IgG serum antibodies. Under certain circumstances, however, passive antibody-mediated immunity is inefficient (tuberculosis).

16. What are the clinical scenarios where evidences of T-cells protection are available?

Bacillus Calmette-Guérin is the only currently used human vaccine for which there is conclusive evidence that T cells are the main effectors. However, there is indirect evidence that vaccine-induced T cells contribute to the protection conferred by other vaccines. $CD4^+$ T cells seem to support the persistence of protection against clinical pertussis in children primed in infancy, after vaccine-induced antibodies have waned. Another example is that of measles immunization in 6-month-old infants. These infants fail to raise antibody responses because of immune immaturity and/or the residual presence of inhibitory maternal antibodies, but generate significant IFN-γ producing $CD4^+$ T cells. These children remain susceptible to measles infection, but are protected against severe disease and death, presumably because of the viral clearance capacity of their vaccine-induced T-cell effectors. Thus, prevention of infection may only be achieved by vaccine-induced antibodies, whereas disease attenuation and protection against complications may be supported by T cells even in the absence of specific antibodies. The understanding of vaccine immunology, thus, requires appraising how B- and T-cell responses are elicited, supported, maintained, and/or reactivated by vaccine antigens.

17. What happens once a vaccine is administered to a vaccinee?

Following injection, the vaccine antigens attract local and systemic DCs, monocytes, and neutrophils. These activated cells change their surface receptors and migrate along lymphatic vessels to the draining lymph nodes where the activation of T and B lymphocytes takes place. In case of killed vaccines, there is only local and unilateral lymph node activation. Conversely, for live vaccines, there is multifocal lymph node vaccination due to microbial replication and dissemination. Consequently, the immunogenicity of killed vaccines is lower than the live vaccines; killed vaccines require adjuvants which improve the immune response by producing local inflammation and recruiting DCs/monocytes to the injection site. Secondly, the site of administration of killed vaccines is of importance; the intramuscular route which is well-vascularized and has a large number of patrolling DCs is preferred over the subcutaneous route. The site of administration is usually of little significance for live vaccines. Finally, due to focal lymph node activation, multiple killed vaccines may be administered at different sites with little immunologic interference. Immunologic interference may occur with multiple live vaccines, unless they are given on the same day, at least 4 weeks apart or at different sites.

18. What are the immune responses of T cell-independent antigens (i.e., polysaccharide vaccines) at the cellular level?

On being released from the injection site, these antigens usually nonprotein, PSs in nature, reach the marginal zone of the spleen/nodes, and bind to the specific immunoglobulin surface receptors of B cells. In the absence of antigen-specific T cell help, B cells are activated, proliferated, and differentiated in plasma cells without undergoing affinity maturation in GCs. The antibody response, sets in 2-4 weeks following immunization, is predominantly IgM with low titers of low affinity IgG. The half-life of the plasma cells is short and antibody titers decline rapidly. Additionally, the PS antigens are unable to evoke an immune response in those aged <2 years due to immaturity of the marginal zones. As PS antigens do not induce GCs, bonafide memory B cells are not elicited. Consequently, subsequent reexposure to the same PS results in a repeat primary response that follows the same kinetics in previously vaccinated as in naïve individuals.

19. What is hyporesponsiveness of repeated doses of a vaccine referring to?

Revaccination with certain bacterial PSs, of which group C meningococcus is a prototype—may even induce lower antibody responses than the first immunization, a phenomenon referred to as hyporesponsiveness whose molecular and cellular bases are not yet fully understood.

20. What are the immune responses of T cell-dependent antigens at the cellular level?

T cell-dependent antigens include protein antigens which may consist of either pure proteins [hepatitis B, hepatitis A, human papillomavirus (HPV), and toxoids] or conjugated protein carrier with PS antigens (Hib, meningococcal, and pneumococcal). The initial response to these antigens is similar to PS antigens. However, the antigen-specific helper T cells that have been activated by antigen-bearing DCs trigger some antigen-specific B cells to migrate toward follicular dendritic cells (FDCs), initiating the GC reaction. In GCs, B cells receive additional signals from follicular T cells and undergo massive clonal proliferation, switch from IgM toward IgG/IgA, undergo affinity maturation, and differentiate into plasma cells secreting large amounts of antigen-specific antibodies. Most of the plasma cells die at the end of GC reaction and thus decline in antibody levels is noted 4-8 weeks after vaccination. However, a few plasma cells exit nodes/spleen and migrate to survival niches mostly located in the bone marrow, where they survive through signals provided by supporting stromal cells and this results in prolonged persistence of antibodies in the serum.

21. What are "memory B cells"?

Memory B cells are those B lymphocytes that generate in response to T-dependent antigens, during the GC reaction, in parallel to plasma cells. They persist there as resting cells until reexposed to their specific antigens when they readily proliferate and differentiate into plasma cells secreting large amounts of high-affinity antibodies that may be detected in the serum within a few days after boosting.

22. What are the characteristics of immune response to live vaccines?

The live vaccines induce an immune response similar to that seen with protein vaccines. However, the uptake of live vaccines is not 100% with the first dose. Hence, more than one dose is recommended with most live vaccines. Once the vaccine has been taken up, immunity is robust and lifelong or at least for several decades. This is because of continuous replication of the organism that is a constant source of the antigen. The second dose of the vaccine is, therefore, mostly for primary vaccine failures (no uptake of vaccine) and not for secondary vaccine failures (decline in antibodies overtime).

23. What determines the intensity and duration of immune responses?

The nature of antigen is the primary determinant; broadly speaking, live vaccines are superior (exception BCG, OPV) to protein antigens, which, in turn, are superior to PS vaccines. Adjuvants improve immune responses to inactivated vaccines. Immune response is usually better with higher antigen dose (e.g., hepatitis B). The immune response improves with increasing number of doses and increased spacing between doses. Technically, 0, 1, and 6 months are the best immunization schedule; the first two doses are for induction and the long gap between the second and third doses allows for affinity maturation of B cells and clonal selection of the fittest B cells for booster and memory response. Extremes of age and disease conditions lower immune response.

24. What are the limitations of young age immunization?

Young age limits antibody responses to most vaccine antigens since maternal antibodies inhibit antibodies responses, but not T-cell response and due to limitation of B-cell response.

Immunoglobulin G antibodies are actively transferred through the placenta, via the FcRn receptor, from the maternal to the fetal circulation. Upon immunization, maternal antibodies bind to their specific epitopes at the antigen surface, competing with infant B cells and thus limiting B-cell activation, proliferation, and differentiation. The inhibitory influence of maternal antibodies on infant B-cell responses affects all vaccine types, although its influence is more marked for live attenuated viral vaccines that may be neutralized by even minute amounts of passive antibodies. Hence, antibody responses elicited in early life are short lasting. However, even during early life, induction of memory B cells is not limited.

Early life immune responses are characterized by age-dependent limitations of the magnitude of responses to all vaccines. Antibody responses to most PS antigens are not elicited during the first 2 years of life, which is likely to reflect numerous factors including: the slow maturation of the spleen marginal zone, limited expression of CD21 on B cells, and limited availability of the complement factors. Although this may be circumvented in part by the use of glycol-conjugate vaccines, even the most potent glycoconjugate vaccines elicit markedly lower primary IgG responses in young infants.

Although maternal antibodies interfere with the induction of infant antibody responses, they may allow a certain degree of priming, i.e., induction of memory B cells. This likely reflects the fact that limited amounts of unmasked vaccine antigens may be sufficient for priming of memory B cells, but not for full-blown GC activation, although direct evidence is lacking. Importantly, however, antibodies of maternal origin do not exert their inhibitory influence on infant T-cell responses, which remain largely unaffected or even enhanced.

The extent and duration of the inhibitory influence of maternal antibodies increase with gestational age, e.g., with the amount of transferred immunoglobulins and declines with postnatal age, as maternal antibodies wane.

25. Maternal antibodies interfere with neonatal immune responses, why hepatitis B, Bacillus Calmette-Guérin (BCG), and oral polio vaccine (OPV) are recommended at birth?

The first dose of hepatitis B, which is administered at birth, acts as "priming dose" while subsequent doses provide an immune response even in presence of maternal antibodies. As mentioned above, maternal antibodies do not interfere with induction of memory B cells, certain degree of priming is allowed. However, hepatitis B vaccine induces lower primary IFN-γ responses and higher secondary Th2 responses in early life than adults. Similarly, antibodies of maternal origin do not exert their inhibitory influence on infant T-cell responses. Since, BCG mainly works by inducing T-cell immune response hence it can be given in the presence of maternal antibodies which may even enhance T-cell responses. OPV is given at birth, since there are no maternal IgA in the gut to neutralize the virus. However, IFN-γ responses to OPV are significantly lower in infants than in adults.

26. How maternal antibodies can sometimes enhance T-cell responses of Bacillus Calmette-Guérin (BCG) vaccine administered at birth?

After administration of BCG, the maternal antibodies form immune complexes with the vaccine antigens. These immune complexes are taken up by more and more number of macrophages and DCs, which, in turn, are dissociated into their acidic phagolysosome compartment and are processed into small peptides. These peptides are displayed at the surface of APCs, thus available for binding by more number of $CD4^+$ and $CD8^+$ T cells.

27. Considering the numerous limitations of young age immunization, why still vaccines are administered at much younger age in developing countries than in developed world?

This can be explained on the basis of disease epidemiology of vaccine-preventable diseases (VPDs). Since, majority of childhood infectious diseases cause early morbidity and mortality in poor, developing countries, hence the need to protect the children before wild organisms infect them. This is the reason why early, accelerated schedules are practiced in developing countries. According to the World Health Organization (WHO) estimates, 2.5–3 million infants are born healthy but succumb to acute infections between the age of 1 and 12 months. These early deaths are caused by a limited number of pathogens, such that the availability of a few additional vaccines that would be immunogenic soon after birth would make a huge difference on this disease burden.

28. How limitations of young age immunization can be taken care of?

They can be countered by increasing the number of vaccine doses for better induction, use of adjuvants to improve immunogenicity of vaccines, and by use of boosters at later age when immune system has shown more maturity than at the time of induction. Increasing the dose of vaccine antigen may also be sufficient to circumvent the inhibitory influence of maternal antibodies, as illustrated for hepatitis A or measles vaccines.

29. Which is the best vaccination schedule for nonlive vaccines acting on the principal of "prime-boost" mechanism?

Traditionally, 0–1–6 months schedule is considered as a most immunogenic schedule than 6–10–14 weeks or 2–3–5 months schedule for nonlive T cell-dependent vaccines like hepatitis B vaccine. This is mainly due to proper spacing of the vaccine doses and adequate time interval between first few doses which act by inducing immune responses and last dose that works as boosters. Since, affinity maturation of B cells in GCs and formation of memory B cells take at least 4–6 months, this schedule quite well fulfills these requirements. More than one dose is needed for better induction and recruitment of more number of GCs in young age considering young age limitations of immune system (**Fig. 4**).

Immunization schedules commencing at 2 months and having 2 months spacing between the doses are technically superior to that at 6, 10, and 14 weeks. However, for operational reasons and for early completion of immunization and attainment of protection, the 6, 10, 14 and weeks schedule is chosen in developing countries.

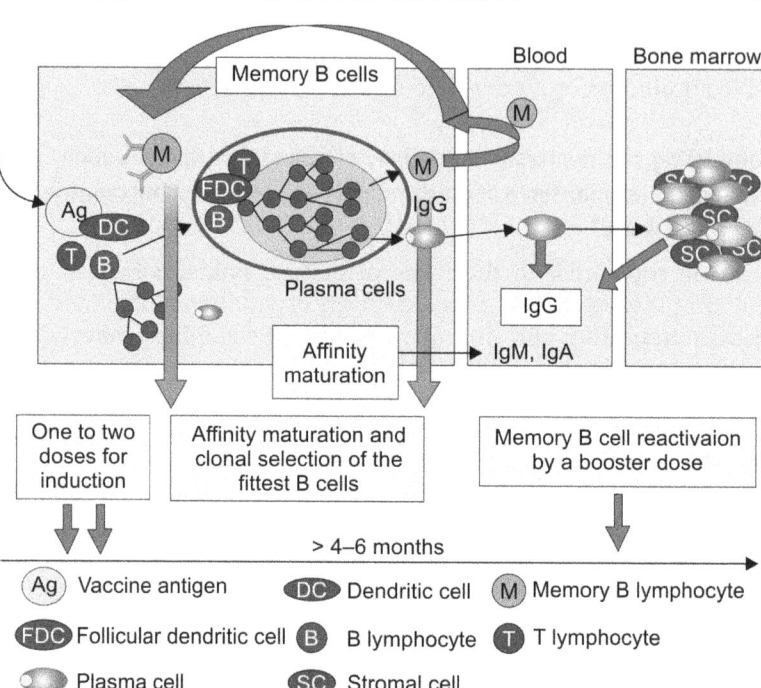

Fig 4: Schematic presentation of various components of 0, 1, and 6 months immunization schedule at cellular level.
(IgA: immunoglobulin A; IgG: immunoglobulin G; IgM: immunoglobulin M)
Source: Siegrist CA. Vaccine immunology. Presentation delivered at 20th Advanced Course of Vaccinology, Annecy, France 2019. Available from: https://www.advac.org/images/files/members/files_presentations/2019/0900_SIEGRIST_ADVAC_2019_Immunology_slides_-_9h-11h30.pdf

Accelerated infant vaccine schedules in which three vaccine doses are given at a 1-month interval (2, 3, 4 months or 3, 4, 5 months) result into lower responses than schedules in which more time elapses between doses (2, 4, and 6 months) or between the priming and boosting dose (3, 5, and 12 months). However, the magnitude of infant antibody responses to multiple dose schedules reflects both the time interval between doses, with longer intervals eliciting stronger responses and the age at which the last vaccine dose is administered.

30. What is a primary and secondary immune response?

When an antigen is introduced for the first time, the immune system responds primarily after a lag phase of up to 10 days. This is called the primary response. Subsequently, upon reintroduction of the same antigen, there is no lag phase and the immune system responds by producing antibodies immediately and this is called the secondary response. However, there are some differences in both these responses—primary response is short-lived, has a lag phase, predominantly IgM type, and antibodies titers are low, whereas secondary response is almost immediate without a lag phase, titers persist for a long

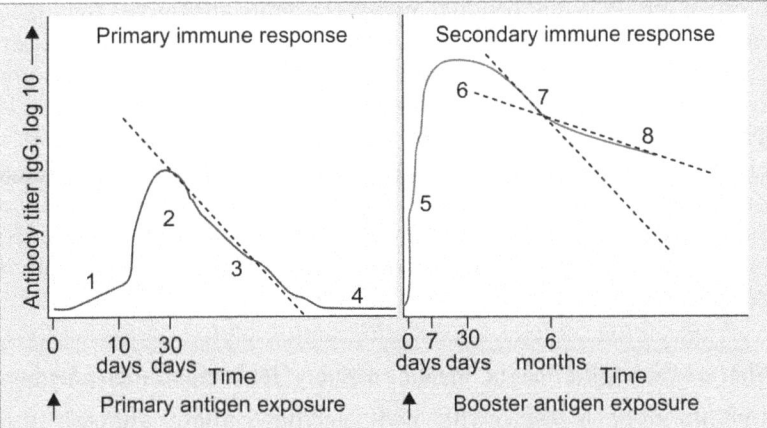

Fig. 5: Correlation of antibody titers to various phases of the vaccine response. The initial antigen exposure elicits an extrafollicular response (1) that results in the rapid appearance of low immunoglobulin G (IgG) antibody titers. As B cells proliferate in germinal centers and differentiate into plasma cells, IgG antibody titers increase up to a peak value (2) usually reached 4 weeks after immunization. The short lifespan of these plasma cells results in a rapid decline of antibody titers (3) which eventually return to baseline levels (4). In secondary immune responses, booster exposure to antigen reactivates immune memory and results in a rapid (<7 days) increase (5) of IgG antibody titer. Short-lived plasma cells maintain antibody (6) during a few weeks—after which serum antibody titers decline initially with the same rapid kinetics as following primary (7) immunization. Long-lived plasma cells that have reached survival niches in the bone marrow continue to produce antigen-specific antibodies, which then decline with slower (8) kinetics.

Note: This generic pattern may not apply to live vaccines triggering long-term IgG antibodies for extended periods of time.

Source: With permission from Siegrist CA. Vaccine immunology. In: Plotkin SA, Orenstein W, Offit P (Eds). Vaccines, 5th edition. Philadelphia: Saunders Elsevier; 2008. pp. 17-36.

time, predominantly of IgG type, and antibodies titers are very high. **Figure 5** describes the background developments at the cellular level and interactions of B cells, memory B cells, and T cells at the follicular level in a lymph node. The secondary response is mainly due to booster response and is seen with vaccines that work on a "prime-boost" mechanism inducing T cells such as conjugate vaccines. On the other hand, nonconjugate, polysaccharide vaccines mainly induce primary response and the repeat dose produces another wave of primary response and not acts as a booster since they do not induce T cells.

31. What are the hallmarks of "memory B cell" responses?

These cells are only generated during T cell-dependent responses inducing GCs responses. These cells are resting cells that do not produce antibodies. Memory B cells undergo affinity maturation during several (4-6) months. A minimal interval of 4-6 months is required for optimal affinity maturation of memory B cells. Memory B cells rapidly (days) differentiate into antibody-secreting plasma cells upon reexposure to antigen. Memory B cells differentiate into PCs that produce high(er) affinity antibodies than primary plasma cells. As plasma cells and memory responses are generated in parallel in GCs, higher postprimary antibody titers reflect stronger GC reactions and generally predict higher secondary responses. During induction, a lower antigen dose at priming results in inducing B cells differentiation away from PCs, toward memory B cells. This phenomenon can be exploited by using small amount of expensive conjugate vaccines such as pneumococcal conjugate vaccine (PCV) followed by use of less expensive pneumococcal polysaccharide vaccine (PPV) as booster. Exposure to exogenous antigens may reactivate or favor the persistence of memory B cells.

32. What are the implications of "immune memory" for immunization programs?

Immune memory is seen with live vaccines/protein antigens due to generation of memory B cells which are activated on repeat vaccination/natural exposure. Immune memory allows one to complete an interrupted vaccine schedule without restarting the schedule. Hence, immunization schedule should never be started all over again regardless of duration of interruption. Regular boosters are not required to maintain immune memory during low risk periods (travelers). Certain immunization schedules may not need boosters, if exposure provides regular natural boosters. Activation of immune memory and generation of protective antibodies usually take 4–7 days. Diseases which have incubation periods shorter than this period such as Hib, tetanus, diphtheria, and pertussis require regular boosters to maintain protective antibody levels. However, diseases such as hepatitis A and hepatitis B do not need regular boosters as the long incubation period of the disease allows for activation of immune memory cells. This is to be noted that memory B cells do not produce antibodies unless reexposed to antigen which drives their differentiation into antibody-producing plasma cells.

33. Why is number of doses for each vaccine different?

Live attenuated vaccines replicate (in case of viruses) or multiply (in case of bacteria) in the body thus, the number of vaccine particles increases many folds which are capable of generating antibodies in large quantity to reach seroprotective levels. Due to some reasons, not fully understood, multiple doses of OPV are needed. On the other hand, inactivated vaccines do not multiply in the body and quantity of vaccine (antigens) required to provide full protection is large; fever and local reactions such as swelling, tenderness, and pain may be very severe, if the required quantity of vaccine is administered at a time, so the quantity of vaccine is generally divided in two or more doses. Diphtheria, pertussis, and tetanus (DPT) is divided in three doses while rabies vaccine is divided in four or five doses.

34. Why do we need booster (booster doses)?

The body starts antibody generation after administration of vaccines, which reach a peak after a period of time which is different for different vaccines.

As already stated, multiple doses of some vaccines have to be administered to attain optimal level of immunity. Over a period of time, which also varies for different vaccines, antibody level declines and revaccination or booster dose(s) is/are required to raise the antibody levels above the required protective levels.

In most cases, subclinical infection acts as a booster dose. As the percentage of vaccinated and immune population increases, circulation of the causative organisms declines in the community. This decline in circulation of organisms lessens the chances of nonimmune individuals in coming in contact with organisms (which is a beneficial for nonimmune people), but those immune following vaccination may be deprived of the benefit of repeated subclinical exposure leading to boosting effect. This is the reason that booster dose for varicella vaccine has been introduced in those countries where vaccine coverage is very high.

35. Why we need to give only one dose of a particular vaccine while multiple doses are needed for another vaccine?

In general, live vaccines generate antibodies to protective levels after administration while antigens need multiple doses because the quantity required to generate antibodies to protective levels is very large, so multiple doses are required.

It has been observed that natural infection with viral diseases provides very long or lifelong protection while infections by bacteria do not provide any long-lasting protection. Typhoid disease, skin infections, and other infections caused by bacteria can recur again and again while second attack of measles or chickenpox occurs rarely, if at all. Similarly, antibodies produced by antiviral vaccines persist for much longer period as compared to antibodies produced by antibacterial vaccines.

36. Do all inactivated vaccines need booster doses? How long after the primary doses are boosters advised? Why?

- No, certain vaccines such as hepatitis A, hepatitis B, HPV, etc., do not require frequent boosters.
- To believe that a single dose or a primary course of vaccination provides a lifelong immunity is a utopian thought. It does not exist because it could not exist. Not only inactivated, but even most live vaccines do need extra doses! Even for some of the highly efficacious live vaccines like measles, we need extra doses.
- The need and timing of boosters further depend on three factors: (1) related to the agent (microbe), (2) host, and (3) vaccine characteristics.
    1. *Agent (microbe)*: If the incubation period of a disease is short than the time required for reactivation of memory B cells, plasma cells secrete antibodies. Boosters needed as incubation period is short in diseases such as diphtheria, tetanus, Hib, and pneumococcus, but not needed as incubation period is long such as in hepatitis B, hepatitis A, HPV, etc. It is generally considered that protection by

toxoid-based vaccines requires the presence of antitoxin antibodies at time of toxin exposure. This is supported by the observation that despite the occurrence of many adult cases of diphtheria during a large outbreak in the former Soviet Union, a single vaccine dose raised strong antibody responses to this relatively poor immunogen. This confirmed that most patients had been immunized in childhood and had lost vaccine antibodies over time, but had persistent immune memory. This immune memory was however not sufficient to protect against diphtheria, a disease characterized by a short incubation period (1–5 days).

2. *Vaccine characteristics*: It depends on the quality of immunogen and the vaccine-elicited immune responses. Take the case of another vaccine like flu vaccines. The immunity persists only for few months. Pertussis vaccines: you need frequent boosters. Japanese encephalitis (JE) vaccines: Old mouse brain: frequent boosters but new generation: only infrequently needed. We are now developing more new technology to have more durable immunity like use of nanoparticles, better adjuvants such as TLRs agonists, new delivery techniques, etc.

3. *Host*: For example, in immunocompromised host with congenital/acquired immunodeficiency states (such as HIV, asplenia, complement deficiency, chronic illnesses, immunosuppressive drugs, malignancy, etc.), one needs frequent boosters to maintain a baseline antibodies level to accord protections.

37. Why cannot we have an "all-in-one vaccine"?

There are very strong scientific and logistic reasons against "all-in-one vaccine". Scientific reasons are: (i) different ideal ages for different vaccines, e.g., OPV, BCG, and hepatitis B vaccines can be administered soon after birth, other vaccines cannot be administered at this age; (ii) different routes of administration, e.g., some are administered orally, others are administered parentally, some are administered intradermally (BCG), some are administered subcutaneously [measles, measles, mumps, and rubella (MMR), and varicella vaccines], and other vaccines are administered intramuscularly. Logistic reasons are: (i) some vaccines need to be administered as a single dose (BCG and varicella vaccines), some vaccines need two doses (such as measles, MMR, hepatitis A, and rotavirus vaccine), some vaccines need three doses (hepatitis B and HPV vaccines) while other vaccines have to be administered at different intervals and (ii) quantity of such an "all-in-one vaccine" would be too large. Certainly, the idea appears to be very attractive, but does not appear feasible in foreseeable future.

38. Few vaccines such as diphtheria, tetanus, and pertussis (DTP) vaccine causes higher incidence of fever, pain, tenderness, and other local reactions. Should antipyretics such as paracetamol, ibuprofen, etc., be prescribed prophylactically routinely?

Prophylactic antipyretic administration decreases the postvaccination adverse reactions. Recent study finds that they may also decrease the antibody responses to several vaccine antigens.

Though prophylactic antipyretic administration leads to relief of the local and systemic symptoms after primary vaccinations, there is a reduction in antibody responses to some vaccine antigens without any effect on the nasopharyngeal carriage rates of *S. pneumoniae* and *H. influenzae* serotypes. Immunologically, this can be explained by reductions in "danger signals" due to anti-inflammatory effects of these compounds that "blunt" the antibodies production (**Fig. 6**). The development of fever or increase in the temperature postvaccination is due to the release of endogenous cytokines (IL-1 and TNF-α).

However, since the antibody response [geometric mean concentration (GMC)] was not reduced below seroprotection level, it is unlikely that prophylactic paracetamol (PCM) would have any detrimental effect for individual child concerned. Future trials and surveillance programs should also aim at assessing the effectiveness of programs where prophylactic administration of PCM is given. The timing of administration of antipyretics should be discussed with the parents after explaining the benefits and risks.

39. Immune memory is the function of adaptive immune system. Do innate immune systems also display memory responses?

Unlike the "adaptive" immunity, the "innate" immune system is supposed to have no memory responses. Recently, the phenomenon of vertebrate innate memory has experienced a renewed interest. This phenomenon is best exemplified by in vivo vaccination with the BCG that could induce a more effective host immune response to subsequent challenges, with a concomitant increase in resistance to unrelated infections. BCG, which can remain alive in the human skin for up to several months, triggers not only *Mycobacterium*-specific memory B and T cells but also stimulates the cells of the innate system (monocytes, neutrophils, macrophages, natural killer, DCs, etc.) for a prolonged period. The process by which BCG imparts immune memory to the innate system is known as "trained innate immunity", which, in turn, is elicited by a phenomenon known as "epigenetic effect".

"Epigenetic effect" is produced by the modification of gene expression rather than alteration of the genetic code or nucleotide sequencing. This effect is brought about by two main mechanisms, DNA methylation and histone modifications that alter innate immunity. BCG does epigenetic reprogramming in the training of innate cells, particularly monocytes. Upon pathogen X recognition by a receptor, "naïve" monocytes undergo epigenetic reprogramming and a metabolic shift and convert into "trained" monocytes, primed to respond more vigorously to nonspecific (pathogens X, Y, and Z) secondary stimulation. Unlike antigen-specific memory of the adaptive immune system, the second stimulation does not have to be with the same pathogen or antigen. Later on, these "trained" monocytes have a

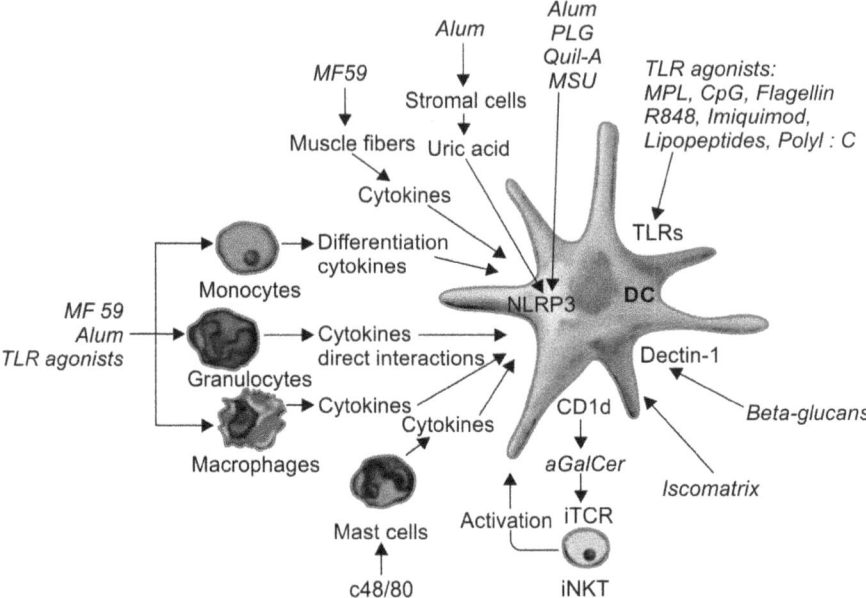

Fig. 6: "Danger signals"/adjuvants activate dendritic cells (DCs) directly or indirectly.
(iNKT: invariant natural killer T; iTCR: invariant T-cell receptor; MPL: monophosphoryl lipid A; MSU: monosodium urate; PLG: poly-α-L-glutamine; TLRs: Toll-like receptors)
Source: De Gregorio E, D'Oro U, Wack A. Immunology of TLR-independent vaccine adjuvants. Curr Opin Immunol. 2009;21(3):339-45.

significantly higher production of several proinflammatory cytokines [such as IFN-γ, TNF-α, interleukins (IL-1β, IL-6, etc.] upon heterologous challenges, particularly T helper cell type 1 polarizing and typically monocyte-derived proinflammatory cytokines that help in rapid clearance of infection (**Fig. 7**). These modified, activated, and "trained" cells can be stimulated by various nonrelated infectious (viruses, bacteria, fungi and their components, parasites) or noninfectious agents such as nanoparticles which lead to potent immune memory responses. This response explains the BCGs nonspecific protection against sepsis, pneumonia, and other pathogens. Both epigenetic changes and increased nonspecific immune responses could be detected up to 1 year after BCG vaccination.

40. What are the differentiating features of adaptive and innate memory responses?

Innate immune memory differs from adaptive memory for many aspects, including the lack of gene rearrangements, the involvement of epigenetic reprogramming, the type of cells involved (innate cells vs. T and B lymphocytes), and the receptors engaged in pathogen/antigen recognition (selective PRRs vs. antigen-specific T-cell and B-cell receptors). In general, innate memory is considered as a nonspecific short-lived phenomenon, as opposed to adaptive memory that is long-lived and highly specific.

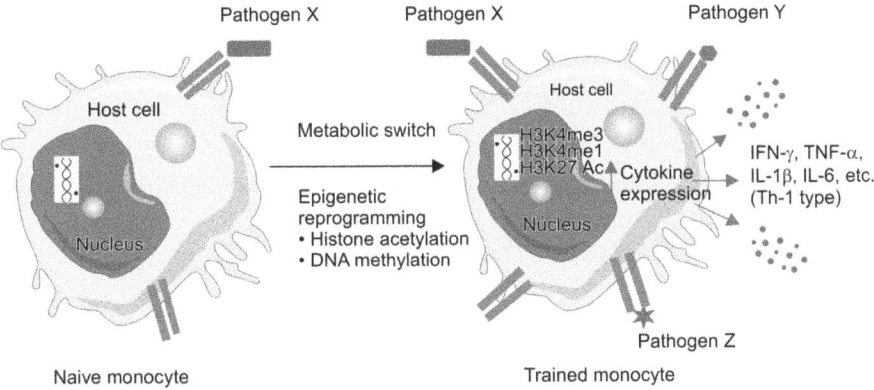

Fig. 7: "Trained innate immunity"—epigenetic reprogramming of monocytes. Upon pathogen X recognition by a receptor, naïve monocytes undergo epigenetic reprogramming and a metabolic shift and become primed to respond more robustly to nonspecific (pathogens X, Y, and Z) secondary stimulation.

(DNA: deoxyribonucleic acid; IFN-γ: interferon-γ; IL-6: interleukin-6; TNF-α: tumor necrosis factor-α)

Source: Vashishtha VM. Are BCG-induced non-specific effects adequate to provide protection against COVID-19? Hum Vaccin Immunother. 2020;7:1-4.

41. Can trained immunity may offer some protection against ongoing coronavirus disease 2019 (COVID-19) pandemic or other future viral pandemics?

Theoretically, the nonspecific, innate immunity shall provide some temporary protection against an unrelated viral pathogen through trained immunity. BCG is the vaccine to be tried for this purpose. It may have some utility owing to induction of strong, nonspecific, and innate immune responses in the vaccinated subjects. One should not expect significant inhibitory responses against the severe acute respiratory syndrome coronavirus 2 (SARS-CoV-2) virus, but even "stop gap" protection and some attenuation of the disease may be expected against coronavirus disease 2019 (COVID-19). An extra dose of BCG to the healthcare workers and elderly people with comorbid conditions would be worth trying till a specific vaccine is developed (**Figs. 8A to C**).

Bacillus Calmette-Guérin is generally safe and well-tolerated. However, it is contraindicated in immunocompromised individuals, so one needs to be extra careful while administering BCG to these individuals. Whether the heterologous immunity would be adequate to neutralize the virus at its first portal of entry? Would the quantum of innate immune responses elicited in adults and elderly be at par with those produced in young children? Would BCG revaccination be safe in *Mycobacterium tuberculosis*-infected and uninfected populations? Would it be safe to administer a live vaccine to elderly with comorbidities? Which BCG strain would elicit the greatest nonspecific immunity? These are some of the queries that need urgent resolution. As discussed above, the main argument against the ecological studies linking universal BCG use with protection against COVID-19 is the waning of

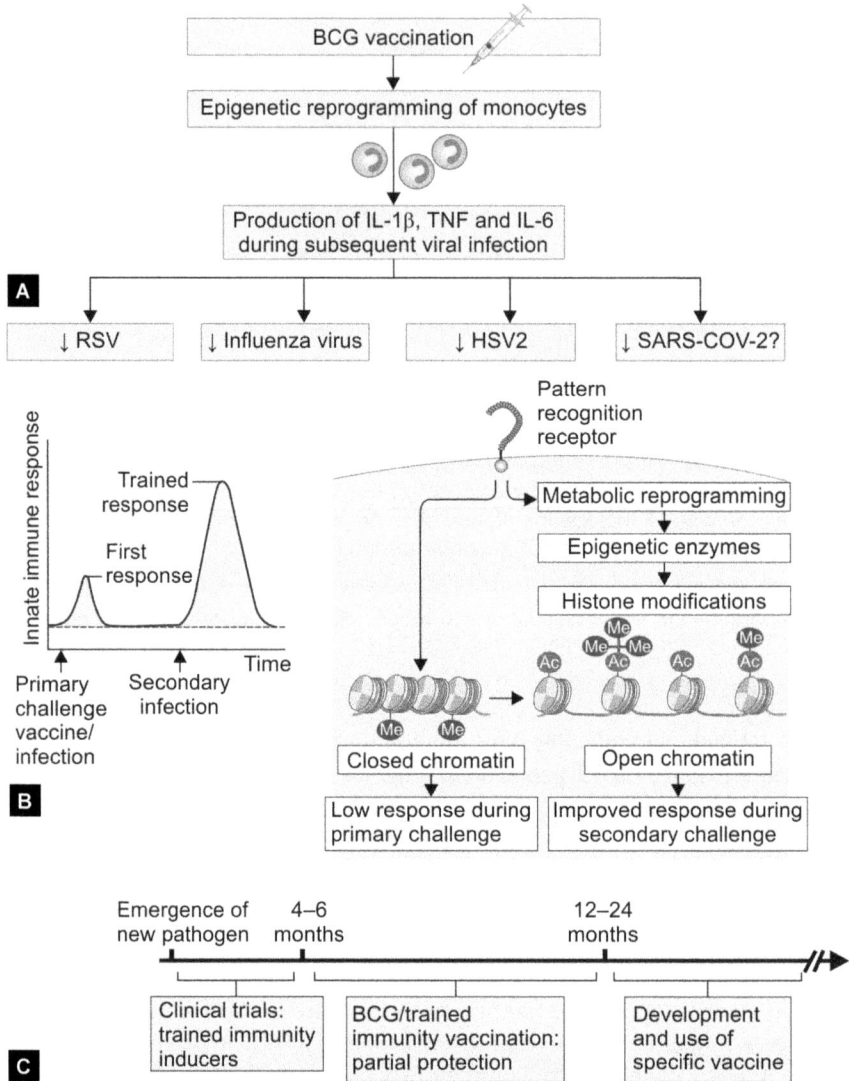

Figs. 8A to C: Trained immunity antiviral host defense and its role in a new viral pandemic. (A) BCG vaccination has been shown to protect against multiple viral pathogens; (B) Trained immunity leading to enhanced innate immune responses to different pathogens after a vaccination is mediated by metabolic and epigenetic rewiring in innate immune cells, which lead to increased gene transcription and improved host defense; and (C). Trained immunity as a tool for enhancing population immunity during a pandemic ahead of the availability of a specific vaccine.

(BCG: Bacillus Calmette-Guérin; HSV: herpes simplex virus; IL-6: interleukin-6; RSV: respiratory syncytial virus; SARS-CoV-2: severe acute respiratory syndrome coronavirus 2; TNF: tumor necrosis factor)

Source: O'Neill LAJ, Netea MG. BCG-induced trained immunity: can it offer protection against COVID-19? Nat Rev Immunol. 2020;20(6):335-7.

BCG-induced immunity. But even if heterologous immune responses persist for a few weeks to few months, they should be able to provide some protection to the frontline health workers by immunomodulation.

SUGGESTED READING

1. Advanced Course of Vaccinology (ADVAC). Presentation delivered at ADVAC. France: Springer; 2019.
2. Das RR, Panigrahi I, Naik SS. The effect of prophylactic antipyretic administration on post-vaccination adverse reactions and antibody response in children: a systematic review. PLoS One. 2014;9(9):e106629.
3. Netea MG, Joosten LAB, Latz E, Mills KHG, Natoli G, Stunnenberg HG, et al. Trained immunity: a program of innate immune memory in health and disease. Science. 2016;352(6284):aaf1098.
4. O'Neill LAJ, Netea MG. BCG-induced trained immunity: can it offer protection against COVID-19? Nat Rev Immunol. 2020;20(6):335-7.
5. Siegrist CA. Vaccine immunology. In: Plotkin SA, Orenstein W, Offit P (Eds). Vaccines, 5th edition. Philadelphia: Saunders Elsevier; 2008. pp. 17-36.
6. Singhal T, Amdekar YK, Agarwal RK. IAP Guidebook on Immunization, 4th edition. New Delhi: Jaypee Brothers Medical Publishers (P) Ltd; 2009.
7. Thacker N, Shendurkar N. Childhood Immunization: Issues and Options, 1st edition. New Delhi: Incal Communications; 2005.
8. Vashishtha M. Manual of Advancing Science of Vaccinology. Mumbai: Indian Academy of Pediatrics; 2009.
9. Vashishtha VM. Are BCG-induced non-specific effects adequate to provide protection against COVID-19? Hum Vaccin Immunother. 2020;7:1-4.

CHAPTER 2

Elementary Epidemiology in Vaccination

Vipin M Vashishtha, Yash Paul

1. What is epidemiology?

The study (observation, measurement, analysis, correlation, and interpretation) of distribution [how many? in whom? (age group) where? when? season and determinants (why there, why then?)] of diseases (etiology and risk factors) is termed as "epidemiology". Epidemiology is the study of the distribution and determinants of disease frequency in man. It is foundation science of public health. It provided insights for applying intervention. It informs if intervention is succeeding. It is the systematic study of the pathogen amplification and transmission systems. Epidemiology can often pin-point the weak links in the chains of the source and transmission pathways of the pathogen so that interventions can be directed at those points. Vaccination is one such intervention.

2. Why is it important to learn epidemiology?

From vaccinology perspective, there are three reasons to learn epidemiology. They are for the rational choice of vaccines for vaccination programs; to design appropriate intervention program including vaccinations; and to monitor and measure the progress and impact of any vaccination program. Knowledge of epidemiology helps in choosing the appropriate vaccines for inclusion in public health programs after carefully assessing disease burden and economic factors. It also helps in designing disease specific control/elimination/eradication strategies after acquiring exact epidemiological data on prevalence, incidence, and transmission characteristics of target pathogens, and their transmission pathways. In the last, it also helps in monitoring intervention success/failure in order to improve performance/efficiency of the vaccination programs.

3. What are the basic measures of disease frequency? What do the terms "incidence" and "prevalence" refer to?

Basic measures of disease frequency are done by incidence and prevalence; incidence relates to the number of new cases of the disease which occur during a particular period of time (e.g., new TB cases). Prevalence relates to total number of cases of a disease in a specified period of time usually during a survey. Often it is expressed as rate which is misnomer and it is actually proportion. In the long run, incidence should be more than the deaths and recoveries for prevalence to accumulate; prevalence of various diseases is a good indicator of the load on health services.

4. What is disease estimation? What are its merits and demerits?

Where measuring of exact incidence and/or prevalence of a disease is not practical, estimates are developed to have a rough idea about the burden of that particular disease in the community at a given geographic region. Hence, where incidence/prevalence is not "measured" estimation is better than nothing. Estimates are for comparative purpose—intercountry and interdisease. Comparison is for choice also, e.g., intervention versus none; or vaccination versus other. An estimate is by definition inaccurate, but may be valid/invalid; reliable/unreliable. It is usually expressed in round figures, e.g., 200,000 rabies; 2 million malaria; 3 million human immunodeficiency virus (HIV) infected; 40 million hepatitis B carriers, etc. No estimate is accurate for the actual burden—therefore, arguments against hepatitis B vaccination program for the reason the estimate is inaccurate and is an obvious misjudgment. For global leadership in specific diseases gross estimates are used. This is such an example for tuberculosis (TB) **(Fig. 1)**.

5. What are the differences between endemic, epidemic, and pandemic patterns of diseases?

Endemic refers to normal occurrence of disease in defined population, e.g., cholera, malaria, TB, etc. Epidemics/outbreaks are the occurrence of more cases of disease than expected in a given area or among a specific

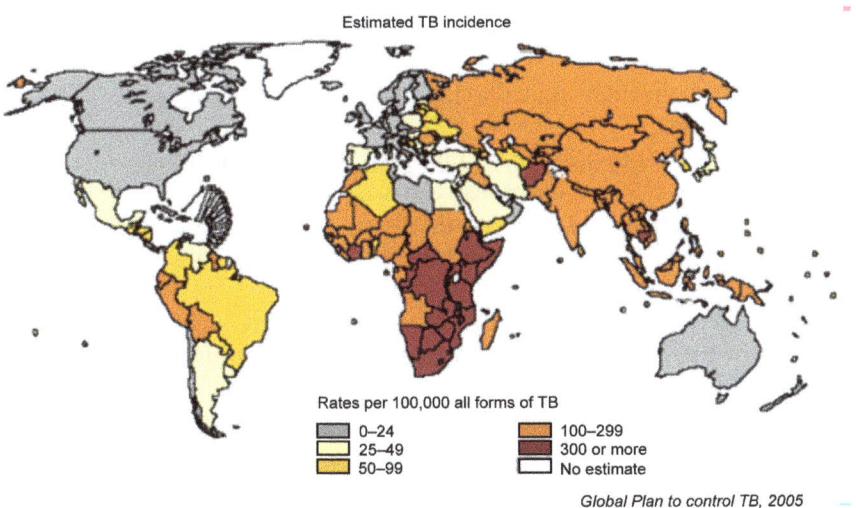

Fig. 1: Global estimate of TB burden (estimate of TB incidence).
Source: Manual of IAP Advancing Science of Vaccinology; 2009.

group of people over a particular period of time, e.g., measles, influenza, meningococcal disease. Epidemic/outbreaks: Spreading rapidly and extensively by infection and affecting many individuals in an area or a population at the same time. The difference between epidemic and outbreak is arbitrary. The terms "epidemic" and "outbreaks" are often used similarly; however, former usually indicates less intensity, e.g., outbreak of salmonella in a neonatal unit. A community-based outbreak meningococcal disease is defined as the occurrence of >3 cases in <3 months in the same area who are not close contacts of each other with a primary disease attack rate of >10 primary cases/100,000 persons.

In terms of the flu, the difference between an epidemic and an outbreak is the percentage of overall deaths caused by the disease. Every week, if the number of flu caused deaths exceeds 7.7% of the total, then the United States of America officially has an epidemic on its hands [Centers for Disease Control and Prevention (CDC)]. Currently it is 7.2, so there is no epidemic yet. The 7.7% figure is not static from year to year. During the flu epidemic of 1990, e.g., the CDC's threshold was 6.7% of total deaths.

Pandemic is global epidemic. Disease originates in one country and then spreads to a number of countries, e.g., acquired immunodeficiency syndrome (AIDS), H1N1, etc.

6. **What the terms such as vaccine immunogenicity, vaccine efficacy, and vaccine effectiveness refer to?**

Vaccine immunogenicity is the ability of a vaccine to induce antibodies which may or may not be protective. These antibodies may be of no use in offering protection against the desired disease. The protective threshold for most vaccines is defined. However, there is often controversy about the cutoffs (pneumococcus/Hib). Levels below the limits may be protective due to other reasons such as immune memory/T-cell immunity.

Vaccine efficacy is the ability of the vaccine to protect an individual. It can be assessed through clinical trials, cohort studies, or case control studies. It is calculated as:

$$VE = \frac{\text{Disease in unvaccinated} - \text{Disease in vaccinated}}{\text{Disease in unvaccinated}}$$

Vaccine effectiveness (VE) is the ability of the vaccine to protect the community and is a sum of the vaccine efficacy and herd effect. It is revealed after a vaccine is introduced in a program. VE is a combination of vaccine efficacy, coverage and herd effect. Hence, vaccine efficacy is the protection at the individual level while effectiveness is at the community level. Higher the force of transmission, younger the age at risk greater the need for VE to reduce $R = 1$ to $R < 1$.

7. **What do you mean by cost-effectiveness of a vaccine or vaccination program?**

Cost-effectiveness is a method of economic evaluation which is carried out by mathematical modeling usually prior to introduction of a vaccine in a national program. It is expressed as cost per infections/deaths/hospitalizations prevented/life years gained.

8. **What do the terms "force of transmission" and "reproductive rate" denote to? What is the significance of "basic reproductive number (R_0)"?**

The key determinant of incidence and prevalence of infection depends on force of transmission which is determined by "reproductive rate". Reproductive rate is a simple concept in disease epidemiology. Incidence and prevalence of infection depend on reproductive rate. R_0 measures the average number of secondary cases generated by one primary case in a susceptible population. Suppose all others were susceptible—then how many will be infected? That is basic reproductive number, R_0. Since population is a mix of susceptible and immune persons, one case must attempt to infect more than one person.

In the long term, pathogen can survive only if one case reproduces another case (effective reproductive rate, R = 1). If R < 1, the disease is declining (e.g., herd effect). If R > 1, an outbreak is occurring. For endemic diseases with periodic fluctuations, R may swing from <1 to >1 but in the long term the average may remain 1. Pathogen can survive if it reproduces. For all endemic infectious diseases (IDs), R = 1 for steady state or for long-term endemicity. The community benefit of a vaccination program is to reduce R to <1 and sustain it for long periods. Such beneficial effect, measured as the degree of disease reduction due to a vaccination program, is sometimes called vaccine effectiveness to distinguish it from vaccine efficacy which refers to only the direct benefit of immunity in vaccinated individuals.

R_0 is not a static entity and changes according at different time period even at a same geographic region.

9. **How can one calculate the magnitude of "basic reproductive number"?**

A series of simple relationships exist between key epidemiological, demographic, and vaccination program-related parameters. The magnitude of R_0 and the average at infection prior to mass vaccination, A, plus life expectancy in the population are related as follows:

$$R/ \approx (L\,A)/(A\,M)$$

Here, "M" is the average duration of maternal antibody protection (6 months) and "L" is life expectancy.

10. **How does vaccination impact natural epidemiology of an infectious disease?**

Vaccination perturbs epidemiology by removing the vaccinated individual from susceptible pool: so, one less disease case, and by removing individuals from chain of transmission: so, lower incidence/prevalence of the disease. In other words, vaccination program interferes with natural epidemiology of the target disease.

11. What is epidemiological shift?

Epidemiological shift refers to an upward shift in age of infection/disease in communities with partial immunization coverage. Owing to vaccination the natural circulation of the pathogen decreases and the age of acquisition of infection advances. This is especially important for diseases such as rubella, varicella, and hepatitis A wherein severity of disease worsens with advancing age.

12. What is herd immunity?

The term "herd immunity" has been in use since 1920s, i.e., for about 90 years. In fact, it denotes resistance of a population to the spread of vaccine preventable diseases where causative organisms spread from human to human. Because immune individuals act as a barrier in spread of infection and lessen the chances of an individual with the disease to come in contact of vulnerable person. Instead of the terms "herd immunity" or "herd effect" terms contact immunity and herd protection are being used now.

Herd immunity is the proportion immune in a herd. This can be deduced from the vaccination coverage. Herd effect is the protection offered to unvaccinated members when good proportion (usually >85%) of the herd is vaccinated. Herd effect is due to reduced carriage of the causative microorganism by the vaccinated cohort and thus is seen only with vaccines against those diseases where humans are the only source (there is no herd effect for tetanus). An effective vaccine is a prerequisite for good herd effect; oral poliovirus vaccine (OPV) in India, bacillus Calmette–Guérin (BCG) and unconjugated polysaccharide vaccines have no herd effect.

13. What is contact immunity?

Following administration live vaccine particles multiply in the body, induce immunity by generating antibodies, and are excreted in body fluids such as nasal secretions or passed out in feces. In case a sufficient number of these live-vaccine particles reach unvaccinated, close contact may induce immunity in this person. As this person has developed immunity without taking the vaccine, benefit has occurred because of secondary spread so this is called contact immunity.

14. Which vaccines can cause contact immunity?

Any live-attenuated vaccine may reach close contact through droplet infection, in case vaccine is administered as a nasal spray, ruptured pustule may result in spread of live vaccines as may happen in case of varicella vaccine, or the vaccine viruses shed in feces may reach close contact through feco-oral route. Thus, theoretically any live vaccine can induce contact immunity.

15. How commonly does this contact immunity occur?

Very rarely. There are only three documented cases where close contacts have developed immunity because of varicella vaccine.

16. How commonly does this contact immunity occur in case of OPV, because vaccine recipients continue to shed live polio vaccine viruses for up to a period of 6 weeks?

It is correct that polio vaccine viruses contained in OPV replicate in the gut are shed in feces and may infect the close contacts, and it was assumed that these vaccine viruses will provide protection. Now it is known that this secondary spread of polio vaccine viruses does not induce immunity because of two reasons: (i) attenuated polioviruses contained in OPV have markedly reduced infectivity, and (ii) low load of vaccine viruses spread through feces. There are about 1,000,000 type 1 polioviruses, about 100,000 type 2 polioviruses, and about 600,000 type 3 polioviruses in each dose of two drops of OPV, i.e., each dose of OPV contains about 1,700,000 polioviruses. On the other hand, 1 g of fecal matter of vaccine recipient contains about 100 vaccine polioviruses. Thus, 17 kg of fecal matter may provide same quantity of vaccine polioviruses as are contained in one dose of OPV. How much antibodies would be generated by few 1,000 vaccine polioviruses spread through feces while many doses of OPV, each dose containing about 17 lac vaccine polioviruses have failed to generate protective immunity in many children? This secondary spread of vaccine viruses may enhance the already existing antibodies.

17. What is herd protection?

Immunized people provide protection to the unimmunized individuals without inducing immunity, virtually by breaking the transmission of the infection or lessening the chances of susceptible individuals coming in contact with infective individual.

In clinical practice, contact immunity does not play significant role, while herd protection plays a major role, though to a limited extent, because unimmunized individuals do not develop immunity, but enjoy the protection because of break in spread of infection. Thus, the herd protection is the major beneficial component of immunization for unimmunized population for the infections which spread from person to person. It should be remembered that these unimmunized individuals enjoy protection till they are among immunized and resistant people. As they have not developed immunity, may develop disease if come in direct contact with infected person, in case they shift to the milieu where there is the outbreak of the disease.

18. How effective is herd protection in real life?

It is not only a relevant question, but is very important to understand the phenomenon of herd protection. It is generally stated that when vaccine coverage is high, say 80% or more in the community, unvaccinated persons get benefit of herd protection. In certain situation such benefit may occur, in other situations this benefit may not be provided. If susceptible person does not come in direct contact of infected person because of presence of immune population, such person will escape infection, so higher the percentage of immune population, lesser are the chances of vulnerable person getting infection. In case a vulnerable individual comes in contact of infective person, such person may develop infection despite presence of very high percentage of immune population. Following example is cited for better understanding of the phenomenon.

One hundred persons go to a restaurant where all are served food which had been accidentally contaminated with *Salmonella typhi*. 99 persons in this group had received typhoid vaccine recently and have developed antibodies and thus resistance against typhoid disease, so, would not develop active disease despite being infected by *Salmonella typhi* from the infected food. But, one individual who had not received the typhoid vaccine may develop typhoid disease from this food. Thus, in this case even 99% vaccine coverage may fail to protect this single unvaccinated individual.

Can BCG vaccine administered to 90% persons of a large family from tubercular endemic area provide effective protection to the 10% unvaccinated persons, if all are exposed to some infective persons? Should we advise 90% vaccine coverage with diphtheria vaccine in a family and expect 10% unvaccinated will be protected against diphtheria disease? The answer for both situations is no. In other words, there is no "free ride" even in case of the vaccines which prevent diseases where the causative organism spreads from person to person.

Thus, this so-called additional benefit to the community or presumptive public good does not provide any real benefit to an individual, except that it reduces the circulation of causative organisms in the community. As the proportion of vaccinated population increases, proportion of unvaccinated (susceptible) population decreases and their chances of coming in contact with infective individual reduce.

19. Do all vaccines provide some benefit to the community in form of contact immunity or herd protection?

The so-called "common good" may be provided by the vaccines which prevent infections where causative organism spreads from person to person, because some vaccines may provide contact immunity (by inducing immunity or by enhancing the existing immunity) as well as herd protection, while some vaccines may provide herd protection by lessening the chances of susceptible individual in coming in contact with infective persons. In case of vaccine preventable diseases where causative organism does not spread from person to person as happens in case of rabies and tetanus, immune people do not provide any benefit to unimmunized people in the community.

Depending upon whether the additional benefit(s) being provided to the community or not, the vaccines may be placed in three groups:
1. Vaccines which can provide contact immunity and herd protection— OPV varicella vaccine, any live vaccine (theoretically possible).
2. Vaccines which can provide herd protection only—inactivate polio vaccine (IPV), diphtheria, pertussis, measles, mumps, rubella, pneumococcal, *Haemophilus influenzae* type b (Hib), rotavirus, meningococcal, hepatitis A, typhoid, and BCG.

3. Vaccines which do not provide any additional benefit to the unimmunized persons—tetanus, rabies, Japanese encephalitis, hepatitis B, and yellow fever.

20. How can the degree of herd immunity and the magnitude of R_0 be assessed?

Various methods are employed to measure these parameters. Few include the following:
- Cross-sectional and longitudinal serological surveys
- Serum and saliva (viral infections)
- Activated T-cells (bacteria and protozoa)
- Quantitative assays

Scientific methods in the study of herd immunity include immunological and disease surveillance methods (provide the empirical base for analysis and interpretation), mathematical and statistical methods (play an important role in the analysis of infectious disease transmission and control). They help to define both what needs to be measured, and how best to measure define epidemiological quantities.

21. What are the "R_0" values of few key, well-known infectious diseases?

Table 1 and **Figure 2** provide R_0 values of some important infectious diseases.

TABLE 1: Values of "R_0" and route of transmission of well-known infectious diseases.

Disease	Route of transmission	Basic reproduction number (R_0)
Measles	Airborne droplet	11–18
Diphtheria	Saliva	6–7
Smallpox	Airborne droplet	5–7
Polio	Feco-oral	5–7
Rubella	Airborne droplet	5–7
Mumps	Airborne droplet	4–7
Pertussis	Airborne droplet	5–6
HIV/AIDS	Sexual contact	2–5
SARS (2003–04)	Airborne droplet	2–5
Influenza	Airborne droplet	1–2
Ebola	Bodily fluids	1.5–2.5
Zika	Mosquito bites	3.0–6.6
Norovirus	Fecal-oral route	1.6–3.7
MERS-CoV (Saudi Arabia and South Korea)	?Close contact/?respiratory secretions	0.6–0.7 and 2–5 (nosocomial)
SARS-CoV-2	Respiratory droplets	2–3.1

(SARS-CoV-2: severe acute respiratory syndrome coronavirus 2; MERS-CoV: middle east respiratory syndrome coronavirus)

36 SECTION 1 General Vaccination

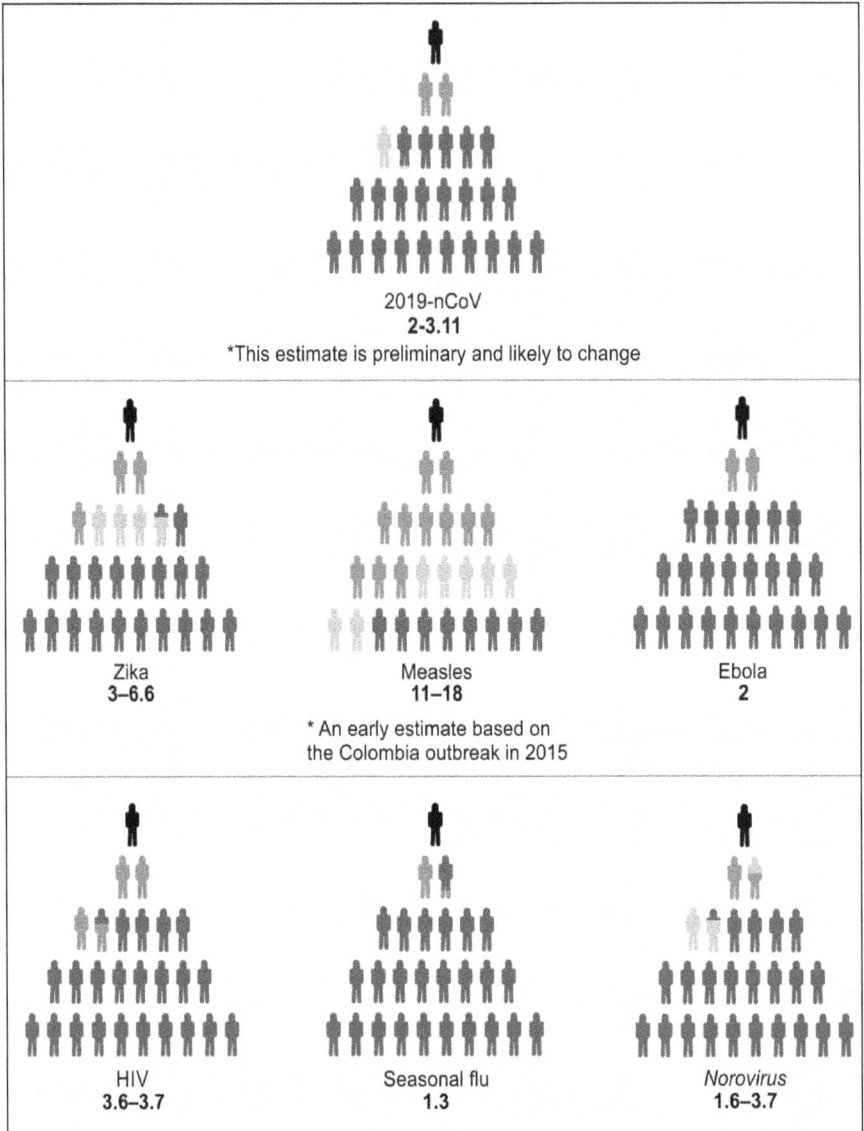

Fig. 2: A graphical display of contagiousness of different infectious diseases based on reproduction numbers ("R_0" values).

22. Can herd protection be achieved without a vaccine? Do we hope that herd protection is effective in saving people during a pandemic such as ongoing coronavirus disease 2019 (COVID-19) outbreak?

It is hard to predict things in a pandemic. Things are changing so fast that even the solid certainties that we thought we were sure of—the reproductive rate, the symptoms of the infection, the key to making a good quarantine—are suspect and need to be re-evaluated.

CHAPTER 2 Elementary Epidemiology in Vaccination

While this is a common approach underlying mass vaccination campaigns for diseases such as measles, which rely on safe and tested vaccines—trying it with a deadly, new, and untreatable disease is a massive risk. In its cruelest form, it is a version of survival of the fittest.

Herd protection without a vaccine is by definition not a preventative measure. Herd protection is an epidemiological concept that describes the state where a population—usually of people—is sufficiently immune to a disease that the infection will not spread within that group. In other words, enough people cannot get the disease—either through vaccination or natural immunity—that the people who are vulnerable are protected.

For example, let us analyze mumps. Mumps is a very infectious disease that, while relatively benign, is extremely uncomfortable and sometimes causes nasty life-long complications. It is also vaccine-preventable, with a highly effective vaccine that has made the disease incredibly rare in the modern age.

Mumps has a basic reproductive rate (R_0) of 10–12, which means that in a population which is entirely susceptible—meaning no one is immune to the virus—every person who is infected will pass the disease on to 10–12 people.

This means that without vaccination roughly 95% of the population gets infected over time. But even with something that is infectious, there are still some people—5% of the population—who do not get sick, because once everyone else is immune there is no one to catch the disease from.

We can increase that number by vaccinating, because vaccination makes people immune to infection, but it also stops infected people passing on the disease to everyone that they otherwise would. If we can get enough people immune to the disease, then it will stop spreading in the population.

For mumps, you need 92% of the population to be immune for the disease to stop spreading entirely. This is what is known as the herd protection threshold. COVID-19 is, fortunately, much less infectious than mumps, with an estimated "R_0" of roughly 3.

With this number, the proportion of people who need to be infected is lower but still high, sitting at around 70% of the entire population. Which brings us to why herd protection could never be considered a preventative measure?

If 70% of the population is infected with a disease, it is by definition not prevention. Most of the people in the country are sick! And hoping that one can reach that 70% by just infecting young people is simply irrational. If only young people are immune, one would have clusters of older people with no immunity at all, making it incredibly risky for anyone over a certain age to leave their house lest they get infected, forever.

It is also worth thinking about the repercussions of this disastrous scenario—the best estimates put COVID-19 infection fatality rate at around 0.5–1%. If 70% of an entire population gets sick, that means that between 0.35% and 0.7% of everyone in a country could die, which is a catastrophic outcome.

With something like 10% of all infections needing to be hospitalized, one would also see an enormous number of people very sick, which has huge implications for the country as well.

The sad fact is that herd protection just is not a solution to our pandemic distresses. Yes, it may eventually happen anyway, but hoping that it will save us all is just not realistic. The time to discuss herd immunity is when we have a vaccine developed, and not one second earlier, because at that point we will be able to really stop the epidemic in its tracks.

Until we have a vaccine, anyone talking about herd protection as a preventative strategy for COVID-19 is simply wrong. Fortunately, there are other ways of preventing infections from spreading, the nonpharmaceutical measures such as physical distancing, using face masks, and adhering to personal hygiene.

SUGGESTED READING

1. Chen RT, Hausinger S, Dajani AS, Hanfling M, Baughman AL, Pallansch MA, et al. Seroprevalence of antibody against poliovirus in inner city preschool children. JAMA. 1996;275:1639-45.
2. Halsey NA, Moulton LH, O'Donovan C, Walcher JR, Thoms ML, Margolis HS, et al. Hepatitis B vaccine administered to children and adolescents at yearly intervals. Pediatrics. 1999;103:1243-7.
3. Manual of Advancing Science of Vaccinology. Nerul, Navi Mumbai: Indian Academy of Pediatrics; 2009.
4. Paul Y. Herd immunity and herd protection. Vaccine. 2004;22:301-2.
5. Paul Y. Vaccines for whose benefit? Indian J Med Ethics. 2010;7:30-1.
6. Paul Y. Herd immunity and herd protection. IAP Textbook of Vaccines. Vashishtha VM, Kalra A (Eds). Second Edition 2020, Jaypee Brothers Medical Publishers, New Delhi
7. Presentations delivered at 9th ADVAC at Annecy, France, 2008 in May 10, 2010.
8. Singhal T, Amdekar YK, Agarval RK (Eds). IAP Guidebook on Immunization, 4th edition. IAP Committee on Immunization. New Delhi: Jaypee Brothers Medical Publishers; 2009.
9. Thacker N, Shendurkar N. Childhood Immunization: Issues and Options, 1st edition. New Delhi: Incal Communications; 2005.

CHAPTER 3

Vaccination Schedules

Yash Paul, Satish V Pandya

1. What is the purpose of immunization?

Immunization alters the host's susceptibility to disease, while all other risk factors remain same; it protects the individual from disease in spite of exposure or even infection. This is for individual benefit. If many are immune, the community may have benefit above and beyond the total number of immune persons. If a large proportion is immune, that may affect the epidemiology of that particular disease. For control of disease burden or eradication of disease we need to immunize a large number in a population or all individuals in a population.

2. What should be the ideal immunization schedule?

Ideal immunization schedule should be epidemiologically relevant, immunologically competent, technologically feasible, socially acceptable, affordable, and sustainable. It will vary from country to country and from time to time. In order to choose vaccines for vaccination program at government funding, not only incidence/prevalence/disease burden but their implications should be known. For government programs, usually it is cost first, efficacy next, and safety last. For an individual, it is safety first, efficacy next, and cost last. Though what is not in the best interests of the individual cannot be in the best interests of the community and what is in the best interests of the community is also in the best interests of the individual **(Table 1)**.

3. What are the determinants of optimal immunization schedules?

They can be summarized in three heads:
1. *Immunological:*
   - Minimum age at which vaccines elicit immune response
   - Number of doses required
   - Interval between doses, if multiple doses are required
2. *Epidemiological*:
   - Susceptibility for infection and disease
   - Disease severity and mortality

TABLE 1: Key differences in the vaccination schedules devise for community and individual protection.

Attributes	Community/Public health	Individual/Private healthcare
Focus	*Community*: Vaccination in public health is in the best interests of community.	*Individual child*: Vaccination in healthcare is in the best interests of each child.
Need	Determined by the epidemiology and disease burden in the community	Determined by the risk (probability of disease) to an individual child
Objective	To control a set of infectious diseases from the community Control = reduce *incidence* and *monitor* reduction	To protect the individual who is vaccinated
Ownership	Government	Consulting physician/pediatrician or individual health facility
Volume	Large	Small
AEFI	Mainly *coincidental* and *programmatic* since large volume is used.	Mainly *vaccine reactions* and *coincidental*
Funding	By the government or international donor agencies	Individual parents
Logistic issues	Major determinants	Not so important
Considerations	Cost first, efficacy next, and safety last	Safety first, efficacy next, and cost last
Examples	EPI and Universal Immunization Program (UIP)	IAP immunization schedule

(AEFI: adverse event following immunization; EPI: expanded program of immunization; IAP: Indian Academy of Pediatrics)

3. *Programmatic*:
   - Opportunity to deliver with other scheduled intervention
   - Increase coverage by limiting the required contacts.

Balance between immunological and epidemiological determinants is mandatory.

One should aim for achieving protective immune response prior to the age when children are most vulnerable. There should be a balance between inducing reasonable protection prior to vulnerable age versus inducing optimal immune response. One should also take care of impact of pre-existing maternal antibodies that may interfere with the take of many antigens **(Fig. 1)**. For example, starting late might induce a higher response, but miss the vulnerable age. Wider intervals between doses give a better response, but delays induction of immunity, leaving children vulnerable in a crucial period of life. Further, the disease epidemiology varies in different population. A schedule that is used in one population may not be the best for another; need to individualize and tailor to suit local needs.

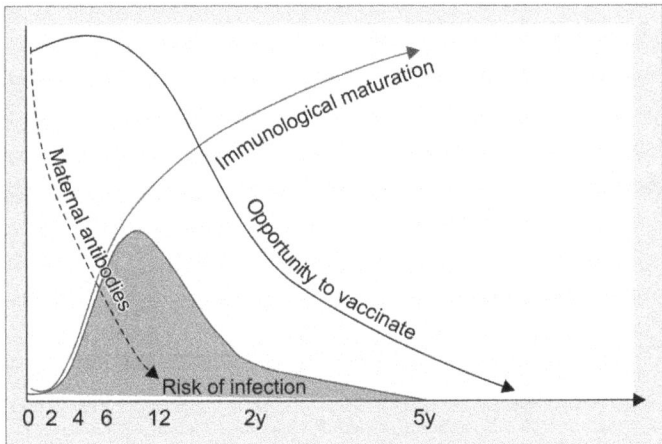

Fig. 1: Elements used to design an optimal schedule for the primary series in infants.

4. How do maternal antibodies influence an infant immunization schedule?

The maternal antibodies may exert inhibitory influence against all vaccine types, particularly against live viral vaccines that can last up to 1 year of age. The inhibitory maternal antibodies affect mainly the infant B-cell responses. Although its influence is more marked for live-attenuated viral vaccines that may be neutralized by even minute amounts of passive antibodies, e.g., the live-attenuated measles vaccine is strongly inhibited by the presence of antibodies coming from the mother, so it is only given at 12 months of age in industrialized countries and at 9 months in developing countries (the rationale of giving it at 9 months in developing countries is again to cover the vulnerable age-group while balancing it with the decreased immunological response to maternal antibodies) **(Fig. 2)**.

However, antibodies of maternal origin do not exert their inhibitory influences on infant T-cell responses, which remain largely unaffected or even enhanced. Therefore, bacillus Calmette–Guérin (BCG) vaccine can be given at birth and is not influenced by maternal antibodies as it elicits T-cell immune responses. Polio and rotavirus (RV) vaccines are also least affected by maternal antibodies.

5. What are the determinants for requirement of doses of different vaccines?

The number of doses required varies by vaccine: Live vaccines induce immunity with a single dose; inactivated vaccines require multiple doses (initial doses to prime and later doses to boost).
- Some live vaccines induce immunity in small proportion of vaccines, requiring multiple doses to induce good immunity, e.g., oral poliovirus vaccine (OPV).
- *Number of doses required may also vary by age*: More doses of conjugate vaccines are required in young infants.

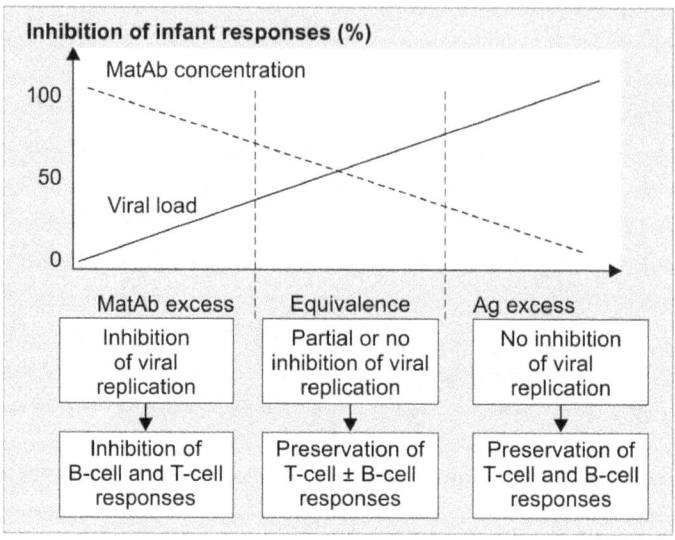

Fig. 2: Expected influence of maternal antibodies on infant responses to live viral vaccines.

- In general, a larger interval between doses induces a higher level of antibody (though not provide better immunity).
- Duration of immunity and requirement for additional doses is needed either to boost or to re-induce immunity (for T-cell independent antigens). But one needs to differentiate between decay in antibody level and immunity.
- Designing of vaccination schedules is indeed a trade-off which can be traded off on efficacy, safety, or cost.
- First aim of vaccination program is to prevent serious disease (in absolute numbers, severity, or both). Second aim is to reduce spread of infection.

6. What are the vaccination schedules in different developing countries?

Vaccination schedules in developing countries are as follows:
- 6, 10, and 14 weeks, e.g., India, Kenya, Madagascar, Mozambique, Philippines, Rwanda, and South Africa
- 2, 4, and 6 months, e.g., Egypt, Chile, Mexico, Thailand, Uruguay, Argentina, and Brazil
- 2, 3, and 4 months, e.g., Gambia, Indonesia, Turkey, and Vietnam
- 2, 3, and 5 months, e.g., Malaysia
- 3, 4, and 5 months, e.g., China.

7. What is the Indian Academy of Pediatrics (IAP) immunization schedule?

Present National Immunization Schedule as proposed by IAP is given in **Table 2**.

TABLE 2: Indian Academy of Pediatrics recommendations for routine immunization (2018–19).

Age (completed weeks/months/years)	Vaccines	Comments
At birth	BCG, OPV_0, HB_1	HB within 24 hours of birth
6 weeks	IPV_1, DTP_1, HB_2, PCV_1, $Rota_1$	DTWP/DTaP, if combination of DTP, Hib, HB, and IPV available should be preferred
10 weeks	IPV_2, DTP_2, HB_3, HIB_2, PCV_2, $Rota_2$	Third dose of Rota vaccine not required, catch-up vaccination up to 1 year of age
14 weeks	IPV_3, DTP_3, HB_4, HIB_3, PCV_3	
6 months	Typhoid conjugate vaccine Influenza vaccine	Influenza vaccine at 6 months or 2–4 weeks before influenza season, 2 doses at 4 weeks during 1st year and single dose yearly till 15 years of age
9 months	Measles/MMR	
12 months	Hepatitis A_1	Live-attenuated HA single dose only
15 months	PCV booster MMR_2, $Varicella_1$	
16–18 months	• IPV, DTP, HiB 1st booster. • HA booster	
4–6 years	DTP 2nd booster, MMR_3/MMRV $Varicella_2$	
9–14 years	Tdap, HPV two doses	Second dose after 6 months
15–18 years	Td, HPV three doses (if not given earlier)	At 0, 1–2, and 6 months
In case IPV is not available or not feasible offer bOPV three doses, in such cases two doses of fractional IPV are given at 6 and 14 weeks of age.		

(BCG: bacillus Calmette–Guérin; bOPV: bivalent-oral poliovirus vaccine; DTP: diphtheria, tetanus, and pertussis; DTWP: diphtheria, tetanus, and whole cell pertussis; DTaP: diphtheria, tetanus, and acellular pertussis; HA: hepatitis A; HB: hepatitis B; HiB: *Haemophilus influenza* type B; HPV: human papillomavirus; IPV: inactivated polio vaccine; MMR_3/MMRV: measles, mumps, and rubella vaccine; PCV: pneumococcal conjugate vaccine; Rota: rotavirus; Td: tetanus and diphtheria; Tdap: diphtheria toxoid and acellular pertussis)

8. Why is national schedule different from IAP schedule?

Perhaps it would be wrong to label it a National Immunization Schedule **(Table 3)**, because a national schedule is applicable for the whole country to be followed by all. At best, it can be called "Government Immunization Schedule" because vaccines recommended under this schedule are provided free. But, due to limited resources, government cannot provide all the vaccines which are required. On the other hand, IAP recommends vaccines depending upon availability of vaccines and disease burden. Depending upon perceptions regarding some diseases and need to prevent these diseases and also cost

TABLE 3: National Immunization Schedule, India, 2020.	
Age	Vaccines given
Birth	Bacillus Calmette–Guérin (BCG), oral polio vaccine (OPV)-0 dose, hepatitis B birth dose
6 weeks	OPV-1, pentavalent-1, rotavirus vaccine (RVV)-1***, fractional dose of inactivated polio vaccine (fIPV)-1, pneumococcal conjugate vaccine (PCV)-1***
10 weeks	OPV-2, pentavalent-2, RVV-2***
14 weeks	OPV-3, pentavatent-3, fIPV-2, RVV-3***, PCV-2***
9–12 months	Measles and rubella (MR)-1, Japanese encephalitis (JE)-1*, PCV-booster***
16–24 months	MR-2, JE-2*, diphtheria, pertussis and tetanus (DPT)-booster-1, OPV-booster
5–6 years	DPT-booster-2
10 years	Tetanus toxoid (TT)/tetanus and adult diphtheria (Td)
16 years	TT/Td
Pregnant mother	TT/Td1, 2 or TT/Td booster**

*JE in 231 endemic districts
** One dose if previously vaccinated with 3 years
***Rotavirus vaccine and PCV in selected states/districts as per details below:
- *Rotavirus*: Andhra Pradesh, Assam, Haryana, Himachal Pradesh, Jharkhand, Madhya Pradesh, Odisha, Rajasthan, Tamil Nadu, Tripura, and Uttar Pradesh.
- PCV: Bihar, Himachal Pradesh, Madhya Pradesh, Uttar Pradesh (12 districts), and Rajasthan (9 districts).

factors, parents have to decide which vaccines they would like to or can afford to provide to their children. Because of some wrong perceptions there are many parents who feel that chickenpox should not be prevented, we need to educate them, but should not coerce them to get their child vaccinated.

9. What are the considerations in deciding the age of administration of vaccines?

This may vary from place to place and country to country. Optimal response to a vaccine depends on a number of factors:
- Nature of the vaccine—killed, live, and polysaccharide
- Age and immune status of the recipient, i.e., ability of persons of a certain age to respond to the vaccine and potential interference with the immune response by passively transferred maternal antibody or previously administered antibody containing blood products
- Age-specific risks for disease and its complications
- Vaccines usually are recommended for members of the youngest age group at risk for experiencing the disease for which efficacy and safety have been demonstrated.

10. Why does vaccination schedule vary from country to country?

Vaccination schedules for different countries may be different primarily due to prevalence of different communicable diseases in different countries.

In India, Yellow fever disease is not prevalent, so there is no need to administer vaccine against yellow fever disease. This vaccine is recommended to those persons who have to travel to those countries where this disease occurs, e.g., sub-Saharan countries in Africa and Saudi Arabia during Haj pilgrimage. Similarly, typhoid disease does not occur in many developed countries because of good sanitation and clean drinking water, so typhoid vaccine is not administered in routine, but people are advised to take typhoid vaccine prior to traveling to a place where typhoid disease occurs. Even BCG vaccine is not administered in routine at birth in most of the developed countries.

Thus, vaccines are recommended to prevent the vaccine preventable diseases according to the disease burden in a population, so some vaccines may be discontinued while new vaccines may be introduced from time to time as epidemiology of diseases changes. Some vaccines are administered universally, e.g., vaccines against polio, diphtheria, tetanus, pertussis, measles, and hepatitis B diseases.

11. If a western/nonresident Indian (NRI) child comes and settles in India, which schedule to follow—native or Indian?

Such a child should be provided vaccines according to the Indian schedule, because this child would be exposed to those infections which are prevalent in India. For example, a 6-year-old child who has migrated from the United Kingdom or the United States of America, where BCG vaccine is not administered as a routine vaccine, should be administered BCG vaccine on a priority basis, after a Mantoux test.

12. With so many vaccines available, what schedule should one follow?

Different countries have their own recommended schedule according to epidemiology of the diseases and other logistic considerations. In India, we have mainly two schedules: (1) National Immunization Schedule and (2) the one suggested by IAP (see above).

National Immunization Schedule comprises those vaccines which are given free of cost to all children of country under expanded program of immunization (EPI).

The IAP schedule is based on the recommendations of the IAP Advisory Committee on Vaccines and Immunization Practices (ACVIP). The committee submits its position on vaccines not included in the national schedule on a periodic basis as they are introduced in the private market. The process of issuing recommendations involves an exhaustive review of published literature including standard textbooks, vaccine trials, recommendations of various countries, World Health Organization (WHO) position papers (*see* Annexure 1), literature from the vaccine industry, postmarketing surveillance reports, cost-effective analysis, epidemiology of disease in India and, if available, Indian studies on vaccine efficacy, immunogenicity, and safety. These recommendations of ACVIP are primarily for pediatricians in office practice.

46 SECTION 1 General Vaccination

13. What are the different vaccines categories formed by IAP and how are the vaccines categorized?

There are now only two vaccines categories:
1. *Category 1*: IAP recommended vaccines for routine use (*see* **Table 2**).
2. *Category 2*: IAP recommended vaccines for high-risk children (vaccines under special circumstances) **(Table 4)**.

TABLE 4: Indian Academy of Pediatrics recommendations for high-risk children/area (2018–19).

Vaccine	Age and doses
Meningococcal vaccine (MCV)	• 9 months through 23 months two doses at least 3 months apart • 2 years through 55 years single dose only
Japanese encephalitis (JE)	For individuals living in endemic areas and for travelers to JE endemic areas, provided their expected stay is for a minimum period of 4 weeks
Cholera vaccine	Two doses 2 weeks apart for >1 year old

14. How do we plan for a child who has not received any vaccination?

Depending on the age of the child at the first contact, we can plan to catch up with the immunization. An accelerated schedule may be planned if required **(Table 5)**.

TABLE 5: Catch-up immunization schedule for an unimmunized child.

Visit	Suggested schedule
First	• Measles (MMR if >12 months) • $DTwP_1/DTaP_1$ (Tdap if 7 years or more) • OPV_1/IPV_1 (only if <6 years) • Hib_1 (only if <6 years) • $Hep\ B_1$ • BCG (only in <5 years)
Second (after 1 month of first visit)	• $DTwP_2/DTaP_2$ (Td if 7 years or more) • OPV_2 (if OPV given earlier) • $Hep\ B_2$ • Hib_2 (if <7 years)
Third (after 1 month of second visit)	• OPV_3/IPV_2 • MMR (if >12 months) • Typhoid (if >6 months)
Fourth (6 months after first visit)	$DTwP_3/DTaP_3$ (Td if 7 years or more), $OPV_4/IPVB_1$, and $Hep\ B_3$

(BCG: bacillus Calmette–Guérin; DTwP/DTaP: diphtheria, tetanus, and whole cell pertussis/diphtheria, tetanus, and acellular pertussis; Hib: *Haemophilus influenza* type b; IPV: inactivated poliovirus vaccine; MMR: measles-mumps-rubella (vaccine); OPV: oral poliovirus vaccine; td: tetanus-diphtheria)

15. How about adolescent immunization?

This is an important period for "top-up" immunization. Additionally, some of the vaccines might not have been available when these adolescents were in their early childhood. The catch-up immunization may be done up to 18 years of age (For details, please *see* Chapter 52).

SUGGESTED READING

1. Balasubramanian S, Shah A, Pemde HK, Chatterjee P, Shivananda S, Guduru VK. Indian Academy of Pediatrics (IAP) Advisory Committee on Vaccines and Immunization Practices (ACVIP) Recommended Immunization Schedule (2018–19) and Update on Immunization for children aged 0 through 18 years. Indian Pediatr. 2018;55:1066-74.
2. Choudhury P, Bang G, Vashishtha VM. Scheduling of vaccines. In: Vashishtha VM (Ed). IAP Textbook of Vaccines, 2nd edition. New Delhi: Jaypee Brothers Medical Publishers (P) Ltd.; 2020. pp. 78-87.

CHAPTER 4

Practice of Vaccination

Yash Paul, Satish V Pandya, Atul K Agarwal

1. What are the safe injection practices?

The hands should be washed with soap and water or cleaned with an alcohol-based waterless handrub before each patient contact to prevent contamination. Skin at the injection site should be prepared with 70% isopropyl alcohol or another disinfecting agent and allowed to dry before injection. Separate disposable syringes and needles should be used for each injection. One should not deviate from the recommended route of administration in the product label. Prefilling of syringe should be avoided as most vaccines appear similar and administration error can occur.

2. How can we alleviate pain associated with vaccination?

Several methods are used for this purpose but they have not been tested widely. Superficial anesthesia can be induced by application of topical lidocaine-prilocaine emulsion cream or patch. However, drug interactions regarding development of methemoglobinemia should be kept in mind. Paracetamol or ibuprofen can be used as analgesic when required. Breastfeeding is a potent analgesic. Sweet fluids just before injection may also help. Distraction techniques, such as music can help children cope with discomfort.

3. What are the roles of preservatives, stabilizers, and antimicrobial agents in a vaccine?

Trace amounts of chemicals (e.g., mercurials, such as thimerosal) and certain antimicrobial agents (such as neomycin or streptomycin sulfate) are commonly included to prevent bacterial growth or to stabilize an antigen. Allergic reactions may occur if the recipient is sensitive to one or more of these additives.

4. What are the general instructions for vaccination?

Following instructions should be strictly followed while providing vaccination services at your practice:

- To prevent accidental needle-sticks or reuse, a needle should not be recapped after use.
- Disposable needles and syringes should be discarded promptly in puncture-proof, labeled containers.
- Changing needles between drawing vaccine into the syringe and injecting it into the child is not necessary.
- Different vaccines should not be mixed in the same syringe unless specifically licensed and labeled for such use.

Whenever possible, patients should be observed for an allergic reaction for 15–20 minutes after receiving immunization.

5. What are the instructions one should follow on orally administered vaccines?

The vaccine must be swallowed and retained. Oral poliovirus vaccines (OPV) should be repeated immediately if a child spits it out, fails to swallow, or regurgitates a dose within 10 minutes after administration. If the second dose is not retained, neither dose should be counted, and vaccine should be re-administered. Breastfeeding does not interfere with successful immunization with oral vaccines (e.g., OPV, rotavirus).

Regarding rotavirus vaccines, instructions given by the manufacturer should be followed if the child spits out the vaccine.

6. What are the general instructions on administration of parenteral vaccines?

Injectable vaccines should be administered in a site as free as possible from risk of local neural, vascular, or tissue injury. Data do not warrant recommendation of a single preferred site for all injections.

Preferred sites for vaccines administered subcutaneously or intramuscularly include the anterolateral aspect of the upper thigh and the deltoid area of the upper arm.

Ordinarily, the upper, outer aspect of the buttocks should not be used for active immunization because:
- The gluteal region is covered by a significant layer of subcutaneous fat, and
- The possibility of damaging the sciatic nerve
- Due to diminished immunogenicity, hepatitis B and rabies vaccines should not be given in the buttocks at any age.

People who were given hepatitis B vaccine in the buttocks should be tested for immunity and reimmunized if antibody concentrations are inadequate.

7. What are general instructions for administration of vaccines intramuscularly?

When the upper, outer quadrant of the buttocks is used for large-volume passive immunization, such as intramuscular (IM) administration of large volumes of immunoglobulin (IG), care must be taken to avoid injury to the sciatic nerve.

- The site selected should be well into the upper, outer mass of the gluteus maximus, away from the central region of the buttocks, and the needle should be directed anteriorly, that is, if the patient is lying prone, the needle is directed perpendicular to the table's surface, not perpendicular to the skin plane.
- The ventrogluteal site may be less hazardous for IM injection, because it is free of major nerves and vessels. This site is the center of a triangle for which the boundaries are the anterior superior iliac spine, the tubercle of the iliac crest, and the upper border of the greater trochanter.

Vaccines containing adjuvants [e.g., aluminum-adsorbed diphtheria and tetanus toxoids, and acellular pertussis (DTaP), diphtheria and tetanus toxoids, and whole-cell pertussis (DTwP), diphtheria and tetanus toxoids (DT), hepatitis B, and hepatitis A] must be injected deep into the muscle mass. These vaccines should not be administered subcutaneously or intracutaneously, because they can cause local irritation, inflammation, granuloma formation, and tissue necrosis.

8. Can two vaccines be administered in the same limb at a single visit? What should be the minimum distance between two injections?

Yes, they can be. When necessary, two vaccines can be given in the same limb at a single visit. The anterolateral aspect of the thigh is the preferred site for two simultaneous IM injections because of its greater muscle mass. The distance separating the two injections is arbitrary but should be at least 1 inch so that local reactions are unlikely to overlap.

9. Should one perform gentle aspiration by pulling back on the syringe while administering vaccine by IM route?

Although most experts recommend "aspiration" by gently pulling back on the syringe before the injection is given, there are no data to document the necessity for this procedure. If blood appears after negative pressure, the needle should be withdrawn and another site should be selected using a new needle.

10. What are the guidelines for site, route of administration and length and gauge of needles?

Table 1 lists details about route, site, and needle length. If more than one vaccine is given at the same anatomic site they should be separated by a distance of at least one inch. Gluteal region should never be used as site of injection. In infants and younger children anterolateral aspect of thigh is preferred whereas deltoid is preferred site for older children and adolescents. If vaccine and an immunoglobulin preparation are administered simultaneously, two different anatomic sites should be used.

TABLE 1: Injection site, type of needle, and technique.			
Age	Site	Type of needle	Comments
Intramuscular injections (needle should enter at 90° angle)			
Preterms and neonates	Anterolateral thigh (junction of middle and lower third)	22–25 gauge, 5/8 inch	Skin should be stretched between thumb and forefinger
Infants (1 to <12 months)	Anterolateral thigh	22–25 gauge, 1 inch	Bunch the skin, subcutaneous tissue and muscle to prevent striking the bone
Toddlers and older children (12 months–10 years)	Deltoid or Anterolateral thigh	22–25 G, 5/8 inch 22–25 gauge 1 inch	Skin should be stretched between thumb and forefinger Bunch the skin, subcutaneous tissue, and muscle
Adolescents and adults (11 years onward)	Deltoid or anterolateral thigh	<60 kg, 1 inch >60 kg, 1.5 inch	
Subcutaneous injections (needle should enter at 45° to the skin)			
Infants >12 months	Thigh Outer triceps	22–25 G, 5/8 inch 22–25 G, 5/8 inch	
Intradermal injections			
All ages	Left deltoid	26/27 G, 0.5 inch	A 5-mm wheal should be raised

Needles used for IM injections
- For newborn infants, especially preterm infants, a 5/8-inch long needle usually is adequate
- A 7/8–1 inch long needle is recommended to ensure penetration of the thigh muscle of full-term infants 2–12 months of age
- For injection into the thigh or deltoid muscle in toddlers and older children, a 7/8–1.25 inch long needle is suggested, depending on the size of the muscle
- The deltoid is preferred for immunization of adolescents and young adults. The needle length should be 1–2 inches, depending on the vaccine recipient's weight
- A 22–25 gauge needle is appropriate for injection of most IM vaccines.

11. What should be the ideal spacing between multiple doses of same vaccine?

Killed vaccines require multiple doses to boost the immune response and develop a protective antibody titer to last for the age till the individual is susceptible for the disease. Though live-attenuated vaccines such as Bacillus Calmette–Guérin (BCG) and rubella require only one dose as the attenuated organism multiplies in the body for a lasting immune response and formation of memory cells. Multiple doses of some live vaccines are recommended to stimulate an immune response to different types of the same virus, such as poliovirus types 1, 2, and 3, or to induce immunity in persons who failed to mount an immune response to an earlier dose of vaccine, such as measles.

These multiple doses constitute a primary vaccination series and are not "booster doses".

Because of immunologic memory, intervals longer than routinely recommended between doses do not impair the immunologic response to live and inactivated vaccines that require more than one dose to achieve primary immunity. As a result, interruption of a recommended primary series or an extended interval between booster doses does not necessitate reinitiation of the entire vaccination series.

Minimum interval is usually 4 weeks. Interval of 8 weeks between multiple doses of diphtheria, pertussis, and tetanus (DPT), injectable polio vaccine (IPV), etc. have the best response in terms of antibody titers but the expanded program on immunization (EPI) schedule of 4 weeks between multiple doses of primary immunization is also effective.

Administration of doses of a vaccine at intervals less than the minimum intervals or earlier than the minimum age may result in a reduced immune response with diminished vaccine efficacy and should be avoided.

12. What should be the spacing of different vaccines?

Two or more inactivated vaccines can be given simultaneously or at any interval between doses. Inactivated and live vaccines can be given at any interval between doses or simultaneously. But two or more live injectable or nasal vaccines should have an interval of 4 weeks if not administered simultaneously. There is a possibility that two doses of the same or different live virus vaccines administered within too short an interval may inhibit the immunologic response to the second dose which is based on evidence from both animal and human studies. If parenterally or nasally administered live virus vaccines are separated by <4 weeks, readministration of the live virus vaccine given second should also be considered. As exception OPV, rotavirus, and oral typhoid vaccines may be given at any time in relation to any live/inactivated vaccine. These guidelines are important for planning catch-up immunization.

This interval between two doses of a vaccine is different for different vaccines, where multiple doses are to be administered. This time interval can be divided in three groups: (1) ideal interval, (2) minimum interval and (3) maximum interval.

In case of rabies vaccine, number of doses and gaps are different for preexposure and postexposure schedules. In pre-exposure schedule, three doses are given on days 0, 7, and 21 or 28. In postexposure schedule, five doses are administered on days 0, 3, 7, 14, and 28/30. In case of DPT vaccine, minimum interval between two doses should be 4 weeks, ideal interval is 8 weeks, and maximum interval between two doses can be 1 year. In case of hepatitis B vaccine, variable intervals between 1st and 2nd, and 2nd and 3rd doses are recommended. In case of pre-exposure schedule recommendations for low-risk individuals and high-risk individuals are different. Ideal schedule for low-risk population is 0, 1, and 6 months, for high-risk population is 0, 1, 2, and 12 months.

> **BOX 1:** Scheduling immunizations.
> - Most vaccines are safe and effective when administered simultaneously.
> - This information is particularly important for scheduling immunizations for children with lapsed or missed immunizations and for people preparing for international travel.
> - Inactivated vaccines do not interfere with the immune response to other inactivated vaccines or to live vaccines.
> - Limited data indicate possible impaired immune responses and increased incidence of a breakthrough illness, when two or more live-virus vaccines are given nonsimultaneously but within 28 days of each other. Therefore, parenterally administered live-virus vaccines not administered on the same day should be given at least 28 days (4 weeks) apart whenever possible, such as measles-mumps-rubella (MMR) and varicella vaccines.
> - Combination vaccine products may be given whenever any component of the combination is indicated and its other components are not contraindicated.
> - The use of combination vaccines is preferred over separate injection of their component vaccines.

13. How many different vaccines can be administered simultaneously?

Any number of vaccines can be given simultaneously on the same day but at different anatomic sites. All vaccines indicated as per schedule should be given together (**Box 1**). Simultaneous administration of different vaccines is particularly important when return of the recipient for further vaccination is uncertain, when imminent exposure to several vaccine-preventable diseases is expected, or when preparing for international travel on short notice.

Vaccines licensed for injection in the same syringe can be given together. If more than one vaccine has to be administered, a single limb of an infant or young child, the thigh usually is preferred because of its large muscle mass. The distance separating two injections in the same limb should be sufficient (e.g., 1–2 inches) to minimize the chance of overlapping local reactions. Studies have shown that two injections on the same day do not increase stress or severity of reactions or immunological interference.

14. What does "simultaneous administration" of vaccines mean?

Simultaneous means the same day—the same clinic day. If someone receives a vaccine in the morning and then another that same afternoon, it would be considered simultaneous administration. It does not mean that the vaccines should be given at the same hour.

15. Why IM route is preferred for certain vaccines and subcutaneously (SC)/intradermal (ID) for some other and vice-versa?

The vaccines, which contain adjuvants, generally cause local reactions such as pain and swelling, induration, irritation, skin discoloration, inflammation, and granuloma formation. For this reason, such vaccines should be administered intramuscular. BCG is administered intradermal. Most of the inactivated vaccines are given IM, with a few exceptions (such as IPV and pneumococcal polysaccharide vaccines, which may be given either

SC or IM). If BCG is administered subcutaneously or intramuscularly, it could result in lower efficacy as well as some local abscess.

16. A 5-year-old child with a plastered arm in cast has come to you for his preschool vaccines, which include MMR, varicella, and diphtheria, tetanus toxoids, and pertussis (DTP) booster. Can the anterolateral thigh be used to administer a subcutaneous vaccine in a 5-year-old child?

Yes. There is no age limit for use of the anterolateral thigh for either subcutaneous or intramuscular vaccines.

17. A 6-week-old child with hip dysplasia with cast covering his both anterolateral thigh on both legs which is supposed to be there for next 2–3 months. How would you vaccinate such a child?

You can ask the orthopedician to provide a space on the anterolateral thighs after cutting the plaster to administer vaccines. If that is not feasible, the gluteal region can be used if not covered by the cast. There are no other sites recommended for vaccination; however, the IPV could be given subcutaneously in either arm.

18. Do immunoglobulins acquired passively or administered IM/intravenously (IV) as available preparations interfere with immune response to live vaccines?

Passively acquired antibodies can interfere with the immune response leading to either absence of seroconversion or a blunting of the immune response with lower final antibody concentrations in the vaccinee. Passively acquired antibody does not affect the immune response to all vaccines. Maternal antibodies affect measles and rubella uptake not varicella, rotavirus, and influenza.

Intramuscular or intravenous administration of immunoglobulin-containing preparations (e.g., serum immunoglobulin, hyperimmunoglobulins, intravenous immunoglobulin, and blood) before or simultaneous with certain vaccines also can affect the immune response to live virus vaccines. Blunting of responses to measles and rubella has been demonstrated. Though low dose of anti-Rh(D) globulin administered to postpartum women has not been demonstrated to inhibit the immune response to RA27/3 strain rubella vaccine. Polio and yellow fever are not affected. Data are insufficient to determine the extent to which passively acquired antibodies interfere with the immune response varicella, mumps, and typhoid (Ty21a strain) (**Box 2**).

19. Do immunoglobulins interfere with immune response to inactivated and component vaccines?

Response to inactivated and component vaccines is less affected with live vaccines and requires exposure to large doses of passively acquired

> **BOX 2:** Minimum ages and minimum intervals between doses.
>
> *Vaccine doses:*
> - Vaccines should not be administered at intervals less than the recommended minimum or at an earlier age than the recommended minimum (e.g., accelerated schedules). Two exceptions to this may occur:
>   - The first is for measles vaccine during a measles outbreak, in which case the vaccine may be administered before 9 months of age. However, if a measles-containing vaccine is administered before 9 months of age, the child should be reimmunized at 12–15 months of age with MMR vaccine.
>   - The second consideration involves administering a dose a few days earlier than the minimum interval or age, which is unlikely to have a substantially negative effect on the immune response to that dose.
> - Vaccine doses administered 4 days or fewer before the minimum interval or age can be counted as valid.
> - This 4-day recommendation does not apply to rabies vaccine because of the unique schedule for this vaccine.
> - Doses administered 5 days or more before the minimum interval or age should not be counted as valid doses and should be repeated as age appropriate.

(MMR: measles-mumps-rubella)

antibodies. Moderate doses of parenterally administered immunoglobulins have not inhibited development of a protective immune response to DTP, tetanus toxoid, hepatitis B vaccines, and *Haemophilus influenzae* type b (Hib) conjugate vaccines. Administration of inactivated hepatitis A vaccine and immunoglobulin simultaneously does not affect seroconversion. Maternal antibody to hepatitis A virus does not affect seroconversion.

20. What is the recommendation regarding spacing with respect to administration of immunoglobulins or antibody-containing products?

Antibody-containing products and inactivated antigen can be administered simultaneously at different sites or at any time interval between doses. Nonsimultaneous administration can also be done at any interval.

Antibody-containing products and live-antigen should not be administered simultaneously. If simultaneous administration of measles-containing vaccine or varicella vaccine is unavoidable, administer at different sites and revaccinate or test for seroconversion after the recommended interval. If live-antigen is administered after antibody-containing products, interval should be dose related. Antibody-containing products can be administered after 2 weeks of live-antigen without any interference with seroconversion. Measles and varicella-containing vaccines should be administered 3–6 months after immunoglobulins or blood transfusion (**Box 3**).

21. Suppose expiry date of a vaccine is June 2021. Can it be used till June 30, 2021 or till May 31, 2021?

It can be used till June 30, 2021. To avoid any confusion, the manufacturers should state: "use till...." information.

> **BOX 3:** Vaccine dose.
> - Reduced or divided doses of DTP or any other vaccine, including those given to premature or low-birthweight infants, should not be administered. The efficacy of this practice in decreasing the frequency of adverse events has not been demonstrated.
> - A previous immunization with a dose that was less than the standard dose or one administered by a nonstandard route should not be counted, and the person should be reimmunized as appropriate for age.
> - Exceeding recommended doses also may be hazardous.
> - Excessive local concentrations of injectable inactivated vaccines might result in enhanced tissue or systemic reactions, whereas administering an increased dose of a live vaccine constitutes a theoretic but unproven risk.

> **BOX 4:** Simultaneous administration of multiple vaccines.
> - Most vaccines can be safely and effectively administered simultaneously.
> - No contraindications to the simultaneous administration of multiple vaccines routinely recommended for infants and children are known.
> - Immune responses to one vaccine generally do not interfere with those to other vaccines.
> - An exception is a decrease in immunogenicity when cholera and yellow fever vaccines are given together or 1–3 weeks apart.
>   - When simultaneous vaccines are administered, separate syringes and sites should be used, and injections into the same extremity should be separated by at least 1 inch so that any local reactions can be differentiated.
>   - Individual vaccines should never be mixed in the syringe unless they are specifically licensed and labeled for administration in one syringe.

22. Are vaccines of different manufacturers interchangeable?

Yes, these are interchangeable. Change of brand may be necessary in case of nonavailability of the same brand or if previous records are not clear about the brand used. Change of brand is acceptable. However, as far as possible one should use the same brand in a given patient (**Box 4**).

23. Can two vaccines (to be given on the same day) be mixed in a single syringe?

Some vaccines are prepared as premixed vaccines such as measles, mumps, and rubella as MMR, diphtheria, tetanus, and pertussis whole cell or acellular component are available as DPT or DaPT. Some manufacturers provide additional vaccines with DPT or DaPT such as Hib or hepatitis B vaccines to be mixed together. In these vaccines, some component is provided as fluid and other component as solid or powder, the final quantity of all these vaccines remains 0.5 mL. Only such preparations should be mixed in a syringe, which are recommended by the manufacturers.

24. Do we need to wait for the vaccine to reach room temperature before we administer it to a patient?

No such recommendation is there from any authority. The vaccine should be administered as soon as it is prepared.

CHAPTER 4 Practice of Vaccination

25. Some single-dose manufacturer-filled vaccines come with an air pocket in the syringe chamber. Do we need to expel the air pocket before vaccinating?

No. You do not need to expel the air pocket. The air will be absorbed. This is not true for syringes that you fill yourself; you should expel air bubbles from these syringes prior to vaccination to the extent that you can do so.

26. For how long can you store the syringe with the needle attached once one has placed a needle on a manufacturer-filled syringe?

In general, a vaccine should not be prepared until the provider is ready to administer it to a patient. This is because once the syringe cap is removed or a needle is attached, the sterile seal is broken. However, if a sterile seal has been broken, one should be sure to maintain the syringe at the appropriate temperature and either use it or discard it at the end of the session day.

27. Should you allow alcohol to dry completely on patients' skin prior to administering a vaccine injection?

It is wise to allow the alcohol to evaporate, but it is unlikely that the small amount residual alcohol on the skin will affect the vaccine's response or increase the risk of an adverse reaction.

28. Is there any recommendation to change needles after a vaccine dose has been drawn into a syringe?

No. It is also unnecessary to change the needle if it has passed through two stoppers, which is done when a lyophilized vaccine is reconstituted. Changing needle is a waste of resources and increases the risk of needle stick injury.

29. Should whole series of vaccination be repeated if one dose is missed/delayed?

The answer cannot be simple no or yes. It needs to be elaborated. Two doses of rotavirus vaccines are recommended, ideally to be administered at 6 and 10 weeks. Second dose should be administered before 24 weeks of age, but if delayed beyond 24 weeks it should not be administered. In case of hepatitis B vaccine, second dose should be administered after 4 weeks, but if the vaccinee comes in <12 months after first dose, second dose can be administered. If vaccinee comes for the second dose after >1 year of the first dose, then this second dose should be considered as first dose. In case of third dose, if interval is >2 years then two doses at interval of 6 months should be advised. Same schedule can be applied for DPT/DaPT and polio vaccines.

30. What precaution is required in a child with bleeding tendency?

Unless contraindicated, subcutaneous route should be used. For those vaccines (aluminum adjuvanted) which need to be given only intramuscularly, vaccination should be planned after factor replacement. A sustained pressure for at least 5 minutes should be applied following injection.

31. Is it necessary to withhold vaccination in a sick child?

Vaccination may be withheld only if child is seriously ill. However, in case of minor illnesses such as upper respiratory tract infection (URTI) and mild diarrhea, vaccination need not be postponed.

32. What precaution should be undertaken in immunizing a child who is also advised tuberculin skin test?

A tuberculin skin test can be applied at the same visit during which live viral vaccines, such as MMR, measles, varicella, etc., are administered. Because measles vaccine temporarily can suppress tuberculin reactivity, if tuberculin testing is indicated and cannot be done at the same time as measles immunization, tuberculin testing should be postponed for 4–6 weeks.

The effect of other live-virus vaccines on tuberculin skin test reactivity is not known.

33. How should a serious anaphylaxis reaction to a vaccine be managed?

Following protocol should be followed immediately:
- Administer epinephrine (1:1,000 solution) 0.01 mL/kg/dose (max 0.5 mL) intramuscular in anterolateral thigh.
- Set up IV access.
- Lay patient flat and elevate legs if tolerated. Give high flow oxygen and airway/ventilation, if needed.
- If hypotensive also, set up additional wide bore access and give IV normal saline 20 mL/kg under pressure over 1–2 minutes.
- Intramuscular adrenaline may be repeated after 3–5 minutes if required.
- Oral antihistaminics may be given to ameliorate skin symptoms but IV antihistaminics are not recommended. Oral or injectable corticosteroids equivalent to prednisone 1–2 mg/kg may be given but benefit is yet unproven.

34. What precautions should be observed for proper storage and handling of vaccines?

Handling vaccines at the recommended temperature at all the time is very important to prevent loss of potency. Vaccines can be damaged by both excessive heat and excessive cold.

Vaccines differ in their sensitivity to heat. Loss of potency cannot be restored by putting them back to correct temperature. With every exposure to improper temperature there is loss of potency and the damage is cumulative. Live vaccines are more sensitive to heat exposure and aluminum adjuvanted vaccines are more damaged by cold injury (**Table 2**).

TABLE 2: Recommendation for storage.	
Vaccines which should not be frozen	Vaccines which can be frozen
DTwP, DTaP, TT, DT, Td, Hep B, combination vaccines, rotavirus, typhoid, and Hib	OPV-I, lyophilized measles, MMR, BCG, LAIV, certain brands of varicella, and MMRV

(BCG: Bacillus Calmette–Guérin; DT: diphtheria tetanus (vaccine); DTwP/DTaP: diphtheria and tetanus toxoids, and whole-cell pertussis/diphtheria and tetanus toxoids, and acellular pertussis (vaccine); Hep: hepatitis; Hib: *Haemophilus influenzae* type b; LAIV: live-attenuated influenza vaccine; MMR: measles-mumps-rubella (vaccine); MMRV: measles-mumps-rubella and variable (vaccine); OPV: oral poliovirus vaccine; Td: tetanus-diphtheria; TT: tetanus toxoids)

Lyophilized and reconstituted BCG, measles, MMR, varicella, rotavirus, HPV and most DTaP containing vaccines are susceptible to exposure to light and need to be protected from strong light, sunlight, ultraviolet, and fluorescent neon lights.

35. What storage equipment is required for office practice and how best one should use it?

A domestic refrigerator with combination of refrigerator and freezer is acceptable. Refrigerator and freezer should have separate external door. The recommended temperature for the main compartment is 2–8°C and for the freezer compartment is 5–15°C. A thermometer to monitor the temperature is must.

The appropriate places for different vaccines are given in **Table 3**.

36. What are the do's and dont's for use of refrigerator?

Following instructions should be followed:
- Do not open the door unnecessarily.
- Do not use for storage of any other items.
- Keep ice packs and bottles filled with water in the freezer and door to maintain cold temperature in case of power failure.
- The power plug should have a sticker saying "Do Not Unplug" or "Do Not Turn Off".
- In case of frequent power failure, an alternative power source should be arranged.
- Use principles of first expired first out (FEFO) and first in first out (FIFO).

37. How should one maintain record of immunization?

Complete and accurate records are mandatory. Failure to do so poses lot of difficulty and confusion as to how to complete the schedule. Ideally one should record date of vaccination, name of the vaccine, manufacturer, lot number, expiry date, site and route of administration and name, and title and address of the healthcare provider.

TABLE 3: Storage at different levels in a refrigerator.

Compartment	Vaccines
Freezer	Unopened vials of BCG and OPV
Top shelf	OPV, measles, MMR, varicella, rotavirus, typhoid (live vaccine), hepatitis A (live vaccine), Swine flu (live)
Middle shelf	TT, dt, DPT, DaPT, pneumococcal, meningococcal, hepatitis A (inactivated), typhoid (inactivated), Japanese encephalitis, yellow fever, hepatitis B vaccines, rabies, HiB, human papilloma, cholera, fly, Swine flu (inactivated), Avian flu
Lower shelf	TT, dt, DPT, DaPT, pneumococcal, meningococcal, hepatitis A (inactivated), typhoid (inactivated), Japanese encephalitis, yellow fever, hepatitis B vaccines, rabies, HiB, human papilloma, cholera, fly, Swine flu (inactivated), Avian flu
Crispator	Diluents
Baffle tray	No vaccines
Doors	No vaccines

(BCG: Bacillus Calmette–Guérin; DaPT/DPT: diphtheria, tetanus and pertussis; dt: diphtheria tetanus (vaccine); HiB: *Haemophillus influenzae* type b; MMR: measles-mumps-rubella (vaccine); OPV: oral poliovirus vaccine; TT: tetanus toxoids)

38. What are the ethical issues of immunization?

With several new vaccines flooding the market, parents find it difficult to decide on which vaccines should be given to their child. The onus is on the pediatrician to give a balanced scientific advice to parents. One has to keep oneself updated with knowledge regarding the vaccines. Special communication skills need to be developed to address many issues related to the decision-making process. Some of the aspects which need to be clearly explained to parents are: risk of developing disease and need for vaccination, efficacy of vaccine, safety issues, cost of vaccine and affordability. The dynamic nature of recommendations should also be emphasized.

39. Should we encourage advertisements of various vaccines in lay press?

No advertisement of any sort should be permitted. I would like to quote what I had stated earlier (Paul Y. Vaccines for whose benefit? Indian Journal of Medical Ethics. 2010;7:30-1).

These days, some of the new vaccines are advertised in the electronic media on the pretext of creating public awareness. Consumer products are advertised, but no new medicine is advertised in similar manner. Some of these vaccines are not recommended for universal immunization but are recommended for specific conditions, but this is not mentioned in the advertisement. So, when parents ask their doctors about such vaccines, doctors find themselves in a piquant situation. For example, the influenza vaccine is recommended when a vaccinee is suffering from chronic pulmonary and cardiac disease, immunodeficiency, HIV infection, etc. On the other hand, the absence of such indications is no contraindication for this vaccine, and no harm is expected to occur. The doctor may choose to explain the true situation and spend a lot of time to convince the parents that the vaccine is not required for that child. Two questions may be asked. First, will any harm occur to the child if this vaccine is administered? The answer is "No". Second, is there any possibility, although it is not likely, that this child could suffer from a severe form of influenza in future? The answer is "Yes", as this possibility is always there. Thus, through advertisements, a sort of fear is created to increase sales of this vaccine. Under these circumstances, doctors cannot be blamed for administering such a vaccine. Such advertisements should not be permitted.

40. Should school administration be allowed to insist on vaccination of any particular vaccine even for hostellers?

In India no vaccine has been declared compulsory. Even for compulsory vaccines, the vaccine recipient or caretakers can refuse vaccination with the undertaking to be responsible for any harm to self or ward. Some schools had insisted on varicella vaccine and hepatitis A vaccine administration to those children seeking admission especially as hostellers. It is for the doctors to suggest vaccines but ultimate decision to administer or not to administer any vaccine rests with the individuals or caretakers in case of children.

SUGGESTED READING

1. Immunization action Coalition. Ask the expert. Administering Vaccines. [online] Available from: https://www.immunize.org/askexperts/administering-vaccines.asp [Last accessed June, 2020].
2. Manual of Advancing Science of Vaccinology. Indian Academy of Pediatrics; 2009.
3. Pickering LK, Baker CJ, Long SS, McMillan JA (Eds). Red Book: 2006 Report of the Committee on Infectious Diseases, 27th edition. Elk Grove Village, IL: American Academy of Pediatrics; 2006.

CHAPTER 5

Vaccine-preventable Diseases Surveillance

Meeta Dhaval Vashi

1. What is vaccine-preventable disease?

Vaccine-preventable diseases (VPDs) are the diseases which can be prevented by vaccines.

2. What is surveillance?

Definitions: Systematic ongoing collection, collation, and analysis of data and the timely dissemination of information to those who need to know so that action can be taken. (World Health Organization)

The ongoing systematic collection, analysis, and interpretation of health data, essential to the planning, implementation, and evaluation of public health practice, closely integrated with the timely dissemination of these data to those who need to know. (US Centers for Disease Control and Prevention)

3. What is "not surveillance"?

The mere collection and compilation of disease-related data without analyzing them and taking appropriate action is "not surveillance".

4. What are the purposes of disease surveillance?

- Establish disease burden
- Monitor progress toward disease eradication, elimination and/or control goals
- Assure rapid detection and response to disease events of public health concern
- Document short-term and long-term effects of vaccination on disease burden and epidemiology, thereby monitoring program effectiveness
- Detect shifts in types or subtypes of organisms causing disease.

5. What is VPD surveillance?

Vaccine-preventable disease surveillance is collection of data on incidence and prevalence of VPDs in population and utilization of this data for focused actions and interventions.

6. Which diseases are included as VPD?

Vaccine-preventable disease includes diphtheria, pertussis, tetanus, polio, severe childhood tuberculosis, measles, rubella, hepatitis B, pneumonia, and meningitis due to *Haemophilus influenza* B type, pneumococcal pneumonia, rotavirus, diarrhea, Japanese encephalitis, cholera, typhoid, hepatitis A, rabies, mumps, yellow fever, and *Varicella zoster*.

7. Is VPD surveillance done for all VPDs?

All VPDs are reported to health system by network of Integrated Disease Surveillance Program (IDSP) and few specific targeted VPDs are included for laboratory-based VPD surveillance system wherein each and every case is investigated and samples are collected.

8. Why is VPD surveillance necessary?

Vaccine-preventable disease surveillance is necessary to detect areas of transmission for focused intervention (such as mission "Indradhanush"), extent of outbreaks, measure impact and quality of immunization programs, and progress toward control/elimination/eradication. The type of surveillance for a specific VPD depends on the attributes of the disease and the objectives of the disease control program—control, elimination or eradication. These factors direct the surveillance activities to be implemented.

9. What is the purpose of surveillance of specific VPDs?

Specific VPDs are prioritized based on public health problem of the disease and for elimination/eradication such as National Tuberculosis Elimination Program (NTEP), measles and rubella elimination, polio eradication, etc.

10. What is the mechanism of VPD surveillance?

Integrated health information platform (IHIP) which includes:
- National Center for Disease Control (NCDC) which includes IDSP and national viral hepatitis surveillance program
- National Public health Surveillance Project (NPSP)
- National Tuberculosis Elimination Program (NTEP).

11. What are S, P, and L forms of Integrated Disease Surveillance Program (IDSP)?

- *S form*: Reporting formats for syndromic surveillance, filled by health worker.
- *P form*: Reporting format for presumptive surveillance, filled by medical officer.
- *L form*: Reporting format for laboratory surveillance.

TABLE 1: Surveillance: Terminologies

Surveillance terminologies	Example of disease
Active surveillance	AFP, measles rubella (MR), pertussis, diphtheria surveillance
Passive surveillance	IDSurv and IDSP
Sentinel surveillance	CRS, rotavirus, Hib, pneumococcal and meningoccal
Population-based surveillance	CDC's active bacterial core surveillance (ABCs)
Outbreak surveillance	Measles control and IDSP
Case-based surveillance	AFP, AES, measles rubella, pertussis, diphtheria
"Zero"/"Nil" reporting	AFP, measles rubella, pertussis, diphtheria surveillamce

(AES: acute encephalitis syndrome; AFP: acute flaccid paralysis; CDC: Center for Disease Control and Prevention; Hib: *Haemophilus influenzae* type b; IDSP: Integrated Disease Surveillance Program; CRS: congenital rubella syndrome)

12. Describe the types of VPD surveillance.

- Outbreak based or case-based surveillance
- Sentinel surveillance
- Nationwide or subnational surveillance
- Facility based or community-based surveillance
- Active/Passive surveillance (**Table 1**).

13. What is sentinel surveillance?

Sentinel surveillance system has reporting sites (usually referral hospitals) with high probability of seeing cases of disease under surveillance, having good laboratory facility and well-qualified staff which reports and investigates specific disease, for example, congenital rubella syndrome (CRS) surveillance (**Fig. 1**).

14. What is active surveillance?

Active surveillance means actively searching for cases (in case of diseases targeted for eradication/elimination) in health facilities and in community. It is a labor-intensive system and is required for diseases targeted for elimination. It involves regular training, reporting, and feedback system.

15. What is passive surveillance?

Passive surveillance involves reporting from health facility passively.

16. What was the role of acute flaccid paralysis (AFP) surveillance in polio elimination from India?

Acute flaccid paralysis surveillance is an important pillar for polio eradication activities. Highly sensitive AFP surveillance with intensified immunization

Types of surveillance

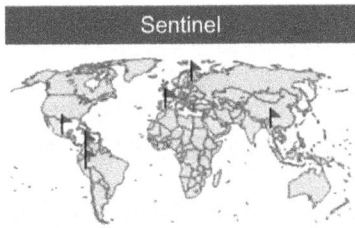

Sentinel
- Reporting from a sample of sources (e.g. hospital, laboratory but without a known population denominator
- Assesses trends
  - Less resource intensive, can be limited to sites with adequate facilities
  - Incidence cannot be estimated

Population-based
- Reporting from a defined catchment population
  - Allows incidence to be estimated
  - Cost, logistics and long implementation timelines

WHO 2012. Measuring impact of *Streptococcus pneumoniae* and *Hemophiles influenzae* type b conjugate vaccination. Available at http://apps.who.int/iris/bitstream/10555/75835/1/WHO IVB 12.08 eng.pdf Accessed: in May 2016;. Thacker et al, MMWR 2012; 61: 3–14

Fig. 1: Difference between sentinel and population-based surveillance.
Source: World Health Organization. (2012). Measuring impact of *Streptococcus pneumoniae* and *Haemophilus influenzae* type b conjugate vaccination. [online] Available from: https://apps.who.int/iris/handle/10665/75835 [Last accessed May, 2020].; Thacker SB, Qualters JR, Lee LM, Centers for Disease Control and Prevention. Public Health Surveillance in the United States: Evolution and Challenges. MMWR Suppl. 2012;61(3):3-9.

efforts has contributed immensely to India for achieving polio elimination. Maintaining sensitive AFP surveillance system is a crucial step to ensure what we detect polio importations/vaccine-derived polioviruses (VDPVs), if any, at the earliest.

17. What should be done when one comes across patient with acute flaccid paralysis?

It should be immediately reported to district immunization officer (DIO) or surveillance medical officer (SMO)-NPSP for further investigation and sample collection.

18. What is the mechanism to report?

It should be reported immediately telephonically to avoid delays as it is important to collect stool samples within 14 days of onset of paralysis. It should be further added in weekly report which is sent by all reporting sites every Monday to district authorities.

19. What are reporting sites?

Reporting sites (RS) are government and private health facilities which are sensitized to report AFP cases. Reporting site network is constantly prioritized and expanded to include new sites and sensitize those who miss case. Reporting sites include reporting units (RUs) and informer units (IUs).

20. What is difference between reporting unit and informer unit?

When reporting sites come across any AFP cases, they report immediately telephonically to government health authority but reporting units additionally send weekly report (H002) to district authorities even if there are no cases reported during the week. Informer units do not send weekly report.

21. What is standard case definition?

Standard case definitions are definitions used for surveillance purpose so that there is uniformity in reporting cases. Each disease has suspect, probable, and confirmed case definitions.

22. What are different surveillance systems in India?

Table 2 provides a brief overview of key surveillance systems in India.

23. Explain suspect definitions of VPDs for surveillance.

- *Acute flaccid paralysis*: Sudden onset weakness and floppiness in any part of the body in a child <15 years of age or paralysis in a person of any age in which polio is suspected.
- *Diphtheria*: A suspected case of diphtheria is defined as: "An illness of upper respiratory tract characterized by laryngitis or pharyngitis or nasopharyngitis or tonsillitis and adherent membranes of tonsils, pharynx and/or nose".
- *Pertussis*: A suspected case of pertussis is defined as a person of any age with a cough lasting two or more weeks, or of any duration in an infant or in any person in an outbreak setting, without a more likely diagnosis and with at least one of the following symptoms on observation or parental report: paroxysms (i.e., fits) of coughing, inspiratory whoop, post-tussive vomiting or vomiting without other apparent causes, apnea in infants (<1 year of age) or clinician suspicion of pertussis.
- *Neonatal tetanus*: Any neonate who could suck and cry normally during the first 2 days of life and who between 3 and 28 days of age cannot suck normally, and becomes stiff or has convulsions/spasms (i.e., jerking of the muscles) or both or any neonate who died of an unknown cause during the 1st month of life.
- *Measles and rubella*: Any person having fever and maculopapular rash with cough or coryza or conjunctivitis.
- *Tuberculosis*: A child with fever and/or cough for >2 weeks, with loss of weight/no weight gain and history of contact with a suspected or diagnosed case of active TB disease within the last 2 years. (World Health Organization).

TABLE 2: A brief overview of the different surveillance systems in India.

System	Description/Salient features	Remarks
IDSP (integrated disease surveillance project)	Nationwide outbreak surveillance system including measles, diphtheria, pertussis, AFP, hepatitis, and AES	Sustainable system but variable state ownership. Data does not capture age and immunization status. Laboratory component weak
CBHI/SBHI (Central and state bureaus of health intelligence)	Nationwide passive reporting system of suspected cases	All VPDs under traditional EPI are reportable. Extremely variable completeness, data quality, and reliability. Annual updates
Measles: ICMR	Selected practitioners and institutions provide clinical samples to NIV-Pune for measles virus isolation and genotyping	Strong laboratory component. Case definition and case inclusion may not be standardized. Not population based
AES/JE: NVBDCP and ICMR	Facility-based surveillance for acute encephalitis syndrome in endemic areas. ICMR provides laboratory support. Laboratory-based surveillance by NIV in Gorakhpur	Variable sensitivity. Many cases of AES without laboratory diagnosis
Multicenter pneumonia and meningitis surveillance	Established in preparation for Hib vaccine probe study in Chandigarh, Kolkata, and Vellore	Established in preparation for Hib vaccine probe study in Chandigarh, Kolkata, and Vellore
Rotavirus surveillance network (India)	The Indian Rotavirus strain Surveillance Network: Sentinel site based	A fecal specimen is tested for rotavirus using a commercial enzyme immunoassay, and strains characterized using rtPCR
VPD surveillance supported by NPSP, India	• *AFP reporting system*: Nationwide, one of the most efficient systems globally; Functional reporting systems in place • *Health facility-based surveillance for DPT*: Most patients with diphtheria, pertussis and tetanus are likely to seek health from hospital or healthcare providers; Laboratory backed system	Expanded to diphtheria, pertussis and neonatal tetanus; MR surveillance is based on this platform Increases the credibility of data generated
WHO-NPSP supported MR surveillance system	Uses AFP surveillance system as a platform; Backed by laboratory support; Scaled up in a phased manner– currently nationwide	Initially outbreak based surveillance system; Transitioning to case based MR surveillance system

(AES: acute encephalitis syndrome; AFP: acute flaccid paralysis; EPI: expanded program on immunization; Hib: *Haemophilus influenzae* type b; ICMR: Indian Council of Medical Research; JE: Japanese encephalitis; NIV: National Institute of Virology; NVBDCP: National Vector Borne Disease Control Program; rtPCR: real-time polymerase chain reaction; VPD: vaccine-preventable disease)

- *Bacterial meningitis*: Any person with sudden onset of fever (>38.5°C rectal or 38.0°C axillary) and one of the following signs: neck-stiffness, altered consciousness, or other meningeal sign. (Integrated Disease Surveillance Program).
- *Hepatitis B*: An acute illness typically including acute jaundice, dark urine, anorexia, malaise, extreme fatigue, and right upper quadrant tenderness. Biological signs include increased urine urobilinogen and >2.5 times the upper limit of serum alanine aminotransferase. *Note*: Most infections occur during early childhood. A variable proportion of adult infections are asymptomatic. (Integrated Disease Surveillance Program).
- *Japanese encephalitis*: A person of any age, at any time of the year with acute onset of fever and change in mental status (including symptoms such as confusion, disorientation, coma or inability to talk), and/or new onset of seizures (excluding simple febrile seizures). Other early clinical findings may include an increase in irritability, somnolence or abnormal behavior greater than that seen with usual febrile illness. (Integrated Disease Surveillance Program).

24. Who is responsible for reporting?

Every reporting site has nodal officer who is responsible for compiling reports from different consultants/departments and sending reports to DIO/SMO.

25. What is weekly report?

Weekly report (H002) is sent by all reporting units (even nil reporting) to DIO/SMO every week on Monday which is compiled at district level in D001 form and sent to state and then in S001 from state to national level.

26. Should we wait to report in weekly report or VPD should be immediately reported?

No, VPD should be telephonically reported and then included in weekly report to facilitate timely investigation and sample collection.

27. What is being done for measles and rubella elimination from surveillance point of view?

Modified case-based surveillance for measles and rubella expanded throughout country. Each and every case of measles and rubella is reported, investigated, and samples collected for virology and serology. This helps in identifying areas of transmission for focused efforts of strengthening routine immunization.

Fever and rash surveillance initiated in three states on pilot basis namely Madhya Pradesh, Odisha, and Karnataka, results will guide on expansion throughout the country.

TABLE 3: Surveillance for different vaccine-preventable diseases (VPDs) in India.

Disease under surveillance	Age group	Date of onset	Sample collection		Sample shipment
Acute flaccid paralysis	<15 years	Date of onset of weakness	*Stool:* Two sample within 14 days of onset of weakness	Sample can be collected till 2 months of onset	
Measles-Rubella	All age groups	Date of onset of rash	*Serum:* 4 – 28 days from onset of rash	*Throat swab/urine:* Within 5 days of onset of rash	To WHO accredited laboratories – through DIO office/SMO office
Diphtheria	All age groups	Date of onset of sore throat	*Throat swab:* 4 weeks		
Pertussis	All age groups	Date of onset of cough	*Naospharyngeal swab/Serum:* 2–4 weeks from onset of cough	*Serum:* > 4 week – 8 weeks of onset of cough	
Neonatal tetanus	Neonate	Date of onset of inability of suck	No sample		NA

Note: AFP can be reported till 6 months from onset while MR/DPT till 3 months of their onset.
(AFP: acute flaccid paralysis; DIO: district immunization officer; SMO: surveillance medical officer; WHO: World Health Organization)

28. When will we say that country/region/world have eliminated measles and rubella?

Elimination of measles and rubella is defined as "absence of endemic measles and rubella transmission for a period of 12 months or more in presence of adequate surveillance indicators" (**Table 3**).

29. What is DPT surveillance?

Laboratory supported surveillance for diphtheria, pertussis, and tetanus (DPT) is initiated in majority of states of India and is being expanded all throughout. It is named as VPD surveillance. NPSP supported AFP and measles and rubella surveillance network is being utilized for surveillance of DPT.

30. What actions are taken after case of VPD is reported?

Each case of diphtheria, pertussis, and neonatal tetanus is investigated using standard case investigation form (CIF) and samples are collected as per guidelines.

- *Diphtheria*: Throat swab or pieces of membrane or nasopharyngeal swab (within 4 weeks)
- *Pertussis*: Nasopharyngeal swab (2–4 weeks) and serum (2–12 weeks)
- *Neonatal tetanus*: No samples.

31. Are we supposed to report tuberculosis cases to government?

Notification of tuberculosis cases is made mandatory by Ministry of Health and Family Welfare, Government of India.

To facilitate TB notification, "case-based web-based TB surveillance system" called "NIKSHAY" is developed by National Tuberculosis Elimination Program https://www.nikshay.in/.

"NIKSHAY" is an integrated integral communication technology (ICT) system for TB patient management and care in India, launched in 2012. NIKSHAY version 2 has been launched in September 2018. It provides a unified interface for public and private sector healthcare providers.

32. What is the meaning of performance indicators?

Performance indicators are used to measure standard of surveillance system and gives indication about performance such as timeliness, investigation, sample collection (% adequate samples, % investigated on time, nonmeasles, nonrubella rate, nonpolio AFP rate, etc.).

33. How is the surveillance quality monitored?

Performance indicators:
- Completeness of weekly or monthly reporting (including "zero" reports)
- Timeliness of weekly or monthly reporting (including "zero" reports)
- Investigation of cases within 48 hours of being reported
- Proportion of cases for which specimens were collected and sent to a laboratory
- Mapping of reporting sites to ensure that all areas are covered.

34. What is meant by EPID number?

The EPID number is a unique case identification code which is allotted by DIO/SMO to each case. It is a 16-character alpha-numeric code allotted to each case of VPD.

MR for measles and rubella, MOB for measles-rubella outbreak, DTH for diphtheria, PTS for pertussis, and NNT for neonatal tetanus.

For example, if Mumbai district of Maharashtra is reporting the first diphtheria case of 2020, the identification code allotted will be *DTH-IND-MH-BMC-20-001*, where:

DTH: suspected diphtheria code, *IND*: country code, *MH*: state code, *BMC*: district code, *20*: year of onset, *001*: serial number of diphtheria case of the district having onset in 2020.

35. What is CIF?

The CIF means case investigation form, which is a standard form having basic personal, demographic, immunization, clinical, health contact, and sample collection information. There are separate CIFs for AFP, MR, and DPT surveillance.

36. What is LRF?

The LRF is a laboratory request form which needs to be sent to laboratory with sample and contains basic information on onset of disease, dates of sample collection, type of sample collection, and person sending samples.

37. Which samples are collected?

- *Acute flaccid paralysis*: Stool sample (preferably within 14 days of onset but can be collected within 60 days)
- *Measles and rubella*: Serum (within 28 days of onset) and virology sample (throat/urine) (within 7 days of onset)
- *Diphtheria*: Throat swab or pieces of membrane or nasopharyngeal swab (within 4 weeks of onset)
- *Pertussis*: Nasopharyngeal swab (2–4 weeks) and serum (2–12 weeks)
- *Neonatal tetanus*: No samples.

38. Which laboratories can test samples collected under VPD surveillance?

Specific WHO accredited laboratory network is established at various places throughout country for surveillance purpose, for example, AFP laboratory network, measles-rubella laboratory network, and VPD laboratory network for diphtheria and pertussis samples.

Only listed laboratories can test samples under VPD program to maintain quality of surveillance data.

39. What is line-list?

The *line-list* is an epidemiologic database made in spreadsheet with rows and columns. Complete information of a case of disease is put in each row. Line-list is used for epidemiological analysis which helps in finding out key performance indicators.

40. How is surveillance data analyzed?

Surveillance data is analyzed using surveillance indicators against minimum standard namely:
- % adequacy of samples (at least 80% of samples)
- % timeliness of weekly report (at least 80% of weekly report should be received timely)

- % notification within 10 days of onset (at least 80%)
- % investigation within 48 hours of reporting (at least 80%)
- % samples reaching laboratory within 5 days of collection (at least 80%)
- Nonpolio AFP rate (at least two AFP cases should be reported per 1 lac under 15 population in absence of polio)
- Nonmeasles, nonrubella discard rate (at least two nonmeasles and nonrubella cases should be reported per 1 lac population).

41. What is public health response when VPD is reported?

Public health response is in form of:
- Active case search in the area for more cases
- Preliminary and detailed survey in case of outbreak
- Vitamin A in recommended dosage to all suspect patients of measles in area during survey
- Outbreak response immunization (ORI) in case of AFP
- Immunization response in form of efforts to track dropouts and organizing special RI sessions.

42. What is an outbreak?

Outbreak of disease is defined in terms of place and time. Measles-rubella outbreak is defined as five cases of suspected measles/rubella in defined geographical area in 4 weeks.

43. What is an outbreak investigation?

Outbreak investigation is investigation in field and on desk describing outbreak in detail using standard outbreak investigation format (OB003

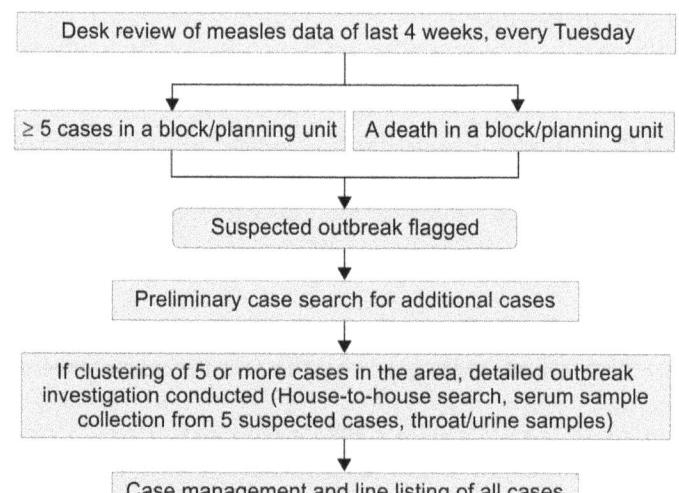

Flowchart 1: Measles-rubella (MR) outbreak investigation algorithm.

CHAPTER 5 Vaccine-preventable Diseases Surveillance **73**

Flowchart 2: Serum specimen testing protocol of measles-rubella (MR) surveillance project.

```
         Suspected  ──▶  Measles IgM serum
       measles case              │
                      ┌──────────┴──────────┐
                      ▼                     ▼
                  Positive               Negative
                      │                     │
                      ▼                     ▼
             Confirmed measles         Rubella IgM
                                            │
                                 ┌──────────┴──────────┐
                                 ▼                     ▼
                             Negative               Positive
                                 │                     │
                                 ▼                     ▼
                             Discard            Confirmed rubella
```

(IgM: immunoglobulin M)

for MR outbreak) and looking for new cases, outbreak investigation leads to specific interventions in the community. **Flowcharts 1 and 2** display outbreak investigation algorithm and testing protocol in measles-rubella (MR) case.

44. What is control, elimination, and eradication?

Control: Reduction in the incidence, prevalence, morbidity or mortality of an infectious disease to a locally acceptable level.

Elimination: Reduction to zero of the incidence of disease or infection in a defined geographical area, for example, polio elimination achieved in India.

Eradication: Permanent reduction to zero of the worldwide incidence of infection, for example, smallpox is eradicated.

TABLE 4: Global surveillance and network links.	
Surveillance name	Link
Dengue net	http://apps.who.int/globalatlas/default.asp
Rotavirus laboratory network	http://www.who.int/immunization/monitoring_surveillance/burden/laboratory/Rotavirus/en/
FluNet	http://www.who.int/influenza/gisrs_laboratory/flunet/en/
Europe–surveillance ATLAS of infectious diseases	http://ecdc.europa.eu/en/surveillance-and-disease-data
Measles and rubella surveillance data	http://www.who.int/immunization/monitoring_surveillance/burden/vpd/surveillance_type/active/measles_monthlydata/en/
Global disease detection program	https://www.cdc.gov/globalhealth/healthprotection.gdd/about.html

45. Provide a brief information about the key global VPD surveillance network links.

Table 4 displays links to the sites of key global surveillance and network links.

46. What is an environmental surveillance?

The environmental surveillance is the collection of environmental samples (sewage samples) for presence of wild/vaccine poliovirus. It complements AFP surveillance to give information about importations/presence of virus in community.

SUGGESTED READING

1. https://idsp.nic.in/
2. https://cbhidghs.gov.in/
3. https://mohfw.gov.in/sites/default/files/Unit10VaccinePreventableDiseasesandVPDsurveillance.pdf
4. https://www.nhp.gov.in/revised-national-tuberculosis-control-programme_pg
5. World Health Organization. (2019). Immunization, Vaccines, and Biologicals: Surveillance for Vaccine Preventable Diseases (VPDs). [online] Available from: https://www.who.int/immunization/monitoring_surveillance/burden/VPDs/en/ [Last accessed June, 2020].
6. World Health Organization. (2018). Overview of VPD Surveillance Principles. [online] Available from: https://www.who.int/immunization/monitoring_surveillance/burden/vpd/WHO_SurveillanceVaccinePreventable_01_Overview_BW_R2.pdf?ua=1 [Last accessed June, 2020].

CHAPTER 6

Vaccination in Special Situations

Abhay K Shah

1. What do you mean by a special situation in reference to vaccinations?

A special situation is a condition in which administration of a vaccine may result in suboptimal efficacy and/or increase the chance of a serious or nonserious adverse effect of immunization.

They include the following:
- Immunocompromised child
- Preterm/low birth weight infants
- Immunization in chronic diseases
- Immunization in bone marrow/organ transplant
- Immunization in asplenia/hyposplenia/splenectomized children
- Immunization in corticosteroid/immunosuppressive therapy
- Transfusion of antibody containing products
- Immunization in the presence of history of allergy
- Immunization in bleeding disorders/anticoagulant therapy
- Immunization during illness
- Lapsed/postponed/unknown immune status
- Immunization in pregnancy/lactation
- Immunization for travelers.

2. What are not special situations?
- Mild illnesses, febrile or afebrile
- Current antimicrobial therapy
- Recent exposure to an infectious disease
- Convalescent phase of illness
- Pregnant or immunosuppressed person in household
- Allergy to products not present in vaccine
- Family history of adverse effects.

3. What are the issues faced by the clinicians in vaccinating an immunocompromised individual?

The need to protect the individual against serious infections is the primary goal. However, the public health point of view is also significant because it is important not to have an increasing number of individuals vulnerable to

serious infectious agents (e.g., poliovirus). Both aspects require an analysis of risks and benefits for the individual patient. The dilemma is because of the following issues:
- Increased susceptibility of an immunocompromised child to infection
- Increased severity of the disease
- Poor immune response to the vaccine
- Safety of vaccination would also be an issue
- Efficacy of vaccination is doubtful.

4. Why are vaccinations not optimally used in immunocompromised patients?
- Ignorance/minor interest for "old" preventive strategies
- Fear of vaccine-associated risks
- Perception of insufficient efficacy and hence a worry sets in regarding the stimulation of a compromised immune system.

5. What are general principles for vaccinating immunocompromised children?
- In severe immunodeficiency all live vaccines contraindicated
- All inactivated vaccines may be given but immunogenicity and efficacy low
- Higher doses, more number of doses may be required (Hepatitis B)
- Antibody titers should be checked post-immunization
- Regular boosters may be needed.

6. What are the recommendations for vaccination of *contacts of persons* with altered immunocompetence?
- MMR, varicella, rotavirus and annual influenza vaccines to all susceptible contacts
- Direct contact should be avoided with susceptible household contact, who has developed a rash after varicella vaccine, until the rash resolves
- Hand hygiene measures should be employed by all members of the household, after contact with feces of a rotavirus-vaccinated infant, for at least 1 week.

7. How is immunosuppression differentiated on the basis of CD4+ count?
Immune response in case of immune-deficient subjects is based on the CD4 counts and the response to any vaccination and the plan to vaccinate the child also depends on the same. If the CD4 count is >25% the immunity is conserved and hence vaccination with live vaccines based on risk benefit ratio can be given.
- Conserved—no immunosuppression: CD4+ T lymphocytes >25%
- Moderate immunosuppression: CD4+ T lymphocytes 15–24%
- Severe immunosuppression (Impaired, absent): CD4+ T lymphocytes <15%.

8. Name various types of immunocompromised conditions.

Various immunocompromised conditions, which require special attention in planning vaccinations, are:

Congenital:
- B cell disorders
- T cell disorders
- Phagocytosis defects
- Complement disorders.

Acquired:
- Children on oral steroids
- Children on chemotherapy for malignancies
- HSCT recipients
- SOT recipients
- Infant of a HIV+ve mother/ HIV+ve child
- Asplenia/Splenectomy, etc.

9. What are the recommendations for vaccination of individuals having primary B lymphocyte defects?

- In B-lymphocyte defects, there is abnormal humoral response to infections
- All live bacterial (BCG and oral typhoid) and live viral (MMR, OPV, measles and varicella) vaccines—contraindicated
- Agammaglobulinemia: Consider pertussis, influenza
- Selective IgG and IgA defects: All live vaccines other than OPV can be considered.

10. What are the recommendations for vaccination of individuals having primary T-lymphocyte defects?

All live vaccines are contraindicated. No vaccine is useful.

11. What are the recommendations for vaccination of individuals having primary phagocytic function disorders?

- All live bacterial vaccines are contraindicated
- Live viral vaccines can be administered
- Consider influenza vaccine to prevent secondary bacterial infections.

12. What are the recommendations for vaccination of individuals having primary complement deficiency?

- All vaccines can be safely administered
- More prone to infections with encapsulated organisms such as pneumococcal and meningococcal infections

- C1, C4, C2, and C3 deficiency: All vaccines are effective; pneumococcal and meningococcal vaccines recommended
- C5-9, Properdin, factor B deficiency: All vaccines are effective; meningococcal vaccine recommended.

13. Which are the issues associated with vaccinations in HIV infected individual?

The HIV is a T-cell defect and is associated with progressive decline in CD4+T lymphocytes count resulting in
- Increased risk of complications from infections
- Impaired effectiveness of vaccines
- Risk of serious adverse events from live vaccines
- Loss of prior immunity (lack of CMI).

14. What are the risks associated with vaccination of HIV infected patients?

In HIV infection, the chances of enhancement of certain diseases and their complications increase many folds. Hence, one needs to weigh the risk benefit ratio of the diseases and plan the vaccination. Various studies have shown the increased chances of the following diseases:
- Risk of tuberculosis enhances by 10–300 times
- *Streptococcus pneumoniae* by 5–50 times
- The chronicity increases in case of hepatitis B exposure
- Hepatitis A also has a severe duration of action
- In case of measles the condition can be life-threatening
- Similarly, the risk enhances in case of influenza, varicella and zoster infection.

15. What are ACIP recommendations for HIV positive children?

Figure 1 shows the Advisory Committee on Immunization Practices (ACIP) recommendations for HIV infected individuals.

16. What is current ACVIP-IAP recommendation for vaccination in HIV infected cases?

Table 1 describes the current Advisory Committee on Vaccines and Immunization Practices (ACVIP) recommendations for HIV infected cases.

17. What about BCG vaccine for a neonate born to HIV mother? Why?

The World Health Organization (WHO) currently recommends administering a single dose of BCG vaccine to all infants living in areas where tuberculosis is highly endemic as well as to infants and children at particular risk of exposure to tuberculosis in countries with low endemicity. BCG vaccine is contraindicated in people with impaired immunity, and WHO does not recommend BCG vaccination for children with symptomatic HIV infection.

As per Global Advisory Committee on Vaccine Safety there is difficulty in identifying infants infected with HIV at birth especially in the areas where

CHAPTER 6 Vaccination in Special Situations

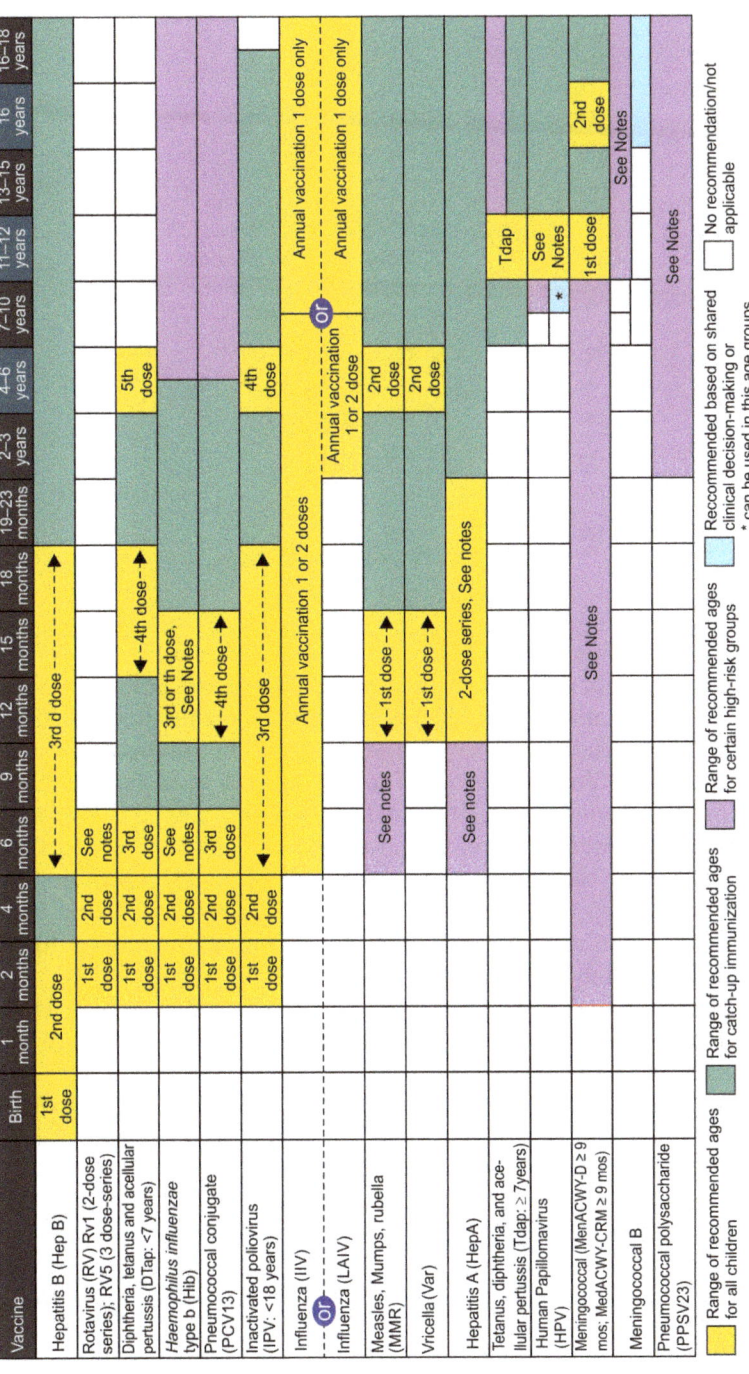

Fig. 1: Recommended child and adolescent immunization schedule for ages 18 years or younger, United States, 2020
Source: Available from: https://www.cdc.gov/vaccines/schedules/downloads/child/0-18yrs-child-combined-schedule.pdf
Note: These recommendations must be read with the notes the follow. For those who fall behind or start late, provide catch-up vaccination at the earliest opportunity as indicated by the green bars.

TABLE 1: Current ACVIP recommendations for HIV infected cases

Vaccine	Asymptomatic	Symptomatic	Comments
BCG	Yes ???	No	
DPT/DT/Tdap	Yes	Yes	
OPV	Yes	No	IPV preferred
IPV	Yes	Yes	Also immunize household contacts
Measles/MMR	Yes	Yes, if CD4 >15%	
HEP B	Yes	Yes, 4 doses, double dose, Antibody levels to be checked, regular boosters needed	
Hib, Pneumonia, killed Influenza	Yes	Yes	
Varicella	Yes, 2 doses,	Yes, 2 doses if CD4>15%	
Typhoid	Yes	Yes	
Rota	??	??	Insufficient data
HEP A Inactivated	Yes	Yes, Check antibody levels, regular boosters	

diagnostic and treatment services for mothers and infants are limited. In such situations, BCG vaccination should be given at birth to all infants regardless of HIV exposure considering the high endemicity of tuberculosis with high HIV prevalence. Close follow-up of infants known to be born to HIV-infected mothers and who received BCG at birth is recommended in order to provide early identification and treatment of any BCG-related complication. If adequate HIV services for early identification and administration of antiretroviral therapy to HIV-infected children are available, delaying BCG vaccination may be considered in infants born to mothers known to be infected with HIV until these infants are confirmed to be HIV negative.

- Risk of disseminated BCG disease in non-HIV-infected infants is <5 per 1 million vaccines and in HIV-infected infants it is 1,100–4,170 per 1 million vaccines.
- Following recommendation is based on the risk of disseminated BCG diseases:
    - Maternal HIV status unknown + Baby asymptomatic = Give BCG
    - Maternal HIV positive
        ✧ Baby asymptomatic, virologic tests not available: Give BCG and close follow-up
        ✧ Baby asymptomatic, virologic tests available but not done: Defer BCG till results
        ✧ Baby symptomatic, virologic tests not available: Do not give BCG
        ✧ Baby asymptomatic, virologic tests available and positive: Do not give BCG

18. Outline the various issues of vaccination of patients receiving steroids.

The immune status and the response to vaccine would depend on the dose and duration of steroid.

There will be absence of immunosuppression if the dose is <20 mg/day (prednisone) or <2 mg/kg in children and the duration of administration is <2 weeks. In these situations, killed vaccines are safe but less efficacious. All vaccines are safe and efficacious during inhalation and topical therapy.

Outside of these conditions no live vaccines (until 1 month after discontinuation of corticosteroids) should be given and the individual vaccine responses should be assessed after vaccination.

19. What about new categories of immunosuppressive agents?

This includes following agents:
- Immune mediators
  - Colony stimulating factors, interferons, interleukins
- Immune modulators
  - Levamisole, cyclosporine, tacrolimus
- Isoantibodies
  - Tumor necrosis factor inhibitors.

Effect of these agents on the safety of live vaccine is not certain as on date. But it is prudent to vaccinate 3 months after stopping therapy. For Rituximab™: Vaccinate after 6 months.

20. What are the recommendations for cancer patients?

Immunization for vaccine preventable diseases is important in children with cancer as it can reduce noncancer related morbidity/mortality and contribute favorably to the overall outcome in these children. Immune suppression in cancer patients varies greatly and depends on many factors such as type of cancer, chemotherapy, radiotherapy, their stages and dosages. Vaccine uptake during chemotherapy and for some time thereafter may be erratic. Acquired immunity through previous infections or immunization also wanes due to effect of chemotherapy on immune system and needs boosting on recovery of immunity following end of chemotherapy.

General Principles
- Children on chemotherapy and radiotherapy for malignancy should avoid all live vaccines during therapy and for at least 6 months after stopping treatment.
  - Exception: Varicella vaccine in children with acute lymphoblastic leukemia (ALL)
    - Children with ALL on maintenance chemotherapy: Can receive varicella vaccine provided
    - Remission > 1 year
    - Platelets >100,000
    - Lymphocyte count >700/mm^3

✧ May need to stop chemotherapy for 1 week before and after vaccination.
- Vaccination schedule for patients 6 months after completion of standard-dose chemotherapy is as under
  - After 3–6 months: Inactivated influenza vaccine
    ✧ After 6 months: Diphtheria, tetanus, acellular pertussis, IPV, Hib-conjugate, PCV13, MCV4-CV, HepA, HepB.
    ✧ After 12 months: MMR
    ✧ For children age 10 years and more give Tdap, IPV, Hib, HPV.

Tables 2 and 3 describe the general recommendations.

TABLE 2: Recommendations for live vaccines.

Vaccine	During chemotherapy	After end of chemotherapy	
		Previously unimmunized children	Children with completed immunization
BCG	Not recommended, contact vaccination not discouraged	Single dose BCG at 6 months after completion of chemotherapy	Not recommended in previously immunized children with visible BCG scar
OPV	Not recommended, contact vaccination contraindicated	IPV preferred, when unavailable 3 doses of bOPV 1 month apart (maximum age 5 year)	IPV preferred, when unavailable 2 doses of bOPV 1 month apart (maximum age 5 year)
MMR	Not recommended, contact vaccination not discouraged	Two doses of MMR (1–3 months apart) should be given to all children after at least 6 months of completion of chemotherapy	Single dose of MMR should be given to all children after at least 6 months of completion of chemotherapy
Varicella vaccine	Not recommended, contact vaccination encouraged.	2 doses of vaccine 1–3 months apart (after 6 months of completing chemotherapy)	Single booster dose 6 months after stopping chemotherapy
Live attenuated HAV	Not recommended	Single dose after 6 months of completing chemotherapy	Single dose after 6 months of completing chemotherapy
Rotavirus vaccine	Not recommended, contact vaccination not discouraged	Generally child outgrows the maximum permissible age, therefore not indicated	Generally child outgrows the maximum permissible age, therefore not indicated

(BCG: Bacillus Calmette–Guérin; OPV: oral polio vaccine; MMR: mumps measles rubella; HAV: hepatitis A vaccine)

Source: Moulik NR, Mandal P, Chandra J, Bansal S, Jog P, Sanjay S, et al. Immunization of Children with Cancer in India Treated with Chemotherapy – Consensus Guideline from the Pediatric Hematology-Oncology Chapter and the Advisory Committee on Vaccination and Immunization Practices of the Indian Academy of Pediatrics. Indian Pediatr. 2019;15:1041-9.

TABLE 3: Recommendations for non-live vaccines.

Vaccine	During chemotherapy	After end of chemotherapy	
		Previously unimmunized children	Children with completed immunization
DPT (age appropriate preparation-DwPT/DaPT/TdaP/Td)	Not recommended during chemotherapy	3 doses at 0, 1 and 6 mo (6 mo after stopping chemotherapy)	Single booster dose (6 mo after stopping chemotherapy)
Hib	Not recommended during ongoing chemotherapy	Age >6 mo 2 doses 8 week apart, followed by booster at 12 mo; 12–15 mo single dose followed by booster at 18 mo; 15–60 mo single dose (6 mo after stopping chemotherapy)	Single booster dose (6 mo after ongoing chemotherapy
IPV	Not recommended during ongoing chemotherapy	2 doses of IPV 2 mo apart and 3rd dose after 6 mo (6 mo after stopping chemotherapy)	Single booster dose (6 mo after ongoing chemotherapy). Two doses for children who received OPV as primary immunization
HBV	4 doses of vaccine (0, 1, 2 and OPV as primary immunization recommended for previously unimmunized children, no further doses for children who completed primary schedule prior to diagnosis	3 doses at 0, 1 and 6 mo (6 mo after stopping chemotherapy)	Single booster dose (6 mo after stopping chemotherapy)
HAV	Not recommended during ongoing chemotherapy	2 doses 6 mo apart (6 mo after stopping chemotherapy)	Single booster dose (6 mo after stopping chemotherapy)

Contd...

Contd...

Vaccine	During chemotherapy	After end of chemotherapy	
		Previously unimmunized children	Children with completed immunization
Inactivated Influenza vaccine	Recommended single dose annually during chemotherapy	Not recommended routinely beyond 1 y from the end of chemotherapy	Not recommended routinely beyond 1 y from the end of chemotherapy
Pneumococcal vaccine	Not recommended during ongoing chemotherapy	(6 mo after stopping chemotherapy) Age <1 yr: 2 doses of PCV-7/13 at 4–8 wk interval followed by a booster dose at 12–15 mo age Age 1–2 y: 2 doses of PCV-7/13, 4–8 wk apart; Age > 2 y: 1 dose of PCV-7/13. PPV-23 booster is not recommended for this group of children	Single booster dose (6 mo after stopping chemotherapy)
Inactivated typhoid vaccine	Single booster dose (6 mo after stopping chemotherapy)	Single dose typhoid conjugate vaccine 6 mo after stopping chemotherapy	Single dose typhoid conjugate vaccine 6 mo after stopping chemotherapy
HPV	Not recommended during ongoing chemotherapy	Age 9–14 y - 2 doses 6 mo apart in females, age >14 y - 3 doses at 0,1 and 6 mo (HPV2) or 0,2 and 6 mo (HPV4) in females (6 mo after stopping chemotherapy)	Insufficient data on booster dose but single booster dose may be considered in females

(DPT: diphtheria pertussis tetanus; wP: whole cell pertussis; aP: acellular pertussis; HiB: *Haemophilus influenzae* Type B; IPV: Inactivated polio vaccine; HBV: hepatitis B vaccine; HAV: hepatitis A vaccine; HPV: human papilloma virus; HPV2: bivalent HPV, HPV4: quadrivalent HPV; mo: month; y: year; wk: week)

Source: Moulik NR, Mandal P, Chandra J, Bansal S, Jog P, Sanjay S, et al. Immunization of Children with Cancer in India Treated with Chemotherapy: Consensus Guideline from the Pediatric Hematology-Oncology Chapter and the Advisory Committee on Vaccination and Immunization Practices of the Indian Academy of Pediatrics. Indian Pediatr. 2019;15:1041-9.

21. Should hematopoietic stem cell transplant (HSCT) donors be vaccinated before transplantation?

The HSCT donor should be current with routinely recommended vaccines based on age, vaccination history, and exposure history. However, administration of MMR, MMRV, varicella, and zoster vaccines should be avoided within 4 weeks of stem cell harvest. Vaccination of the donor for the benefit of the recipient is not recommended.

22. What are the important issues in relation to vaccination of recipients of HSCT patients?

Infections have been major obstacles for successful transplantations. Thus, infection prevention is very important. Immunizations can protect the recipient against serious inections that may occur during the early or late post-transplant period.

There is going to be a total marrow ablation with loss of all the memory response and an individual is considered immunologically naïve.

23. What are the recommendations for HSCT recipients?

Table 4 provides the details of such recommendations.

TABLE 4: Recommendations for HSCT recipients.

Vaccine	When	Comments
All inactivated DPT, DT, dT, Hib, IPV	>12 months later	
Influenza vaccine	> 3–6 months later	>24 months if GVHD
MMR, Varicella	>24 months later	Poor response if on IVIG or has GVHD
Pneumococcal	>12 months later	Poor response if GVHD 2 doses of PCV at 8 week interval, followed by PPV 8 weeks later

24. What are the recommendations for solid organ transplants (SOT)?

Pretransplant
- Should complete all immunizations prior to transplant in accelerated schedules if needed
- Vaccination with live vaccines should be completed at least 4 weeks prior to transplant
- MMR and varicella vaccines can be administered to 6–11 months infants, at least 4 weeks before transplant
- Desirable that seroconversion be documented.

Post-transplant
- Vaccination with inactivated vaccines can recommence 6 months post-transplant when immunosuppression has been lowered

- Inactivated influenza vaccine (IIV) can be given as early as 1–2 months post-transplant, during community outbreaks
- Boosters for inactivated vaccines should be given as per schedule/when antibody levels wane (Hepatitis A and B) starting 6 months post-transplant
- No live vaccines post-transplant.

25. What are the risks associated with graft rejection through immunization?

There is always a perception of increased risk in graft rejection following immunization but not a single study showing increased rates of graft rejection episodes following immunizations was seen. On the contrary, it has been demonstrated that there is increased evidence of rates of rejection after viral infections such as influenza.

26. What about immunization of children with anatomical or functional asplenia and splenectomized children?

- Risk of mortality from septicemia increases by about 50 times in post-traumatic splenectomy cases and it increases greatly to about 350 times in sickle cell disease and thalassemia.
- Risk is higher in younger (<5 years) than older children/adults.
- They are having high risk for serious infections with encapsulated organism.
- All live and inactivated vaccines are indicated and especially pneumococcal, Hib, influenza and meningococcal vaccine is a must.
- Complete age appropriate schedule at least 2 weeks prior to splenectomy.
- If emergency splenectomy is planned vaccination can be started 2 weeks after the surgery.
- Special need for pneumococcal (PCV13 followed 8 weeks later by PPSV23), Hib, meningococcal and typhoid vaccines.

27. What are the recommendations for individuals who have recently received antibody-containing products?

- Inactivated vaccines can be administered safely
- Live vaccines including MMR and varicella should be avoided for 3 months
- Antibody containing products should be avoided for 2 weeks after these vaccinations
- Oral typhoid vaccine, LAIV, OPV and yellow fever vaccine may be given at any time
- Rotavirus vaccine should be avoided for 6 weeks.

Table 5 describes the interval of vaccination in relation to dose of antibody.

TABLE 5: The interval of vaccination in relation to dose of antibody.

Recommended intervals between administration of immuje globulin preparations and measles or varicella-containing vaccine

Product/indication	Doses, including mg immunoglobulin G (IgG)/kg body weight	Recommended interval before measles or varicella-containing[1] vaccine administration
Botutinum immune Golublin intravenous (Human)	1.5 mL/kg (75 mg IgG/kg) IV	6 months
Tetanus IG (TIG)	250 units 10 mg IgG/kg) IM	3 months
Hepatatis A IG		
• Contact prophylaxis	0.02 mL/kg (3.3 mg IgG/kg) IM	3 months
• International travel	0.06 mL/kg (10 mg IgG/kg) IM	3 months
Hepatitis B IG (HBIG)	0.6 mL/kg (10 mg igG/kg) IM	3 months
Rabies IG (RIG	20 IU/kg (22 mg IgG/kg) IM	4 months
Measles prophylaxis IG		
• Standard (i.e. nonimmunocompromised) contact	0.25 mL/kg (40 mg iGG/kg) IM	5 months
• Immunocompromised contact	0.5 mL/kg (80 mg IgG/kg) IM	6 months
Blood transfusion		
• Red blood cells (RBCs) washed	10 mL/kg (negligible IgG/Kg) IV	None
• RBCs, adenine-satine added	10 mL/kg (10 mg IgG/kg) IV	3 months
• Packed RBCs (hematocrit 65%)[2]	10 mL/kg (60 mg IgG/kg) IV	6 months
• Whole blood (hematocrit 35–50%)[2]	10 mL/kg (80–100 mg IgG/kg) IV	6 months
• Plasma/platelet products	10 mL/kg (160 mg IgG/kg)IV	7 months
Cytomegalovirus IGIV	150 mg/kg maximum	6 moths

Contd...

Contd...

Prodct/indication	Doses, including mg immunoglobulin G (IkgG)/kg body weight	Recommended intervall before measless or varicells-containing vaccine administration
IGIV		
• Replacement therapy for immune deficiencies[3]	300–400 mg/kg IV	8 months
• Immune thrombocytopenic purpura treatment	400 mg/kg IV	8 months
• Immune thrombocytopenic purpura treatment	1,000 mg/kg IV	10 months
• Kawasaki disease	2 g/kg IV	11 months
• Postexposure varicella prophylaxis[4]	400 mg/kg IV	8 months
Monoclonal antibody to respiratory syncytial virus F protein (Synagis ™)[5]	15 mg/kg (IM)	None

This table is not intended for determining the correct indications and dosages for using antibody-containing products. Unvaccinated persons might not be fully protected against measles during the entire recommended interval, and additional doses of IG or measles vaccine might be indicated after measles exposure. Concentrations of measles antibody in an IG preparation can vary by manufacturer's lot. Rates of antibody clearance after receipt of an IG preparation also might vary. Recommended intervals are extrapolated from an estimated half-life of 30 days for passively acquired antibody and an observed interference with the immune response to measles vaccine for 5 months after a dose of 80 mg IgG/kg.

1. Does not include zoster vaccine. Zoster vaccine may be given with antibody-containing blood products.
2. Assume a serum IgG concentration of 16 mg/mL.
3. Measles and varicella vaccinations are recommended for children with asymptomatic or mildly symptomatic human immunodeficiency virus (HIV) infections, but are contraindicated for persons with severe immunosuppression form HIV or any other immunosuppressive disorder.
4. This investigational product variZIG, similar to scensed VZIG, is a purified human IG preparation made from plasma containing high levels of anti-varicella antibodies (IgG). The interval between VariZIG and varicella vaccine (Var or MMRV) is 5 months.
5. Contains antibody only to respiratory syncytial virus

Source: CDC. (2019). ACIP General Best Practice Guidelines. [online] Available from: https://www.cdc.gov/vaccines/pubs/pinkbook/downloads/appendices/a/mmr_ig.pdf. [Last Accessed August, 2020].

28. What are the recommendations for vaccination in the presence of chronic diseases?

Chronic diseases may make children more susceptible to the severe manifestations and complications of common infections. Unless specifically contraindicated, immunizations recommended for healthy children should be administered to children with chronic diseases. It is very important to document antibody responses in such cases.

Chronic liver diseases
- Prevention of hepatitis A:
    - It has been seen before cirrhosis the seroconversion to 2 doses is >95% but the antibody titers are lower. But when cirrhosis sets in, the seroconversion ranges from 0% to 66% with low antibody titers, and may transient responses. Hence, antibody titers measurements and need for boosters are crucial.
- Prevention of hepatitis B:
    - Poorer results are due to the lower immunogenicity of hepatitis B vaccine. In advanced liver disease (cirrhosis), better immunogenicity is achieved by double dose vaccines, i.e., adult dose in children. Also better immunogenicity may be achieved with additional doses as needed after standard (0, 1, 6 months) schedule.

Chronic kidney diseases
Document response to Hepatitis B vaccine, yearly titers and revaccinate if suboptimal titers.

Chronic rheumatic diseases
Document response/antibody titters, revaccinate if suboptimal, before starting biologicals.

29. What about patient going for cochlear implants?

- The rate of bacterial meningitis was 189 cases per 100,000 person-years, a more than 30-fold increased risk compared with that in the overall population.
- 13-valent pneumococcal conjugate (PCV13) followed at least 8 weeks by the
    - 23-valent pneumococcal polysaccharide (PPSV23)
- *Haemophilus influenzae* type b conjugate
- The schedule should be completed at least 2 weeks before surgery
- There is no evidence that people with cochlear implants are more likely to get meningococcal meningitis (caused by *Neisseria meningitidis*) than people without cochlear implants.

30. What are the general recommendations for immunizing individuals with history of allergy?

Yellow fever is contraindicated for people who have a history of a severe (anaphylactic) allergy to eggs. People with a history of egg allergy who have experienced only hives after exposure to egg should receive any influenza vaccine (inactivated, recombinant or live attenuated) without specific precautions (except a 15-minute observation period for syncope). People who report having had an anaphylactic reaction to egg (more severe than hives) may also receive any age- and condition-appropriate influenza vaccine (inactivated, recombinant or live-attenuated) in a medical setting and should be supervised by a healthcare provider who is able to recognize and manage severe allergic condition.

People with a history of anaphylactic reactions to latex should generally not be given vaccines that have been in contact with natural rubber or latex, either in the vial or in the syringe, unless the benefit of vaccination outweighs the risk of a potential allergic reaction. People with latex allergies that are not anaphylactic in nature may be vaccinated as usual. Children who have had a serious hypersensitivity reaction or anaphylaxis to a particular vaccine must never receive it again. A mild reaction is not a contraindication to vaccination. In any case, all children should be watched for at least 15 minutes after vaccination for allergy and resuscitation equipment should be kept standby.

31. What are the general recommendations for immunizing individuals with bleeding disorders?

Preferred route is subcutaneous (unless contraindicated). Aluminum-adjuvanted vaccines should be avoided. Vaccination should be offered after factor replacement therapy.

32. What are the general recommendations for immunizing pregnant women?

All live vaccines in pregnancy are contraindicated. Yellow fever vaccine is contraindicated during pregnancy, but if traveling cannot be postponed it is better to take yellow fever vaccine as the disease carries a greater risk. MMR and varicella are also contraindicated and if administered, pregnancy should be avoided for next 4 weeks. However, if it is administered inadvertently termination of pregnancy is not indicated.

Inactivated vaccines are safe. Td, Tdap, inactivated flu vaccines are recommended. Rabies vaccine is also permitted when indicated.

33. What are the general recommendations for immunizing lactating woman?

All inactivated and live vaccines are safe during lactation. Only exception is yellow fever vaccine as it causes meningoencephalitis in baby. If it is administered inadvertently if mandatory, breastfeeding should be omitted for 10 days.

34. What are the general recommendations for immunizing preterm/low birth weight infant?

Vaccinations of premature infants are often delayed despite being at an increased risk of contracting vaccine preventable diseases. Vaccines are immunogenic, safe and well tolerated in preterm infants. Preterm infants should be vaccinated using the same schedules as those usually recommended for full-term infants, with the exception of the hepatitis B vaccine, where additional doses should be administered in infants receiving the first dose during the first days of life if they weighed less than 2,000 g because of a documented reduced immune response.

BCG and birth dose of OPV can be safely and effectively given to low birth weight/preterm babies after stabilization and preferably at the time of discharge.

The birth dose of hepatitis B vaccine can be administered at any time after birth in babies weighing ≥2 kg.

In babies less than 2 kg, the birth dose of hepatitis B vaccine should be delayed for 1 month after birth as immunogenicity is lower if given earlier.

In babies less than 2 kg born to a hepatitis B positive mother, hepatitis B vaccine should be given along with HBIG within 12 hours of birth and 3 more doses at 1, 2 and 6 months are recommended.

Since preterm, low birth weight babies have increased susceptibility to infections, vaccines such as pneumococcal conjugate vaccines, rotavirus and influenza should be offered if resources permit.

35. What are the general recommendations on "Catch up immunization"?

For catch up immunization, doses should preferably be given at the minimum possible interval to entail early protection.

Any number of vaccines live/inactivated may be given on the same day either singly or as combination vaccines maintaining a gap of 5 cm between different vaccines.
- Inactivated vaccines can be given at any time in relation to any other live/inactivated vaccines.
- If not given on the same day a gap of 4 weeks should be maintained between two live vaccines.

OPV, rotavirus and oral typhoid vaccines may be given at any time in relation to any live/inactivated vaccine.

36. What are the general recommendations on "lapsed immunization"?

A lapse in the immunization schedule does not require reinitiating the entire series or addition of doses to the series for any vaccine in the recommended schedule. This is because of immune memory. Vaccine is to be offered at the next available opportunity. Vaccine doses must not be offered 4 or less days from the minimum desired interval.

37. What are the general recommendations on interchangeability of vaccine brands?

When possible, effort should be made to complete a series with vaccine made by the same manufacturer. Similar vaccines made by different manufacturers can differ in the number and amount of their specific antigenic components and formulation of adjuvants and conjugating agents, thereby eliciting different immune responses. However, if previous brand is not known or no longer available, any brand may be used and vaccination should not be delayed/canceled.

There is sufficient data that brands of hepatitis, hepatitis B and hepatitis A may be safely interchanged with no compromise on immunogenicity and efficacy. However robust data for immunogenicity of vaccination with different brands of DTaP is lacking. Hence, vaccination with DTaP should be completed with the same brand. Interchangeability for HPV vaccines brand is not permissible.

SUGGESTED READING

1. AAP Committee on Infectious Diseases. Red Book: 2018–2021. Report of the Committee on Infectious Diseases, 31st edition. Illinois: American Academy of Pediatrics; 2018.
2. CDC. (2019). ACIP General Best Practice Guidelines. [online] Available from: https://www.cdc.gov/vaccines/pubs/pinkbook/downloads/appendices/a/mmr_ig.pdf. [Last Accessed August, 2020].
3. CDC. Epidemiology and Prevention of Vaccine-Preventable Diseases. The Pink Book: Course Textbook,13th edition. Grorgia: CDC; 2015.
4. IAP. IAP Guidebook on Immunizations (2013-2014, 2018-19). New Delhi: IAP; 2018.
5. Moulik NR, Mandal P, Chandra J, Bansal S, Jog P, Sanjay S, et al. Immunization of Children with Cancer in India Treated with Chemotherapy – Consensus Guideline from the Pediatric Hematology- Oncology Chapter and the Advisory Committee on Vaccination and Immunization Practices of the Indian Academy of Pediatrics. Indian Pediatr. 2019;15:1041-9.
6. NIH. (2019). Guidelines for the Prevention and Treatment of Opportunistic Infections in HIV-Exposed and HIV-Infected Children. [online] Available from: https://aidsinfo.nih.gov/guidelines/html/5/pediatric-opportunistic-infection/431/figure-1--recommended-immunization-schedule-for-children-with-hiv-infection-aged-0-through-18-years--united-states--2019. [Last Accessed August, 2020].
7. Reefhis J, Honein MA, Whitney CG, Chamany S, Mann EA, Biernath KR, et al. Risk of bacterial meningitis in children with cochlear implants. N Engl J Med. 2003;349:435-45.
8. Rubin LG, Levin MJ, Ljungman P, Davies EG, Avery R, Tomblyn M, et al. 2013 IDSA clinical practice guideline for vaccination of the immunocompromised host clinical infectious diseases. Clin Infect Dis. 2014;58(3):309-18.
9. WHO. Extract from report of GACVS meeting (November 2006). Wkly Epidemiol Rec. 2007;82:181-96.

CHAPTER 7

Adverse Events following Immunization, Vaccine Safety and Misinformation against Vaccination

Meeta Dhaval Vashi, Vivek R Pardeshi

1. What are the adverse events following immunizations (AEFIs)?

Adverse events following immunization is any untoward medical occurrence which follows immunization and which does not necessarily have a causal relationship with the usage of vaccines. These events may include one or more unfavorable or unintended signs, symptoms, or laboratory findings which raise concern among immunization program managers, policy makers, family of beneficiary and the community.

2. What is an AEFI surveillance?

Adverse events following immunization surveillance is a system to detect report and respond to any actual or perceived untoward event following immunization. Purpose of the AEFI surveillance is to maintain public and stakeholder's confidence in immunization. In India, the AEFI surveillance system has been in place since 1988. The national AEFI guidelines are revised in 2015. The National AEFI Guidelines Handbook provides complete guidance and other details for reporting, investigating, and conducting the causality assessment of cases reported as AEFIs.

3. What is necessity of an AEFI surveillance?

Immunization is intended to protect the individuals and the public from vaccine preventable diseases. Vaccines are safe and effective but, like any other pharmaceutical product, vaccines are not completely risk-free and adverse reactions may occur. A well-developed AEFI surveillance system is needed to build up and sustain confidence of the individuals, caregivers, health workers, and manufacturers in immunization.

4. What is revised Council for International Organizations of Medical Sciences (CIOMS) and World Health Organization (WHO) classification of AEFIs?

Revised CIOMS and WHO cause-specific categorization of AEFIs **(Table 1)**.

TABLE 1: Cause-specific categorization of adverse events following immunization (AEFIs).

Cause-specific type of AEFI	Definition
Vaccine product-related reaction	An AEFI that is caused or precipitated by a vaccine due to one or more of the inherent properties of the vaccine product
Vaccine quality defect-related reaction	An AEFI that is caused or precipitated by a vaccine due to one or more quality defects of the vaccine product, including its administration device as provided by the manufacturer
Immunization error-related reaction (formerly "programmatic error")	An AEFI that is caused by inappropriate vaccine handling, prescribing or administration and thus by its nature is preventable
Immunization anxiety-related reaction	An AEFI arising from anxiety about the immunization
Coincidental event	An AEFI that is caused by something other than the vaccine product, immunization error, or immunization anxiety

Source: Operational Guidelines for AEFI surveillance, India; 2015.

5. What are different types of AEFIs?

Adverse events following immunizations can be:
- *Common and minor*: Such as fever, local pain, and swelling
- *Serious*: Conditions requiring hospitalization or leading to death or disability or clusters
- *Severe*: Conditions which are not minor and not serious fall under severe type such as convulsions or anaphylaxis managed in casualty and did not need hospitalization.

6. What are common minor AEFIs?

These are the events occur because vaccine induces immunity by causing the recipient's immune system to react to it. Local reaction, fever, and systemic symptoms may result as a part of the immune reaction. In addition, some of the vaccine's components (e.g., adjuvant, stabilizers, or preservatives) can lead to reactions. These are categorized as common minor AEFIs.

7. What are severe AEFIs?

Severe AEFIs are the events that are not minor but do not result in death, hospitalization, or disabilities are categorized as severe. The term "severe" describes the intensity of a specific event (as in mild, moderate, or severe). The event itself, however, could also be of relatively minor medical significance.

8. What is serious AEFI?

Serious AEFI is the event which results in death, requires hospitalization, or results in persistent or significant disability/incapacity. If there is a cluster of AEFIs (two or more cases) occur in a geographical area, it is considered as serious AEFI.

9. Who can notify AEFI cases?

Parents of the beneficiary of the vaccine, adult beneficiaries themselves, vaccinator, treating healthcare provider, immunization supervisor, pharmacy dispensing the vaccine, adverse drug reactions (ADR) monitoring centers or anyone who comes across an AEFI case, including local media can notify the case to local government health authority.

10. What are different channels of reporting AEFI in the government system?

- Serious and severe AEFI cases should be immediately reported using case reporting form (CRF).
- *Monthly progress reports*: This is done using currently available monthly immunization reporting formats such as the formats used for National Health Mission (NHM), Health Management Information System (HMIS), etc. Peripheral health staff must submit a NIL monthly report in case no AEFI is detected from their area during the month. For minor AEFI cases brought to the notice of the health staff as a concern (from parents/community) should be reported and documented in a line-list.
- Adverse events following immunization serious and severe are also included in weekly report (H002) form of reporting sites.

11. Who should report AEFI?

Any healthcare worker, auxiliary nurse midwives (ANMs) public health nurses (PHNs), supervisors, vaccinators, medical officers, and private medical practitioners, who come across any AEFI case, should report AEFI case to the district health authority.

12. Which AEFIs should be reported? Why?

All the events including minor, severe, and serious events must be reported. Reporting of minor events on monthly basis is equally important as it helps to estimate and compare background rates of events which are significant to identify product quality defects, immunization errors or increased susceptibility to vaccine reactions among the population.

13. What is mechanism of reporting AEFI cases?

Medical officer of the primary health center (PHC)/health post or the reporting person reports serious/severe AEFI using case reporting format (CRF).

After completion of the CRF, he/she sends to the district immunization officer within 24 hours of getting the information of the case.

14. What process is followed after notification of serious/severe AEFI cases?

There are following steps:
- Immediate reporting of serious/severe AEFI to the appropriate authority
- District level investigation of reported AEFI cases such as:
  - Serious AEFIs (death, disability, hospitalization, and cluster)
  - Signals and events associated with a newly introduced vaccine
  - Adverse events following immunization that may have been occurred by an immunization error related reaction
  - Significant events of unexplained cause occurring within 30 days of vaccination
  - Events causing significant parents/community concern
- These cases are further studied by members of AEFI committees at district, state, and national level, causality assessment is done and if indicated, remedial actions are taken.

15. Enlist key serious/severe reportable AEFI cases.

- Anaphylactoid reaction (acute hypersensitivity reaction)
- Anaphylaxis
- Persistent inconsolable crying (>3 hours)
- Hypotonic-hyporesponsive episode (HHE)
- Toxic shock syndrome (TSS)
- Severe local reaction
- Sepsis
- Injection site abscess (sterile/bacterial)
- Seizures such as febrile seizures
- Encephalopathy
- Acute flaccid paralysis (AFP)
- Brachial neuritis
- Intussusception
- Thrombocytopenia
- Lymphadenitis
- Disseminated bacillus Calmette-Guérin (BCG) infection
- Osteitis/osteomyelitis
- Death due to any reason other above
- Hospitalization due to any reason other than above
- Disability
- Cluster
- Any other severe and unusual events that are thought by health workers or public to be related to immunization.

16. **Sixty one cases of paralytic poliomyelitis were reported after the administration of inactivated polio vaccine (IPV) (cutter incident). Investigations revealed that the wild poliovirus (WPV) underwent inadequate inactivation. What type of AEFI is it?**

This is an instance of "vaccine quality defect-related reaction" since the vaccine did not undergo a proper inactivation process.

17. **A 14-week-old infant develops a thigh abscess following the third dose of penta vaccine. What is the type of vaccine reaction?**

This reaction is "immunization error-related reaction" (formerly "program error") because there may be some fault during the administration of the vaccine such as the needle may be contaminated hence nonsterile injection was given **(Box 1)**.

BOX 1: Program errors leading to adverse events and causes of nonsterile injection.
• Reuse of disposable syringes or needles
• Improperly sterilized syringes or needles
• Contaminated vaccines or diluents
• Reuse of reconstituted vaccine at subsequent session
• Local suppuration at injection site, abscess, cellulitis
• Systemic infection
• Sepsis
• Toxic shock syndrome
• Transmission of blood born infections such as HIV, HBV, HCV, etc.

(HBV: hepatitis B virus; HCV: hepatitis C virus; HIV: human immunodeficiency virus)

18. **A 5-year-old girl developed syncopal episode during a college HPV vaccine session. What types of AEFIs are we dealing with?**

It is immunization anxiety-related reaction. Fainting is relatively common, but usually only affects older children and adults. It does not require any management beyond giving the injection while the children are seated (to avoid injury caused by falling) and placing the patient in a recumbent position after the injection.

19. **What are the other examples of anxiety-related reaction?**
- *Hyperventilation*: Can cause light-headedness, dizziness, tingling around the mouth and in the hands.
- *Vomiting*:
  - Younger children tend to react differently, with vomiting a common anxiety symptom

- Breathholding may occur, which can end in a brief period of unconsciousness, during which breathing resumes
- They may also scream to prevent the injection or run away
- *Convulsions*:
  - Convulsions in rare cases
  - These children do not need to be investigated but should be reassured.

20. How can we reduce the incidence of anxiety-related AEFI?

The likelihood of anxiety from these reactions can be reduced by:
- Clear explanations about the immunization, and
- Calm, confident administration.

21. A normal 5-month-old infant develops pneumonia 3 weeks after liquid pentavalent vaccine. What types of AEFIs are we dealing with?

Coincidental type since the adverse event is caused by something other than the vaccine product, immunization error, or immunization anxiety.

22. How to conduct AEFI case investigation?

The ultimate goal of a case investigation is to make a clinical diagnosis based on the chronology of medical events, detailed medical history, and other available evidence. On receipt of a report on AEFI:
- The District Immunization Officer (DIO) along with the members of the District AEFI Committee visits the immunization site, vaccine storage points, residence and locality of the patient, and the treatment center to collect information regarding the prevaccination health status, treatment taken, hospitalization or postmortem reports, details of vaccination and cold chain. The epidemiological investigation is also an important aspect while investigating an AEFI. DIO ensures that the filled preliminary case investigation format (PCIF) is submitted to the state and the national level simultaneously within 10 days of notification.
- The District AEFI Committee meets and discusses the case and summarizes the findings of the investigation in the final CIF (FCIF) and gives its opinion on the probable diagnosis. The FCIF is sent within 70 days of notification to the State AEFI Committee and the "immunization division" along with all the relevant documents of the case.

Note: In case of reported AEFI death and cluster (two or more cases of the same adverse event related in time, place, or vaccine administration), the investigation should be conducted without any delay. It is recommended that an autopsy in a death suspected to be due to an AEFI be performed as soon as possible (within 72 hours) to avoid tissue damage, development of postmortem artifacts and lysis of the adrenal glands, which can alter diagnosis.

23. What are the guidelines on samples collection during AEFI investigation?

It is important to collect appropriate specimens in adequate quantities. Important documents such as laboratory request form (LRF), CRF, CIF with proper epidemiological number are *must* with the specimen under investigation. For local AEFI: abscess swab and blood, for CNS-related AEFI: CSF, blood (stool, in case of AFP), and for anaphylaxis, TSS, death: blood, blood culture, postmortem tissue (as per the physician) and urine samples are needed. If indicated, vaccines, diluents, and logistics should also be tested. In case of AEF Japanese encephalitis (JE) immunization, samples should be sent to National Institute of Virology Pune or Gorakhpur. *Please note*: Specimen collection is *not* needed for all cases. Only if appropriate, CSF, serum (or other biological products), the implicated vaccine, and logistic samples should be collected and dispatched to appropriate laboratories with LRF.

24. Are there any designated laboratories for sample testing?

Yes, biological samples should be sent to laboratories identified by the district/state AEFI committees. Autopsy samples should be sent to approved and accredited state forensic laboratories. Central Drug Standard Control Organization has designated Central Drugs Laboratory (CDL), Kasauli, for vaccines and diluents. Syringes and needles are sent to CDL, Kolkata.

25. Is there any special procedure to investigate reported sudden unexplained deaths following vaccination?

Unexplained deaths following immunization must be investigated completely as it has a big impact on the immunization program. It is important to differentiate between vaccine-related deaths and deaths due to other causes. A special document, verbal autopsy form has been designed, based on the WHO and Centers for Disease Control and Prevention (CDC) sudden infant death investigation (SUIDI) form should be used.

26. What are the guidelines on conduction autopsy in case of sudden unexplained deaths following vaccination?

The guidance on conducting autopsy has been developed by a committee of leading experts in the field of immunology. Use of "verbal autopsy" form in case of unexplained death/home death is a new addition in the guidelines. The format collects information regarding history, circumstances of death, medical examination, feeding history, etc. to rule out causes of death. These formats should be filled by the investigating team while investigating the reports of AEFI deaths where information regarding the event is inadequate. For example, brought dead to OPD, home death, insufficient medical records regarding the event, death in nonhospitalized case or if clinical diagnosis cannot be established. An autopsy must be performed in every case of an AEFI death within 72 hours of death, ideally by forensic specialist or medical officer.

27. What is causality assessment of an AEFI?

"Causality assessment" is a critical part of the AEFI monitoring which enhances confidence in the National Immunization Program. It is a systematic evaluation of the information obtained about an AEFI to determine the likelihood of the event having been caused by the vaccine/s received.

28. Are there any standard guidelines to conduct causality assessment of AEFIs?

There are revised WHO/CIOMS causality assessment guidelines (2014). The guidelines encourage the states to conduct "causality assessment" for reported AEFI cases. The AEFI report must have investigation formats, relevant documents, and a diagnosis for being eligible for "causality assessment".

29. What are steps for causality assessment?

The "causality assessment" process has four steps:
1. *Eligibility*: To determine if the reported AEFI case satisfies the minimum criteria for "causality assessment" as mentioned above.
2. *Checklist*: To systematically review the relevant and available information to address possible causal aspects of the AEFI.
3. *Algorithm*: To obtain a direction as to the "causality" with the information gathered in the checklist.
4. *Classification*: To categorize the AEFI's association to the vaccine/vaccination based on direction determined in the algorithm. All the cases being investigated by the district should be assessed by the causality assessment experts of the state AEFI committee after discussing all the investigation formats and reports available. The results of causality assessment should be disseminated so that others can learn from the experience.

30. What are guidelines about formation and function of AEFI committee?

The AEFI committees are formed at district/state/national levels. Standard guidelines are revised along with the terms of reference of the committee members. The AEFI committees provide technical inputs to review the factors leading to the adverse event and provide inputs to improve the system to provide safe and effective immunization. The committee should include members from various departments such as pediatrician, microbiologist, pathologist, epidemiologist, neurologist, forensic expert, cold-chain officer, representatives from Integrated Disease Surveillance Program (IDSP), drug authority, and municipal corporation and partner agencies.

31. What are the ways to handle media in case of an AEFI?

As any AEFI causes scare in public and other stakeholders, effective communication is needed to manage public reactions. Guidelines include strategic communication plan to address the short-term crisis in cases of the AEFI and long-term support that the immunization program requires at the national and local level. The plan focuses on regular communication with the community, print and electronic media on routine immunization (RI) activities to encourage use of vaccines and thus help in improving the vaccine coverage levels.

An AEFI response protocol has standardized procedures for communication to assist a prompt crisis management. It identifies the spokesperson who will respond in crisis situations at all the levels. The protocol recommends that in case of media interest in an AEFI crisis, a press note should be issued as early as possible (preferably within first 6 hours).

32. What is the role of NRA in an AEFI surveillance program?

The National Drug Regulatory Authority (NRA) and Pharmacovigilance Program of India (PVPI) have prime role in coordination between the Central Drug Standard Control Organization (CDSCO) and the Immunization Division, Ministry of Health and Family Welfare (MoHFW). The results of the causality assessment approved by the National AEFI Committee are shared with the CDSCO which analyzes the results to conduct further necessary regulatory actions such as inspections, amendments to product inserts, reporting by manufacturers, etc.). The Indian Pharmacopoeia Commission (IPC) has established a knowledge-sharing arrangement with the AEFI secretariat for ensuring convergence in vaccine safety reports and their adequate investigations.

33. What is the necessity of vaccination?

Vaccines are necessary to develop immunity against multiple vaccine preventable diseases. In fact, it is the biggest gift of modern medicine that has been given to mankind. It provides protection to the vaccinated individual and helps to increase "herd immunity" in the susceptible population. Deadly disease such as smallpox eradication was possible just because of mass vaccination. Not only communicable diseases but also noncommunicable diseases such as cervical cancer and liver cancer can be controlled. If vaccination is stopped, the diseases which are prevented by vaccination return in the population. Diphtheria, pertussis (whooping cough), polio, and measles are such diseases which have potential to quickly reappear in a disease-free population.

34. Are vaccines safe?

Vaccines are very safe. Like any new medicine, vaccines also go through multiple rigorous tests in multiple phases of trials before it is approved and licenced for use. Even postmarketing, vaccines are frequently reassessed to ensure safety. Vaccines are generally given to healthy individuals and it becomes imperative to ensure vaccine safety thus, pharmacovigilance mechanism is constantly on and any perceived or actual signal against vaccine safety is taken very seriously. Constant monitoring is done through information from several sources for any sign that a vaccine may cause an adverse event. Some beneficiaries may present with minor and temporary vaccine reactions, such as pain at injection site or mild fever. Rarely, if any serious side effect is reported, it is immediately investigated through adverse events following surveillance. Risks and complications of getting infected by vaccine preventable diseases and risks of dying due to them are very high as compared with very few and risks of vaccination and benefits are too many.

35. Is vaccine immunity better than natural immunity from infections?

It is very risky to acquire immunity through natural infection; it may lead to complications or deaths. For example, death from complication due to measles, birth defects from rubella, liver cancer from hepatitis B virus, etc. in unimmunized individuals. On the other hand, vaccines interact with the immune system to mimic an immune response similar to that produced by the natural infection, but they do not cause the disease or put the immunized person at risk of its potential complications.

36. Does MMR vaccination lead to autism?

The study published in the year 1998 had raised concerns about a possible link between measles-mumps-rubella (MMR) vaccine and autism. Later, it was found that the study had many flaws and results were manipulated. The research paper was retracted by the journal that published it after confirming the flaws and manipulations. This paper created a lot of panic which led to dropping immunization coverage, leading to outbreaks of these diseases. It is proved beyond doubt and there is no evidence of a link between MMR vaccine and autism or autistic disorders.

37. Does polio vaccine cause impotence?

There is absolutely no evidence ever published that the polio vaccine (either oral or parenteral) leads to impotency or erectile dysfunction. The vaccine contains live-attenuated strains (oral poliovirus vaccine) and killed strains (inactivated poliovirus vaccine). It does not contain any antifertility agents. The vaccine has played very vital role in eliminating the disease from all the countries in the world, now only two countries are struggling to eliminate the disease with the use of oral poliovirus vaccine.

38. What is vaccine confidence?

Vaccine confidence is when parents, caregivers or the community understand the value of vaccination and voluntarily demand vaccination services as a right, whether these vaccinations are part of the RI schedule for their children or part of adult vaccinations such as tetanus toxoid (TT) for pregnant women. Vaccine confidence comes from adequate awareness about the benefits of vaccines, both to the individual and to the community, and the trust in the immunization service delivery system to be able to provide quality vaccination.

39. What is vaccine hesitancy?

Vaccine hesitancy is the behavior of parents, caregivers, or the community, who hesitate to get their children vaccinated in spite of immunization services being available and accessible. Inadequate immunization services due to nonavailability of vaccines, absenteeism of vaccinators and long distances to vaccination centers contribute to this hesitancy. Other reasons for vaccine hesitancy are low perception of the benefits of vaccines, loss of wages, social beliefs, fear of AEFIs, inadequate IPC skills of health workers, and geographical barriers.

40. How to tackle vaccine hesitancy behavior in the population?

Vaccine hesitancy behavior is experienced in many sectors of the population. It adversely affects vaccination coverage in given population. It is important to take steps to understand the extent and nature of hesitancy at a local level, regularly. A concrete social mobilization and vaccine advocacy strategy is needed to increase acceptance and demand for vaccination, which should include ongoing community engagement and trust-building, active hesitancy prevention, regular national assessments of concerns, and crisis response planning. There are many local and international organizations who constantly strive to address vaccine hesitancy behavior of the population.

SUGGESTED READING

1. Adverse Events Following Immunization—Surveillance and Response Operational Guidelines, MOHFW; 2015.
2. World Health Organization (2020). Global Vaccine Safety: Six common misconceptions about immunization. [online] Available from: http://itsu.org.in/repository-resources/AEFI-Surveillance-and-Response-Operational-Guidelines-2015.pdfhttps://www.who.int/vaccine_safety/initiative/detection/immunization_misconceptions/en/ [Last accessed June, 2020].
3. World Health Organization (2020). Immunization, Vaccines and Biologicals. [online] Available from: https://www.who.int/immunization/programmes_systems/vaccine_hesitancy/en/ [Last accessed June, 2020].

CHAPTER 8

Cold Chain and Vaccine Storage

Digant D Shastri

INTRODUCTION

An effective logistics system and a well-maintained cold chain are essential for safe and effective immunization service delivery, and it is a shared responsibility from the time the vaccine is manufactured until it is administered. The cold chain has three main components: (i) transport and storage equipment, (ii) trained personnel, and (iii) efficient management procedures. All three elements must combine to ensure safe vaccine transport and storage.

An improperly functioning of cold chain can lead to wastage of vaccines, missed opportunities to immunize due to shortage of vaccines, and children receiving vaccines that do not protect them as intended due to loss of potency or that actually make them sick. Cold chain breaches can occur even in well-designed and well-managed systems as a result of technical malfunctions but if there are good procedures in place, problems will be detected and effectively managed. Efficient vaccine storage management is an essential quality assurance measure for vaccine service providers. Majority of vaccine storage and handling mistakes are easily avoidable.

1. What is cold chain?

The "cold chain" is the system of transporting and storing vaccines within the within temperature range from the place of manufacture to the point of administration. Immunization service providers should maintain their vaccine refrigerators as close as possible to 5°C, as this gives a safety margin of ± 3°C **(Table 1)**.

2. What is the importance of cold chain?

The vaccines which are exposed to the highest temperature cause degradation and consequently total or partial loss of potency, while vaccine which is exposed to freezing increases the local reactivity with or without loss of potency. Commonly the degradation rate of a vaccine is determined by the storage temperature: the higher the temperature, the more rapid and extensive is the degradation. There are considerable differences between degradation rates for different vaccines. An effective logistics system and a well-maintained cold chain are essential for safe and effective immunization service delivery.

CHAPTER 8 Cold Chain and Vaccine Storage

TABLE 1: World Health Organization (WHO) recommended vaccine storage conditions.

	National	Intermediate		Primary health center	Subcenter/ session site
		Regional	District		
OPV	−15°C to −25°C				
BCG	WHO no longer recommends that freeze-dried vaccines can be stored at −20°C. Storing them at −20°C is not harmful but is unnecessary. Instead, these vaccines should be kept in refrigeration and transported at +2°C to 8°C.			+2°C to +8°C	
Hep B					
DT					
DPT					
TT					
Diluent vials must *never* be frozen. If the manufacturer supplies a freeze-dried vaccine packed with its diluent, *always* store the product at between +2°C and +8°C. If space permits, diluents supplied separately from vaccine may safely be stored in the cold chain between +2°C and +8°C.					

(BCG: bacillus Calmette–Guérin; DPT: diphtheria, pertussis and tetanus; DT: diphtheria and tetanus; Hep B: hepatitis B; OPV: oral poliovirus vaccine; TT: tetanus toxoid)

3. What are the drawbacks of improper cold chain?

An improperly functioning of cold chain can lead to increased chances of adverse events, wastage of vaccines, missed opportunities to immunize due to lack of vaccines, and inability to provide immunity to recipient of vaccines and that may ultimately lead to loss of confidence in parents.

4. What are the important components of cold chain?

The cold chain has three main components:
1. Vaccine transport and storage equipment, and temperature monitoring tools
2. Trained personnel
3. Efficient vaccine storage and handling protocols.

All the three elements must combine to ensure safe vaccine transport and storage.

5. Which is the vaccine storage equipment used in the immunization program?

There is equipment of different capacity for storage of vaccines at different levels. They are:
- Walk-in freezer
- Walk-in coolers
- Deep freezer

- Ice-lined refrigerator (ILR)
- Purpose-built refrigerator
- Domestic refrigerator
- Isothermic cold boxes
- Vaccine carrier.

6. Which is the most ideal vaccine storage device in vaccination clinic and why?

Purpose-built vaccine refrigerator is the most ideal refrigerator for vaccine storage in vaccination clinic **(Fig. 1)**. The purpose-built refrigerators have following advantages over the domestic refrigerator:

- They are programmed to maintain an internal temperature between 2°C and 8°C
- Good temperature recovery—when the fridge is open to access the vaccines
- Cabinet temperature is not affected by an ambient temperature and is stable and uniform all across the refrigerator
- Have an external temperature display and have continuous display of maximum/minimum temperature, and an alarm for deviations outside the programmed temperature range
- Defrost cycle allowing defrosting without rise in cabinet temperature
- They automatically defrost
- Do not require to be modified for vaccine storage
- Nearly all internal space can be used to store the vaccines, so the size of the purpose built refrigerator may be smaller than the previously used domestic refrigerator.

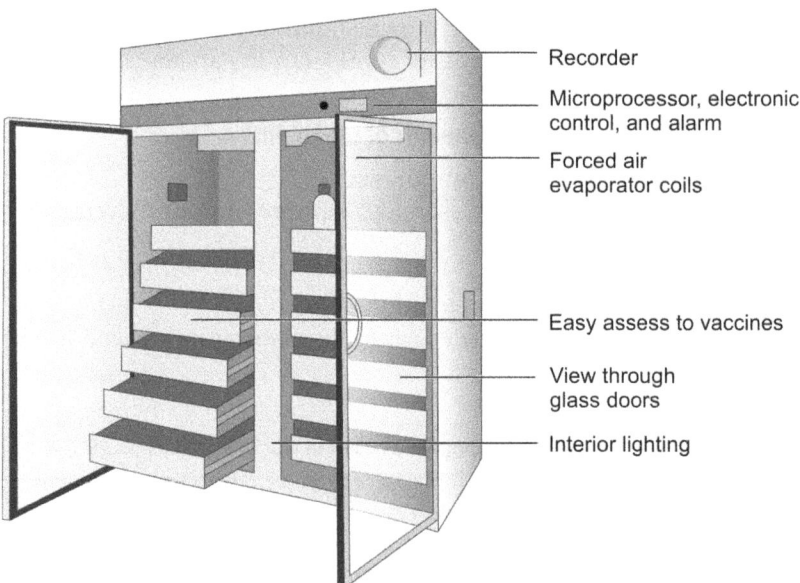

Fig. 1: Purpose-built refrigerator.

7. What are the drawbacks of domestic refrigerator in storage of vaccines?

Domestic refrigerators used for the vaccine storage are basically designed for the storage of food and drink and usually have different temperature zones to meet the requirements of different foods **(Figs. 2A to C)**. Since they are not designed for the special temperature needs of vaccines if not used properly can put the safety of vaccines at risk. From the angle of vaccine storage the domestic refrigerator suffer from following drawbacks:

- Cabinet temperature varies significantly every time when the door is opened.
- Cabinet temperature rises during defrosting in cycle in cyclic defrost and frost-free refrigerator
- Cabinet temperature is easily affected by the ambient temperature
- Temperature setting using dial is crude and inaccurate
- Whole inner space cannot be used to store the vaccines.

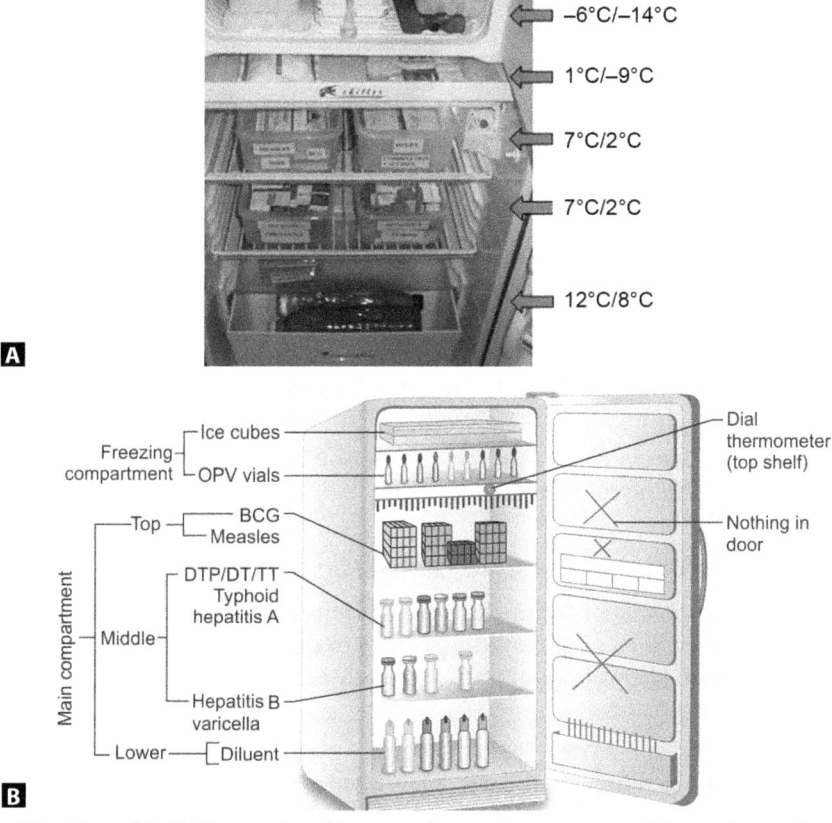

Fig. 2A and B: (A) Domestic refrigerator for vaccines storage—"thermal zones"; (B) Domestic refrigerator—suggested placement of different vaccines.

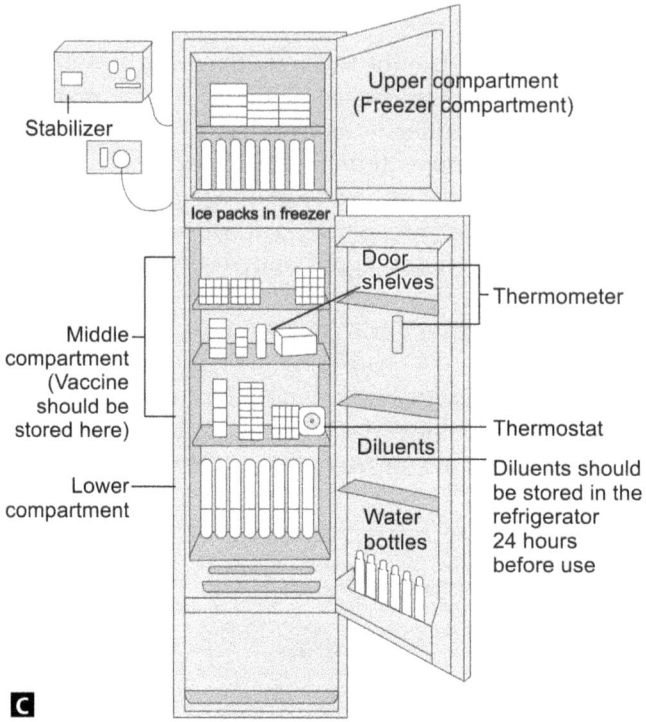

Fig. 2 C: Domestic refrigerator—storage protocol for different vaccines and diluent storage. Double-door fridge should be preferred.

8. What are the different types of domestic refrigerator?
The different types of domestic refrigerator are:
- *Dormitory/bar style refrigerator*: Single door with common freezer and cabinet compartment
- Cyclic type refrigerator
- Frost-free refrigerator
- *Chest type refrigerator*: Front opening door refrigerator
- Top lid opening refrigerator.

9. Why bar refrigerators are not recommended to use to store vaccines?
There are high chances of temperature instability and freezing injury to stored vaccines as well, it has higher susceptibility to the ambient temperature. For all these reasons *bar* refrigerators are strongly not recommended to store the vaccines.

10. Why frost-free refrigerators are recommended to use to store vaccines?
Frost-free refrigerators do not have heating cycles but have low-level warming cycles and hence there are less chances of fluctuation of cabinet temperature

outside 2–8°C range. The cyclic refrigerators have regular internal heating and that can cause wide fluctuation in the internal temperature. Hence, "frost-free" rather than cyclic-type domestic refrigerators are recommended for storage of vaccines. Frost-free refrigerators usually have several temperature zones.

11. What are the prerequisites in domestic refrigerators for safe vaccine storage?
- Should have a separate freezer compartment.
- Should exclusively be used to store the vaccines only.
- Should maintain temperatures without fluctuating into the danger zones:
  - The refrigerator compartment should maintain temperatures between 2°C and 8°C
  - The freezer compartment should maintain temperatures at or below 5°F (–15°C).
- Should not have required repairing for last 2 years.
- Should be free of any water or coolant leaks.
- The door seals should be in good condition and should seal tightly.
- The door should close properly automatically on leaving it free.
- The refrigerator compressor should be quiet and does not make sound.
- The refrigerator is of an adequate size for the individual storage needs.

12. What are the points to be considered in placement of refrigerator?
- Refrigerator should be placed out of direct sunlight and away from heat.
- It should be at least 10 cm away from wall.
- *It should be placed in* secure area *so that the accessibility to* the vaccine refrigerator is restricted to identified staff only. This can minimize the risk of unnecessary door opening, accidental switched off of power at the power point.

13. What precautions should be observed while storing vaccines in domestic refrigerator?
- Vaccines must never be stored in the door of the refrigerator.
- Place *freeze-tolerant vaccines* [measles, mumps, rubella, oral poliomyelitis vaccine (OPV) and bacillus Calmette–Guérin (BCG)] in the shelves identified as being the coldest and *freeze-sensitive vaccines* [DTP containing vaccines; Hib, pneumococcal, influenza, hepatitis, inactivated polio vaccine (IPV), and some varicella vaccines] on shelves identified as having more stable temperatures (e.g., no "cold spots").
- Store the vaccines in enclosed plastic containers/labeled baskets:
  - This will allow easy identification of vaccines and minimize time spent with the door opened searching for vaccines.
  - Enclosed plastic containers will help to stabilize temperatures a little and provide some protection in borderline freezing episodes as well as against effects from the cooling plate and blasts of cold air from outlets.

- Do not crowd the vaccines by overfilling the shelves. Allow space between containers for air circulation.
- Storage of vaccine against refrigerator walls increases the risk of freezing. Ensure a gap of at least 4 cm from all walls of refrigerator and between two large packs of vaccines.
- Keep a distance of at least 4 cm above and below the vaccine container to allow free air circulation.
- Rotate stock so vaccines with the shortest expiry date are used first.

14. Can we straight away start using the refrigerator/freezer unit that is new or has just repaired?

If the refrigerator/freezer unit is new or just repaired, allow 1 week of recorded temperature checks within normal ranges before placing vaccines into the unit.

15. What is the importance of placing ice packs/gel packs in the freezer and water bottles in lower drawer and door?

- This will assist in stabilizing the temperature in refrigerator compartment, as in most frost-free refrigerators, cold air is distributed from the freezer to the fresh food compartment.
- It reduces warming periods when the refrigerator is opened. This is particularly useful if there is a power cut or other cause of refrigerator failure.
- It will be available for vaccine transport in isothermal box or in vaccine carrier for outreach immunization.

16. What are the protocols for maintenance of the vaccine refrigerator?

- Refrigerator breakdowns should be repaired immediately.
- Regularly check the door seals to ensure that a good seal is maintained. Replace the seals if they are damaged or cold air is leaking from the refrigerator.
- Refrigerators that are not "frost-free" should be defrosted regularly to prevent ice build-up. If the freezer is not frost-free, ice should not be allowed to build up more than 1/4 inch. Ice build-up reduces the efficiency and performance of a refrigerator. During defrosting or cleaning of the refrigerator, move the vaccines to a second refrigerator.
- If there are exposed coils on the back of the refrigerator keep them clean and dust free to improve operating efficiency.
- A summary of preventive maintenance of the vaccine refrigerator is described in **Table 2**.

17. Which are cold-sensitive vaccines?

- Diphtheria-tetanus-pertussis containing vaccines
- *Haemophilus influenzae* type B [the exception being the lyophilized polyribosyl-ribitol-phosphate (PRP)-T vaccines]

TABLE 2: Checklist for preventive maintenance.		
External	*Internal*	*Technical*
• The exterior is clean • It is firm on the floor • It is properly leveled • Its sides are at least 10 cm away from walls • It is away from direct sunlight • Room is well-ventilated • It is opened only when necessary	• Doors seal properly without gap • The door seal is clean • Ice packs are in proper position • Vaccines are neatly placed with space for air circulation • DPT, TT, Hep B, and DT are not touching the cooling surface • Thermometer has been kept among the vaccine • Temperature is recorded twice a day	• Temperature is within prescribed limit (if not, set the thermostat) • Voltage stabilizer is working properly and equipment is connected through it • Plug of the voltage stabilizer is fitted properly to the power line • There is no abnormal noise • Compressor mounting bolts are tight

(DPT: diphtheria, pertussis, and tetanus; DT: diphtheria and tetanus; Hep B: hepatitis B; TT: tetanus toxoid)

- Hepatitis B-containing vaccines
- Hepatitis A vaccine
- Influenza vaccine
- Pneumococcal (polysaccharide and conjugate) vaccines
- Meningococcal C conjugate vaccines
- Japanese encephalitis vaccine.

18. Which vaccines are heat sensitive?

- Bacille Calmette–Guérin vaccine
- Measles-mumps-rubella (MMR) vaccine
- Oral poliomyelitis vaccine
- Varicella zoster vaccine
- Yellow fever vaccine
- All reconstituted vaccines.
  A summary of vaccine sensitivities is described in **Table 3**.

19. Which are light sensitive vaccines?

Following vaccines are sensitive to strong light, sunlight, ultraviolet, fluorescents (neon), and exposure to light should be avoided **(Fig. 3)**.
- Bacillus Calmette–Guérin
- Measles
- Rubella
- Measles-mumps-rubella
- Varicella.

20. What is ice-lined refrigerator (ILR)?

Ice-lined refrigerators are used to store vaccines at +2°C to +8°C. ILR operates on electricity, it has specifically microprocessor for controlling temperature

TABLE 3: Summary of vaccine sensitivities.

Vaccine	Exposure to heat/light	Exposure to cold	Recommended temperature range
Heat- and light-sensitive vaccines			
BCG	Relatively heat stable, but sensitive to light	Not damaged by freezing	+2°C to +8°C
OPV	Heat sensitive	Not damaged by freezing	+2°C to +8°C
Measles	Sensitive to heat and light	Not damaged by freezing	+2°C to +8°C
Freeze-sensitive vaccines			
DPT	Relatively heat stable	Freezes at −3°C	+2°C to +8°C
Hep B	Relatively heat stable	Freezes at −0.5°C	+2°C to +8°C
DT	Relatively heat stable	Freezes at −3°C	+2°C to +8°C
TT	Relatively heat stable	Freezes at −0.5°C	+2°C to +8°C

(BCG: bacillus Calmette–Guérin; DPT: diphtheria, pertussis, and tetanus; DT: diphtheria and tetanus; Hep B: hepatitis B; OPV: oral poliovirus vaccine; TT: tetanus toxoid)

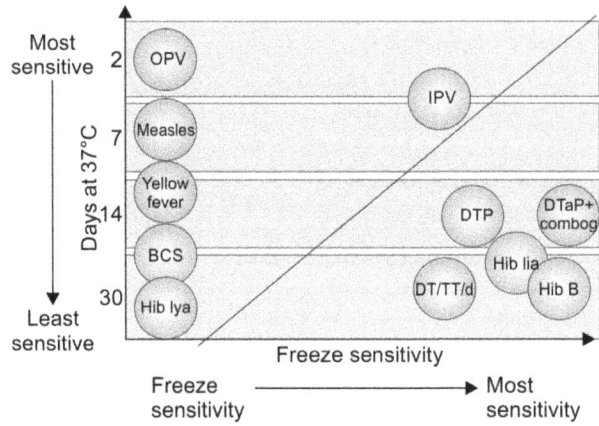

Fig. 3: Graphical depiction of heat and freeze sensitivities of commonly used vaccines.
(BCG: bacillus Calmette–Guérin; DPT: diphtheria, pertussis, and tetanus; DT: diphtheria and tetanus; DTaP: diphtheria, tetanus acellular, and pertussis; DTP: diphtheria, tetanus toxoids, and pertussis; Hep B: hepatitis B; Hib: *Haemophilus influenzae* type b; IPV: inactivated polio vaccine; OPV: oral poliovirus vaccine; TT: tetanus toxoid)

designed evaporator and condenser to provide maximum refrigeration. It can maintain the temperature up to 16–24 hours without power. They are ideal for vaccine storage, but are more expensive than domestic refrigerators, costing INR 75,000–150,000.

21. Where one should use ice-lined refrigerator?

Ice-lined refrigerators are most suited for the facility/clinics where continuous power supply is not available, or power-cut are long and frequent.

CHAPTER 8 Cold Chain and Vaccine Storage   **113**

22. How should vaccines be stored in an ILR? What precautions should be taken while storing vaccines in ILR?

In an ILR, the upper half of the cabinet (which has the baskets) has a higher temperature than the lower half **(Figs. 4 and 5)**. This is because cold air sinks and ILRs are top opening.

The ILR has got two sections: the top and bottom. The bottom of the refrigerator is the coldest place. The DPT, DT, TT, and hepatitis B vaccines should not be kept directly on the floor of the refrigerator, as they can freeze and get damaged. The DPT, DT, TT, and hepatitis B vaccine along with diluents are to be placed in basket. If frozen T-series vaccines are seen in an ILR, they should be immediately discarded. Therefore, to prevent accidental freezing, it is recommended that vaccines should be stored in the following order in layers from the base of the baskets—OPV, BCG, and measles, followed by DPT, DT, TT, and then hepatitis B with diluents on the topmost layer **(Fig. 4)**.

A thermometer should also be placed in the basket along with the vaccines, as this gives the correct temperature. If no basket is available, place two rows of empty/water filled with ice packs on the floor of the ILR.

23. From where can one buy a good quality ILR?

There are only very few vendors manufacturing and supplying ILRs in India. **Table 4** summarizes some key vendors supplying ILRs in India along with specifications of different models, cost, and contact details of the same.

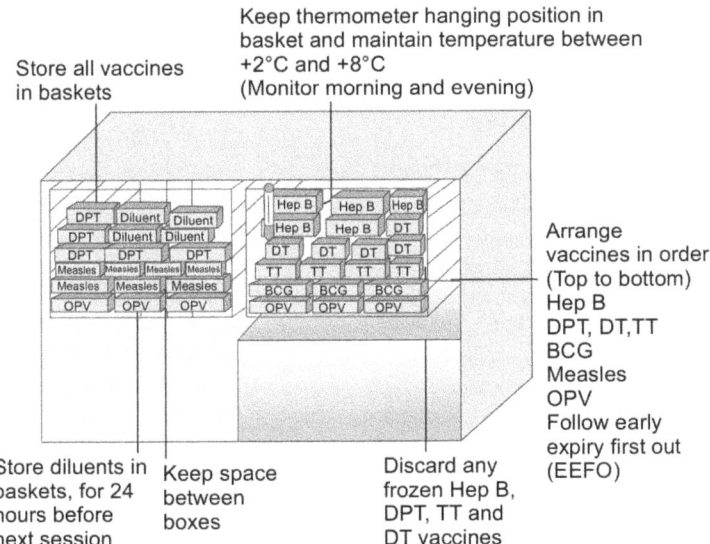

Fig. 4: Schematic representation of storage of vaccines in an ice-lined refrigerator (ILR).
(BCG: bacillus Calmette–Guérin; DPT: diphtheria, pertussis, and tetanus; DT: diphtheria and tetanus; Hep B: hepatitis B; OPV: oral poliovirus vaccine; TT: tetanus toxoid)

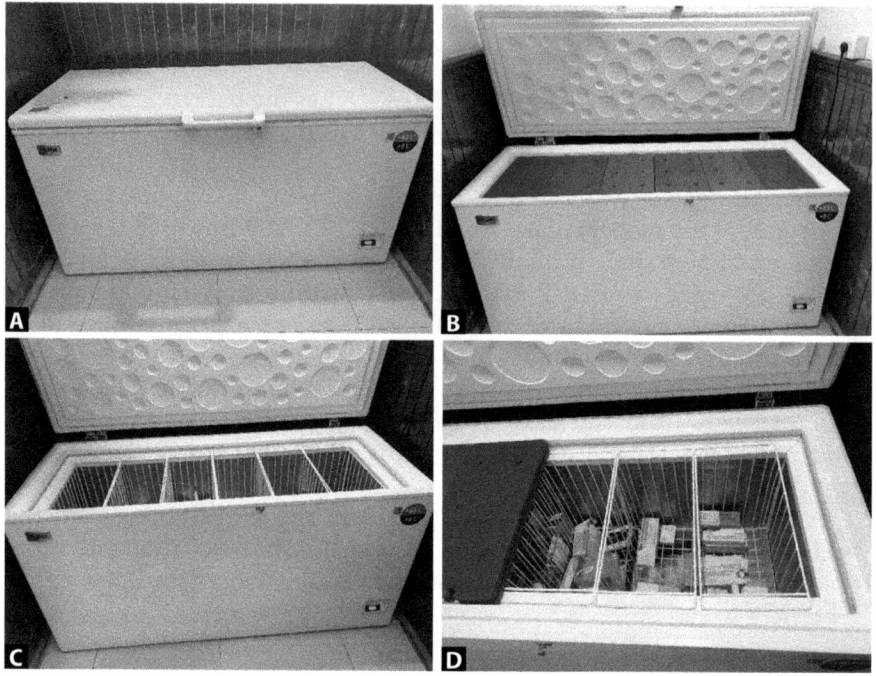

Figs. 5A to D: Ice-lined refrigerator of Haier Bioline company.

TABLE 4: Ice-lined refrigerators (ILRs) manufacturers and suppliers in India.		
ILR vendors in India		
Specifications	*Haier*	*Cold-chain controls*
Models with price	Model HBC-70 Model HBC-200 Model HBC-340	VC-200 Lit VC-300 Lit VC-500 Lit
Hold over time	More than 25 hours	Up to 28–34 hours
Accreditations/certificate	WHO-PQ, CE, ISO 13485, MoHFW	NABL accredited certificate MoHFW, GoI
Voltage stabilizer	On payment	One unit free
Office/contact details	Thane, MS info@bioline.in	Coimbatore, TN coldchaincontrols@gmails.com

(GoI: Government of India; MoHFW: Ministry of Health and Family Welfare; NABL: National Accreditation Board for Testing and Calibration Laboratories)

24. How to pack vaccines in isothermic cold boxes?

Before the vaccines are placed in the cold boxes, fully frozen ice packs should be placed at the bottom and sides of the cold box. The vaccines should be placed in cartons or polythene bags and then placed in the cold box.

The vaccines are to be covered with a layer of fully frozen ice packs and the cold box is then closed. The vials of DPT, DT, Hep B, and TT vaccines should not be placed in direct contact with frozen ice packs and should be surrounded by OPV vials. Hard frozen ice packs (frozen at -20°C) should be conditioned before laying out in the cold box. This will protect "T" series vaccine from getting frozen.

25. What precautions should be taken while storing vaccines in vaccine carriers?

Vaccine carriers are used by health workers for carrying vaccines (16–20 vials) to subcenters or to villages or for delivery of vaccines from the supplier's shop to vaccination clinic. They maintain the cold chain during transport and for 1 day's use in the field. The inside temperature of a vaccine carrier is maintained between 2°C and 8°C with four frozen ice packs for 1 day (if not opened frequently).

- Only vaccine carriers with four ice packs should be used.
- Do not leave vaccine carriers in the sun light.
- Do not open the lid unnecessarily, as this can allow heat and light into the carrier, which may spoil vaccines.
- Do not drop or sit on the vaccine carrier, this can damage the carrier.

26. How to safeguard vaccines during immunization sessions?

- Keep domestic refrigerator/ILR door openings to a minimum
- Reconstitute vaccines immediately prior to administering
- When the vaccines are outside the vaccine carrier, keep them out of direct sunlight and away from other sources of heat and ultraviolet light (e.g., fluorescent light)
- Avoid handling vaccines any more than absolutely necessary. Take vaccine (and diluents if needed) from the cooler only as required.

27. How to safeguard vaccines during power failure?

- During a power failure of 4 hours or less, the refrigerator door should be kept closed.
- *During power failures >4 hours*: If the backup generator facility is lacking, identify an available unit at another nearby site and shift the vaccines to the alternative storage site.
- If a refrigerator with a backup generator has not been located or is not working, and for power failures >4 hours, store vaccines in a cooler with conditioned ice packs/gel packs.
- Continue to monitor the temperature of the vaccines by placing the thermometer probe inside a vaccine box inside the cooler.

28. What should be line of action when cold chain breach is found?

- Immediately isolate the vaccines until you have been in touch with the relevant authority.

- Keep vaccines refrigerated between 2°C and 8°C and label them "Do Not Use".
- Do not discard any vaccine until advice has been sought. Depending on manufacturer specifications, the vaccine may still be viable.
- For privately purchased vaccines contact the manufacturer for advice.

29. What are the different temperature monitoring devices?

To measure the temperature during storage of vaccines, different types of thermometers are used. The different types of thermometers commonly used are:
- *Standard fluid-filled*: Very easy to see and read temperature.
- *Dial*: The most common, but not the most accurate.
- *Minimum/maximum*: It shows the current temperature and the minimum and maximum temperatures achieved. Temperature fluctuations outside the recommended range can also be detected. Available in fluid-filled and digital forms of which digital type with a probe is most effective type and is recommended for use in vaccination clinics.
- *Digital*: Very easy to read and some come with an alarm, but the temperature probe must be placed in the proper location inside the unit in order to get an accurate reading.
- *Continuous reading*: It will record the temperature inside the unit at all times, 24 hours a day, on a sheet of paper, but the paper must be changed when it is running low. Using this thermometer is the most effective method of tracking the refrigerator/freezer temperature over time.

30. How to use them?

- *Digital minimum/maximum*: It should be placed outside the refrigerator. Place the probe directly in contact with a vaccine vial or package. Minimum/maximum thermometer must be reset regularly, the thermometer battery must be checked and replaced time-to-time and one should choose a thermometer which records temperature in "Celsius".
- *Digital*: Place the probe directly in contact with vaccine vial or package.
- *Continuous reading*: It will record the temperature inside the unit at all times, 24 hours a day, on a sheet of paper, but the paper must be changed when it is running low. Using this thermometer is the most effective method of tracking the refrigerator/freezer temperature over time.

SUGGESTED READING

1. Centers for Disease Control and Prevention. Safety of vaccines affected by a power outage. Quick Clinical Notes, Disaster management and response. 2004;2:62-3.
2. Galazka A, Milstien J, Zaffran M. Thermostability of Vaccines. WHO (Global Programme for Vaccines and Immunization), Geneva; 1998.
3. Getting started with VVMs. VVM for all, Technical Session on Vaccine Vial Monitors. WHO publication 27/3/2002. Geneva.

4. Gupta SK, Shastri DD. Cold chain and vaccine storage. In: Vashishtha VM (Ed). IAP Textbook of Vaccines, 2nd edition. New Delhi: Jaypee Brothers Medical Publishers; 2020. pp. 116-27.
5. Ketan B, Jariwala V, Kirit S. Target-5: Guide to Vaccine Storage and Handling, 1st edition. Gujarat: IAP Surat Publication; 2006.
6. Shastri DD. Vaccine storage and handling. In: Parthasarathy A (Ed). IAP Textbook of Pediatrics, 5th edition. New Delhi: Jaypee Brothers Medical Publishers; 2013. pp. 1-5.
7. Shastri DD. Vaccine storage and handling. In: Parthasarathy A (Ed). IAP Textbook of Pediatrics Infectious Diseases, 1st edition. New Delhi: Jaypee Brothers Medical Publishers; 2013. pp. 493-501.
8. Shastri DD. Vaccine storage and handling. In: Parthasarathy A (Ed). IAP Textbook of Pediatrics, 7th Edition. New Delhi: Jaypee Brothers Medical Publishers; 2019.

CHAPTER 9

Control and Eradication of Infectious Diseases

Yash Paul, Priya Marwah

1. **How do we define endemic, epidemic, and pandemic?**

Endemic stage of a disease means constant and normal existence of a disease or infectious agent in a locality or area at all times. Typhoid and tuberculosis occurrence in India are examples of endemic diseases. Epidemic stage of a disease means a large number of persons in a community are affected and at the same time, spread occurs to other areas. Pandemic stage of a disease means there is widespread epidemic disease affecting a large number of people at the same time and in many geographical regions, in other words, it becomes global.

2. **What is the difference between control and eradication of an infectious disease?**

Due to some active interventions, there occurs drastic decline in disease incidence, it means disease is under control. On the other hand, when causative organisms, viz., bacteria or viruses have been eliminated, this results in eradication of a particular disease. Smallpox vaccine eliminated variola virus and thus smallpox disease was eradicated.

3. **Bacteria and viruses do not possess locomotive mechanisms like monocellular protozoa, e.g., *Entamoeba* and *Giardia lamblia*. How do these bacteria and viruses travel?**

Microorganisms causing infectious diseases can be transmitted from infectious body including human beings to others in any of the following ways:
- *Direct transmission*: Direct contact, droplet infection, contact with soil, by inoculation into skin or mucosa, and transplacental, i.e., vertical from mother to fetus. These modes of transmission result in quick spread of microorganisms, but occurs in close contact in limited areas, thus overcrowding facilitates spread of microorganisms.
- *Indirect transmission*:
  - Vehicle-borne like water, food, blood, and other body constituents.
  - Vector-borne by flies, mosquitoes, other insects, birds, and animals
  - Airborne by droplet nuclei and dust

- Fomite-borne like soiled clothes, utensils, taps, and other objects
- *Unclean hands*: These modes of transmission may result in spread of disease near as well as far.

4. How does the infectious disease occur?

Entry of disease causing microorganisms in the host may result in disease of varying degree or no disease. Outcome depends on many factors and their combinations:
- Infectivity of the microorganisms.
- Virulence of the microorganisms.
- *Infective dose*: Successful infection requires an adequate number of bacteria or viruses that should gain entry in the host.
- Host should be genetically susceptible to develop a disease; in that case, microorganisms may cause a disease. For example, man does not develop distemper disease, which a pet dog may have developed even on being in close contact.
- Host resistance.

5. Why is severity of disease different and not uniform in the population?

Outcome and severity of disease depend on combination of many factors like infecting dose of microorganisms, immune status of the host, presence of comorbidity, and age of the host.
- *Infecting dose is large*: In case immune status of the host is robust, survival chances are high because of adequate levels of antibody generation for protection against current and future invasion. In case, the immune system is not robust, disease may be severe and in some cases, death may occur. In case of immunodeficiency, chances of death are more, antibody generation may be very low or may not occur, so such host may remain vulnerable in future also.
- *Infecting dose is low*: In case host's immune system is robust, the host may remain asymptomatic and may develop antibodies. In case of immunodeficiency, even small infecting dose of microorganisms may result in severe disease or death.

6. How many types of immunity are present in human beings?

Immunity is a state of resistance to a disease through the defense activities of the immune system. It is of two types: (1) innate or natural immunity and (2) acquired immunity.
- Innate immunity to a disease is species-specific, whereby different species of animal kingdom suffer from different diseases and are resistant to some diseases.
- Acquired immunity can be acquired passively or actively.
  - *Passively acquired immunity*: Maternal antibodies provide protection against some diseases during early childhood and administration of immunoglobulins gives instant but short-lived immunity.

- Active immunity occurs following infections and vaccination. In case antibody level reaches equal to or above the required protective levels, the individual is considered immune or resistant to develop the disease, if infection occurs again. On the other hand, as immunity decreases due to passage of time or due to comorbidity, the probability of an individual developing disease increases if infection occurs again.

7. How do we combat and control infection?

- Administer antibiotics or antiviral drugs if available
- Administer vaccine if available prior to occurrence of infection
- Quarantine of infected persons and sometimes quarantine of noninfected persons especially during epidemics.

8. What is quarantine?

Quarantine is a process to prevent infected persons coming in contact with noninfected persons. In 1340s plague hit Europe, eventually wiping out more than half of the population, it resulted in formal measure to separate the infected from noninfected people. The first isolation stations were made along the coast of Dubrovnik in year 1377. All ships arriving from plague-affected ports had to wait for 30 days to ensure that passengers and cargo were uncontaminated, it was called "trentino". Later this, waiting period was extended to 40 days time for greater safety. The term trentino was changed to "quarantine"—derived from quaranta, Italian for 40. During epidemics or pandemics, sometimes it is imposed on noninfected persons as some infected persons may be in incubation period and may not have developed the signs and symptoms of the disease. During coronavirus disease 2019 (COVID-19) pandemic caused by coronavirus, quarantine was imposed both on infected and noninfected population.

9. Should we target 100% population for vaccination?

Yes. We should vaccinate all so as not to leave any person vulnerable to the disease.

10. We are taught that when 80–90% people in a community are vaccinated, unvaccinated people are safe.

It was presumed that when large sections of a community are vaccinated, they act as barrier to the spread of infection to unvaccinated people. This theory was based on assumptions and not on science. But, it is a myth, which has perpetuated for about a century in medical science. Hypothetical situation is presented here. 100 guests attend a dinner. 99 guests have received typhoid vaccine in recent past, so are immune to develop typhoid disease despite getting infected by *Salmonella typhi*. One guest is unvaccinated. The food gets contaminated, accidentally, with *Salmonella typhi*. The unvaccinated guest can get infected and develop typhoid infection though he/she had been in a group where 99% guests were vaccinated. For more information, please see Chapter 2 "Elementary Epidemiology in Vaccination" regarding role of herd immunity and herd protection.

11. Why are extreme age groups more vulnerable to infectious diseases?

Young age correlates with both an immature immune system and lack of prior exposure to potential pathogens so have not developed postexposure immunity. Older age correlates with declining immunity, increased incidence of comorbid diseases, and in some cases, adverse effects of smoking and alcohol consumption.

12. What message should be given during or at time of impending epidemic or pandemic?

Immunization, prevention of transmission of infection, and quarantine for self-protection. More important is that doctors should act as role models.

13. What message should we give to people to help in reducing incidence of infectious diseases?

Immunization and prevention of transmission of infection to protect others.

14. Epidemics have occurred in the past also. What is the most notable difference between the past and present epidemics?

In past, man had to travel mostly for business or wars. Had to travel on foot, on horse, camel, animal—cart, or by sea, so traveling time used to be very long. Destinations used to be specific and limited. Thus, there used to be time interval for spread of a disease from one area to the other. At present, because of very rapid travel facilities, the disease may spread very fast to other regions of the world because at present people travel to other distant places for many reasons including tours. Centuries earlier epidemics used to kill about a thousand persons in different places. Spanish flu killed 50–100 million people between 1918 and 1920. In recent time, severe acute respiratory syndrome (SARS) epidemic resulted in death of large population all over the world. Currently, COVID-19 epidemic has spread globally in a very short time. On the positive side is the rapid communication facilities and many modes of treatment for the diseases, so means of containment of epidemics are better now. Till the recent past, studies were interrupted but now studies can be continued due to online facilities, a great boon to the students. Similarly, many other business activities can be carried out.

15. I am a practicing doctor, not attached to a big hospital. Can I refuse to attend a patient suffering from epidemic disease?

Yes. As you do not have facilities to manage a serious patient, you should explain the situation and advise the patient to go to any of the hospitals where such facilities are available.

16. At present, no drug or vaccine is available for coronavirus disease 2019 (COVID-19) infection. There are many drugs undergoing trials, some have shown good results. Can I administer any of these drugs, which have shown good results for the disease?

No, no one can experiment with any drug, which is undergoing trial despite showing excellent results. In India, a doctor can administer only those new drugs, which have been approved by the Indian Council of Medical Research (ICMR). Accredited institutions can carry out the studies of the drugs, which have shown good results during the trials, only after obtaining approval from the Ethics Committee.

17. What special advice should a doctor give to his patients, their families, or general public during epidemics?

We should teach all in our contact regarding the problems associated with incubation period of a disease. They should be told that there is some interval between getting infected and development of signs and symptoms of the disease, an infected person may infect other persons before getting ill. In case, any person who had visited a person or a place where infection was reported should immediately contact his/her doctor or the health provider/facilities for the concerned disease and should never hide these facts, so as to get the correct advice. Otherwise, such a person may develop the disease and infect others during the incubation period. Hiding this information may put in danger the life of the individual, family, and the community.

18. Which one step plays most important role in containment of infectious diseases during endemic, epidemic, or pandemic stages?

Diagnosis in time is not only key to survival of the patient, but also helps in containment of the disease. It helps not only in cure and survival of the patient, but also helps in preventing the spread of the infection.

19. What steps should be taken by individuals during epidemic of an infectious disease?

Everyone should follow "social distancing", report to the doctor as and when early symptoms of the disease appear to get diagnosed and treated in time.

20. What steps should be taken by the families during epidemic of an infectious disease?

Families should take extra care of very young, very old, and sick persons in the family.

21. What steps should be taken by the society during an epidemic?

Healthy people should join social groups who are rendering help to the affected people. Every member should actively counter the negative activities of the people or groups. During polio eradication program, many individuals and groups had played negative role by misguiding public that this campaign is harmful. Hence, this action is necessary.

22. Which is the most vulnerable section of the society during epidemics?

Economically, poor people are most vulnerable because of overcrowding, unhygienic surroundings, lack of medical facilities, and financial constraints. During any epidemic, such groups need help on priority basis.

23. What three measures are most important during epidemics for self-protection and protection of others?

Safety, safety, and safety.

SUGGESTED READING

1. Paul Y. Herd immunity and herd protection. Vaccine. 2004;22:301-2.
2. Paul Y. Herd immunity and herd protection. In: Vashishtha VM, Kalra A (Eds). IAP Textbook of Vaccines, 2nd edition. New Delhi: Jaypee Brothers Medical Publishers (P) Ltd; 2020. pp. 99-104.

CHAPTER 10

Development and Licensing of Vaccine

Gautam Rambhad, Canna Jagdish Ghia

DEVELOPMENT OF VACCINES

1. What are the steps involved in vaccine development?

Vaccination is among the few revolutionary inventions that have enormously transformed human life by ensuring healthy living and longevity. Being highly complex, vaccine development involves several stages—including the preclinical and clinical phases, process development, assay development, etc. As per the Indian Academy of Pediatrics (IAP) book on vaccine, 2nd edition, the development of a new vaccine occurs in several broad stages **(Table 1)**:

TABLE 1: Roadmap of vaccine development.

Stage	Initial focus	Stage details	Time frame
Stage I	Clinical proof of concept	This can be made feasible through the identification of an antigen, followed by small-scale production, which is required for: • Initial preclinical and clinical evaluation • Development of several assays • Nonclinical toxicity and safety studies • Application for investigational new vaccine approval	≥2 years
Stage II	Elucidating the product and associated processes before efficacy evaluation	This stage comprises developing protocols on: • Method of preparation • Constituents of formulation • Assays for various evaluations • Regulatory and developmental plans	≥1 year
Stage III	Clinical dose	This stage involves: • Dose-ranging, efficacy and safety evaluation • Corresponding manufacturing of vaccine formulation; technology transfer of the manufacturing process to the final site is required for full-scale manufacturing	≥2 years

Contd...

Contd...

Stage	Initial focus	Stage details	Time frame
Stage IV	Final safety and efficacy evaluation	• The final safety and efficacy evaluation are carried out in large-scale studies • Site validation, consistent manufacturing of vaccine preparation, and scaling up of production are simultaneously carried out • Evidence on shelf life/stability of the product must be generated	3–4 years
Stage V	Regulatory review and approval– licensure	• If the vaccine candidate is found to be safe and effective, a new vaccine application is submitted to the Central Drugs Standard Control Organization (CDSCO) for approval of the vaccine in India • The CDSCO conducts its own testing and also inspects the production of the vaccine candidate and monitors its potency, safety, and purity	Up to 2 years
Stage VI	Production – scaling up	• Large-scale manufacturing takes place at this stage • All products should meet the necessary regulatory requirements, including current Good Manufacturing Processes (cGMP)	
Stage VII	Quality control – Performance review, post-marketing	• The vaccine is continuously tracked and monitored for its performance, safety, and effectiveness through pharmacovigilance conducted after the product is released into the market	

On an average it takes around 10–15 years for developing a vaccine.

2. What are the four phases in the clinical development of vaccines?

Following an extensive preclinical study, i.e. studies on animal models, which may take 1–2 years, safer vaccine candidates with the potential for inducing immunogenicity may proceed forward for clinical study. For licensing purposes, three clinical study phases are to be completed in healthy subjects. The administration of vaccines is typically done in healthy humans, whose tolerance of adverse effects is much lower. Therefore, a few governments have made it compulsory to investigate adverse events following immunization; this requires a comprehensive and systematic investigation and careful evaluation of all possible adverse events of the vaccine before proceeding for licensing. Stepwise testing is commenced in three phases in a clinical trial, and the trial must be stopped in case of any safety concerns. The vaccine's effect is compared with that of placebo to identify the cause of any

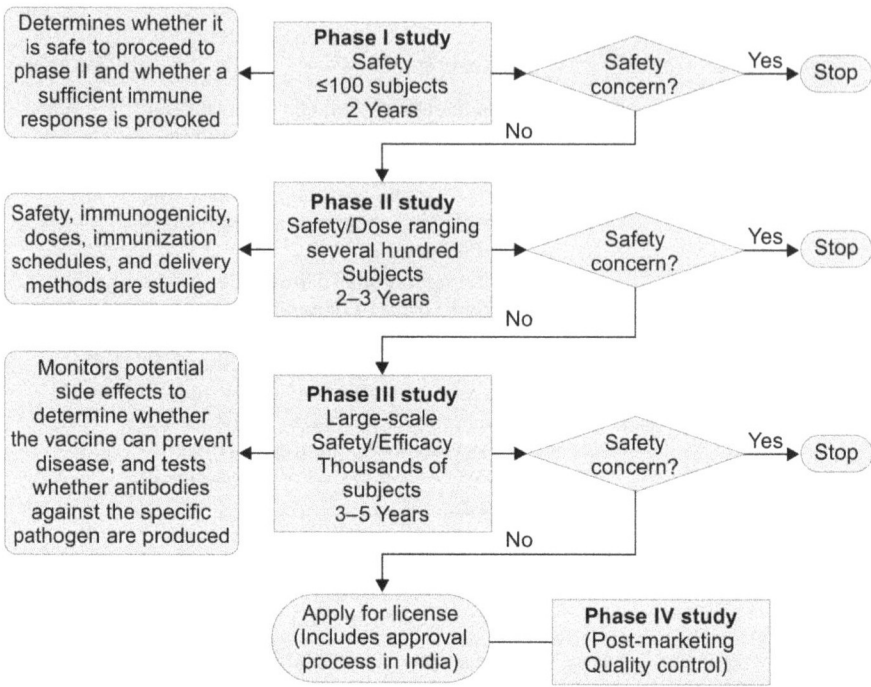

Fig. 1: Safety testing of vaccines in three phases of clinical trials.

adverse events. Both phase III and post-licensure (phase IV) trials are crucial for gathering experience on the efficacy/immunogenicity and safety of vaccines **(Fig. 1)**.

3. What considerations guide vaccine development?

As mentioned in the book Prevention and Therapy of Immunologic Diseases' 2008, multiple considerations largely impact vaccine-development programs **(Fig. 2)**.

4. What are the challenges or roadblocks in vaccine development, and how are they overcome?

Despite being a highly valuable intervention for public health, vaccine development involves numerous challenges, including lack of proper technology and expertise, associated cost burden, political issues, regulatory concerns, etc. Some inescapable consequential adverse events, either related or nonrelated to the vaccine itself, also compound existing challenges.

Vaccines were initially developed based on Pasteur established paradigm i.e., "isolate, inactivate, and inject" the disease-causing microorganism. Despite attaining massive success in developing vaccines against numerous

1. What are the prominent unmet need about medical and public health in current condition?	2. What are the known information on the infection of interest such as natural history and pathogenesis?	3. Is immunity to a given antigen linked with protection against disease following re-exposure in the context of natural infection?	4. If natural immunity shows potential of preventing re-infection following an initial infection, can a specific host immune effector mechanism be identified responsible for immune protection?
5. Can the pathogen be developed in culture? If so, does the pathogen cause such a life-threatening disease that an attenuated version of the virus would face an impossible barrier for demonstration of safety?	6. Whether identification of a specific antigen (or antigens) is possible which may represent the target of protective host immune responses?	7. If the protective immune response is antibody-mediated, can the target antigen be produced in scalable quantities to aid in eliciting antibody responses that can block the key functional role(s) of the target molecule in the pathogen?	8. What will be the best possible way to produce the antigen in large scale following detection of an antigen and presentation system?
9. What could be the most efficient way to introduce the antigens of the pathogen of interest to the host immune system?	10. Whether the antigen of interest is adequately immunogenic on its own or conjugation to a specific carrier is required to have an augmentation of desired immune response?	11. What are the most likely/predictable safety concerns associated with the use of the vaccine in question?	12. What is the epidemiology/prevalence of the concerned infection?
13. If the infection has an overall low prevalence rate, can the high-risk population be identified to hasten the achievement of statistically significant protection?	14. What are the tests that need to be performed on the clinical trial samples to assess the immunogenicity of the vaccine?	15. Will assessment of antibody titers, responses of T-cell, pathogen presence and quantity along with its serotype, and other parameters related to the disease in question demonstrate the primary criteria for vaccine effect?	16. Development and validation of the evaluating tests may be a crucial aspect for the clinical success of the trial vaccine

Fig. 2: Considerations guiding vaccine development.

diseases, such as smallpox, measles, poliomyelitis, etc., several other human infectious diseases remained unprevented using this strategy. Thus, even after the implementation of Pasteur established paradigm, vaccine development was associated with a few challenges. Moreover, vaccine efficacy is impacted/affected by genetic variation that necessitates the development of specific vaccines for different regions of the world.

Despite immense expansion in the understanding of immune response against infections, several hindrances come across the path of vaccine development. The inability to understand the optimal immune response required for conferring the protection, or lack of approved adjuvants and delivery systems to induce the required responses may make vaccine development challenging. Use of inactivated or attenuated organisms may not be applicable to some diseases as few pathogens are not culturable. Selection of appropriate pathogen antigen without culturing the organism is another crucial aspect to be considered while developing a vaccine. Some attenuated vaccine strains may carry a residual risk of producing disease. Inactivated organisms may retain residual virulence that may affect their efficacy in susceptible populations. Moreover, probable dearth of antigen determinants or adjuvant properties in inactivated organisms may elicit a suboptimal stimulation of immune response against the targeted pathogen. An optimal response to antigen administration is impacted by several aspects like the delivery systems, vectors, and adjuvants of choice, which influence different variables such as route of entry and need of multiple doses. Financial aspect is another challenge as the cost associated with development and licensing of new vaccine is significant and may often/sometimes result in premature abandonment.

Based on an article published in New England Journal of Medicine 2020, in the current pandemic, multiple platforms are being examined for developing an appropriate vaccine against severe acute respiratory syndrome coronavirus 2 (SARS-CoV-2). To cope up with the accelerated developmental demand, DNA- and RNA-based platforms, followed by those for developing recombinant-subunit vaccine may have high potential, but are not devoid of several developmental challenges. Few of the current challenges in the path of developing vaccine for SARS-CoV-2 are mentioned below:

- Despite having virus' spike protein as a potential immunogenic target to confer protection, it is critical to optimize the antigen design to ensure optimal immune response. Further, there exists ambiguity over targeting either the full-length protein or only the receptor-binding domain.
- Preclinical studies on SARS vaccine have shown potential of exacerbating lung disease, either directly or as a result of antibody-dependent enhancement, rendering a high necessity of test in a suitable animal model along with rigorous monitoring of safety parameters.
- The lack of established correlates of protection is another critical challenge since the potential duration of immunity is unknown in case of naturally acquired infection. Moreover, ambiguity exists on the necessity of single or multiple-dose vaccine for optimal immune response.
- Conducting clinical trials during a pandemic poses additional challenges. It is difficult to predict where and when outbreaks will occur and to prepare trial sites to coincide with vaccine readiness for testing.

Table 2 Highlights some of the outstanding issues and barriers for successful vaccine development.

The manufacturer may face manufacturing challenges as well. For example, the influenza (flu) vaccine is made in chicken eggs; hence, the manufacturing process demands massive amounts of pathogen-free eggs; this is a huge concern, especially during pandemics. This limitation negatively impacts the production capacity of the seasonal influenza vaccine.

To overcome this challenge, research is ongoing on the use of continuous cell lines (including Vero, PER. C6, and MRC-5) to produce vaccines. This method may ensure delivery of the product on time, as well as high production capacity, without the risk of infection—which is otherwise a concern with egg-based manufacturing processes.

TABLE 2: Challenges and possible overcoming action in vaccine development.	
Challenges/Limitations	Probable action to be taken
Lack of preclinical data and inadequate information on protective correlates of immunity may lead to product failure in clinical trials	Development of more relevant animal models; more human samples to be collected and analyzed
Lack of information on the infectious exposures of intended vaccine recipients	More human samples to be collected and analyzed
Vaccines are to be used in populations with less-responsive immune system	Better understanding of the mechanisms of action of the adjuvants; development of vaccine delivery systems specifically for use in immunocompromised populations
Antigenic variation requires constant updating of vaccine formulations	Monitor genetic variation of infectious organisms in the community
Huge financial commitment associated with vaccine development may lead to premature abandonment of promising products	More investment in vaccine research
Dearth of adequate access to vaccines in poorer countries, especially those for use against tropical diseases	More tiered pricing strategies; facilitate the development of vaccines in developing countries

5. What are the cost drivers for vaccine manufacturing?

Being highly capital-intensive processes, vaccine manufacturing and testing has witnessed a tremendous transformation over time. Sophisticated manufacturing processes, along with hundreds of quality-control tests, have amplified associated developmental costs in the past few decades. Research and development of vaccine may cost more than 500 million USD and cost associated with facilities and equipment may range between 50 and 700 million USD. Starting from discovery to licensure, vaccine development may be highly exorbitant, with substantial chances of failure (~94%). The cost associated with the development of a single vaccine has shown an ascending trend over the years **(Fig. 3)**.

Development of Vaccines: Regulatory Norms Specific to India

6. Which regulatory authority in India approves vaccines?

The Central Drugs Standard Control Organization (CDSCO) is the National Regulatory Authority (NRA) of India. It works under the authority of the Directorate General of Health Services, Ministry of Health and Family Welfare, Government of India. The CDSCO has its headquarters in New Delhi. Under the Drugs and Cosmetics Act, the CDSCO approves new drugs, grants permission for the conduct of clinical trials, lays down standards for drugs,

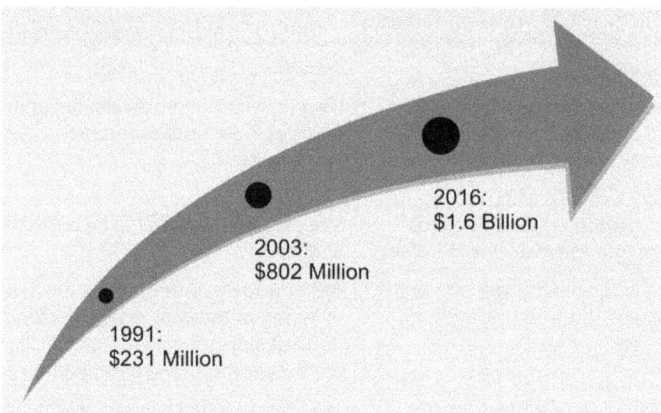

Fig. 3: The rising trend of cost associated with vaccine development.

controls the quality of imported drugs in the country, etc. Additionally, the CDSCO—in coordination with state regulators—is jointly accountable for the granting of licenses for certain specialized categories of critical drugs such as blood and blood products, intravenous fluids, vaccines, and sera.

7. **What is the basic process for vaccine approval in India?**

As per the Indian National Vaccine Policy, the complete vaccine developmental and approval process in India is detailed in **Figure 4**.

Seeking Permission for Conducting Clinical Trials on Vaccines

8. **What are the aspects need to be covered for writing a trial protocol summary?**

A clinical trial protocol summary should contain parameters mentioned in **Table 3**.

Seeking Permission for Conducting Clinical Trials on Vaccines in India

This section highlights information referring Schedule Y and Clinical Trial Rule India' 2019.

9. **What is the requirement for an Ethics Committee in clinical trials, and what are its responsibilities?**

The applicant desirous of conducting a clinical study must obtain approval from an Ethics Committee. The Ethics Committee will apply for registration with the central licensing authority:

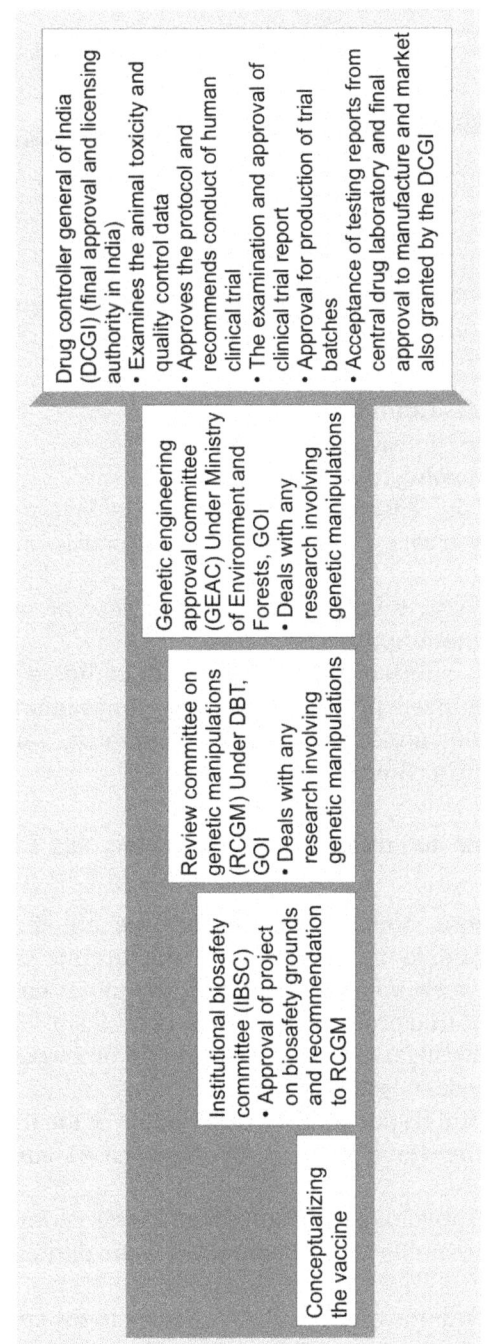

Fig. 4: Vaccine—approval and development path in India.
(DBT: Department of Biotechnology)

TABLE 3: Parameters to be included in the clinical trial protocol summary.

Trial title and protocol number/code	Dosage regimen and rationale for dose selection
Background and rationale	Wash-out period
Objective	Pre-study screening and baseline evaluation
Study design and duration	Treatment/assessment visits
Total number of sites and number of indian sites	Concomitant medication
List of investigators	Rescue medication and risk management
Sample size	Premature withdrawal/Discontinuation criteria
Patient population	Efficacy variables and analysis
Inclusion, exclusion criteria	Safety variables and analysis
Drug formulation	Statistical analysis

Responsibilities of Ethics Committee
- Review and approve clinical trial protocols
- Regular review of ongoing trials
- Communication of the reason for cancelation to the Investigator and the Licensing Authority in case the approved trial protocol is canceled by the Ethics Committee
- Thorough analysis and refurbishing report in case of occurrence of serious adverse events among trial subjects
- Decides whether the subjects must be financially compensated
- Allow officers authorized by the central licensing authority to enter, with or without prior notice, to inspect the premises, any records or documents related to a clinical trial.

10. What are the criteria for choosing the investigators and what are their responsibilities?

Appropriate qualifications, training, and experience are the mandatory criteria to be an investigator for the clinical trial of the vaccine. An investigator should have access to such investigational and treatment facilities as are relevant to the proposed trial protocol. A qualified physician, who will be an investigator or a sub-investigator for the trial, should be responsible for all trial-related medical (or dental) decisions.

The Investigator(s) are responsible for the conduct of the trial according to the protocol and the Good Clinical Practice (GCP) guidelines. The investigators should:
- Document standard operating procedures for the tasks performed by them
- Ensure that adequate medical care is provided to the participants for any adverse events
- Report all serious and unexpected adverse events to the sponsor within 24 hours and the Ethics Committee within 7 working days of their occurrence
- Provide information to subjects through the informed consent process.

11. What are the responsibilities of sponsors in a clinical trial?

As per schedule Y, responsibilities of sponsors in a clinical trial are as follows:
- Implementation and maintenance of quality assurance systems that affirm that the study is conducted and that the data are generated, documented, and reported in compliance with the protocol and GCP guidelines
- Periodic submission of clinical trial status report to the Licensing Authority (LA)
- Submission of a summary report within 3 months of premature study discontinuation (if any)
- Prompt communication (within 14 calendar days) with the LA and the other Investigator(s) regarding any unexpected serious adverse event (as defined in GCP guidelines).

12. How to apply and grant permission to conduct a clinical trial for an investigational vaccine?

Flowchart 1 depicts the application process for seeking permission for conducting a clinical trial on a new investigational vaccine.

The validity of permission for initiating a clinical trial, as granted in Form CT-06, is 2 years from the date of issue, unless extended by the central licensing authority.

13. What additional information must be submitted with the clinical trial application?

Table 4 lists the additional information that must be submitted with the clinical trial application.

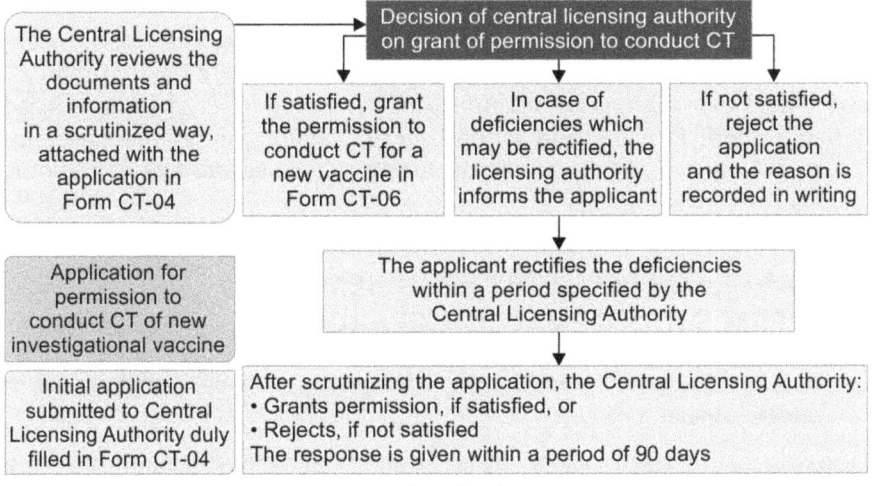

Flowchart 1: Application for permission and grant of permission to conduct clinical trial on new investigational vaccine.

(CT: clinical trial)

TABLE 4: Information to be submitted with clinical trial (CT) application.

Information	Details
RCGM/GEAC approvals	The environmental angle clearance from competent authority in accordance with Environment Protection Act
Physicochemical characterization	Tests for identity and purity
Biological characterization	• Characterization of MCB, WCB, and cell substrate • Purity of the product by a suitable method in case of whole-cell vaccine • Purity of the product by SDS-PAGE and Western blot in case of toxins • Standardization of inactivation process • Immunogenicity of product
Validation studies	Analytical methods
Excipients (animal/human origin)	TSE/BSE compliance
Sample	Sample of product

(RCGM: review committee on genetic manipulation; GEAC: genetic engineering approval committee; MCB: master cell bank; WCB: working cell bank; SDS-PAGE: sodium dodecyl sulfate–polyacrylamide gel electrophoresis; TSE: transmissible spongiform encephalopathy; BSE: bovine spongiform encephalopathy)

14. How to obtain permission to manufacture a new or investigational new vaccine for clinical trial or for examination, testing, and analysis?

Figure 5 depicts the application process for permission for manufacturing new vaccines for conducting clinical trials or for examination, testing, and analysis.

15. How to proceed for the inspection of vaccines manufactured for clinical trial in terms of examination, testing, and analysis?

The license holder is bound to allow the inspection officer authorized by the central licensing authority or the state licensing authority to enter the premises where the new vaccines are manufactured or stored, with or without prior notice. The officer is officially authorized to examine the premises and the records/documents, inspect manufacturing processes, storage conditions, etc.

GUIDANCE FOR INDUSTRY REQUIREMENTS FOR PERMISSION OF VACCINE APPROVAL

16. What is the stepwise process involved for getting a manufacturing license of vaccine in India?

Flowchart 2 highlights the stepwise process for getting a manufacturing license of vaccine in India.

CHAPTER 10 Development and Licensing of Vaccine **135**

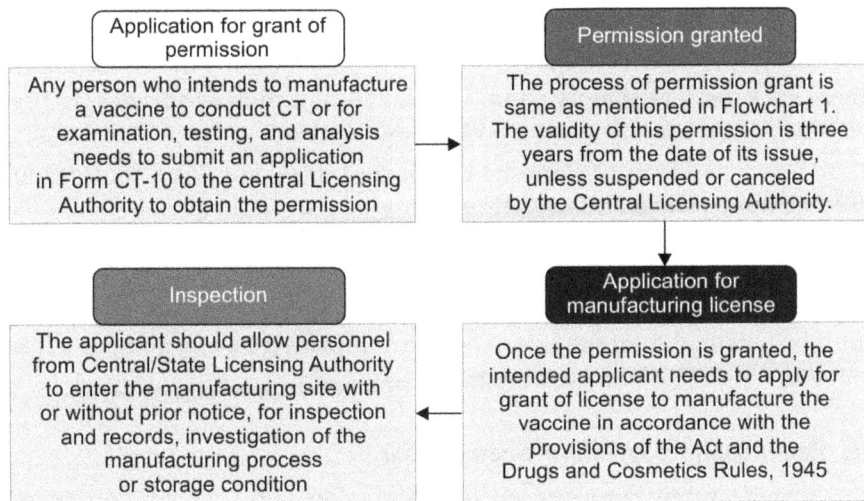

Fig. 5: Application for permission to manufacture new vaccine for clinical trial or examination, testing, and analysis.

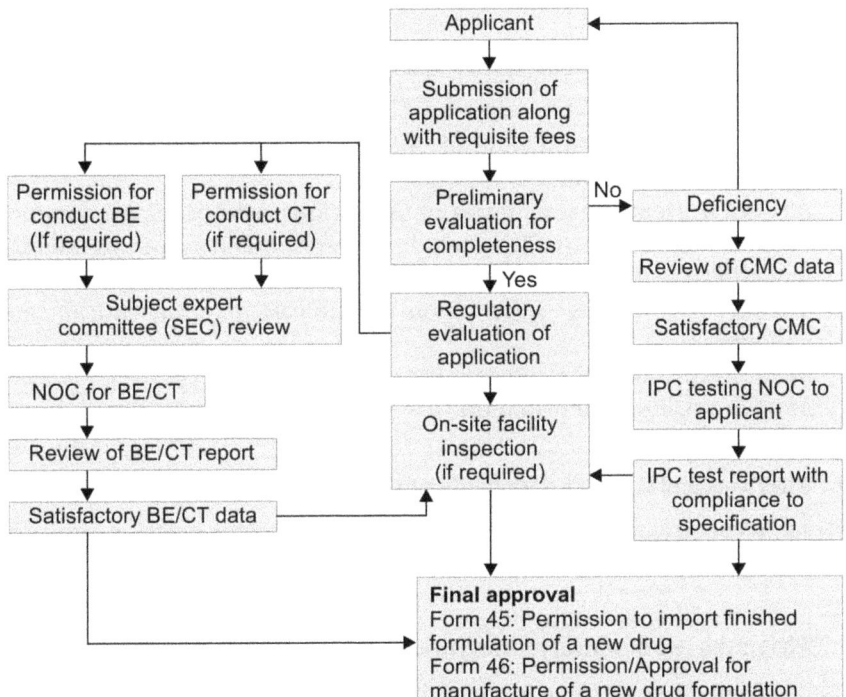

Flowchart 2: DCG(I) approval process for new vaccine or new drug in India.

(DCGI: Drugs Controller General of India; BE: bioequivalence; CMC: chemistry and manufacturing control; CT: clinical trial; NOC: no objection certificate; IPC: Indian Pharmacopoeia Commission)

17. What are the different regulatory approvals and no objection certificates required for manufacturing of vaccines in India?

There are several regulatory approvals and no-objection certificates (NOCs) required for the manufacturing of vaccines in India.

Test License or Form 29: Form 29 is a license to manufacture vaccines for examination, testing, and analysis of a product. An application is submitted using Form 30 to the licensing authority appointed by the State Government. Following that, the approval/license is issued in Form 29.

No-Objection Certificate for Form 29: Before obtaining a test license, an NOC must be obtained from the CDSCO for carrying out tests and analysis of test batches.

18. How to apply for approval of a new vaccine?

The manufacturers/sponsors must apply using Form 44 for permission for new vaccine approval under the provisions of Drugs and Cosmetic Act 1940 and Rules 1945. As Form 44 is an application for grant of permission to import or manufacture a new vaccine or to undertake a clinical trial, the CDSCO prescribes information to be submitted for new vaccine approval (market authorization) in a format, to simplify the submission requirements. The document design is as per the International submission requirements of Common Technical Document (CTD) and has five modules.

19. What modules must be addressed under Form 44 application?

There are total of five modules that must be submitted for vaccine approval:
- *Module I:* Administrative/legal information comprising documents specific to each region.
- *Module II:* Detailed summaries of the various sections of the common technical document (CTD), including overall quality report/summary, nonclinical and clinical overview, etc.
- *Module III:* Quality information (chemical, pharmaceutical, and biological).
- *Module IV:* Nonclinical information.
- *Module V:* Clinical information.

20. What legal and statutory documents must be attached for new vaccine approval?

Several legal documents must be submitted for new vaccine approval application **(Table 5)**.

21. What is the role of stability testing in vaccine formulations?

Stability testing is performed to check the quality of a vaccine and its variation with time under the influence of various environmental factors such as temperature, humidity, and light. Stability testing is crucial to establish the

TABLE 5: Legal document to be attached for vaccine approval.

Required items	Details
License and approval (as applicable)	• Copy of Form 11 for imported vaccine product • Form 29 for indigenous vaccine • Clinical trial no-objection letters/approval • GEAC clearance
Legal documents to be notarized	• A copy of plant registration/approval certificate issued by MOH/NRA of the country of origin • A copy of approval, if any, showing the vaccine is permitted for manufacturing and/or marketing in the country of origin • A copy of PPC as per WHO GMP certification scheme for imported vaccine products • A copy of FSC from the country of origin for imported vaccine products • Certificate of GMP of other manufacturers involved in the vaccine production process • Batch release certificate issued by NRA for imported products • Undertaking to declare
Others	• A copy of site master file • Certificate of analysis from Central Drug Laboratory (India) of three consecutive batches • Product permission document

(MOH: Ministry of Health; NRA: National Regulatory Authority; PPC: pharmaceutical product certificate; WHO: World Health Organization; GMP: good manufacturing practice; FSC: free sale certificate; GEAC: genetic engineering approval committee)

TABLE 6: Stability evaluation at different stages.

Developmental stage	It is important for: • Identification of appropriate stability-indicating parameters • Detection of potential degradation products that could develop over time
Licensing stage	• Shelf life (real-time stability) • Stability profile (accelerated stability testing)
Post-licensure stability monitoring	The objectives are: • To support shelf-life specifications and/or release specifications • To refine the stability profile of a vaccine in question • Identifies manufacturing-related changes (intentional or unintentional) and their impact on stability • Support the conclusion that the vaccine stability profile is still the same as at licensure

shelf life of the formulation and recommended storage conditions. **Table 6** highlights the stability evaluation at different stages of vaccine development as well as after marketing the vaccine.

22. How to get marketing authorization for vaccines?

For availing authorization to market a new vaccine, i.e., an innovative new product, new vaccine application needs to be submitted to the regulatory authority, i.e., CDSCO. As mentioned earlier, to avail this approval, the applicant needs to submit the complete common technical document containing the complete preclinical and clinical test data for evaluating the vaccine information and description of manufacturing trials. On receipt of this application, the regulatory agency screens the technical document to ensure receipt of adequate data and information in each section, required for processing the application further. Based on complete evaluation of the application, three possible actions can be taken:

1. *Not approvable*: Letter contains list of deficiencies and explain the reason.
2. *Approvable*: Letter suggests the changes and possible request commitment to do post-approval studies.
3. *Approval*: Letter states that the vaccine is approved.

In case of the first or second action, the applicant is given an opportunity to meet and discuss the deficiencies with the regulatory authority.

The regulations under Drugs and Cosmetics Act 1940 and its rules 1945, 122A, 122B, and 122D describe the information required for approval of an application to import or manufacture of new vaccine for marketing.

23. What is the role of periodic safety update reports in vaccine approval?

Following approval, once the vaccine is marketed, the response of the vaccines must be monitored in a scrutinized manner, to check the safety of the product. Periodic safety update reports (PSURs) must be established by the applicant to:

- Report all the relevant new information from appropriate sources
- Relate these data to patient exposure
- Summarize the market authorization status in different countries and any significant variations in safety
- Indicate whether changes should be made to product information in order to optimize the use of the product.

For the first 2 years after approval, PSURs must be submitted every 6 months followed by once a year for the next 2 years. Thus, PSURs are submitted to CDSCO for 4 years after getting vaccine approval.

24. What is postmarketing commitment, and when is it required?

Additional information/data generation on a vaccine may be required by the US Food and Drug Administration (FDA) or the European Medicines Agency (EMA) from the sponsoring company to grant approval or to continue marketing of the product. This is called postmarketing commitment (PMC). These commitments are agreed to by a pharmaceutical company with the health-regulatory authority and are used to conduct further studies to generate additional information on the product's safety, effectiveness, and/or optimal use. Postmarketing commitments can be required either before or after the health authority has granted approval to a company to market a medication.

IMPORTING VACCINES INTO INDIA

25. How to apply for permission to import vaccine for clinical trial or for examination, testing, and analysis?

- Any person (or institution or organization) who intends to import a new vaccine for conducting a clinical trial or bioavailability or bioequivalence study or for examination, testing, and analysis should make an application using Form CT-16 to the central licensing authority.
- The application shall be accompanied by a fee specified in the Sixth Schedule, and such other information and documents as specified in Form CT-16.
- Any person or institution or organization that intends to import a new vaccine or any related substances. Following a scrutinized review of the documents, the central licensing authority may either:
  - Grant the permission in Form-17 within 90 days from receipt of the application, or
  - Reject the application.

(In case of deficiencies that can be rectified, the central licensing authority informs the applicant, who can later rectify the deficiencies within a period specified by the central licensing authority.)

26. What is the validity of an import license for a new vaccine obtained for clinical trial or for examination, testing, and analysis?

- The validity of the license granted in Form CT-17 is 3 years from the date of issue, unless suspended or canceled by the central licensing authority.
- In exceptional cases, after considering needs and exigencies, the central licensing authority may extend the validity of the license by 1 year following a written application from the license holder.

27. How to apply for permission to import a vaccine for sale or distribution?

- Any person who intends to import a new vaccine in the form of a pharmaceutical formulation, for sale or distribution in India, should make an application to obtain a permit from the central licensing authority, using Form CT-18.
- The application should be accompanied by other information or documents based on the approval status of the product in the country **(Table 7)**.
- The submission of required documents pertaining to animal toxicology, teratogenic studies, perinatal studies, reproduction studies, mutagenicity, and carcinogenicity may be modified or relaxed:
  - If the vaccine intended to be imported is approved and marketed for more than 2 years in other countries.
  - If the central licensing authority finds the published studies on safety are adequate to grant approval.

TABLE 7: Additional documents for importing vaccine, based on approval status.

Intended to import	Approval status in the country	Additional document to be attached with CT 18
New vaccine proposed to be marketed	Contains unapproved new molecule	Local clinical trial data
New vaccine already approved, but the importer intends to market for new claims (e.g., new indication or new dosage form or new route of administration or new strength)	Already permitted for certain claims	Local clinical trial data
Fixed-dose combination		Results of local clinical trial

- Following a review of the documents, the central licensing authority may:
  - Either grant permission in the form of pharmaceutical formulation in Form CT-20 within 90 working days from receipt of the application, or
  - Reject the application.

(In case of deficiencies that can be rectified, the central licensing authority informs the applicant, who can later rectify the deficiencies within a period specified by the central licensing authority.)

After obtaining permission from central licensing authority to import new vaccine for sale or for distribution, the applicant shall make an application as per provisions of the Drugs and Cosmetics Rules, 1945 for grant of import license to import and market the new vaccine. The application shall be accompanied by the permission in Form CT-20.

28. What are the conditions for importing a vaccine for sale or distribution?

Figure 6 lists the conditions for importing new vaccines for sale or distribution.

The new vaccine shall conform to the specifications approved by the central licensing authority	The labeling of the vaccine shall conform to the requirements specified in the Drugs and Cosmetics Rules 1945	The label on the immediate container of the drug as well as the packing should contain the following warning: "WARNING: to be sold by retail on the prescription of a ....only" which shall be in red box
As post-marketing surveillance, the applicant shall submit periodic safety update report as specified in the fifth schedule	All reported adverse reactions related to vaccine shall be intimated to the central licensing authority, and regulatory action resulting from their review shall be complied with	No claims except those mentioned above shall be made for the vaccine without prior approval of the central licensing authority
Specimen(s) of the carton, labels, and package insert that will be adopted for marketing the drug in the country shall get approved from the central licensing authority before the drugs and marketed	In case of import, each consignment shall be accompanied by a test or analysis report	If long-term stability data submitted do not cover the proposed shelf-life of the product, the stability study shall be continued to firmly establish the shelf-life, and complete stability data shall be submitted

Fig. 6: Condition of permission for import of new vaccine for sale or distribution.

29. How to apply for permission to manufacture a vaccine for sale or distribution?

- Any person who intends to manufacture a new vaccine in the form of pharmaceutical formulation in India should apply using Form CT-21 to obtain permission from the central licensing authority.
- This application should be accompanied with information as specified in the Second Schedule and fee as specified in the Sixth Schedule.
- The application should be accompanied by other information or documents based on the approval status of the product in the country, as mentioned in **Table 7**.
- Following a review of documents, the central licensing authority may:
  - Either grant permission to manufacture the new vaccine in the form of pharmaceutical formulation in Form CT-23, or
  - Reject the application.

(In case of deficiencies that can be rectified, the central licensing authority informs the applicant, who can later rectify the deficiencies within a period specified by the central licensing authority).

30. How to proceed in case of suspension or cancelation of import license for new vaccine for clinical trial or for sale or distribution?

- In case of noncompliance to the respective provisions of the Act, the approved import license of the licensee can be canceled or suspended by the order of the central licensing authority.
- The licensee will be given an opportunity to show and justify the reason behind noncompliance to provision and he will be heard by the central licensing authority before taking this action.
- The licensee can appeal to the Central Government within 45 days from the receipt of the suspension or cancelation order; the government, after necessary inquiry and hearing, may give its decision within 60 working days from the date of filing the appeal.

31. How to renew import licenses for sale and distribution of vaccines?

Applications for import license should be submitted along with the application for re-registration, provided the importer and Indian agent are the same, a minimum of 3 months ahead of the expiry of the import license. If all the documents are in order, the import license can be issued within 4 weeks of application.

32. What are the responsibilities of importers or manufacturers in the marketing of new vaccines?

- The manufacturer or importer should market the new vaccine for approved indication/s only.
- However, if the manufacturer or importer is not involved in the promotion or use of the new vaccine for indication/s other than those approved, they will not be punished for any deleterious consequences resulting from use for unapproved indication/s.

33. How to seek fast-track approvals for vaccines in case of epidemics or pandemics?

In case of a pandemic, to encourage research and development of a vaccine for the prevention or treatment of the pandemic, the CDSCO may consider a series of actions to accelerate the development of vaccines for use in the management of the pandemic. The possible actions are as follows:

- Any firm developing a vaccine for the pandemic can directly approach the DCG(I) through the Public Relations Office for seeking guidance for product approval and regulatory norms.
- Any firm or research institute that seeks to repurpose existing vaccines for the treatment of the pandemic will also be given priority for review and approval.
- Applications for clinical trial permission and applications to import or manufacture vaccine for sale and distribution would be processed on priority through expedited review/accelerated approval.
- Any firm with a vaccine already approved for the pandemic in any other country can directly approach the DCG(I) through the Public Relations Office regarding expedited review/accelerated approval for marketing in India.
- Data requirements for animal toxicity studies, clinical studies, stability studies, etc. may be abbreviated, deferred, or waived on a case-to-case basis—depending on the type of vaccine, nature of the vaccine, plant from which the drug is extracted.
- Applications to manufacture or import a vaccine for testing, analysis, and bioavailability/bioequivalence or clinical trial may be processed within 7 days.
- In case of emergency, an import license (Form 10) would be granted without a registration certificate (Form 41), subject to approval from the Central Government.

Although there is no separate guideline for fast-track approval other than applying for a new product application using Form 44, considering the gravity of the crisis—as well as the need of the hour—the entire approval process may be accelerated.

ACKNOWLEDGMENT

The authors acknowledge Dr Daniel Scott, Vice President, Clinical Research, Pfizer Vaccines for his scientific contribution to the article.

SUGGESTED READING

1. Barbosa T, Barral-Netto M. Challenges in the research and development of new human vaccines. Braz J Med Biol Res. 2013;46:103–8.
2. Central Drugs Standard Control Organization, Directorate General of Health Services, Ministry of Health and Family Welfare, Government of India. Guidance document for test license. [online] Available from: https://searn-isp.org/SEARN/export/sites/SEARN/Pdf_documents/RF/Guidelines/india/test_license_guide_doc_1.pdf. [Last Accessed August, 2020].

3. Central Drugs Standard Control Organization. CDSCO Guidance for industry. [online] Available from: https://www.kem.edu/wp-content/uploads/2019/12/CDSCO-Guidance-For-Industry.pdf. [Last Accessed August, 2020].
4. Central Drugs Standard Control Organization. CDSCO letter X-1026107/2020-PRO. [online] Available from: https://cdsco.gov.in/opencms/opencms/system/modules/CDSCO.WEB/elements/download_file_division.jsp?num_id=NTc2OQ==. [Last Accessed August, 2020].
5. Central Drugs Standard Control Organization. Clinical Trial Rules 2019. [online] Available from: https://cdsco.gov.in/opencms/export/sites/CDSCO_WEB/Pdf-documents/NewDrugs_CTRules_2019.pdf. [Last Accessed August, 2020].
6. Central Drugs Standard Control Organization. Divisions. [online] Available from: https://cdsco.gov.in/opencms/opencms/en/Home/. [Last Accessed August, 2020].
7. Clinical development service agency (CDSA). FAQs. [online] Available from: https://thsti.res.in/cdsa/FAQs+for+New+Drug+Regulation/. [Last Accessed August, 2020].
8. Gouglas D, Thanh Le T, Henderson K, Kaloudis A, Danielsen T, Hammersland N, et al. Estimating the cost of vaccine development against epidemic infectious diseases: a cost minimisation study. Lancet Glob Health. 2018;6(12):e1386-96.
9. Guidance document on Common Submission Format for Import and Registration of bulk drugs and finished formulations in India. Central Drugs Standard Control Organization: Import and Registration Division Guidance Document. Document No. IMP/REG/200711.
10. Gupta NV, Reddy CM, Reddy KP, Kumar A. Process of approval of new drug in India with emphasis on clinical trials. Int J Pharmaceut Sci Rev Res. 2012;13(2):17-23.
11. History of Vaccines. Vaccine development, testing and regulation. [online] Available from: https://www.historyofvaccines.org/content/articles/vaccine-development-testing-and-regulation. [Last Accessed August, 2020].
12. Lurie N, Saville M, Hatchett R, et al. Developing Covid-19 vaccines at pandemic speed. NEJM. 2020:1969–73.
13. Oyston P, Robinson K. The current challenges for vaccine development. J Med Microbiol. 2012; 61:889-94.
14. Pfizer. How Vaccines are developed? [online] Available from: https://www.pfizer.com/news/hot-topics/how_are_vaccines_developed. [Last Accessed August, 2020].
15. Pfizer. Post marketing commitment. [online] Available from: https://www.pfizer.com/purpose/transparency/what-is-pmc#one. [Last Accessed August, 2020].
16. Pharma Research. Vaccine Factbook 2013. Available from: http://phrma-docs.phrma.org/sites/default/files/pdf/PhRMA_Vaccine_FactBook_2013.pdf. [Last Accessed August, 2020].
17. Plotkin S, Robinson JM, Cunningham G, Iqbal R, Larsen S. The complexity and cost of vaccine manufacturing – An overview. Vaccine. 2017;35(33):4064-71.
18. Rajiv Gandhi Centre for Biotechnology. Schedule Y. [online] Available from: https://rgcb.res.in/documents/Schedule-Y.pdf. [Last Accessed August, 2020].
19. Rambhad G, Ghia C. Vaccine industry and manufacturing of vaccines. In: Vashishtha VM (Eds). IAP Textbook of Vaccines, 2nd edition. New Delhi: Jaypee Brothers Medical Publishers (P) Ltd.; 2020.
20. Sawant AM, Mali DP, Bhagwat DA. Regulatory requirements and drug approval process in India, Europe and US. Pharmaceut Reg Affairs. 2018;7:2.
21. Shaw AR, Feinberg MB. Part Ten: Prevention and therapy of immunologic diseases. Vaccines. Clin Immunol. 2008:1353-82.
22. Vashishtha VM. National vaccine policy of India. IAP Textbook of vaccines. https://www.researchgate.net/publication/275153455_National_Vaccine_Policy_of_India Accessed on 16 Sep 2020.

23. WHO. Guidelines on stability evaluation of vaccine by WHO. [online] Available from: https://www.who.int/biologicals/publications/trs/areas/vaccines/stability/Microsoft%20Word%20-%20BS%202049.Stability.final.09_Nov_06.pdf. [Last Accessed August, 2020].
24. WHO. Stability evaluation of a vaccine by WHO: Lessons Learnt. [online] Available from: https://www.who.int/medicines/areas/quality_safety/regulation_legislation/icdra/WI-3_2Dec.pdf. [Last Accessed August, 2020].
25. World Health Organization. WHO finds India's vaccine regulatory authority compliant with international standards. [online] Available from: https://www.who.int/medicines/regulation/india-authority_reg_compliant-int-standards/en/. [Last Accessed August, 2020].

CHAPTER 11

National Immunization Technical Advisory Group

Madhu Gupta, Adarsh Bansal

1. What is National Immunization Technical Advisory Group (NITAG)?

National Immunization Technical Advisory Group (NITAG) is an advisory committee consisting of multidisciplinary groups of experts responsible for providing information to national governments that is used to make evidence-based decisions regarding vaccine and immunization policy.[1,2] It is a balanced group that can aid a national program to resist pressure from any pressure groups including vaccine manufacturing industry, vaccine promoting groups as well as anti-immunization groups. The advantage of such groups is the credibility which leads to transparency and evidence-based processes by which it arrives at its decisions.[3] There are 171 reported NITAGs in the world. In India, we call this group as the NTAGI, i.e., National Technical Advisory Group on Immunization.[4]

2. What is the need of the National Technical Advisory Group on Immunization (NTAGI)?

The NTAGI was established in the year 2001 and is currently the primary advisory committee advising the Ministry of Health and Family Welfare (MoHFW) on all immunization-related issues. The body provides technical advice to inform decision-making on both technical and operational matters pertaining to immunization and choice and scheduling of existing and planning vaccines. The NTAGI is not a policy-making body in its own right and has no regulatory function. It has more of an advisory role. Recommendations made by the NTAGI are generally used by the government to formulate policy relevant to immunization. The NTAGI has to review its recommendation on every vaccine-preventable disease every 5 years.

3. Who all are the members of the National Technical Advisory Group on Immunization (NTAGI)?

The Secretary to Government of India in the MoHFW represents the chair while the Secretary to the Department of Biotechnology represents the cochair. It had representation from a wide spectrum of relevant constituencies. They included national organizations involved in healthcare policy and research such as the Indian Council of Medical Research (ICMR) and the

National Institute of Health and Family Welfare, professional organizations such as the Indian Academy of Pediatrics, the Indian Medical Association, representatives of Government of India agencies such as the Department of Biotechnology, *Niti Aayog*, Drugs Controller General of India, along with representations of state governments. There are technical experts from the field of epidemiology, biotechnology, pharmacology, community medicine, vaccinology, health economics, public health, nursing, clinical research, immunology, pediatrics, bacteriology, and neurology. This is supplemented by technical experts, representatives from the United Nations International Children's Emergency Fund (UNICEF), the World Health Organization (WHO), and World Bank[5] (**Table 1**).

4. What are the responsibilities, structure, and procedures of the National Technical Advisory Group on Immunization (NTAGI)?

The responsibilities, structure, functioning, and procedures of the NTAGI and Standing Technical Subcommittee (STSC) are also known as the Code of Practice. It is prepared after reviewing the best practices at global and national scientific advisory committees and has been ratified by chair and cochairs of the NTAGI with inputs from members of the STSC. All members of the NTAGI and STSC as well as individuals attending meetings

TABLE 1: Composition of the NTAGI, 2018.

Member types	Profile/Description
Chair, ex officio	Secretary, H&FW, and MoHFW
Cochair, ex officio	Secretary, DBT; Secretary, DHR
Core members, ex officio	DGHS; Additional Secretary and Mission Director, NRHM; Directors of NCDC, NII, NIV, and THSTI
Core members, independent experts	16 experts from various vaccine-related disciplines—biotechnology, epidemiology, pediatrics, infectious disease, community medicine, obstetrics and gynecology, pharmacology, vaccinology, health economics, social sciences, and virology
Liaison members	Joint Secretary, RCH, and MoHFW
Representatives from professional organizations	Presidents of the IAP, IMA, and PHFI
Representatives from international partners	Country representatives for the WHO, India and the UNICEF, India
Representatives from states/union territories	Principal Secretaries of four states (on rotation basis) with at least one from the hilly/Northeastern states

(DBT: Department of Biotechnology; DGHS: Directorate General of Health Services; DHR: Department of Health Research; IAP: Indian Academy of Pediatrics; IMA: Indian Medical Association; MoHFW: Ministry of Health and Family Welfare; NCDC: National Center for Disease Control; NII: National Institute of Immunology; NIV: National Institute of Virology; NRHM: National Rural Health Mission; NTAGI: National Technical Advisory Group on Immunization; PHFI: Public Health Foundation of India; RCH: Reproductive and Child Health; THSTI: Translational Health Science and Technology Institute; UNICEF: United Nations International Children's Emergency Fund; WHO: World Health Organization) are required to confirm their acceptance of the provisions set out in this document by signing a declaration. The Code of Practice must be reviewed every 5 years. An earlier review of the Code of Practice may be taken up, if needed, at the discretion of chair and cochairs.[5]

5. What are the major roles and terms of references of the National Technical Advisory Group on Immunization (NTAGI)?

The major roles and terms of references of the NTAGI are described here:[6,7]

Major roles:
- To be an advisory body to assist the Government of India in developing a nationwide policy framework for vaccines and immunization
- To prioritize immunization activities and set attainable targets
- Identify critical gaps in policy and program and identify studies, assessment, and research areas to be addressed
- To review periodic assessment of the National Immunization Program (NIP), including immunization performance and disease incidence.

Terms of reference:
- Identify reasons for the decline in immunization coverage levels, identify bottlenecks, and suggest measures to revitalize the routine immunization activities
- Establish criteria for ensuring a cost-effective expansion/renewal plan for the cold chain
- Set up norms for periodic evaluation of the immunization program (e.g., frequency surveys, methodology to be adopted, and mechanism for data dissemination)
- Examine the current status of surveillance under the Reproductive and Child Health Program and suggest mechanism for integrating the National Polio Surveillance Project network with the existing surveillance system once the polio is eradicated
- Firm up guideline for epidemic/outbreak control measures for vaccine-preventable diseases
- Establish standards and criteria for introduction of newer vaccines under the Universal Immunization Program
- Guide policy for introduction of injection safety technology into the immunization program
- Suggest innovative strategies for introducing demand generation strategies in the program
- Examine the role of private sector vis-à-vis immunization and suggest measures for a more effective program with private sector partnership
- Identify strategies, which would be required under special circumstances for instance: (a) in underserved areas like urban slums and tribal areas and (b) immunization during natural calamities
- Identify areas that need research studies including cost-effectiveness analysis, burden of diseases studies, operations research, etc., and suggest modalities for conducting the same

- Suggest mechanisms and modalities for improving the vaccine quality assurance through the National Regulatory Authority (Drug Controller General of India)
- Examine the need for decentralization of program implementation and suggest the degree and modalities for affecting the same.

6. **What are the considerations that are looked into before introducing newer vaccines in the national immunization program?**

For introducing a new vaccine into the NIP, following questions need to be answered:
- Burden of the disease
- Severity of the disease
- Disease-specific fatality rate
- Morbidity associated with the disease
- Catastrophic health expenditure due to the disease that brings the family below poverty line
- Morbidity and mortality prevented by the vaccine
- Vaccine efficacy and effectiveness
- Cost-effectiveness analysis of introducing the vaccine in NIP
- Any additional data needed for decision-making like safety data of the vaccine, postmarketing surveillance, impact assessment of new vaccine, and technological assessment of new vaccine delivery mechanisms.

7. **What are the preparations that need to be done before the introduction of a new vaccine in Universal Immunization Program (UIP)?**

The NTAGI considers various factors before recommending a new vaccine in the program. The immunization division of the NTAGI decides upon how the process will be implemented. Once it is decided that the new vaccine will be launched, a standard implementation plan (SIP) is prepared in the form of a document with the help of experts in the field. This document includes the modifications in the existing immunization schedule for accommodation of new vaccine. Then the operational guidelines are prepared with the help of experts such as scientists, program managers, cold chain managers, etc. All the stakeholders are identified and provided training for the requisite process.

8. **How new vaccines are introduced in Universal Immunization Program (UIP) and how immunization schedule is decided?**

The decision on inclusion of vaccines is taken by the MoHFW, Government of India, on recommendation of the NTAGI. Schedule for administration of different vaccines is decided based on the operational aspects of the NIP, the recommendations provided by the WHO-recommended schedules, vaccine position papers, as well as the Strategic Advisory Group of Experts (SAGE). The steps of new vaccine introduction are shown in **Figure 1**.[8]

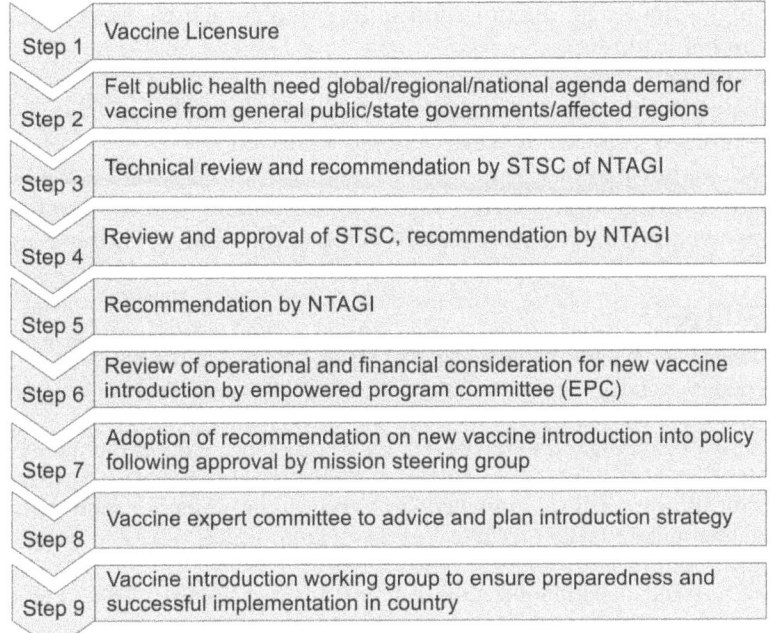

Fig. 1: Steps of introducing new vaccines in India.
(NTAGI: National Technical Advisory Group on Immunization; STSC: Standing Technical Subcommittee)

9. Why the National Technical Advisory Group on Immunization (NTAGI) recommends less vaccine to be included in Universal Immunization Program (UIP) and there are a greater number of vaccines recommended by private sector?

The NTAGI mainly provides recommendations on the vaccines that prevent the diseases of public health significance i.e., the diseases with high mortality and high morbidity rate among the community whereas the private practitioners follow the recommendations of the Indian Academy of Pediatrics (IAP) for pediatric age group. The IAP recommends the use of vaccines based upon not only diseases of public health significance, but also of those diseases, which may affect health at the individual (child) level. Hence, we have more number of vaccine recommendations in the private sector.

10. What are the challenges faced by the National Technical Advisory Group on Immunization (NTAGI) in implementation of the newer vaccines?

The challenges faced by the NTAGI at the national level include:
- Lack of evidence or authentic data on burden of disease
- Nonavailability of the locally manufactured vaccine or if its available, it is not in sufficient quantities
- High cost per dose of the vaccine
- Opportunity cost of introducing the newer vaccine need to be considered
- Limited integration with national decision-making process.

Some of the challenges documented at the global level include:[9,10]
- Unreliable funding
- Insufficient diversity of member expertise
- Inadequate conflicts of interest management procedures
- Insufficient capacity to access and use evidence
- Lack of transparency
- Limited integration with national decision-making process that reduces the recognition and incorporation of recommendations by these groups.

REFERENCES

1. Gessner B, Duclos P, DeRoeck D, Nelson E. Informing decision makers: experience and process of 15 National Immunization Technical Advisory Groups. Vaccine. 2010;28:A1-5.
2. World Health Organization (WHO). (2019). National Immunization Technical Advisory Groups (NITAGs). [online] Available from: http://www.euro.who.int/en/health-topics/disease-prevention/vaccines-and-immunization/activities/national-immunization-technical-advisory-groups-nitags. [Last accessed July, 2020].
3. Duclos P. National Immunization Technical Advisory Groups (NITAGs): guidance for their establishment and strengthening. Vaccine. 2010;28:A18-25.
4. National Immunization Technical Advisory Groups (NITAGs). (2019). The latest news from the NITAG community. [online] Available from: nitag-resource.org. [Last accessed July, 2020].
5. National Technical Advisory Group on Immunization (NTAGI). (2019). Code of Practice. [online] Available from: http://www.nitag-resource.org/media-center/document/3939-code-of-practice. [Last accessed July, 2020].
6. John T. India's National Technical Advisory Group on Immunization. Vaccine. 2010;28:A88-90.
7. National Immunization Technical Advisory Groups (NITAGs). (2019). Major roles and terms of reference of the National Technical Advisory Group on Immunization in India. [online] Available from: http://www.nitag-resource.org/sites/default/files/1dd77ae6d6675b107610c9d180954dc783ab1895_1.pdf. [Last accessed July, 2020].
8. Government of India. Immunization Handbook for Medical Officers. New Delhi: Department of Health and Family Welfare; 2016.
9. Bell S, Blanchard L, Walls H, Mounier-Jack S, Howard N. Value and effectiveness of National Immunization Technical Advisory Groups in low-and middle-income countries: a qualitative study of global and national perspectives. Health Policy Plan. 2019;34:271-81.
10. Mohapatra A, Paul DK, Narendra K Arora NK. National Technical Advisory Group on Immunization (NTAGI) and National Regulatory Authority (NRA) in vaccination programs and practices. In: Vashishtha VM, Kalra A (Eds). IAP Textbook of Vaccines, 2nd edition. New Delhi: Jaypee Brothers Medical Publishers (P) Ltd; 2020. pp. 798-809.

CHAPTER 12

Medicolegal and Ethical Issues in Immunization

Satish Kamtaprasad Tiwari, Yash Paul

1. **Many people think that vaccines outside the Universal Immunization Program (UIP) are only for providing financial benefit to the doctors.**

   All vaccines provide benefit to the vaccine recipients. Due to financial burden, the Government may not be in a position to provide each and every vaccine free under the Universal Immunization Program (UIP).

2. **Some vaccines are not included in the Universal Immunization Program (UIP); is it ethical to deprive poor children from the benefits of vaccines, which are already available in the market?**

   As there should be no death by starvation, likewise it is the responsibility of the government that no one dies of a disease for which treatment is available. Similarly, the Advisory Committee should from time to time decide regarding prioritizing the vaccines, according to the needs at a particular time.[1]

3. **Due to antivaccine lobbies, some people think that vaccinations do more harm than providing benefits. What steps should I take to convince the benefits of vaccination?**

   We should explain in easy to understand language that vaccines are to provide benefit. Doctors should show vaccination records of themselves and family members. This has high impact.

4. **Many people are very enthusiastic about immunization and want all available vaccines to be administered to their children, but some vaccines need to be administered under special circumstances only?**

   Though no harm is expected to occur, it is the doctor's duty to explain which vaccine should be given priority. Yellow fever vaccine is recommended for those who have to travel to South America or Africa.

5. **Should I recommend diphtheria, pertussis, and tetanus (DPT) or diphtheria, acellular pertussis, and tetanus (DaPT) vaccine in routine?**

   Diphtheria, pertussis, and tetanus (DPT) is more effective than diphtheria, acellular pertussis, and tetanus (DaPT) during primary immunization.

DPT should be recommended for primary immunization. In case there is history of febrile convulsions or prolonged crying following administration of DPT in the past, then such children should be administered DaPT.[2]

6. **Many people want tetanus vaccine even for minor and clean injuries although they had been immunized with tetanus vaccine in combination or as Tet-Vac in recent past.**

The doctor should enquire about immunization status of the injured person. In case the person has been vaccinated with tetanus vaccine as part of vaccination recommendations, this should be recorded. In a child if DPT or DaPT vaccines have been administered and next dose is due in next 4–6 weeks, then DPT or DaPT should be given. In case second booster dose has been administered between 4 and 5 years of age, then such a child should not be administered tetanus vaccine till age of 10 years. In children up to age of 6 years, tetanus vaccine alone should not be given if second dose of DPT or DaPT had been missed and this child should be given DPT or DaPT. In adolescents and adults, no tetanus vaccine is needed for 10 years for clean injury and for 5 years for tetanus-prone injury. Only tetanus [tetanus toxoid (TT)] vaccine is not available at present and is now replaced by tetanus and diphtheria (Td) vaccine.

7. **Many people are reluctant to get antirabies vaccine, especially in case it was not a bite but a scratch with the paw.**

We must explain that a dog licks its paws and it is the saliva which carries the infection. So, a doctor must explain the necessity of vaccination. Even if there is no danger of infection from this scratch, the doses administered will act as pre-exposure prophylaxis for future. In case the patient or attendant refuses vaccination, it must be stated or recorded on prescription.

8. **Currently, measles and rubella (MR) vaccine is under the Universal Immunization Program (UIP) or the National Immunization Program. Should I discuss with the parents that MR does not protect against mumps, so they should get children immunized with measles, mumps, and rubella (MMR)?**

Mumps has not been eradicated; mumps vaccine as such is not available. The doctor should recommend that measles, mumps, and rubella (MMR) should be administered in place of measles and rubella (MR), but should leave the decision on the caretaker. Getting scientific, evidence-based information is the right of each and every individual. Our role is to inform the parents, relatives, or patients, whether to take it or not is their decision.

9. **Ideal vaccination schedule for hepatitis B is at birth (0). It is further stated that third or fourth dose should not be administered before the age of 6 months and interval between the second and third and fourth dose should not be <2 months. Is it the right recommendation?**

Any recommendations have to be scientific, evidence-based, and accepted by a group of qualified persons or consultants. According to "Bolam principle", there can be different schools of thoughts accepted as standard recommendations by group of consultants. If you are following any one of these accepted or approved recommendations, you may not be at fault. You may have to justify why you have preferred and followed that particular approach or recommendations.

10. Ideal vaccination schedule of diphtheria, pertussis, and tetanus combination vaccination is 2 months, 4 months, and 6 months. Is it the right recommendation?

Probably yes, again as discussed above you will have to justify as per the Bolam principle and scientific recommendations.

11. I want to provide best schedule to my patients. Should I follow current Indian Academy of Pediatrics (IAP) and the Universal Immunization Program (UIP) schedule where hepatitis B vaccine is administered at birth then at 6 weeks, 10 weeks, and 14 weeks along with diphtheria, pertussis, and tetanus (DPT) or diphtheria, acellular pertussis, and tetanus (DaPT)? Yes or No.

Doctor should explain that this schedule appears to reduce the visits at cost of lower benefits to the child. Also, inform the reasons behind 6–10–14 weeks schedule or 2–4–6 months schedule and let the relatives or parents make informed choice/decision. If they insist on our suggestions, we have to suggest them the schedule which is practically possible or which has better results and these recommendations may vary from patient to patient in a particular situation.[3]

12. If the answer is no, then what schedule should I adopt?

We should recommend second dose of hepatitis B vaccine after 1 month of first dose and rotavirus vaccine at 6 weeks and 10 weeks. DPT + inactivated polio vaccine (IPV) with or without hepatitis B at 8, 16, and 24 weeks, but hepatitis B vaccine should be administered at 6 months of age. The present trend is of giving all the recommended vaccines on same day. Our suggestions are we may give penta, rota on 6–14–22 weeks and pneumococcal, polio on 10–18–26 weeks. This recommendation is based on the reason that ideal interval between two doses of same vaccines is 6–8 weeks and not 4 weeks.

13. In case child has been administered vaccine in gluteal region, should it be administered at proper site soon?

No vaccine should usually be administered in gluteal region because it is less effective. In case of rabies vaccine, dose or doses administered in gluteal region should never be counted and depending on the situation, vaccine dose/doses should be administered in thigh or upper arm as such deficiency in duty may prove fatal. Regarding other vaccines, one extra dose should be administered.

14. Many people may not be able to afford costly vaccine. Is it their constitutional right to get these vaccines through government schemes?

This issue is not simple and any suggestions or discussions will raise lots of debates and controversies. Health is supposed to be one of the fundamental constitutional rights of each and every citizen.[4] But at the same time, government policy or decisions have some practical difficulties/restrictions. If government has schemes for other illnesses like Ayushman Bharat, Rajiv Gandhi/Mahatma Phule schemes, or Mediclaim policies, they should also have immunization-related schemes. Because if children do not receive vaccinations and suffer from vaccine-preventable diseases (VPDs) resulting in malnutrition, long-term disability, or suboptimal development, the entire community will have to suffer.

15. If some parents are unable to get their children immunized, does this amount to child neglect or child abuse?

Unfortunately, this is also debatable issue with lots of ifs and buts. The main controversy will be what is more important for the child; adequate nutrition, proper education, or immunization against some disorders which a child may suffer only in later part of life (40–50 years of age). Whether the life is more important or quality of life? If the parents have adequate resources, not giving vaccines may amounts to neglect or abuse.[5,6] But if they do not have adequate money to buy their daily needs, how we can force them for immunization. If such a case comes to the notice of a doctor, the doctor should stress upon the need for vaccination in a friendly way. Another option is that government should provide immunization under various schemes (as discussed in previous question).

16. Is it true that international or multinational companies are using Indian population as "guinea pigs"?

This statement though sounds very much correct and legally valid, but many will reject it by denying the actual facts. The present situation is that the population in developed country is less while most of the developing countries have population explosion. During any research or scientific study, if there are complications resulting in mortality or morbidity, the compensations are in billions. The implementations of orders or court judgments are strictly followed in some of the countries while in most of the developing countries, there are lots of loopholes or excuses while taking legal actions. This is the reason many of us believe that the peoples from developing countries (including India) are used as "guinea pigs" during clinical trials for any drugs or vaccines.

17. Should we take consent before vaccination?

Many of us feel that consent is not required before vaccination. If a patient or parents have come for vaccination, there is implied consent and they are willing for all the vaccines. But in the present era of human rights and judicial activism, the concept of implied consent is outdated. The Article 21 of the Indian Constitution protects the right of the individual to get proper knowledge and benefits for the health and life of the individual. As per the judiciary, the citizen should get proper information regarding the effects, side effects, complications related to investigation, or treatments (including the costs). After knowing the pros and cons of the available remedies, then the concerned person shall make informed choice.[7] Hence, an informed consent is preferable over implied consent. In case patient or parents do not want to take any particular vaccine, a "negative consent" or refusal shall also be recorded in writing.

18. If you inject expiry date vaccine, is it negligence?

Negligence has "four Ds"; a *duty* toward patients, *deficiency* in that duty which *directly* results in *damage* to the patient or family. Inadvertent injection of expiry date vaccine if does not result in any damage, it cannot be labeled as negligence.[8] If there is allegation of deficiency in duty, we can repeat the dose after 4–6 weeks of giving expiry date vaccine. If there are financial considerations in such cases, the repeat dose can be given free of cost. All the events should be properly documented for any possible litigation in future. Such mishaps can be prevented by following the principle of "first in-first out" and checking the expiry date at the time of vaccination.

19. If the child develops the disease despite being vaccinated against it, is it negligence?

No, if vaccine has been properly maintained, has been properly given in right dose, and administered properly. Such an allegation can be minimized by informing the relatives or parents that no vaccine provides 100% protections to everybody.

20. Can an AYUSH doctor do vaccination?

This issue will be decided depending upon the fact that whether immunization is there in the curriculum which was taught to them. If they have learned vaccination during their undergraduate (UG) or postgraduate (PG) courses, then it is not negligence. Otherwise, this amounts to "crosspathy".[9]

21. Should regular immunization be deferred during a pandemic?

May or may not, depends upon cause of epidemic and what we are going to achieve by deferring the regular immunization. During the corona pandemic, initially it was advised to defer the routine vaccines by many consultants in order to maintain the social distancing and to prevent exposure to undiagnosed asymptomatic carriers of corona. But subsequently, it was thought that this will result in collapse of immunization program and child may suffer from so many VPDs. So, the present suggestion is to continue the routine schedule. Emergency lifesaving vaccines like antirabies vaccination should not be deferred under any circumstances.

22. Can an immunization certificate be issued even if parents do not have immunization record?

If you are very much sure and remember that the child was immunized with you, then only you should issue the certificate. If any age-related dose is pending, you can give that dose and then issue the certificate. One should always avoid issuing false certificates.

23. Can a politician, government official, or celebrity do the immunization?

Ideally not. Orally administered vaccines like oral polio vaccine (OPV) and rotavirus vaccine may be given as a token to send a message to public or as a part of inauguration of some project or program. Injectable vaccines can be given by a celebrity in case he or she is a qualified person like a doctor or a nurse.

24. How to regulate the exorbitant cost of vaccines?

In case a vaccine of similar quality is marketed by different manufacturers, one should go for the vaccine which has a lower price. The control of price is the responsibility of government or the regulatory authorities. Many times, manufacturers increase the cost of vaccines under the pretext that this is a better vaccine because of some innovative technique or combinations (injectable polio). The regulatory bodies should understand all these publicity gimmicks or biased scientific reasoning. There is need to take bold steps or decisions in these regard, so that the low cost vaccines are available for financially weaker section of the society or such vaccines can be included in the UIP schedule.

25. What are the conflicts of interest in the vaccination schedules?

As discussed in various preceding questions, there are different schedules by government and academic organizations. While finalizing these schedules, the vaccines are divided in different groups like essential or mandatory vaccines, affordable or costly vaccines, vaccines with one-to-one discussions with parents, newer vaccines, etc. We have already discussed that the vaccines are needed to prevent the VPD and it is the right of every child to get this preventive benefits irrespective of his religion, caste, color, or financial status. How there can be different schedule for the children in the same country? If vaccines are essential as per recommendations of the academic organizations, then why government should not provide the same to weaker section of society by including it under some of the schemes. All these facts raise the eyebrows that there are some conflicts of interest among the stakeholders. There is need to identify these conflicts of interest, so that there is "one country: one schedule" for all the children in the entire country.

26. What is the vaccine-related adverse event following immunization (AEFI)? How to prevent and protect?

Adverse event following immunization (AEFI) results following administration of any vaccine. Mild adverse effects are swelling at the site of injection, local pain, and fever. Serious adverse effects are anaphylaxis, encephalopathy, shock, and seizures (the details about AEFI are discussed in Chapter number 7). Fever and pain can be reduced by administration of proper dose of paracetamol about 45 minutes before administration of injection. History of seizures or breath-holding should be elicited and managed accordingly. In case of a patient who had been vaccinated in past elsewhere, history regarding any adverse reactions should be enquired into. In case of serious adverse reactions, they should be managed accordingly and if need, be transferred to centers with higher facilities.[10] Such adverse reactions should be reported to appropriate authorities.

REFERENCES

1. Tiwari S. Consumer problems and the pediatrician. In: Suraj G (Ed). Recent Advances in Pediatrics—19: Hot Topics. New Delhi: Jaypee Brothers Medical Publishers (P) Ltd; 2010. pp. 72-84.
2. Lavin J, Broutin H, Harvill ET, Bjornstad ON. Imperfect vaccine-induced immunity and whooping cough transmission to infants. Vaccine. 2010;29:11-6.
3. Mittal SK, Mathew JL. Expanded program of immunization in India: time to rethink and revamp. J Pediatr Sci. 2010;5:e43.
4. Paul Y, Tiwari S. Ethical issues in immunization. In: Vashishta VM, Kalra A (Eds). IAP Textbook of Vaccines, 2nd edition. New Delhi: Jaypee Brothers Medical Publishers (P) Ltd; 2020. pp. 819-23.
5. Nair MKC. Child abuse. Indian Pediatr. 2004;41:319-20.
6. Baldwa M, Tiwari S. Punishment for refusing OPV. Indian Pediatr. 2009:46:540-1.
7. Centers for Disease Control and Prevention (CDC). (2020). Vaccine Information Statements (VISs). [online] Available from: https://www.cdc.gov/vaccines/hcp/vis/index.html?CDC_AA_refVal=https%3A%2F%2Fwww.cdc.gov%2Fvaccines%2Fpubs%2Fvis%2Fdefault.htm. [Last accessed August, 2020].
8. Phatnani P, Lele RD. The Medical Profession and the Law, 1st edition. Mumbai: Sajjan & Sons; 1992. pp. 11-22.
9. Tiwari S. Legal issues related to vaccinology today. In: Vashishta VM, Kalra A (Eds). IAP Textbook of Vaccines, 2nd edition. New Delhi: Jaypee Brothers Medical Publishers (P) Ltd; 2020. pp. 810-8.
10. Indian Academy of Pediatrics Committee on Immunization (IAPCOI). Consensus recommendations on immunization and IAP immunization timetable 2012. Indian Pediatr. 2012;49:549-64.

CHAPTER 13

Vaccine Schedules including National Immunization Program

Meeta Dhaval Vashi, Vivek R Pardeshi

1. What is National Immunization Schedule (NIS) under Universal Immunization Program (UIP)?

National Immunization Schedule is a vaccination plan that all children and pregnant women should take to ensure protection against vaccine-preventable diseases. This schedule includes name of vaccine, recommended age/s of administration, dose, diluents, route and site of administration.

2. Which vaccines are included in NIS?

Nationally, vaccines are provided against 9 diseases namely diphtheria, pertussis, tetanus, polio, measles, rubella, severe form of childhood tuberculosis, hepatitis B, meningitis, and pneumonia caused by *Haemophilus influenzae* type B.

Sub-nationally, vaccination against 3 more diseases namely rotavirus diarrhea, pneumococcal pneumonia and Japanese encephalitis (JE) is provided.

3. Which additional vaccines are added to NIS in recent years?

Vaccines introduced in Universal Immunization Program during last few years are JE (2006), hepatitis B (2007), Pentavalent (2011), IPV (2015), rotavirus vaccine (2016), pneumococcal conjugate vaccine (PCV) and measles-rubella (MR) vaccine (2017).

4. Why rotavirus vaccine (RVV), pneumococcal vaccine (PCV) and JE vaccine are not given throughout the nation?

Rotavirus vaccine and pneumococcal conjugate vaccine are being introduced in phased manner and it will be expanded throughout India. JE vaccine is provided only in JE endemic districts.

CHAPTER 13 Vaccine Schedules including National Immunization Program

5. What is the current immunization schedule?

Vaccine	Due age	Maximum age	Dose	Diluent	Route	Site
For Pregnant Women						
Td-1	Early in pregnancy	Give as early as possible in pregnancy	0.5 mL	No	Intramuscular	Upper arm
Td-2	4 weeks after TT-1		0.5 mL	No	Intramuscular	Upper arm
Td- Booster If received 2 TT/Td doses in a pregnancy within the last 3 years			0.5 mL	No	Intramuscular	Upper arm
For Infants and Children						
BCG	At birth	Till 1 year of age	(0.05 mL until 1 month) 0.1 mL beyond age 1 month	Yes manufacturer supplied diluent (sodium chloride)	Intradermal	Upper arm *left*
Hepatitis B: Birth dose	At birth	Within 24 hours	0.5 mL	No	Intramuscular	Anterolateral side of mid-thigh - *left*
OPV-0	At birth	Within the first 15 days	2 drops		Oral	Oral
OPV 1, 2 and 3	At 6 weeks, 10 weeks and 14 weeks	Till 5 years of age	2 drops		Oral	Oral
Pentavalent 1, 2 and 3 (Diphtheria + Pertussis + Tetanus + Hepatitis B + Hib)	At 6 weeks, 10 weeks and 14 weeks	Penta 1 can be started till 1 year of age	0.5 mL	No	Intramuscular	Anterolateral side of mid-thigh - *left*
Fractional IPV (inactivated polio vaccine)	At 6 and 14 weeks	IPV1 till 1 year of age	0.1 mL	No	Intradermal	Upper arm - *right*

Contd...

Contd...

Vaccine	Due age	Maximum age	Dose	Diluent	Route	Site
Rotavirus	At 6 weeks, 10 weeks and 14 weeks	1 year of age	5 drops*	No*	Oral	Oral
Pneumococcal conjugate vaccine (PCV) (where applicable)	At 6 weeks and 14 weeks At 9 completed months - booster	1 year of age	0.5 mL	No	Intramuscular	Anterolateral side of mid-thigh - *right*
Measles/Rubella 1st dose	At 9 completed months	5 years of age	0.5 mL	Yes manufacturer supplied diluent (sterile water)	Subcutaneous	Upper arm - *right*
Japanese encephalitis	At 9 months	15 years of age	0.5 mL	Yes manufacturer supplied diluent (phosphate buffer solution)	Subcutaneous	Upper arm - *left*
Vitamin A (1st dose)	At 9 months	5 years of age	100,000 IU	No	Oral	Oral
DPT Booster-1	16–24 months	7 years of age	0.5 mL	No	Intramuscular	Anterolateral side of mid-thigh – *left*
Measles/Rubella 2nd dose	16–24 months	5 years of age	0.5 mL	Yes manufacturer supplied diluent (Sterile water)	Subcutaneous	Upper arm - *right*
OPV Booster	16–24 months	5 years	2 drops	No	Oral	Oral
Japanese encephalitis – 2	16–24 months	Till 15 years of age	0.5 mL	Yes manufacturer supplied diluent (phosphate buffer solution)	Subcutaneous	Upper arm - *left*
Vitamin A (2nd to 9th dose)	At 16 months. Then, one dose every 6 months	Up to the age of 5 years	2 mL (200,000 IU)	No	Oral	Oral
DPT Booster-2	5–6 years	7 years of age	0.5 mL	No	Intramuscular	Upper arm
Td	10 years and 16 years	16 years	0.5 mL	No	Intramuscular	Upper arm

*Exceptions are some states supplied with RotasiilTM vaccine which needs to be reconstituted and dose is 2.5 mL.

6. Explain which vaccine prevents which disease?

Vaccine	Disease prevented
BCG	Severe form of childhood tuberculosis
OPV	Poliomyelitis
Hepatitis B	Hepatitis B
Pentavalent	Diphtheria, pertussis, tetanus, hepatitis B, pneumonia and meningitis due to *Haemophilus influenzae* type b
IPV	Poliomyelitis
RVV	Rotavirus diarrhea
MR/MMR	Measles and rubella
JE	Japanese encephalitis or acute encephalitis syndrome (AES)
DPT	Diphtheria, pertussis, tetanus
Td	Tetanus and diphtheria
PCV	Pneumococcal pneumonia

7. Which are additional vaccines which are not yet given under National Immunization Schedule?

Human papilloma virus (HPV) vaccine, typhoid vaccine, hepatitis A vaccine, meningococcal vaccine and mumps vaccine are some vaccines, which are not yet included as part of national immunization schedule.

8. How many visits are required for immunization?

Total 7 visits are required to immunization session till 5 years of age for complete immunization—at birth, 6 weeks, 10 weeks, 14 weeks, 9 months, 16 months, and 5 years.

9. Who is a fully immunized child?

A child is said to be fully immunized if child receives all due vaccines as per national immunization schedule before completing 1 year. Ministry of Health and Family Welfare (MoHFW) is making intensive efforts to reach to more than 95% fully immunized children. This is to see to it that children receive age appropriate immunization.

10. Who is a completely immunized child?

A child who has received all vaccines recommended for the first and second year in the NIS is said to be completely immunized.

11. Why some vaccines need booster doses after primary immunization?

Immunity generated by some vaccines gradually diminishes over time and increases vulnerability to target infections. For such vaccines, booster doses are administered after primary immunization as it boosts immunity and enhances protection level against specific vaccine-preventable disease. For example, DPT, OPV and PCV.

12. What vaccines are given to newborns?

According to NIS, one dose each of hepatitis B, OPV and BCG should be given to newborns irrespective of the place of delivery. This is recommended for all institutional and non-institutional deliveries, in both public and private sectors.

13. Why hepatitis birth dose is given within 24 hours of birth?

Hepatitis B (known as "birth dose") should be given within 24 hours of birth to protect the newborn from possible hepatitis B infection that gets transferred from mother during delivery. If birth dose of hepatitis B vaccine is given beyond 24 hours, then it will not provide this protection. However, maximum protection against hepatitis B transmission is provided if the vaccine is given within 12 hours of birth.

14. Why OPV dose given at birth is called the "zero dose"

Because it is an "extra" dose that adds to the protection of the individual and the community and it is given before the scheduled three primary doses.

15. BCG is being given to majority of children in India. Still we see cases of tuberculosis. Why?

Bacille Calmette-Guérin (BCG) prevents severe form of childhood tuberculosis.

16. Pentavalent vaccine contains which 5 vaccines?

Diphtheria, pertussis, tetanus, hepatitis B and Hib.

17. Why measles vaccine is replaced by MR vaccine in the immunization schedule?

Addition of rubella containing vaccine in the form of MR campaign followed by replacement of measles vaccine with MR vaccine indicates the country's efforts and commitment to eliminate measles and rubella/congenital rubella syndrome (CRS).

18. What is MRCV/MCV/MR/Measles vaccine?

MCV means measles containing vaccine such as MR or MMR or measles vaccine

MRCV means measles and rubella containing vaccine such as MMR or MR.

19. Why are we continuing giving IPV and OPV even though India has eliminated polio?

Even though India is declared "Polio-free", country is at risk of importation of polio as it is still present in some countries and infected person coming to India can bring the disease and spread occurs if population immunity against disease is low. Also, IPV protects against vaccine derived polio viruses (VDPV).

20. Why TT is replaced by Td in National Immunization Schedule?

The TT vaccine has been replaced with *tetanus and adult diphtheria (Td) vaccine* in NIS to limit the waning immunity against diphtheria in older age groups.

21. What are key messages which need to be given to parents when they bring their children for vaccination?

- Which vaccine is given and which disease it prevents
- What are adverse effects and how to deal it
- When to come for next dose
- Keep immunization card safe and bring card for next visit.

22. Why 30 minutes waiting post vaccination at immunization session necessary?

Some vaccines can lead to an allergic reaction in rare cases. Allergic reactions or anaphylaxis requires early diagnosis and treatment. Anaphylaxis kit is available at all session sites hence it is advised to stay at immunization session for at least 30 minutes after receiving vaccine.

23. How many days gap is necessary between two doses?

There should be minimum 28 days gap between administration of two doses of same multidose vaccine except for PCV which is 2 months and JE vaccine which is 3 months.

Reduced interval between two doses of multidose vaccine may interfere with the antibody response and hence protection.

24. If gap between two doses is long, do we need to restart schedule from beginning?

No, there is no need to restart the schedule from beginning as longer than normally recommended gap between two subsequent doses of multidose vaccines normally does not impair the immunologic response.

If the child is brought late, we should give the next due dose of the vaccine and motivate the parents to bring the child for the remaining doses as per the immunization schedule.

25. Why are vaccines being administered in thigh instead of buttocks?

This site is recommended under UIP because of following reasons:

- Sciatic nerve passing through gluteal region may get accidentally damaged in case of injection leading to weakness of lower limb.
- Anterolateral aspect (front and outer part) of mid-thigh provides the largest muscle mass which facilitates quick absorption of vaccine into the blood capillaries.

26. Is there a definite sequence in which vaccines need to be given?

Yes, multiple vaccines are given on 6th, 10th, 14th weeks and 9 months and sequence is followed for feasibility (considering factors such as oral first, painful injection last) and uniformity:
- 6 weeks: OPV, RVV, IPV, PCV, Penta
- 10 weeks: OPV, RVV, Penta
- 14 weeks: OPV, RVV, IPV, PCV, Penta
- 9 months: Vitamin A, PCV, MR, JE (where applicable).

27. Why are vaccines in NIS administered at specific sites only?

Each vaccine is normally administered at the same specific site on the body to maintain uniformity and to facilitate recall of previous vaccinations in case immunization card is not available (example if we get response, only one vaccine given on right arm at 16 months of age, we can relate to which vaccine is given and which is not).

28. Can multiple injections be given together?

Yes, multiple injections can be safely given together as it does not affect effectiveness of individual vaccines and does not result in higher incidence of adverse events and has benefit of reducing number of visits and dropouts.

29. What precautions are needed while giving multiple vaccines?

- Two or more vaccines should not be mixed in the same syringe
- If two injectable vaccines are given on the same site, they should be given 2.5 cm (1 inch) apart.

30. Can vaccines used in National Immunization Program be stored in domestic refrigerator?

No. Domestic refrigerators have different temperature in different areas and cannot maintain temperature in case of power supply failure.

Ice lined refrigerator and deep freezers are supplied for storage of vaccines under UIP.

However, in certain unavoidable situations domestic refrigerators may be used but vaccine vials should not be stored in freezer, chiller compartment, door, or basket of the refrigerator and no other drugs, injections and non-UIP vaccines should be stored in it.

31. What are the upper age limits for giving vaccine in NIS?

Maximum age for giving vaccines in NIS for all vaccines is defined and vaccine cannot be given beyond this age:

Vaccine	Upper age limit
Hepatitis B birth dose	within 24 hours of birth
OPV 0 dose	15 days
BCG	1 year
OPV	5 years
Pentavalent 1	1 year
IPV1	1 year
MR	5 years
DPT	7 years

For pentavalent, IPV, PCV and rotavirus vaccines, if at least one dose is given before 1 year of age, then remaining doses can be administered and schedule must be completed irrespective of the age of child.

If the first dose is not administered before 1 year of age, then these vaccines cannot be administered to the child under UIP. In that case, instead of Penta, DPT 1, DPT 2 and DPT 3 is given at interval of 1 month and booster at 16 months/6 months after DPT 3 whichever is later.

32. What should be minimum gap between Pentavalent 3 and DPT booster?

Six months.

33. What should be minimum gap between IPV1 and IPV2?

Eight weeks.

34. What should be minimum gap between MRCV1 and MRCV2 if first dose is delayed?

One month.

35. What is minimum gap between two doses of JE vaccine if first dose is delayed?

Three months.

36. What is vitamin A schedule under UIP?

Vitamin A first dose (100,000 IU) is given at 9 months with MR vaccine and 2nd to 9th doses (200,000 IU) are given 6 months apart. 2nd to 9th doses can be administered to 1–5 years children during biannual rounds in collaboration with ICDS.

37. What is left out?

Left outs are those children who have never been vaccinated or reached hence remaining unimmunized. This could be because of problems of access.

38. What is drop-out?

Drop-outs are those children who started vaccination but did not complete the schedule hence are partially immunized. Due listing and tracking every child is important part of Mission Indradhanush (MI) program to reduce drop-outs.

39. What is Mission Indradhanush program of Government of India?

Mission Indradhanush was launched in December 2014 and aims at increasing the full immunization coverage to children to 90%. It focuses on pockets of low immunization coverage and hard to reach areas where the proportion of unvaccinated and partially vaccinated children is highest.

40. Which vaccines are better for children—those provided by private practitioners or those provided at the government health facilities?

All vaccines available in the country are licensed by Drug Controller General of India (DCGI). Therefore, are safe for use. Both government and private sectors procure same vaccines from government-approved and licensed manufacturers. However, complete immunization services are given to all the children and pregnant women free of cost, at government health facility.

SUGGESTED READING

1. Ministry of Health and Family Welfare. Immunization. [online] Available from: https://main.mohfw.gov.in/Organisation/Departments-of-Health-and-Family-Welfare/immunization. [Last Accessed August, 2020].
2. National Health Mission. (2018). Immunization Handbook for Medical Officers. [online] Available from: https://nhm.gov.in/New_Updates_2018/NHM_Components/Immunization/Guildelines_for_immunization/Immunization_Handbook_for_Medical_Officers%202017.pdf. [Last Accessed August, 2020].

CHAPTER 14

Vaccine Hesitancy

Chandrakant Lahariya, Dewesh Kumar

INTRODUCTION

There are a number of licensed vaccines available against nearly 30 odd pathogens. These vaccines are recommended mostly for the children but also for other age groups. Yet, not all target beneficiaries get the full benefit of the available vaccines and one of the reasons of low coverage with vaccines is emerging phenomena of vaccine hesitancy (VH). The relevance and importance of vaccines is becoming highlighted when the entire world is looking for one vaccine: the coronavirus (SARS CoV-2) vaccine to fight against the COVID-19 pandemic. The frequently asked questions (FAQs) in following sections discuss the phenomena of VH and how to tackle it.

1. What is vaccine hesitancy?

Vaccine hesitancy has been defined by the World Health Organization (WHO) Strategic Advisory Group of Experts (SAGE) working group as "delay in acceptance or refusal of vaccination despite availability of vaccination services. VH is complex and context specific, varying across time, place, and vaccines, and including factors such as complacency, convenience, and confidence".

The term "VH" has been carefully selected from various alternatives such as confidence and refusal. Hesitancy is set on a continuum between those who accept all vaccines with no doubts to a complete refusal by the vaccine-hesitant individuals, the heterogeneous group between these two extremes. VH was recognized as one of 10 global health challenges in the year 2019 by the WHO. The WHO SAGE working group identified VH on a spectrum of accept all and refuse all **(Fig. 1)**.

2. Are there different types of vaccine hesitancy?

The VH can be grouped into two broad categories: (1) "baseline" and (2) "reactive". The "baseline" VH refers to the level of refusal or delay in acceptance of vaccinations that is constantly present in the population. Though it may vary, changes are unlikely to be sudden or dramatic. On the other hand, the "reactive" VH, which often occurs because of vaccine-related events, is characterized by a rapid spike in levels of hesitancy, usually subsiding at a slow rate. This understanding of VH is required to design and implement appropriate interventions.

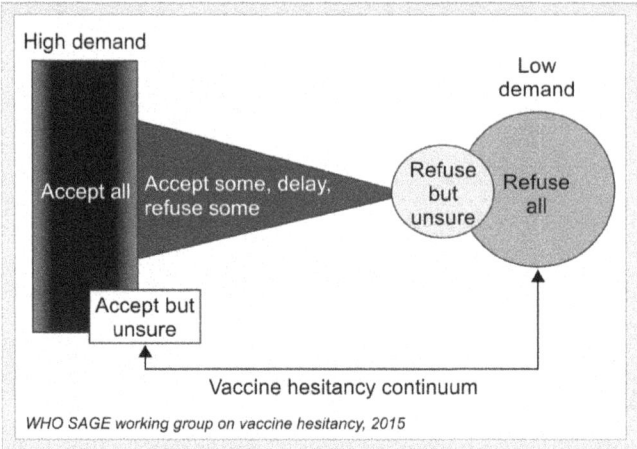

Fig. 1: Vaccine hesitancy spectrum.
Source: World Health Organization (WHO). (2014). SAGE Working Group on Vaccine Hesitancy: Summary of Findings. [online] Available from: http://origin.who.int/immunization/sage/meetings/2014/october/2_Summary_MacDonald_revised_final.pdf. [Last accessed June, 2020].

3. What are the factors which influence vaccine hesitancy?

There are a number of factors including complacency, convenience, and confidence, which contributes to VH. Vaccine complacency is known to be present where the risk of vaccine-preventable diseases is perceived to be low and where vaccination is not considered essential. It has been observed that VH is heavily impacted by lack of confidence in the vaccine's safety and efficacy as well as fears regarding the reliability and competence of health system. Additionally, the quality of vaccination services and their convenience (e.g., physical availability, geographical accessibility, and affordability) as well as the patient's willingness to pay are all factors that affect the decision of whether or not to be (or get a dependent) vaccinated. As health policymaker and the provider, we need to understand these factors, which influence VH, to address the challenges.

4. What are the characteristics of vaccine-hesitant parents?

Vaccine hesitancy is associated with perceived risk. For example, over the years, increased vaccine coverage has reduced the incidence of diseases prevented by the licensed and available vaccines. Many of the parents of current generation have not seen these diseases and often under-estimate the risk associated with these diseases. Any parent, family, and group of people could be vaccine hesitant. However, the hesitation and possible refusal for vaccines are more common among the parents who have concerns about vaccine safety or those who have underimmunized children. Yet, many parents of fully immunized children also express concerns. However, parents and families, which accept one group of vaccines, may be hesitant on other types of vaccines.

5. What is the evidence on factors which makes parents or families vaccine hesitant?

There has been research, which points that vaccine-hesitant parents tend to believe they can control their child's susceptibility to disease, have doubts about the reliability of vaccine information, or rely on herd immunity to protect their child. Studies show that some parents and physicians follow invalid contraindications such as not vaccinating a child with a mild illness (e.g., low-grade fever), leading to undervaccination. Additional characteristics that have been associated with parental hesitance include false beliefs about contraindications, not wanting to deliberately expose healthy children to potential yet minimum adverse events, exposure to negative media messages, and philosophical and religious beliefs.

6. What are the concerns of parents that result in vaccine hesitancy?

The parents have access to various sources of information including internet. These are not always reliable and trustworthy. Some of the information at times is motivated. These result in various concerns among the parents such as the vaccines are far too many given too soon or in a short period of time. Similar, parents often have heard about the use of preservative as an additive in vaccines, e.g., thimerosal. Some parents have expressed concerns about a potential link between health problems, particularly autism and vaccines containing thimerosal. Thimerosal is a preservative that contains a form of mercury (organomercurial). However, there is no evidence that thimerosal in vaccine results in any side effect.

7. Is vaccine hesitancy a new phenomenon?

The reluctance, low acceptance, and refusal have been part of vaccination history since availability of smallpox vaccine. When smallpox vaccine reached India in early 19th century, contrary to what should have happened that people should have demanded for vaccine, the uptake was very low and a section of society was not willing to get vaccinated. The philosophical and religious grounds were used to refuse vaccines and vaccination. As early as in 1879, the Anti-Vaccination Society of America was formed. Soon thereafter, Europe witnessed an anti-vaccination movement which is still active in different forms. In present time, the anti-vaccination movements can be found worldwide. The modern resistance is considered to have started with isolated reports of resistance to smallpox vaccination (around the 1960), for whole-cell pertussis vaccine (in 1970s), and then during the years of polio elimination period (from 1990s onward). VH and refusal became a bigger global challenge when a falsified paper was published linking measles, mumps, and rubella (MMR) vaccine and autism **(Box 1)**. The paper was later on retracted; however, by then, it caused decline in vaccine coverage and outbreaks were reported from many countries, which had nearly eliminated the diseases. The anti-vaccine group received a flip and boost by these reports. The social media, with unvaried sources at times, has also contributed to rise in VH in recent years.

> **BOX 1:** A falsified paper on vaccine side effect which shook faith of people in vaccines.
>
> A falsified research paper published in The Lancet in 1998, which wrongly concluded an association between measles, mumps, and rubella (MMR) vaccine and autism (later retracted by the journal and the authors discredited), did an irreparable damage to the global immunization efforts. As an immediate fallout, measles and rubella vaccine coverage started to decline in many countries in Europe and Americas. The voices of opponents of vaccines became louder and reach amplified by social media platforms with some sort of false legitimacy. This has resulted in decreased coverage for many vaccines with most visible impact on measles and rubella vaccines. During this period, there was an increase of up to 30% measles cases in some parts of the world. A few countries, which were close to elimination, had faced resurgence. Keeping the vaccination coverage high is very essential in current times and being threatened by the reduced confidence or opposition of the vaccines along with what is being now termed as "vaccine hesitancy" which has become a constant and steady threat to immunization programs.

8. What are the status and challenges in vaccine hesitancy in India?

The issue of VH is even bigger challenge for country such as India where coverage with vaccines has traditionally been low. The polio elimination program in India faced many challenges and social mobilization was an integral part of program to increase acceptance and coverage. The measles catch-up campaign from 2010 to 2013 and then 2017 onward—the measles-rubella (MR) vaccination campaigns in a number of Indian states faced similar opposition and challenges. Though, a small number but very organized group of people opposing vaccines had some success in spreading the myths about vaccines.

9. What are the common factors contributing to vaccine hesitancy in India?

As part of polio elimination efforts as well as efforts to increase coverage of vaccines in routine immunization program, a number of studies on vaccine refusal and opposition have been conducted to understand the phenomenon and take corrective actions. A study in two states (Uttar Pradesh and Jharkhand) of India in 2015–2017 found that lack of confidence in a vaccine or a provider, apprehension—about the side effects of the vaccine, lack of full understanding of value the vaccines, and complacency—do not perceive a need for a vaccine were key factors behind low uptake of various vaccines in India. Another research paper published in December 2018, listed hesitancy as an important barrier to vaccination in India. It reported that 31% children remained undervaccinated in selected districts and hesitancy-related factors accounted for 80% of the reasons for missing vaccination among the undervaccinated. The authors of that paper noted that social media platforms aided the rapid dissemination of false beliefs and rumors contributing to hesitancy. The resistance though was localized and context specific; though often reinforced by local social and community connections. The ethnicity and faith-based perceptions informed the lack of trust in vaccine safety, usefulness, and efficacy in some pockets.

10. Why vaccine hesitancy is a challenge for everyone?

Vaccination stands among the most effective measures ever accomplished by medical intervention; however, this is seriously endangered by the growing phenomena of VH, which has become of growing public health challenge. Lack of trust in vaccines is a threat to the success of vaccination programs. VH is believed to be responsible for decreasing vaccine coverage and an increasing risk of vaccine-preventable disease outbreaks and epidemics. Moreover, when coverage go low, the indirect benefit of vaccination—known as herd immunity—results in protection in unprotected individuals—is also reduced. In 2019, the WHO listed VH as one of the 10 threats to public health at global level.

11. How the vaccine hesitancy can be addressed?

Considering the wide prevalence of VH and its actual and future impact on immunization program, there is need for developing appropriate strategy to tackle the challenge. These include communication strategies and trainings of healthcare professionals dealing with vaccination **(Box 2)**, vaccine champions and engagement of religious or other influential leaders to promote vaccination in the community, social mobilization, optimal use of mass media, improving convenience and access to vaccination, employing reminder and follow-up, communications training for healthcare workers,

---

BOX 2: Vaccine hesitancy (VH) communication: A few principles.

Communication is an important strategy in tackling VH. It needs to follow a few basic principles:
- *A balance of content versus process*: The evidence base for VH communication is generally confined to research focused on the content of the message rather than the process of communication. This has important consequences because shifting focus to encompass the process of communicating, and not just on the content of message being conveyed, opens the possibility of greater insight and understanding regarding the conversation of healthcare workers with those who are vaccine hesitant, creating increased chances of acceptance.
- *Reframing of vaccine communication*: While continuing to provide evidence on the efficacy and safety of vaccines, a reframing of vaccine communication that focuses on the positive, emotional values of immunizations could be more effective. This change of perspective requires a strong opening to multidisciplinary collaboration. New and possibly disruptive information strategies can arise from the cross-fertilization among clinicians, vaccine researchers, behavioral scientists, journalists, and communication experts. There is need for focus on how vaccines impact on a person's life, not exclusively in clinical terms, but through the invisible values they generate. Starting from a concept (the positive emotional values of vaccines), the message is spread through different channels (TV, web, social media, radio, etc.) and using different formats (images, videos, infographics, etc.).
- *Regular monitoring of media*: The media news influence shapes the public sentiments and behavior. The recent experiences indicate significant influence of online news and social media on immunization behavior in India. A sizable proportion of news contained negative messages, which may influence public vaccine behavior. Past experiences (pentavalent and measles-rubella) call for regular monitoring of media messages and adopt appropriate communication strategy to retain vaccine confidence and reduce vaccine hesitancy. According to a recently published study on vaccine news in online mass media; measles-rubella vaccine topped the news (23.5%) followed by poliomyelitis (10.4%) and Japanese encephalitis (6.6%) vaccines. While 65.8% of news was positive, 27.9% and 6.35% were negative and neutral, respectively. The negative news comprised of the adverse events, social resistance, vaccine shortage, etc.

> **BOX 3:** Communities, health systems strengthening, and suitable policies can help in tackling VH.
>
> *Communities*: It has been amply documented that VH is dependent upon social norm, which mandates that to tackle the issue effectively; there is essential need to engage with communities and shape the social norms. The evidence-based social and behavioral change activities focus on improving community awareness and knowledge, creating and continually reinforcing positive social norms toward immunization, as well as providing individualized reminders on where/when to go for services and timely motivational "nudges" (e.g., through positive messaging and motivational content through SMS, social media, and interpersonal communication) to help bridge the "intention to action" gap.
>
> *Systems strengthening*: Strengthening various components of health systems such as capacity building of providers in vaccines and translating their messages in compelling ones can help. Providers themselves must also be confident in vaccine safety and efficacy and translate this confidence into a strong recommendation, as a physician's recommendation is frequently cited as the reason parents choose to vaccinate their children. The capacity building should be sufficiently broad based, extending beyond public providers to include pediatric associations and other similar professional groups. Similarly, setting up reliable and public repository of immunization education and evidence would help. Having reliable, trustworthy resources readily available for the providers can help them have their own concerns answered. Education material, in layman language, can also be prepared and shared with parents.
>
> *Policies*: The health policy formulation and involvement of the professional association in these processes are key influencer of VH. The process for policy formulation and adoption could be more transparent and evidence informed. There has to be consistency and continuity in public health policy formulation, especially in federal system, where state governments are key player, their engagement in policy process affects the end outcome. Decision-making processes should be transparent and evidence-based, informed by the recommendations of National Immunization Technical Advisory Groups (NITAGs) or the local equivalent. Civil society organizations can play a key role in channeling information on public needs and priorities to the relevant subnational and national policy and decision-making levels.

(VH: vaccine hesitancy; SMS: short message service)

and actions to increase knowledge, awareness about vaccination. In addition, the strategies targeted at communities, health systems strengthening, and formulation of appropriate policies can contribute to addressing VH **(Box 3)**.

12. What role individual practitioners and professional associations can play in addressing vaccine hesitancy?

The professional association of doctors, nurses, and private sector providers play a key role in addressing VH by sharing the knowledge about vaccines, building capacity of the providers in handling VH, and ensuring effective communication. Removing the conflict of interests in vaccine policy and recommendations can ensure tackling the VH. This need sustained engagement and efforts.

13. What are the ways forward to tackle vaccine hesitancy (VH) in India?

The VH is a widely recognized in India and other parts of the world. Experts worldwide acknowledge that VH is a growing global challenge aggravated by vaccines-related rumors and (mis)information, at times, amplified by various types, including social, media. The individuals unsure about vaccination since the first vaccines were made available, but hesitancy is a relatively new phenomenon. In India, public health system now fully recognizes "VH". The experiences from measles and now MR campaigns have contributed to understanding of VH in India. The determinants of VH are known, the possible strategies have been documented, and there are learning from various initiatives. The stage is fully set to effectively tackle VH to reap the maximum benefit of available vaccines for all age groups. The recognition of problem is first step toward solution and that has been done for the challenge of VH. The earlier sections in this chapter as well as boxes provide information on how to tackle VH in India. This knowledge and understanding would be even more relevant as coronavirus (SARS CoV-2) vaccine would be available. The learnings would be useful for preventing the pandemic as well as to get maximum benefit from licensed vaccines for all age groups. The situation demands continuous efforts to ensure that benefit of proven and safe vaccines continue to reach each and every person/child, everywhere in the world, today, tomorrow, and all the years ahead.

SUGGESTED READING

1. Dubé E, Vivion M, MacDonald NE. Vaccine hesitancy, vaccine refusal and the anti-vaccine movement: influence, impact and implications. Exp Rev Vaccines. 2015;14:99-117.
2. Dubé E, Laberge C, Guay M, Bramadat P, Roy R, Bettinger J. Vaccine hesitancy: an overview. Hum Vaccin Immunother. 2013;9:1763-73.
3. Gowda C, Dempsey AF. The rise (and fall?) of parental vaccine hesitancy. Hum Vaccin Immunother. 2013;9:1755-62.
4. Kumar D, Chandra R, Mathur M, Samdariya S, Kapoor N. Vaccine hesitancy: understanding better to address better. Isr J Health Policy Res. 2016;5:2.
5. Lahariya C. A brief history of vaccines and vaccination in India. Indian J Med Res. 2014;139:491-511.
6. Larson HJ, Jarrett C, Eckersberger E, Smith DMD, Paterson P. Understanding vaccine hesitancy around vaccines and vaccination from a global perspective: a systematic review of published literature, 2007–2012. Vaccine. 2014;32:2150-9.
7. Spier RE. Perception of risk of vaccine adverse events: a historical perspective. Vaccine. 2001;20:S78-84.
8. World Health Organization (WHO). (2014). SAGE Working Group on Vaccine Hesitancy: Summary of Findings. [online] Available from: http://origin.who.int/immunization/sage/meetings/2014/october/2_Summary_MacDonald_revised_final.pdf. [Last accessed June, 2020].

SECTION 2

Licensed Vaccines

15. **Bacillus Calmette-Guérin Vaccine**
    Vipin M Vashishtha, A Parthasarathy, Hitt Sharma
16. **Polio Vaccines**
    Naveen Thacker, Prem Pal Singh, Vipin M Vashishtha
17. **Diphtheria, Tetanus and Pertussis Vaccines**
    Vipin M Vashishtha, Unmesh A Upadhyay
18. **Measles Vaccines**
    Baldev S Prajapati, Arun Wadhwa
19. **Measles, Mumps and Rubella Vaccines**
    Arun Wadhwa, Baldev S Prajapati, Sudhir Kumar Choudhary
20. **Hepatitis B Vaccines**
    Ajay Kalra, Sanjay Verma
21. **Hepatitis A Vaccines**
    Arun Wadhwa, Nigam P Narain
22. **Varicella Vaccines**
    Vijay N Yewale, Dhanya Dharmapalan
23. **Typhoid Vaccines**
    Chandra Mohan Kumar, Vipin M Vashishtha, Ajay Kalra
24. *Haemophilus influenzae* **Type B Vaccines**
    Jaydeep Choudhury
25. **Pneumococcal Diseases Vaccines**
    Shobha Sharma, Neha Goel
26. **Rabies Vaccines**
    Omesh Kumar Bharti, Jaydeep Choudhury, Vipin M Vashishtha
27. **Japanese Encephalitis Vaccines**
    Vipin M Vashishtha, Chandra Mohan Kumar
28. **Rotavirus Vaccines**
    Rakesh Bhatia
29. **Human Papillomavirus Vaccines**
    Jaydeep Choudhury, Srinivas G Kasi
30. **Influenza Vaccines**
    Sanjay Srirampur, Pritesh Nagar, Vipin M Vashishtha
31. **Meningococcal Vaccines**
    Parang N Mehta
32. **Cholera Vaccines**
    Nupur Ganguly
33. **Dengue Vaccines**
    Dipti Agarwal
34. **Malaria Vaccines**
    Abhay K Shah
35. **Combination Vaccines**
    Ashok K Dutta
36. **Yellow Fever Vaccines**
    Chandra Mohan Kumar, Obeid Shafi, Shweta Singh
37. **Ebola Vaccines**
    Arun Wadhwa

CHAPTER 15

Bacillus Calmette-Guérin Vaccine

Vipin M Vashishtha, A Parthasarathy, Hitt Sharma

1. What are the key characteristics of Bacillus Calmette-Guérin (BCG) vaccine?

Bacillus Calmette-Guérin (BCG) is a live attenuated, bacterial vaccine. It contains 0.1–0.4 million live viable bacilli of *Mycobacterium bovis* per dose. The vaccine is very light sensitive. The dose is 0.1 mL intradermal (ID) at insertion of left deltoid. It is modestly effective against pulmonary tuberculosis (TB) (around 50%), but highly efficacious (around 75–86%) against severe disseminated types of TB, the meningeal [tuberculous meningitis (TBM)] and miliary TB.

2. When should one administer Bacillus Calmette-Guérin (BCG) vaccine? What is the current recommendation on administration of BCG?

Bacillus Calmette-Guérin has been recommended at birth in countries with a high TB burden for decades. The World Health Organization (WHO) in its recent position paper has strongly emphasized administration at birth. BCG at birth provides protection in the early years when infection can often lead to devastating widespread disease such as miliary TB or TBM. This is particularly important in high prevalence countries where the chance of being infected in very early life is high. Reducing delays and increasing coverage at birth would substantially reduce global pediatric TB mortality. BCG vaccination at birth is the main component of ongoing "End TB Strategy". Accordingly, it is estimated that high global coverage (90%) and widespread use of the vaccine in vaccination programs could prevent over 115,000 TB deaths per birth cohort in the first 15 years of life.

3. What is the status of Bacillus Calmette-Guérin (BCG) administration rates in different countries? Does a late administration have any deleterious effect on tuberculosis (TB) burden?

Currently, 152 low and middle-income countries (LMICs) have a policy of universal neonatal vaccination at birth or in the first week of life. In these 152 high-burden countries, the estimated BCG coverage in 2016 was 37% at 1 week of age, 67% at 6 weeks of age, and 92% at 3 years of age. According to a recent modeling study (2019), 92% BCG coverage at birth can reduce TB deaths in the global birth cohort by 5,449 or 2.8% by age 15 years and 100% coverage at birth reduced TB deaths by 16.5%.

Later administration increases TB deaths, e.g., BCG vaccination at 6 weeks, the recommended age of diphtheria, tetanus, and pertussis 1 (DTP1) increased TB deaths by 0.2% (0–0.4%), even if BCG reached DTP1 coverage levels (94% at 3 years). Hence, it is of utmost importance to administer BCG at birth.

4. When can we give Bacillus Calmette-Guérin (BCG) vaccine to a newborn who did not receive the same at birth?

Ideally, the BCG should be given at birth or as soon as possible after birth. If the opportunity to give BCG is not available in the neonatal period, it may be given at 6 weeks simultaneously with diphtheria, pertussis, and tetanus (DPT) vaccine and oral polio vaccine (OPV). It is to be given to all children as a part of Expanded Program on Immunization (EPI) schedule.

5. Can we give Bacillus Calmette-Guérin (BCG) vaccine to a preterm/low birth weight (LBW) newborn or should we wait for 2 months or till the baby gains 2 kg weight?

Till quite recently, the common practice was to defer BCG till 34 weeks of age. But now studies are available that show it is safe to administer after 30-week stable newborn infants. According to a recent systematic review and meta-analysis (JAMA Pediatr, 2019), no increase in adverse reactions or infant mortality after BCG vaccination within 7 days of birth was found when compared with vaccination delayed after 7 days in clinically stable infants who were preterm and/or had low birth weight. Meta-analysis revealed no differences for scar formation or tuberculin skin test (TST) conversion. So, currently, evidence from clinically stable infants who were born after >30 weeks' gestational age and/or weighing >1.5 kg seems to support BCG vaccination within 7 days of birth.

Early BCG vaccination of low birth weight infants weighing down to ~1,500 g has a beneficial effect on overall infant mortality as reported from randomized controlled studies conducted in the high TB endemic setting in West Africa. A normal infant dose of BCG should be administered and revaccination is not required.

6. If Bacillus Calmette-Guérin (BCG) is not administered at birth or early infancy, till what age it can be given?

In India, the catch-up vaccination with BCG is recommended till 5 years of age. The WHO estimated that approximately 253,000 children <15 years died from TB in the year 2016. It is estimated that the majority of childhood TB deaths occurred in children younger than 5 years.

7. Live vaccines are more susceptible to maternal antibodies as compared to killed vaccines. Then, why Bacillus Calmette-Guérin (BCG) is given at birth?

Although maternal antibodies interfere with the induction of infant antibody responses, they may allow a certain degree of priming. However, antibodies of maternal origin do not exert their inhibitory influence on infant T-cell responses, which remain largely unaffected or even enhanced. This is best explained by the fate of maternal antibodies-vaccine antigen complexes: immune complexes are taken up by macrophages and dendritic cells, dissociate into their acidic phagolysosome compartment, and are processed into small peptides. These peptides are displayed at the surface of antigen-presenting cells, thus available for binding by CD4+ and CD8+ T cells. BCG may be given as the maternal antibodies that actually enhance T-cell responses.

8. **Mother has come with baby girl aged 6 months for hepatitis B vaccination. On examination of baby, there is no Bacillus Calmette-Guérin (BCG) scar (nothing visible/palpable at BCG vaccination site at left upper arm). However, mother vividly recalls BCG inoculation and having seen a small boil at BCG injection site at 6–7 weeks of age. The family pediatrician does not believe this and repeats BCG injection. Is this possible? Visible BCG takes up at 6 weeks and followed by no scar at 6 months!**

Yes, possible. It is a well-established but poorly documented BCG reaction called "abortive reaction". BCG gives a characteristic local reaction. A sequence of changes has been described after a correct ID injection of a potent vaccine. 2–3 weeks after vaccination, a papule develops at the site of vaccination, which slowly increases in size and reaches a diameter of approximately 4–8 mm in about 5 weeks. It then ulcerates and healing occurs spontaneously within 6–12 weeks leaving a permanent tiny round scar.

In 9.9% of infants, the papule or pustule developed at 6–10 weeks after BCG vaccination, but disappeared at 14 weeks and did not leave any scar at the vaccination site. This phenomenon has been termed as "abortive reaction". Abortive reaction lowered the BCG reaction rate at 12 weeks by 8% as compared to the observations at 8 weeks in that study.

In a recent study, abortive reaction has been seen in 3.2% of twin babies as well. It has been mentioned that a pustule may heal with ulcer formation or may subside. Abortive reaction appears to be of clinical significance because scar failure has been termed as unsuccessful vaccination and revaccination is recommended. The classic description of sequence following BCG vaccination is of a papule or pustule, which ulcerates and culminates in scar formation. At times, the reaction may be arrested at the stage of papule or pustule, which may disappear without scar formation. There is a paucity of literature on whether abortive reaction is a manifestation of local BCG reaction like papule, pustule, ulcer, scab, and scar formation.

9. **Should abortive reactors be considered immunized?**

Evidences like positive in vitro leukocyte migration inhibition test (LMIT) and positive purified protein derivative (PPD) response in babies with scar failure are strong pointers that these infants may have developed immunity to BCG. Further studies are required to evaluate the immunization status of abortive reactors. Babies showing abortive reaction after BCG reaction should be, therefore, considered different from nonreactors where no local reaction has taken place. All healthcare providers and vaccinologists should be sensitized that abortive reaction is one of the local reactions after BCG vaccination. Hence, local BCG reaction may be described as papule, pustule, ulcer, scab, scar, and abortive reaction.

10. **What is the significance of scar formation? If the baby does not develop a scar after Bacillus Calmette-Guérin (BCG) vaccination, what to do? Should we repeat BCG, if scar is not formed?**

There is no specific association of scar formation and added protection against TB. However, recently in few studies, it has been observed that presence of scar may increase the beneficial "nonspecific effects" (NSEs) of BCG **(Fig. 1)**.

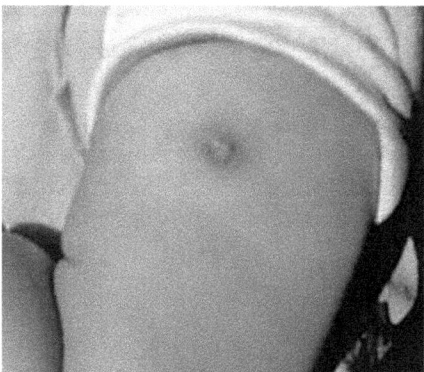

Fig. 1: Bacillus Calmette-Guérin (BCG) scar at left deltoid.

Correct vaccine administration technique by a trained health worker is important to ensure correct dosage and optimal BCG vaccine efficacy and safety. BCG vaccination usually causes a scar at the site of injection due to local inflammatory processes. The presence of a scar is a sign of BCG vaccination. However, scar formation is not a marker for protection and approximately 10% of vaccine recipients do not develop a scar. The absence of a BCG scar after vaccination is not indicative of lack of protection. Studies have shown minimal or no evidence of any additional benefit of repeat BCG vaccination against TB or leprosy. Therefore, revaccination is not recommended even if the TST reaction or result of an interferon-γ release assay (IGRA) is negative.

11. **Few expert associations advice revaccination if scar fails to appear after 3 months of vaccination. Should we follow this guideline? For how long should one wait to see scar formation?**

It has been seen that onset and completion of local BCG reaction may be delayed and scar formation may not occur by 12 weeks of vaccination. It may take 6 months or longer. In a recent study on local BCG reaction in low birth weight and normal birth weight babies, the scar formation was reported in 47.2% infants at 14 weeks, although other stages of local reaction were present. Simultaneous administration of OPV was suggested to be responsible for delayed completion of local BCG reaction. The health worker should be aware that scar formation after vaccination may take 6 months or more. In about 10% of infants, scar formation may not occur after BCG vaccination. So, it would be reasonable to repeat BCG after 6 months of vaccination if no scar is formed.

12. **A 4-month-old girl is presented to you with a swelling in left axilla, which is progressively increasing in size. No constitutional symptoms were present. Fine-needle aspiration cytology (FNAC) was done and report was suggestive of tubercular lymphadenitis with demonstration of Mycobacteria. The lymph node had become fluctuant in next 2–3 days (Fig. 2).**
    - Was there a need for doing FNAC?
    - What treatment do you suggest for this lymph node?
    - Should antitubercular therapy (ATT) be started in this case?

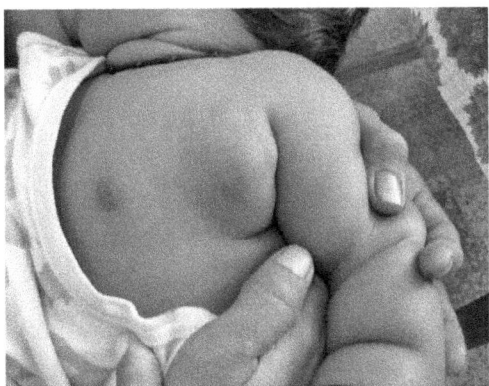

Fig. 2: Left-sided axillary lymph node after Bacillus Calmette-Guérin (BCG) vaccination (BCG adenitis).

Subcutaneous administration of BCG is associated with an increased incidence of BCG adenitis. The injected site usually shows no visible change for several days. Subsequently, a papule develops after 2–3 weeks, which increases to a size of 4–8 mm by the end of 5–6 weeks. This papule often heals with ulceration and results in a scar after 6–12 weeks. The ulcer at vaccination site may persist for a few weeks before formation of the final scar. No treatment is required for this condition. Considering this natural reaction following BCG vaccination, fine-needle aspiration cytology (FNAC) was not needed.

Ipsilateral axillary/cervical lymphadenopathy may develop a few weeks/months after BCG vaccination. Antitubercular therapy (ATT) is of no benefit in such situations and should not be administered. The nodes regress spontaneously after a few months. Secondary infection at the vaccination site may require antimicrobials.

It should also be noted that if FNAC of the nodes is carried out, stain for acid-fast bacilli may be positive. These are bovine vaccine bacilli and should not be misconstrued as being suggestive of tuberculous disease. In some children, the nodes may even liquefy and result in an abscess.

Surgical removal of the nodes or repeated needle aspiration is the treatment of choice; again, ATT is not recommended **(Box 1)**.

BOX 1: Management of Bacillus Calmette-Guérin (BCG) adenitis.

Medical:
- No role for antibiotics like erythromycin
- Antituberculous drugs too are ineffective
- Risk of adverse drug reactions

Needle aspiration:
- Recommended for suppurative BCG lymphadenitis
- Prevents discharge and associated complications
- Shortens the duration of healing
- Safe

Surgical excision:
- Risk of general anesthesia
- Useful in cases with failed needle aspiration, multiloculated or matted lymph nodes, and draining sinuses

---

13. Is there any benefit of scar formation?

Yes, the NSEs of BCG vaccine are greater when there is a scar. Although, the presence of scar does not provide any added benefits against TB and revaccination with BCG confers little or no extra protection against TB, but it may increase the beneficial NSEs of BCG. According to a study, it was found that infants who had received BCG–Moscow vaccine, those with a scar had a 52% lower mortality rate than those with no scar.

14. Does oral polio vaccine (OPV) administration affect scar rates? Is there any difference if Bacillus Calmette-Guérin (BCG) and OPV administered simultaneously or separately at different intervals?

Simultaneous administration of BCG vaccine with trivalent OPV to term infants in early neonatal period prolongs the time of scar formation, but sequence of local reaction is not affected. Sequence of local BCG reaction may be described as papule, pustule, ulcer, scab, scar, and abortive reaction. An observational study from Guinea-Bissau suggested that OPV at birth (OPV0) provided with BCG vaccine was associated with downregulation of the immune response to BCG vaccine 6 weeks later. Receiving OPV^{0} + BCG versus BCG alone was associated with significantly lower prevalence of IFN-γ responses to PPD and reduced interleukin-5 (IL-5) to PPD. Hence, it can be said that OPV attenuates the immune response to coadministered BCG at birth.

15. How does Bacillus Calmette-Guérin (BCG) elicit its antituberculosis (TB) effects?

Bacillus Calmette-Guérin vaccine mainly works through induction of cell-mediated immunity whereas almost all other childhood vaccines offer protection primarily through induction of humoral immunity, i.e., production of antibodies.

Even after almost 100 years of its invention, it is still a mystery how exactly the BCG vaccine works. It would be ironic if we were to discover that BCG protects against TB via an "NSE" mediated by innate immunity.

16. Why Bacillus Calmette-Guérin (BCG) fails to fully protect against pulmonary tuberculosis (TB)?

It could be due to coinfections (e.g., helminths, EM, etc.) preventing the full development of immune responses in the lung or discrepancies between immune responses at the site of vaccine administration versus the natural route of *Mycobacterium tuberculosis (Mtb)* infection through the lungs. Perhaps it is not because BCG is poor at generating effective immune responses, but that the immunosuppressive status of the lung prevents it from doing so. A major question remains: Is BCG poor at stimulating mycobacterial immunity or is *Mtb* simply adept at avoiding immunological responses against it?

17. How can Bacillus Calmette-Guérin (BCG) be made more immunogenic?

Bacillus Calmette-Guérin could be at its saturation point and thus further stimulation of the immune system would yield no added immunity. The answer could simply lie in shifting research efforts toward a more immunogenic route of vaccination. The literature suggests that intranasal and/or intratracheal vaccination with BCG is a more effective method to develop immunity against *Mtb*, yet no human studies have been published on this matter, mainly due to increase in pathology observed in the lungs using this delivery method. Thus, finding a way to decrease this inflammation in the lungs may open new avenues to explore direct mucosal vaccine delivery into the lungs. Efforts directed at exploring immunological events that occur following intranasal/intratracheal BCG vaccination and the status of immune cells within the lung could yield valuable answers in doing so.

18. There are reports that the Bacillus Calmette-Guérin (BCG) can be given intravenous (IV). Is this report correct? What is the exact status?

Very recently, an animal study in Rhesus monkeys has shown that the BCG vaccine has provided almost complete protection when injected intravenously.

The researchers have shown that IV administration of BCG profoundly alters the protective outcome of *Mtb* challenge in nonhuman primates (*Macaca mulatta*). Compared with ID or aerosol delivery, IV immunization induced substantially more antigen responsive CD4+ and CD8+ T-cell responses in blood, spleen, bronchoalveolar lavage, and lung lymph nodes. Moreover, IV immunization induced a high frequency of antigen-responsive T cells across all lung parenchymal tissues. 6 months after BCG vaccination, macaques were challenged with virulent *Mtb*. Notably, nine out of 10 macaques that received IV BCG vaccination were highly protected, with six macaques showing no detectable levels of infection, as determined by positron emission tomography (PET) scans imaging, mycobacterial growth, pathology, and granuloma formation. The finding that IV BCG prevents or substantially limits *Mtb* infection in highly susceptible rhesus macaques has important implications for vaccine delivery and clinical development and provides a model for defining immune correlates and mechanisms of vaccine-elicited protection against TB.

19. Does Bacillus Calmette-Guérin (BCG) provide other positive effects on other diseases apart from protection against tuberculosis (TB)?

Bacillus Calmette-Guérin is only moderately efficacious against pulmonary TB, but it is known to provide "NSEs" (heterologous) protection against certain respiratory infections and sepsis caused by viruses (e.g., vaccinia virus, herpes, and influenza), bacteria (e.g., *Shigella flexneri*), and protozoa (e.g., malaria). These positive NSEs are noticed in both developing and developed countries. In Guinea-Bissau, vaccination with BCG reduced neonatal mortality in low birth weight babies by 48%. In Spain, the BCG vaccine reduced non-TB hospital admissions in infants by 32% for respiratory infections and by 53% for sepsis. Additionally, it has been shown that BCG vaccination was responsible for the reduction of all-cause mortality by approximately 50% among under 5-year-old children.

Additionally, it has been shown that BCG administration enhances immune responses of other vaccines like hepatitis B, poliovirus type 1, inactivated polio vaccine (IPV), and pneumococcal conjugate vaccines (PCVs), with significantly higher production of antibodies.

20. Can Bacillus Calmette-Guérin (BCG) also helps in cases of severe neonatal sepsis?

Yes, the BCG can also help in severe cases of neonatal sepsis by promoting granulocytosis. According to a new trial, within 3 days of administration, the BCG vaccination can reduce mortality from neonatal sepsis in human newborns. However, the underlying mechanism for this rapid protection is unknown. In animal studies, it was found that BCG was also protective in a mouse model of neonatal polymicrobial sepsis, where it induced granulocyte colony-stimulating factor (G-CSF) within hours of administration. This was necessary and sufficient to drive emergency granulopoiesis (EG), resulting in a marked increase in neutrophils. This increase in neutrophils was directly and quantitatively responsible for protection from sepsis.

21. What are the World Health Organization (WHO) views on these nonspecific effects (NSEs) of Bacillus Calmette-Guérin (BCG) vaccines?

Most of the studies on NSEs of BCG were done by Abay P et al. mainly in Guinea-Bissau. Some of these studies were observational, nonrandomized with questionable methodology, hence, with low-level evidence. The WHO had also reviewed these trials and concluded that BCG appeared to lower overall mortality in children, but graded the evidence as "low". It suggested the need for more randomized trials to demonstrate these effects. It was only after a few recent studies mainly by Netea MG et al. that provided evidence on the NSEs of the BCG through human studies with the explanatory mechanism.

22. Does Bacillus Calmette-Guérin (BCG) have nonspecific effects (NSEs) in adults also?

Bacillus Calmette-Guérin is found useful in many non-TB conditions of adults also. This vaccine has been licensed for the treatment of superficial bladder cancer, for which it also exerts NSEs. Thus far, it has not been surpassed by any other drug in terms of its ability to reduce disease recurrence and progression. BCG has also been shown to be useful in some autoimmune disorders such as insulin-dependent diabetes mellitus (IDDM) and multiple sclerosis. In a study from Harvard Medical School, adults with long-standing type 1 diabetes showed a remarkable recovery of serum hemoglobin A1c (HbA1c) levels to near normal with no episodes of severe hypoglycemia at the end of 3 years which remained stable for the next 5 years. Some observational studies suggest that BCG vaccination is associated with some protection against allergies, eczema, and asthma, although these findings have been inconsistent. Additionally, BCG has also been shown to be associated with protection against melanoma and may play a role in its treatment. Recently, a retrospective review has shown a lower risk of development of lung cancer among those who had received BCG vaccination during childhood.

23. How does Bacillus Calmette-Guérin (BCG) produce nonspecific effects (NSEs)?

Unlike the "adaptive" immunity, the "innate" immune system is supposed to have no memory responses. But BCG, which can remain alive in the human skin for up to several months, triggers not only *Mycobacterium*-specific memory B and T cells but also stimulates the cells of the innate system (monocytes, neutrophils, macrophages, natural killer, dendritic cells, etc.) for a prolonged period. The process by which BCG imparts immune memory to the innate system is known as "trained innate immunity" which in turn is elicited by a phenomenon known as "epigenetic effect" **(Fig. 3)**.

24. What do you mean by "epigenetic effects" and "trained immunity"?

The "epigenetic effect" is produced by the modification of gene expression rather than alteration of the genetic code or nucleotide sequencing. This effect is brought about by two main mechanisms, deoxyribonucleic acid (DNA) methylation and histone modifications that alter innate immunity.

Bacillus Calmette-Guérin does epigenetic reprogramming in the training of innate cells, particularly monocytes. Upon pathogen X recognition by a receptor, "naïve" monocytes undergo epigenetic reprogramming and a metabolic shift and convert into "trained" monocytes, primed to respond more vigorously to nonspecific (pathogens X, Y, and Z) secondary stimulation.

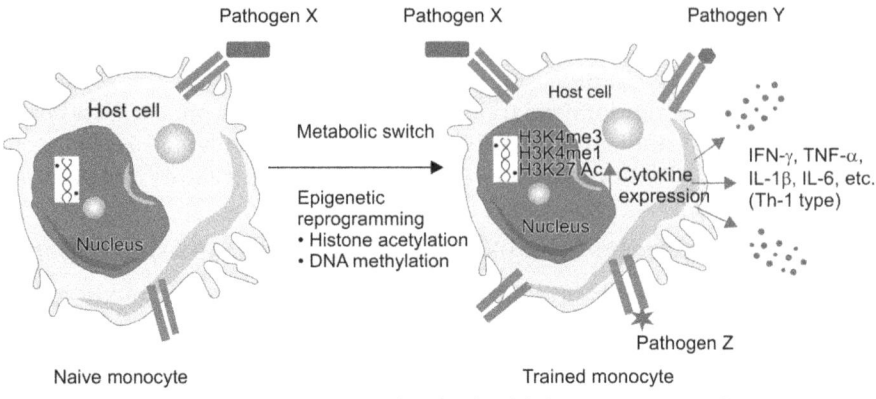

Fig. 3: "Trained innate immunity"—epigenetic reprogramming of monocytes. Upon pathogen X recognition by a receptor, naïve monocytes undergo epigenetic reprogramming and a metabolic shift and become primed to respond more robustly to nonspecific (pathogens X, Y, and Z) secondary stimulation.

(DNA: deoxyribonucleic acid; IFN-γ: interferon-γ; IL-6: interleukin-6; TNF-α: tumor necrosis factor-α)

Unlike antigen-specific memory of the adaptive immune system, the second stimulation does not have to be with the same pathogen or antigen. Later on, these "trained" monocytes have a significantly higher production of several proinflammatory cytokines [like interferon-γ (IFN-γ), tumor necrosis factor-α (TNF-α)], interleukins (IL-1β, IL-6, etc.) upon heterologous challenges, particularly T-helper cell type 1 polarizing and typically monocyte-derived proinflammatory cytokines that help in rapid clearance of infection **(Figs. 3 to 6)**. These modified, activated, and "trained" cells can be stimulated by various nonrelated infectious (viruses, bacteria, fungi, and their components, parasites) or noninfectious agents such as nanoparticles which lead to potent immune memory responses. This response explains the BCGs nonspecific protection against sepsis, pneumonia, and other pathogens. Both epigenetic changes and increased nonspecific immune responses could be detected up to 1 year after BCG vaccination.

25. What are the different strains of Bacillus Calmette-Guérin (BCG)? Do they differ in their efficacy against tuberculosis (TB)? Do different strains of Bacillus Calmette-Guérin (BCG) have different scar formation rates?

The World Health Organization-approved strains of BCG are BCG-Danish, BCG-Tokyo, and BCG-Moscow. Although, there are several more stains that were produced and used earlier. In Kazakhstan, vaccination of neonates reduced the risk of clinically diagnosed TB by 69% after BCG-Tokyo vaccination, by 43% after BCG-Serbia, and only by 22% after BCG-Moscow.

In addition to the important genetic differences between the strains of BCG, there are genetic differences within some strains that can cause major

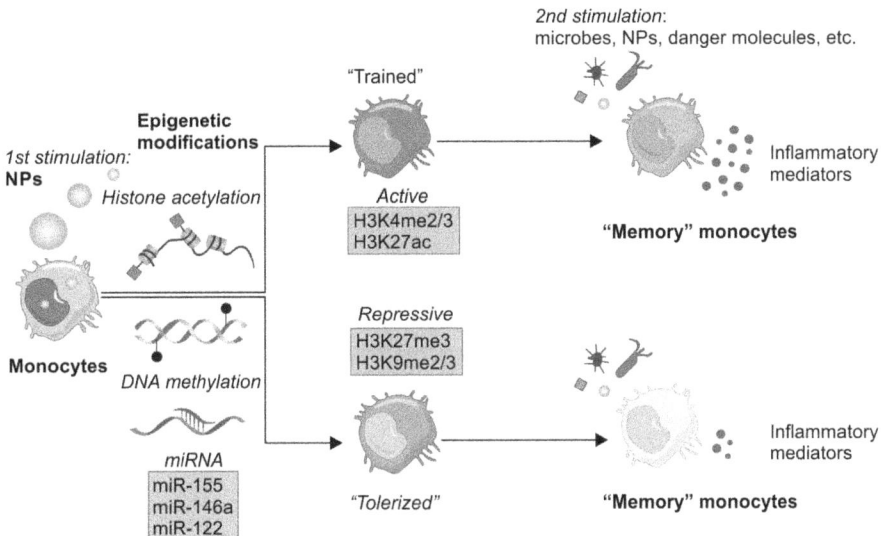

Fig. 4: "Trained innate immunity" (epigenetic reprogramming of monocytes). Nanoparticles (NPs) as possible inducers of innate immune memory. Schematic representation of the putative mechanism of innate memory induction by NPs.
(DNA: deoxyribonucleic acid; miRNA: micro ribonucleic acid)

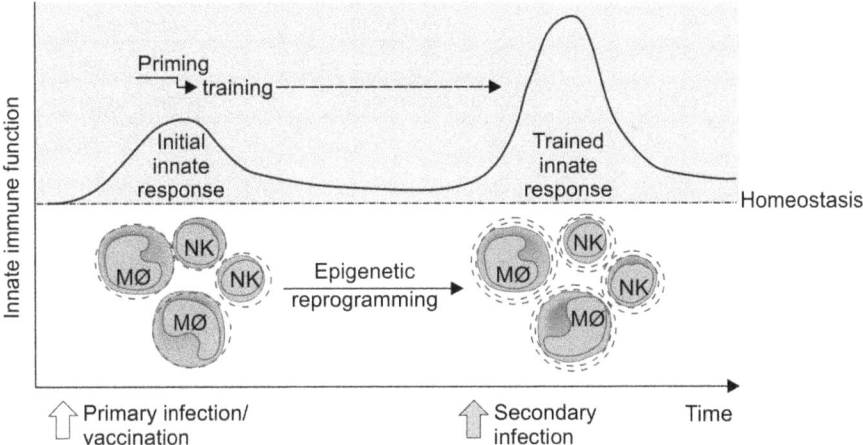

Fig. 5: "Trained innate immunity" (epigenetic reprogramming of monocytes). Second exposure of heterologous exposure leads to a robust immune response.
(NK: natural killer)

differences in the characteristics of BCG vaccine produced from the same seed lot by different manufacturers and between different batches from a single manufacturer. BCG-Tokyo and BCG-Danish vaccines each contain at least 2 genotypes. In 1983, Osborn suggested that BCG vaccines used for routine immunization should be prepared from seed lots derived from single

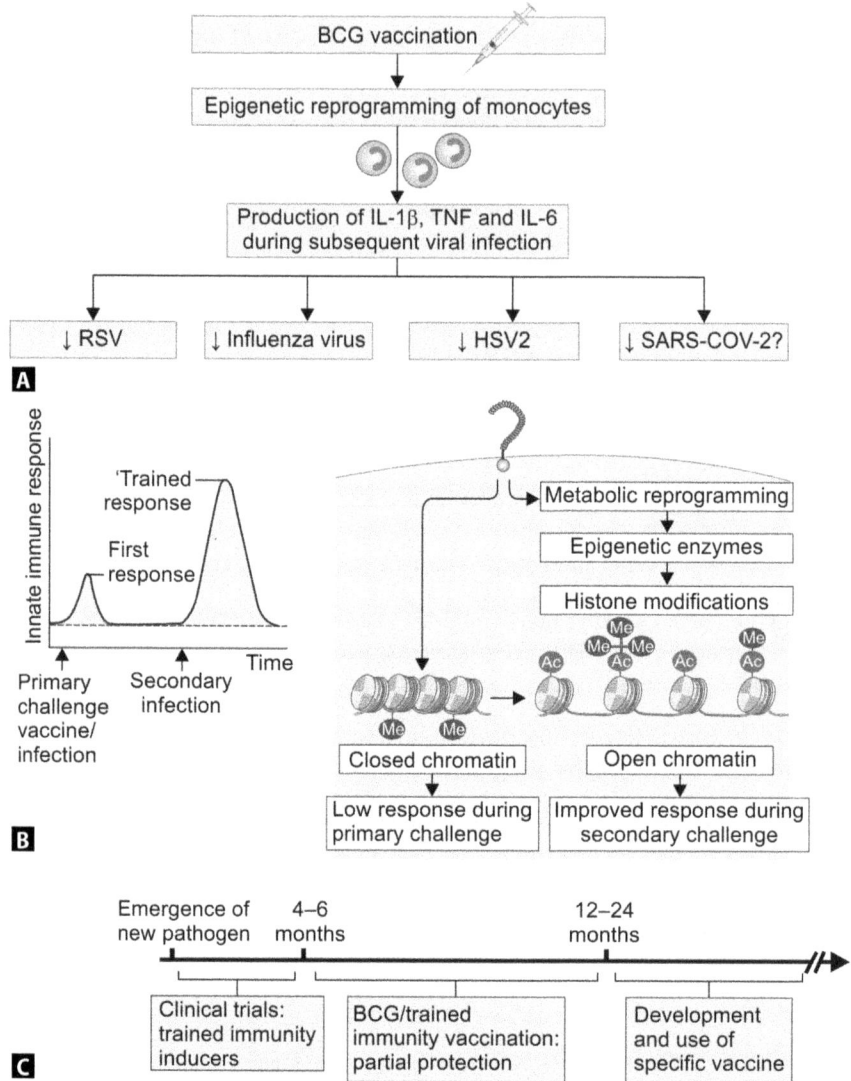

Figs. 6A to C: Trained immunity antiviral host defense and its role in a new viral pandemic. (A) BCG vaccination has been shown to protect against multiple viral pathogens; (B) Trained immunity leading to enhanced innate immune responses to different pathogens after a vaccination is mediated by metabolic and epigenetic rewiring in innate immune cells, which leads to increased gene transcription and improved host defense; (C) Trained immunity as a tool for enhancing population immunity during a pandemic ahead of the availability of a specific vaccine.

(BCG: Bacillus Calmette-Guérin; HSV: herpes simplex virus; IL-6: interlekin-6; RSV: respiratory syncytial virus; SARS-CoV-2: severe acute respiratory syndrome coronavirus 2; TNF: tumor necrosis factor) colonies so that they have stable characteristics. Unfortunately, this has not been done for BCG–Tokyo or BCG–Danish vaccines.

The BCG vaccine is not a single vaccine; the different strains have very different properties, and there are different genotypes within strains. It is likely that we could substantially improve protection against tuberculosis and lower child mortality from other infections by manufacturing each BCG vaccine from a single genotype, comparing these vaccines to find which genotype has the strongest effects against tuberculosis and against other infections, investigating the effect of revaccination on all-cause mortality, and ensuring that a high proportion of neonates are given BCG vaccine in the first few days of life.

The BCG vaccine strains that are employed in the immunization programs of different countries vary widely. Over the years, more than 14 substrains of BCG have been used as BCG vaccine in different parts of the world. Not all strains of BCG have similar potential to induce "trained immunity" in vaccinated individuals; as a result, they have different propensity to induce "NSEs". Most of the studies on beneficial effects of BCG against sepsis and pneumonia were done with Danish strain. Whether other strains do have similar "nonspecific" responses is not yet ascertained.

The "NSEs" of BCG are greater when there is a scar. Different strains of BCG have different scar rates. Scar formation rate is higher around >90% with BCG-Danish and BCG-Tokyo strains whereas it is only 52% with BCG–Moscow. Among BCG-vaccinated children in a setting with low scar prevalence, having a scar is associated with lower mortality and morbidity. Revaccination with BCG confers little or no extra protection against TB, but it may increase the beneficial NSEs of BCG.

26. Can Bacillus Calmette-Guérin (BCG) have some protection against coronavirus disease 2019 (COVID-19) also?

Now we know that BCG elicits heterologous, "NSEs" effects against a variety of infectious diseases and severe acute respiratory syndrome coronavirus 2 (SARS-CoV-2) shall not be an exception. Its beneficial effects are also well-documented in adults albeit with some potential for toxicity. BCG may have some utility owing to induction of these strong NSEs innate immune responses in the vaccinated subjects. BCG may not be able to exert significant inhibitory responses against the SARS-CoV-2 virus, but even "stopgap" protection and some attenuation of the disease may be expected. An extra dose of BCG to the healthcare workers and older people with comorbid conditions would be worth trying. BCG is generally safe and well-tolerated; however, it is contraindicated in immunocompromised individuals, so one needs to be extra careful while administering BCG to these individuals.

Apart from safety, there are other issues like the selection of proper strain of the vaccine and quantum of the immune responses elicited in older and high-risk individuals in comparison to the young and healthy population that need deliberation before employing the vaccine in these groups. One argument against the protective effects of childhood BCG vaccination on coronavirus disease 2019 (COVID-19) susceptibility is the waning of

BCG-induced immunity. However, if the heterologous, "NSEs" persist even for a few months, they should be able to offer some protection through modulation of innate immunity to the frontline health workers and high-risk individuals till a specific anti-SARS-CoV-2 vaccine becomes available.

27. What is the available evidence on Bacillus Calmette-Guérin (BCG) efficacy against coronavirus disease 2019 (COVID-19) infection and severity? What is the World Health Organization (WHO) stand on this issue? Are there any trials going on?

According to some nonpeer reviewed reports, the countries using BCG vaccine in their National Immunization Program are somewhat protected from severe adverse impact of the disease. However, most of these preliminary reports are basically anecdotal, ecological studies. They cannot confirm a "cause-effect" relationship of the vaccine with the disease. Recently, the WHO has issued a statement that there is no evidence of BCG-induced protection against SARS-CoV-2 infection. Few countries like Netherland, Australia, UK, and Germany have started BCG trials among healthcare workers to assess its protective effects, if any. The Indian Council of Medical Research (ICMR) is also conducting trials in this regard.

28. What is the new GlaxoSmithKline (GSK) tuberculosis (TB) vaccine all about?

The new TB vaccine is developed by the GlaxoSmithKline (GSK) and is known as M72/AS01E. The M72/AS01E is a subunit vaccine comprised of an immunogenic fusion protein (M72) derived from two *Mtb* antigens (MTB32A and MTB39A) and the GSK proprietary adjuvant AS01E. AS01E is the same adjuvant used in Shingrix GSK vaccine as well as in the new malaria vaccine RTS,S/AS01E.

29. Is it more efficacious than existing Bacillus Calmétte-Guerin (BCG) vaccine?

The M72/AS01E vaccine was tested in about 3,300 adults in Kenya, South Africa, and Zambia. All of them already had latent TB—a silent infection that might or might not progress to active TB. Of those who got two doses of the GSK vaccine, only 13 developed active TB during 3 years of follow-up, according to the new study published in The New England Journal of Medicine. By contrast, 26 of those who got a placebo progressed to active TB. The results showed that administering two doses of M72/AS01E to human immunodeficiency virus (HIV)-negative adults with evidence of latent TB infection (LTBI) was successful in reducing the development of active TB disease with 54% efficacy [90% confidence interval (CI): 13.9–75.4; 95% CI: 2.9–78.2; $p = 0.04$]. Hence, its efficacy is not superior to existing vaccine (BCG) against TB.

30. How does this new tuberculosis (TB) vaccine work?

The exact mechanism of action of M72/AS01E is not known. Previous studies have showed that this vaccine induces an immune response characterized by the activation of IFN-γ producing CD4+ T cells and the production of antibodies.

31. Can we give Bacillus Calmétte-Guerin (BCG) vaccine to human immunodeficiency virus (HIV)-positive/acquired immunodeficiency syndrome (AIDS) inflicted children or adolescents?

Bacillus Calmétte-Guerin should be avoided in the immunocompromised, especially those with cellular immunodeficiency; it may, however, be given at birth to children born to HIV-positive mothers. Disseminated BCG infection is extremely unusual, but may occur in children with cellular immunodeficiency.

Since severe adverse effects of BCG vaccination are extremely rare in asymptomatic HIV-positive infants, all healthy neonates should be BCG vaccinated in areas endemic for TB. However, where resources permit, long-term follow-up of BCG-vaccinated infants of known HIV-positive mothers is desirable for early treatment should disseminated BCG disease occur in children with rapid development of immunodeficiency.

Infants and children with symptomatic HIV or those known to have other immunodeficiency states should not be BCG vaccinated.

However, if HIV-infected individuals, including children, are receiving antiretroviral therapy (ART), are clinically well and immunologically stable (CD4% >25% for children aged <5 years or CD4+ count ≥200 if aged ≥5 years) and they should be vaccinated with BCG.

Neonates born to women of unknown HIV status should be vaccinated. However, neonates with unknown HIV status born to HIV-infected women should be vaccinated if they have no clinical evidence suggestive of HIV infection, regardless of whether the mother is receiving ART. Additionally, neonates with HIV infection should delay BCG vaccination until ART has been started and are immunologically stable.

32. What are the risks if Bacillus Calmétte-Guerin (BCG) vaccine is given to human immunodeficiency virus (HIV)-infected infants?

Severe adverse event following immunization (AEFI) can occur in HIV-infected infants following BCG vaccination. Evidence shows that children who were HIV infected at birth and vaccinated with BCG at birth and who later developed acquired immunodeficiency syndrome (AIDS) were at increased risk of developing disseminated BCG disease. Early initiation of ART, before immunological and/or clinical HIV progression, has been shown to substantially reduce the risk of BCG-immune reconstitution inflammatory syndrome (IRIS) regional adenitis. However, where resources permit, long-term follow-up of BCG-vaccinated infants of known HIV-positive mothers is desirable for early treatment should disseminated BCG disease occur in children with rapid development of immunodeficiency.

33. What are the recommendations for the travelers?

Bacillus Calmette-Guérin (BCG) vaccine may be considered for travelers in areas of high TB incidence, particularly when serial TST testing and appropriate chemotherapy are not possible or where the prevalence of drug resistance, particularly multidrug resistant (MDR) TB, is high. This decision should be made in consultation with an infectious disease or travel medicine specialist.

Travelers with medical conditions, particularly HIV infection, which may be associated with an increased risk of progression of latent TB infection to active disease, should carefully weigh, with their physician, the risk of travel to a high-incidence area in determining the most appropriate means of prevention.

34. Parents of 14-year-old boy want their son to be given Bacillus Calmette-Guérin (BCG) because his friend has recently diagnosed with pulmonary tuberculosis (TB). The boy has received BCG at birth. What will you do? Will you give BCG to the boy?

No, BCG revaccination is not recommended. The recommended age of administration is at birth (for institutional deliveries) or at 6 weeks with other vaccines, if it was not administered at birth. Catch-up vaccination with BCG is recommended till the age of 5 years.

The WHO also does not recommend revaccination as there is no evidence of usefulness.

35. A health worker had inadvertently injected 0.5 mL of Bacillus Calmette-Guérin (BCG) vaccine intramuscularly in the thigh of a 9-month-old infant confusing it with measles vaccine. After 2 weeks, the child developed large abscess and discharge at the injection site. How this child be managed? Should antitubercular therapy (ATT) be prescribed or not?

One must first exclude secondary infection (pyogenic) at the injection site. Since details are not provided in the query, one has to exclude a pyogenic abscess by pus culture and if positive should receive appropriate antibiotics as per susceptibility test. Incision and drainage can be done if the abscess is large. Local uncontaminated abscess at injection site should not require any specific treatment and should heal within 8–12 weeks' time.

Ipsilateral inguinal lymphadenopathy may be managed as discussed earlier (surgical excision, if large fluctuant node or repeated needle aspirations) but no need to give ATT.

Antitubercular therapy is of no benefit in such situations and should not be administered.

36. What are the precautions to be taken before administering Bacillus Calmette-Guérin (BCG) vaccine?

The precautions include:
- Administering BCG vaccine intradermally and not to inject subcutaneously, intramuscularly, or intravenously.

- Using a separate sterile needle and syringe, or a sterile disposable unit, for each individual patient to prevent disease transmission. All equipment, supplies, and receptacles in contact with BCG vaccine should be handled and disposed off as biohazardous waste.
- The vaccine should not be administered to individuals receiving drugs with antituberculous activity, since these agents may be active against the vaccine strain.
- Bacillus Calmette-Guérin immunization is contraindicated in persons with immune deficiency diseases, altered immune status due to malignant disease, and impaired immune function secondary to treatment with corticosteroids, chemotherapeutic agents, or radiation.
- Extensive skin disease or burns are also contraindications. BCG is contraindicated for individuals with a positive TST, although immunization of tuberculin reactors has frequently occurred without incident.
- A review of each patient's immunization records to include history on reactions to immunizations should be completed prior to vaccination. All precautions should be taken for the prevention of allergic or any other side reactions. Epinephrine injection (1:1,000) for the control of immediate allergic reactions must be available and should an acute anaphylactic reaction occur.

37. What are the adverse effects following Bacillus Calmette-Guérin (BCG) vaccination and how to manage them?

The usual response to ID administration of BCG vaccine is the development of erythema, induration, and either a papule or ulceration, followed by a scar at the immunization site. No treatment is required for this condition. Secondary infection at the vaccination site may require antimicrobials.

Rates of adverse reactions appear to vary with the strain of vaccine, dose and method of immunization, and the age of the recipient. Adverse reactions are more common in young vaccinees (infants vs. older children) and are frequently related to improper technique in administration (mainly improper dilution).

Intradermal administration of BCG vaccine usually results in the development of erythema and either a papule or ulceration (in about 95%), followed by a scar at the immunization site. Keloid formation occurs in 2-4% of vaccine recipients. Nonsuppurative regional lymphadenopathy occurs in 1-10%. Most reactions are generally mild and do not require treatment. ATT is of no benefit in such situations and should not be administered. The nodes regress spontaneously after a few months. It should also be noted that if FNAC of the nodes is carried out, stain for acid-fast bacilli may be positive. These are bovine vaccine bacilli and should not be misconstrued as being suggestive of tuberculous disease. In some children, the nodes may even liquefy and result in an abscess. Surgical removal of the nodes or repeated needle aspiration is the treatment of choice again, ATT is not recommended in this situation also.

Since neonates have a higher risk of vaccine-induced suppurative lymphadenitis than older children, infants aged <30 days should receive a reduced dose of the vaccine.

A review of published and unpublished data, including a survey sponsored by the International Union Against Tuberculosis and Lung Disease, recorded 10,371 complications following almost 1.5 billion BCG vaccinations in adults and children. The most serious complication of BCG vaccination was disseminated BCG infection, which occurred in 3 per 1 million recipients. In that review, dissemination was fatal in 0.02 per 1 million vaccine recipients and occurred in children who had primary immunodeficiencies.

38. Some countries routinely recommend adolescent Bacillus Calmette-Guérin (BCG) vaccination in their National Immunization Program. What is the World Health Organization recommendation?

As per the WHO recommendation, BCG vaccination is recommended for unvaccinated TST- or IGRA-negative older children, adolescents, and adults from settings with high incidence of TB and/or high leprosy burden and those moving from low to high TB incidence/leprosy burden settings. BCG vaccination of adolescents and adults has shown variation in protective efficacy with geographical region, possibly because of differences in previous exposure to environmental mycobacteria. However, given the serious consequences of contracting MDR disease and the low reactogenicity of the vaccine, BCG vaccination should be offered to all unvaccinated, tuberculin-negative persons who are exposed to MDR tuberculous infection.

39. What are the reasons for variable efficacy of Bacillus Calmette-Guérin (BCG) vaccine? Why the World Health Organization (WHO) still recommends BCG vaccination despite variable efficacy?

Though the reasons for the variable efficacy of BCG in different countries are difficult to understand, the following may stand true for the lack of efficacy in both low TB burden countries (US) and high TB burden countries (India):
- *Background frequency of exposure to TB*: It has been hypothesized that in areas with high levels of background exposure to TB, every susceptible individual is already exposed prior to BCG and that the natural immunizing effect of background TB duplicates any benefit of BCG.
- *Genetic variation in BCG strains*: There is genetic variation in the BCG strains used and this may explain the variable efficacy reported in different trials.
- *Genetic variation in populations*: Difference in genetic makeup of different populations may explain the difference in efficacy.
- *Interference by nontuberculous mycobacteria*: Exposure to environmental mycobacteria (especially *Mycobacterium avium*, *Mycobacterium marinum*, and *Mycobacterium intracellulare*) results in a nonspecific immune response against mycobacteria. Administering BCG to someone who already has a nonspecific immune response against mycobacteria

does not augment the response that is already there. BCG will, therefore, appear not to be efficacious because that person already has a level of immunity and BCG is not adding to that immunity.
- *Interference by concurrent parasitic infection*: Another hypothesis is that simultaneous infection with parasites changes the immune response to BCG, making it less effective. A T-helper type 1 (Th1) cell response is required for an effective immune response to tuberculous infection; one hypothesis is that concurrent infection with various parasites produces a simultaneous Th2 response, which blunts the effect of BCG.
- Despite the variable efficacy, the WHO still recommends BCG vaccination as BCG is known to prevent life-threatening forms of TB such as meningitis and disseminated disease in infants and young children. Vaccination with BCG remains the standard for TB prevention in most countries because it is available, is inexpensive, and requires only one encounter with the patient; in addition, it rarely causes serious complications and systems for early diagnosis and effective treatment of TB are lacking in many areas of the world.

40. Is Bacillus Calmette-Guérin (BCG) vaccine given routinely in developed countries as per the World Health Organization (WHO) recommendation? If so, what are the countries, which have included BCG vaccine in their national schedule?

The WHO recommends that BCG be given to all children born in countries highly endemic for TB because it protects against miliary TB and TB meningitis. However, developed countries like the US and the UK have not introduced the vaccine in their National Immunization Program. They rely more on the detection and treatment rather than universal immunization of all children. The age of the patient and the frequency with which BCG is given have always varied from country to country.
- *US*: The US has never used mass immunization of BCG, relying instead on the detection and treatment of latent TB.
- *UK*: The UK introduced universal BCG immunization in 1953 and until 2005; the UK policy was to immunize all school children at the age of 13 years and all neonates born into high-risk groups. The injection was only given once during an individual's lifetime (as there is no evidence of additional protection from more than one vaccination). BCG was also given to protect people who had been exposed to TB. The peak of TB incidence is in adolescence and early adulthood and the evidence from the Medical Research Council (MRC) trial was that efficacy lasted only 15 years at most. Styblo and Meijer argued that neonatal immunization protected against miliary TB and other noncontagious forms of TB and not pulmonary TB, which was a disease of adults, and that mass immunization campaigns with BCG would, therefore, not be expected to have a significant public health impact. For these and other reasons, BCG was, therefore, given to time with the peak incidence of pulmonary disease. Routine immunization with BCG was withdrawn in 2005 because of falling cost-effectiveness whereas in 1953, 94 children would have to

be immunized to prevent one case of TB; by 1988, the annual incidence of TB in the UK had fallen so much that 12,000 children would have to be immunized to prevent one case of TB.
- *France*: The BCG was mandatory for school children between 1950 and 2007 and for healthcare professionals between 1947 and 2010. Vaccination is still available for French healthcare professionals and social workers, but is now decided on a case-by-case basis.
- *India*: India introduced BCG mass immunization in 1948, the first non-European country to do so.
- *Brazil*: Brazil introduced universal BCG immunization in 1967–1968 and the practice continues until the present day. According to Brazilian law, BCG is given again to professionals of the health sector and to people close to patients with TB or leprosy.
- *Norway*: In Norway, the BCG vaccine was mandatory from 1947 to 1995. It is still available and recommended for high-risk groups.
- *South Africa*: In South Africa, the BCG vaccine is given routinely at birth, to all newborns, except those with clinically symptomatic AIDS.
- *Other countries*: In the UK, BCG was only ever given once (as there is no evidence of additional protection from more than one vaccination), but in some countries, such as the former Union of Soviet Socialist Republics (USSR), BCG was given regularly throughout life. In South Korea, Singapore, Taiwan, and Malaysia, BCG was given at birth and again at the age of 12 years. But in Malaysia and Singapore, from 2001, this policy was changed to once only at birth and it was discontinued in South Korea.

41. What are the results of recent meta-analysis on Bacillus Calmette-Guérin (BCG) vaccination? Despite repeated passages over many years, do the BCG strains retain their immunogenicity?

Meta-analysis of 10 randomized and controlled studies showed that the average protection against TB meningitis and disseminated disease was 86%; the corresponding result of case–control studies was 75%. In another analysis that included 15 prospective and 12 case–control studies, the BCG-induced protection against TB disease was 51% and 50%, respectively. The protection against TB-related death was 65%, against TB meningitis was 64%, and against disseminated TB was 78%. Few reports show high protective efficacy following BCG vaccination of adults. However, in the late 1920s, BCG vaccination of tuberculin-negative Norwegian nursing students before entering TB wards reduced the development of tuberculous disease by >80% during a 3-year observation period.

The current vaccine strains are all descendants of the original *Mycobacterium bovis* isolate that Calmette and Guérin passaged through numerous cycles during the 13-year period 1909–1921. Subsequent passages under different laboratory conditions resulted in a variety of new BCG strains showing phenotypic as well as genotypic differences. Though, a number of BCG vaccine strains are available, in terms of efficacy, no BCG strain is demonstrably better than another and there is no global consensus as to which strain of BCG is optimal for general use.

For instance, in India, BCG vaccine manufactured by Serum Institute of India Pvt. Ltd., Pune, India was developed using Moscow BCG-I (Russian) strain. This vaccine was licensed in India in October 2001 and subsequently prequalified by the WHO in June, 2003 for purchase by United Nations (UN) agencies for developing countries. Since then, millions of doses have been administered worldwide clearly indicating that this vaccine is safe and can be used effectively for prevention of miliary TB and tubercular meningitis. Apart from the BCG vaccines manufactured by BCG Vaccine Laboratory, Guindy, Chennai, India and Green Signal Bio Pharma Pvt. Ltd., Chennai, India, the only WHO prequalified BCG vaccine being used by Government of India (GoI) in its National Immunization Program is by Serum Institute of India Pvt. Ltd., Pune, India.

42. In view of the closure of public sector undertakings (PSUs) in India, only Bacillus Calmette-Guérin (BCG) vaccine manufactured by private sector is available. Are they the World Health Organization (WHO) prequalified laboratories? Are there any efficacy studies available on the indigenous BCG vaccine formulations? Can we use them freely?

Bacillus Calmette-Guérin vaccine in India is manufactured by Serum Institute of India Pvt. Ltd., Pune, India, BCG Vaccine Laboratory, Guindy, Chennai, India, and Green Signal Bio Pharma Pvt. Ltd., Chennai, India. BCG Vaccine Laboratory, Guindy, Chennai, India has since resumed production after the public sector undertaking (PSU) revival.

The only private sector, the WHO prequalified vaccine used in India, is by Serum Institute of India Pvt. Ltd., Pune, India. The vaccine meets all the quality requirements and has been prequalified by the WHO for purchase by UN agencies. Millions of doses of this vaccine have been administered worldwide. Numerous clinical studies conducted with the vaccine and number of doses administered over the years clearly indicate that this vaccine is safe and can be used effectively for prevention of serious TB infection and tubercular meningitis.

SUGGESTED READING

1. Aaby P, Roth A, Ravn H, Napirna BM, Rodrigues A, Lisse IM, et al. Randomized trial of BCG vaccination at birth to low-birth-weight children: beneficial nonspecific effects in the neonatal period? J Infect Dis. 2011;204:245-52.
2. Arts RJW, Moorlag SJCFM, Novakovic B, Li Y, Wang SY, Oosting M, et al. BCG vaccination protects against experimental viral infection in humans through the induction of cytokines associated with trained immunity. Cell Host Microbe. 2018;23:89-100.e5.
3. Badurdeen S, Marshall A, Daish H, Hatherill M, Berkley JA. Safety and immunogenicity of early Bacillus Calmette-Guérin vaccination in infants who are preterm and/or have low birth weights: a systematic review and meta-analysis. JAMA Pediatr. 2019;173:75-85.

4. BCG Vaccines: WHO Position Paper—February 2018. Wkly Epidemiol Rec. 2018;93:73-96.
5. Manerikar SS, Malaviya AN, Singh MB, Rajgopalan P, Kumar R. Immune status and BCG vaccination in newborns with intra-uterine growth retardation. Clin Exp Immunol. 1997;26:173-5.
6. Moliva JI, Turner J, Torrelles JB. Immune responses to Bacillus Calmette-Guérin vaccination: why do they Fail to protect against Mycobacterium tuberculosis? Front Immunol. 2017;8:407.
7. Public Health Agency of Canada. (2016). Canadian Immunization Guide: Part 4—Active Vaccines. [online] Available from: https://www.canada.ca/en/public-health/services/publications/healthy-living/canadian-immunization-guide-part-4-active-vaccines.html. [Last accessed July, 2020].
8. Sedaghatian MR, Kardouni K. Tuberculin response in preterm infants after BCG vaccination at birth. Arch Dis Child. 1993;69:309-11.
9. Shann F. Editorial commentary: different strains of Bacillus Calmette-Guérin vaccine have very different effects on tuberculosis and on unrelated infections. Clin Infect Dis. 2015;61:960-2.
10. Uthayakumar D, Paris S, Chapat L, Freyburger L, Poulet H, De Luca K. Non-specific effects of vaccines illustrated through the BCG example: from observations to demonstrations. Front Immunol. 2018;9:2869.
11. World Health Organization (WHO) and SAGE Working Group on BCG Vaccines and WHO Secretariat. (2017). Report on BCG vaccine use for protection against mycobacterial infections including tuberculosis, leprosy, and other nontuberculous mycobacteria (NTM) infections. [online] Available from: https://www.who.int/immunization/sage/meetings/2017/october/1_BCG_report_revised_version_online.pdf. [Last accessed July, 2020].

CHAPTER 16

Polio Vaccines

Naveen Thacker, Prem Pal Singh, Vipin M Vashishtha

1. What is the clinical spectrum of poliomyelitis?

Table 1 summarizes various types of clinical features and syndrome seen with a wild poliovirus infection.

2. What are the different vaccines available for polio?

There are two types of polio vaccines, first the inactivated polio vaccine (IPV) by Jonas Salk and other the live oral polio vaccine (OPV) by Albert Sabin. Earlier, both these vaccines contained all the three types of polioviruses but, after the switch from trivalent oral polio vaccine (tOPV) to bivalent oral polio vaccine (bOPV), only type 1 and 3 strains are present in OPV.

3. What are the different types of oral polio vaccine (OPV)?

Different types of OPV are:
- *Trivalent oral polio vaccine*: tOPV is no more in use after its withdrawal and its replacement with bOPV (type 1 and 3) since April 2016.

TABLE 1: Clinical spectrum of poliomyelitis.

S. No.	Presentation	Frequency	Clinical features
1.	Asymptomatic	Up to 95%	Inapparent infection without symptoms
2.	Minor illness ("abortive")	4–8%	• No central nervous system (CNS) involvement • Three syndromes: (1) upper respiratory tract infection, (2) gastrointestinal disturbances, and (3) influenza-like illness
3.	Major illness	3%	With CNS involvement
3.1.	Nonparalytic	1–2%	Aseptic meningitis
3.2.	Paralytic	<1%	–
3.2.1.	Spinal	79% of paralytic cases	Asymmetric paralysis that most often involves cases of the legs
3.2.2.	Bulbar	2% of paralytic cases	Weakness of muscles innervated by bulbar cranial nerves
3.2.3.	Bulbospinal	19% of paralytic cases	A combination of bulbar and spinal paralysis

The ratio of paralytic cases to infections was estimated per 100 infections at approximately 0.5 for serotype 1, 0.05 for serotype 2, and 0.08 for serotype 3

- *Monovalent oral polio vaccine (mOPV)*: mOPV (mOPV1 for type 1 and mOPV3 for type 3), licensed in 2005 to enhance the impact of supplementary immunization activities (SIAs), is the key remaining reservoirs of wild poliovirus (WPV).
- *Bivalent oral polio vaccine (bOPV)*: bOPV (for type 1 and type 3), licensed in 2010 and used effectively in selective SIAs campaigns in pulse polio program, National Immunization Days (NIDs) to sustain the immunity against both type 1 and type 3 virus together in certain areas. After the withdrawal of tOPV (April 2016), bOPV is used in national routine immunization (RI) program for polio vaccination.

4. What are the features of bivalent oral polio vaccine (bOPV)?

Bivalent oral polio vaccine is a bivalent vaccine consisting of a suspension of live attenuated poliovirus types 1 and 3 grown in monkey kidney cell cultures and stabilized with magnesium chloride. It is presented in a buffered salt solution, with light pink color indicating the right pH. OPV is available as vial containing multidose. The dose is two drops (0.1 mL) per dose orally. It is a very safe vaccine.

5. What is the shelf-life of oral polio vaccine (OPV)?

Oral polio vaccine is a very heat sensitive vaccine having a shelf-life of 2 years at a temperature of –20°C, 6 months at 2–8°C, and 1–3 days at room temperature (depending upon the season and room temperature). OPV should be stored at –20°C at the state and district level and in the freezer at the clinic level. The vaccine must reach the outreach facility at 2–8°C in vaccine carriers with ice packs.

6. What is the impact of thawing on oral polio vaccine (OPV)?

Multiple freeze-thaw cycles should be avoided as the virus loses its potency. After thawing, it should be kept at temperatures between 2°C and 8°C for a maximum of 6 months.

7. Is there any difference in the vaccine if it is of a different color?

Usually, the color of an OPV is pink. However, sometimes the color may also be yellow or white. All the vaccines are same and this color difference in no way affects the quality or type of vaccine.

8. If a child is given more than two drops at the time of immunization, then what will be the harm to the child?

If more than two drops are given to the child, due to any reason, then there will be no harm to the child as OPV is among very safe vaccines.

9. If a child is vaccinated with an oral polio vaccine (OPV) vial having third stage of vaccine vial monitor (VVM), what will be the harm to the child?

Third stage of vaccine vial monitor (VVM) on OPV vial indicates that vaccine in the vial has lost its potency due to breech in cold chain. If any child is immunized with such vial, then it will not produce the immunity in the child and such child will remain unprotected from disease, but there will be no harm to the child.

10. What are the contraindications of oral polio vaccine (OPV)?

Oral polio vaccine is contraindicated in severely immunocompromised patients with known underlying conditions such as primary immunodeficiencies, disorders of the thymus, symptomatic human immunodeficiency virus (HIV) infection or low CD4+ T-cell values, malignant neoplasm treated with chemotherapy, recent hematopoietic stem cell transplantation, drugs with known immunosuppressive or immunomodulatory properties [e.g., high-dose systemic corticosteroids, alkylating drugs, antimetabolites, tumor necrosis factor-α (TNF-α) inhibitors, interleukin-1 (IL-1) blocking agent, or other monoclonal antibodies targeting immune cells], and current or recent radiation therapies targeting immune cells. These populations can safely receive IPV. OPV can be given to a patient with diarrhea, but that dose should not be counted and should be followed by an extra dose.

11. What are the side effects of oral polio vaccine (OPV)?

Oral polio vaccine is very safe vaccine and has minimum side effects. It can lead to gastrointestinal (GI) upset like diarrhea and vomiting. It does not lead to fever. The most important but rare side effect with OPV is vaccine-associated paralytic poliomyelitis (VAPP). Massive benefits of OPV far outweigh the rare risk of paralysis.

12. What is vaccine-associated paralytic poliomyelitis (VAPP)?

Vaccine-associated paralytic poliomyelitis is serious adverse effect associated with OPV. It is defined as those cases of acute flaccid paralysis (AFP), which have residual weakness 60 days after the onset of paralysis and from whose stool samples, vaccine-related poliovirus but no WPV is isolated. VAPP may occur in the vaccine recipient (recipient VAPP, occurring within 4–40 days of receiving OPV) or contact of the vaccine recipient (contact of VAPP). VAPP occurs due to loss of attenuating mutations and reversion to neurovirulence during replication of the vaccine virus in the gut.

13. What is the incidence rate of vaccine-associated paralytic poliomyelitis (VAPP)?

The incidence of VAPP has been estimated about 1 in 2.7 million doses of OPV. The incidence of VAPP in developed countries, such as USA, has been reported to be 1 per 2.4 million doses distributed and 1 per 750,000 with first dose.

Available data suggest differences in the epidemiology of VAPP in developing and industrialized countries. In the latter, VAPP occurs mainly in early infancy associated with the first dose of OPV and decreases sharply (>10-fold) with subsequent OPV doses. In lower-income countries, which experience relatively lower rates of vaccine seroconversion, this decline is more gradual and VAPP may occur with second or subsequent doses of OPV, with the age distribution concentrated among children aged 1–4 years. The main factors contributing to this difference are believed to be lower immune responsiveness to OPV and higher prevalence of maternally-derived antibody in populations in low-income settings. The risk of VAPP in India has been estimated to be 1 per 4.1–4.6 million doses distributed and 1 per 2.8 million first-dose recipient risks.

14. Is it true that Indian kids are immune against vaccine-associated paralytic poliomyelitis (VAPP)? If yes, why is it so?

The lower risk of VAPP in India might be attributed to high prevalence and titer of maternal antibodies, birth dose of OPV, and early immunization with OPV in the RI schedule.

15. What is vaccine-derived poliovirus? What is its importance?

Vaccine-derived polioviruses (VDPVs) are rare but well-documented strains of poliovirus, which emerge after prolonged multiplication of attenuated strains of the virus, contained in the OPV in the guts of children with immunodeficiency or in populations with very low immunity. After prolonged multiplication, these vaccine viruses-derived strains change and revert to a form that can cause paralysis in humans. Some VDPVs have shown a capacity for sustained circulation in communities.

In July 2015, the Global Polio Eradication Initiative (GPEI) revised the definition of circulating vaccine-derived polioviruses (cVDPVs) to enhance its sensitivity. In the new guidelines, cVDPVs are defined as genetically linked VDPVs isolated from: (i) at least two individuals—not necessarily AFP cases—who are not household contacts; (ii) one individual and one or more environmental surveillance (ES) samples; or (iii) at least two ES samples if they were collected at more than one distinct ES collection site (no overlapping of catchment areas) or from one site if collection was >2 months apart or a single VDPV isolate with genetic features indicating prolonged circulation [i.e., a number of nucleotide (nt) changes from parent Sabin strains suggesting ≥1.5 years of circulation or 15 nt changes].

16. How vaccine-derived poliovirus (VDPV) differs from original Sabin strain?

Vaccine-derived poliovirus arises due to mutation and recombination in the human gut and is 1–15% divergent of VP1 nucleotide from the parent vaccine virus. They are capable of both neurovirulence and transmissibility. VDPVs have caused outbreaks including in the neighboring countries of China, Myanmar and Indonesia, and huge outbreak in Nigeria. Since 2009 globally, earlier the Sabin type 2 in the tOPV had been responsible for >90% of all cVDPV cases and 40% VAPP cases due to low immunity against type 2 hence for VDPV type 2, cases with ≥6th difference from the Sabin in VP1 (>0.6% genetic divergence or >6 nt changes) and for VDPV types 1 and 3 cases with ≥10th difference from Sabin in VP1 (>1% genetic divergence or >10 nt changes) are considered as VDPV.

17. What are the types of vaccine-derived poliovirus (VDPV)?

They have been classified into three groups:
1. *Circulating vaccine-derived poliovirus*: VDPV with evidence of person-to-person virus circulation in the community causing two or more paralytic cases.
2. *Immunodeficiency-related vaccine-derived poliovirus (iVDPV)*: VDPV in the immunodeficient person isolated from some people with primary B-cell or combined immunodeficiency disorders (with defects in antibody production) who may have prolonged VDPV infections (in individual cases, excretion has been reported to persist for 10 years or more).
3. *Ambiguous vaccine-derived poliovirus (aVDPV)*: VDPV isolated from environmental sources or evidence of circulation not established.

Till 2017, about 24 outbreaks counting about 760 cases of cVDPVs were reported. Since 2006, majority (>90%) of cVDPV cases are due to type 2.

18. What is persistent circulating vaccine-derived poliovirus (cVDPV)?

The term "persistent cVDPV" refers to cVDPVs that continue to circulate for >6 months following detection. Persistent cVDPVs represent programmatic failures to contain the cVDPV outbreak within 6 months of detection.

19. How can a vaccine-derived poliovirus (VDPV) circulation be stopped?

The management of VDPVs is a necessary part of the global polio eradication effort and is similar to management of WPV outbreaks, i.e., by rapid implementation of large-scale, high-quality SIAs. Global experience with VDPVs shows that they are less virulent than WPV strains and can be rapidly stopped with two to three rounds of high-quality, large-scale SIAs.

20. Is there a difference in a disease caused by a vaccine-derived poliovirus (VDPV) and one caused by wild poliovirus?

No, there is no clinical difference between paralytic polio caused by WPV or a VDPV.

21. What are the salient features of inactivated polio vaccine (IPV)?

Inactivated polio vaccine is formaldehyde-killed poliovirus, grown in monkey kidney cell or human diploid cells. Old IPV contained 20, 8, and 32 D antigen units of types 1, 2, and 3 polioviruses, respectively. All currently used IPV vaccines are enhanced potency inactivated polio vaccine (eIPV) which contains 40, 8, and 32 D antigen units of types 1, 2, and 3, respectively. Currently, the term IPV means eIPV. The vaccine should be stored at 2–8°C. It is highly immunogenic. Its immunogenicity is dampened by the presence of maternal antibody in the very young infant, especially up to the age of 8 weeks. IPV based on the attenuated Sabin virus strain [Sabin inactivated polio vaccine (sIPV)] was developed and licensed in Japan in 2012. The advantages of sIPV are that biocontainment requirements are less stringent than for wild viruses and the consequences of any release of Sabin strains into populations would be less serious than with release of wild strains.

Inactivated polio vaccine is made from selected WPV strains—Mahoney or Brunhilde (type 1), Middle East Forces-1 (MEF-1) (type 2), and Saukett (type 3)—or from Sabin strains and are now grown in Vero cell culture or in human diploid cells. IPV may contain formaldehyde as well as traces of streptomycin, neomycin, or polymyxin B. Some formulations of IPV contain 2-phenoxyethanol (0.5%) as a preservative for multi-dose vials. IPV formulations do not contain thiomersal, which is incompatible with IPV antigenicity.

22. How inactivated polio vaccine (IPV) is to be given?

Inactivated polio vaccine should be given intramuscularly (preferably) or subcutaneously and may be offered as a component of fixed combinations of vaccines. The dose is 0.5 mL. IPV is available as single-dose vial containing 0.5 mL of vaccine. It is also available in combination with other vaccines.

Current 10-dose and five-dose IPV vials can be used according to the World Health Organization (WHO) multi-dose vial policy and kept for up to 28 days after opening. IPV is available either as a stand-alone product or in combination with one or more other vaccine antigens including diphtheria, tetanus, and pertussis (DTP), hepatitis B, or *Haemophilus influenzae* type b (Hib). According to manufacturer specifications, IPV can be administered by subcutaneous or intramuscular (IM) injection. When combined with an adjuvanted vaccine, the injection must be IM. A fractional dose of stand-alone IPV can also be administered via the intradermal route. IPV is considered very safe, whether given alone or in combination with other vaccines.

23. How efficacious is inactivated polio vaccine (IPV)?

Seroconversion rates (SCRs) of IPV are >90% after two doses. A third dose, given after a suitable interval, boosts the antibody levels and effective up to 99% or 100% and ensures the perpetuation of immunity for decades and more.

Single fractional dose of inactivated polio vaccine (fIPV)—one-fifth of the full dose gives lower SCRs than a full dose but after two doses, the rates are almost similar to those after two full doses but lower than with the two full doses. Also, two fractional doses of IPV, given intradermally at 6 and 14 weeks, provide higher SCRs than a single full dose (IM) given at 14 weeks. A schedule of fractional intradermal doses administered at 6 and 14 weeks ensures early and appropriately-timed protection. The two fractional doses should be separated by a minimum interval of 4 weeks. One fIPV may be suitable for outbreak response, if supplies are limited. The immunogenicity of IPV schedules depends on the age at administration and number of doses due to interference by maternal antibodies.

24. What are the benefits of fractional dose of inactivated polio vaccine (fIPV) over inactivated polio vaccine (IPV) in the Expanded Program on Immunization (EPI)?

Intradermal IPV administration with fIPV (0.1 mL or one-fifth of a full dose) offers potential cost reduction and allows immunization of a larger number of persons with a given vaccine supply.

Table 2 describes the comparison between IPV and fIPV.

TABLE 2: Comparing IPV and fIPV.		
	IPV	*Fractional dose of IPV (fIPV)*
Volume per dose	0.5 mL	0.1 mL
Schedule	One dose: 14 weeks	Two doses: 6 and 14 weeks
Administration	Intramuscular (IM) injection	Intradermal (ID) injection
Site of administration	Thigh	Upper arm
Syringe	0.5 mL AD syringe	0.1 mL AD syringe
Are two fractional doses as effective as a single standard dose?	Two fractional doses of IPV given ID at 6 and 14 weeks produce better immunogenicity than a single standard IM dose given at 14 weeks	

(AD: auto-disable; IPV: inactivated polio vaccine)

25. Can inactivated polio vaccine (IPV) be given with other vaccines?

Inactivated polio vaccine can be administered along with all other childhood vaccines and can be used in combination with DTP [diphtheria, tetanus, and whole-cell pertussis (DTwP)/diphtheria, tetanus, and acellular pertussis (DTaP)], Hib, and hepatitis B vaccines without compromising seroconversion or increasing side effects. The vaccine is very safe.

26. What are the demerits of inactivated polio vaccine (IPV)?

High cost, scarce availability, and injectable route—extra injections are needed (monovalent use).

27. Can polio vaccine be given to a child who has received immunoglobulin?

The administration of polio vaccine should be delayed by at least 6 weeks after administration of immunoglobulin.

28. Can polio vaccines be administered to immunocompromised subjects?

Inactivated polio vaccine is the vaccine recommended for vaccination of immunodeficient persons and their household contacts. Many immunodeficient persons are immune to polioviruses as a result of previous vaccination or exposure to wild virus when they were immunocompetent. While OPV is contraindicated in such subjects, IPV is the vaccine of choice. Although a protective immune response in these persons cannot be ensured, IPV might confer a significant protection.

29. What should be schedule for polio immunization in children with human immunodeficiency virus (HIV)?

Polio vaccine (IPV or bOPV) may be administered safely to asymptomatic HIV-infected infants. HIV testing is not a prerequisite for vaccination. In HIV children, IPV is preferred and to be given at 6, 10, 14 weeks, 16–18 months, and 5 years. If indicated, IPV is to be given to household contact. If IPV is not affordable or available, OPV should be given as it has been found to be generally safe in HIV-infected infant, especially in early stages.

30. What is the risk of serious reactions following inactivated polio vaccine (IPV)?

There is no proven causal relationship with any adverse events other than transient minor local erythema (0.5–1%), induration (3–11%), and tenderness (14–29%). Poor aseptic precautions are the main cause of local reactions and rarely serious problems such as a severe allergic reaction. It can lead to fever which is mild and lasts for 24–48 hours. As IPV contains trace amounts of streptomycin, neomycin, and polymyxin B, allergic reactions may be seen in individuals with hypersensitivity to these antimicrobials. IPV should not be administered to persons who have experienced a severe allergic reaction after a previous dose of IPV or to streptomycin, polymyxin B, and neomycin.

31. What is the minimum age for inactivated polio vaccine (IPV) vaccination?

Minimum age for primary vaccination of IPV is 6 weeks.

32. What is the National Immunization Schedule for polio vaccination?

As per the National Immunization Schedule, five doses of bOPV are to be given; zero dose at birth, three primary doses at 6, 10, and 14 weeks, and one booster dose at 16–24 months of age. Along with bOPV, two fIPV are also given at the age of 6 weeks and 14 weeks.

Another dose of bOPV is given at the age of 5 years. Apart from this, OPV is to be given to every child till the age of 5 years in every SIA being conducted in the area.

33. What is the primary schedule for polio vaccination as per recent Indian Academy of Pediatrics (IAP) Advisory Committee on Vaccines and Immunization Practices (ACVIP) recommendation 2018–2019?

As per the recommendation of the Advisory Committee on Vaccines and Immunization Practices (ACVIP) timetable 2012, the polio vaccination schedule is depicted in **Table 3**.

TABLE 3: Indian Academy of Pediatrics Advisory Committee on Vaccines and Immunization Practices (ACVIP) timetable 2018–2019: the polio vaccination schedule.

Birth	OPV0
6 weeks	IPV1
10 weeks	IPV2
14 weeks	IPV3
16–18 months	IPV B1

(OPV: oral polio vaccine; IPV: inactivated polio vaccine)

In case IPV is not available or feasible, the child should be offered bOPV (three doses) at 6, 10, and 14 weeks. In such cases, give two fIPV at 6 weeks and 14 weeks at government facility.

Similarly, if IPV is not available or feasible for booster (stand-alone or combination), bOPV is to be given.

In addition to this, all OPV doses (mono- or bi-) offered through SIAs should also be provided.

34. What are the major changes for polio immunization recommendation in the Indian Academy of Pediatrics (IAP) timetable 2018–2019?

In place of sequential IPV-OPV schedule, apart from birth dose of OPV, IPV is recommended for primary polio immunization. But, due to poor availability of IPV in the market, OPV is recommended, if IPV is not available or feasible.

35. What are the reasons for these changes in recommendation?

This policy is in accordance with the decision taken by GPEI where phased removal of Sabin viruses would be undertaken. This will pave the way to ultimate adoption of all-IPV schedule in future considering the inevitable cessation of OPV from immunization schedules owing to its safety issues (VAPP and cVDPVs). This will result in elimination of VDPV type 2 in "parallel" with eradication.

36. What is the rationale of oral polio vaccine (OPV) plus inactivated polio vaccine (IPV) schedule?

For all countries using OPV in the National Immunization Program, the WHO continues to recommend the inclusion of at least one dose of IPV in the vaccination schedule. The primary purpose of this IPV dose is to induce an immunity base that could be rapidly boosted due to poliovirus outbreak after type 2 after the removal of type 2 component from OPV. Inclusion of IPV may reduce risks for the development of VAPP and could boost both humoral and mucosal immunity against poliovirus types 1 and 3 in vaccine recipients. In polio-endemic countries and in countries at high risk for importation and subsequent spread of poliovirus, the WHO recommends a bOPV birth dose (zero dose) followed by a primary series of three bOPV doses and at least one IPV dose. If one dose of IPV is used, it should be given IM at 14 weeks of age or later (when maternal antibodies have diminished and immunogenicity is significantly higher) and can be coadministered with a bOPV dose. In India, two intradermal fIPV are given in the Expanded Program on Immunization (EPI) at 6 and 14 weeks in place of single IM IPV at 14 weeks.

For infants starting the routine immunization schedule late (age > 3 months), the IPV dose should be administered at the first immunization contact along with bOPV and the other routinely recommended vaccines.

37. What is birth dose or zero dose of oral polio vaccine (OPV)?

The birth or zero dose of bOPV should be administered as soon as possible or within 15 days after birth to maximize SCRs following subsequent doses and to induce mucosal protection before enteric pathogens may interfere with the immune response. Also, a first dose of bOPV given while infants are still protected by maternally-derived antibodies that may, at least theoretically, prevent VAPP. Even in cases of perinatal HIV infection, early bOPV vaccination seems to be well-tolerated and no additional risk of VAPP has been documented in such children.

38. In the schedule recommended by the Advisory Committee on Vaccines and Immunization Practices (ACVIP), can oral polio vaccine (OPV) be used in place of inactivated polio vaccine (IPV)?

All doses of IPV may be replaced with OPV, if IPV is unaffordable or unavailable. The primary schedule must be completed with three doses of OPV given at 6, 10, and 14 weeks. No child should be left without adequate protection against WPV (i.e., three doses of either vaccine).

39. If inactivated polio vaccine (IPV) first followed by oral polio vaccine (OPV) can prevent vaccine-associated paralytic poliomyelitis (VAPP), then why the Advisory Committee on Vaccines and Immunization Practices (ACVIP) has retained birth dose of OPV before IPV in immunization timetable 2018–2019?

Providing the first OPV dose at a time when the infant is still protected by maternally-derived antibodies may, at least theoretically, also prevent VAPP. A birth dose of OPV is considered necessary to induce gut immunity in countries where the risk of poliovirus transmission is high. Also, zero dose of OPV is retained as studies have proved that immunogenicity with IPV is better, if there is prior priming with OPV.

40. Why booster of inactivated polio vaccine (IPV) is required?

Since IPV administered to infants in immunization schedule (i.e., 6, 10, and 14 weeks) results in suboptimal seroconversion, hence, a supplementary dose of IPV is recommended at 16–18 months.

41. What is catch-up schedule of polio vaccination as per the Advisory Committee on Vaccines and Immunization Practices (ACVIP)?

Inactivated polio vaccine may be offered as "catch-up vaccination" for children <5 years of age who have completed primary immunization with OPV. IPV can be given as three doses; two doses at 2 months interval followed by a third dose after 6 months. This schedule will ensure a long-lasting protection against poliovirus disease.

42. What are the recommendations for polio vaccination for travelers?

The recommendations for travelers to polio-endemic countries are:
- Some polio-free countries may require resident travelers from polio-infected countries to be vaccinated against polio in order to obtain an entry visa or they may require that travelers receive an additional dose on arrival or both. Travelers to infected areas should be vaccinated according to their national schedules.
- Nonimmunized individuals should complete a primary schedule of polio vaccine, using either IPV or OPV. Primary series includes at least three doses of either vaccine.
- For people who travel frequently to polio-endemic areas but who stay only for brief periods, a one-time only additional dose of a polio vaccine after the primary series should be sufficient to prevent disease.

43. What are the schedule and dose in preterm and low birth weight (LBW) babies?

Dose and schedule are the same in preterm or low birth weight (LBW) babies as after birth dose of OPV, vaccination starts at the age of 6 weeks. Birth dose of OPV can be given safely in these children.

44. What should be the schedule for polio immunization if a child comes late?

Polio immunization is given to any child presents till 5 years of age. Such a child should receive three primary doses followed by first booster 1 year after third primary dose and a second booster 3–4 years after the first booster dose, provided the child is <5-year-old. As per the WHO recommendation, infants starting the routine immunization schedule late (age > 3 months), the IPV dose should be administered at the first immunization contact.

45. What are the merits/demerits of oral polio vaccine (OPV) and inactivated polio vaccine (IPV)?

The differences of both vaccines are given in **Table 4**.

46. What are the programmatic benefits of inactivated polio vaccine (IPV)?

- Reduce risks associated with type 2 poliovirus—As oral polio vaccine type 2 (OPV2) has now been withdrawn from use, the provision of IPV in strengthened routine settings will raise population immunity against

TABLE 4: Merits and demerits of OPV and IPV.

OPV	IPV
Oral, ease of administration, and suitable for mass campaigns	Necessity of skilled personnel for injection
High systemic immunity except in developing countries	High systemic immunity
High gut immunity, pharyngeal immunity	Lower gut immunity, but good oropharyngeal immunity
High efficacy (but suboptimal efficacy in tropical countries)	High efficacy
Risk of VAPP	No risk of VAPP
Risk of VDPVs	No risk of VDPVs
Contraindicated in immunodeficient individuals	The only polio vaccine recommended for immunodeficient individuals

(IPV: inactivated polio vaccine; OPV: oral polio vaccine; VAPP: vaccine-associated paralytic poliomyelitis; VDPV: vaccine-derived poliovirus)

type 2 poliovirus. A region immunized with IPV would have a lower risk of re-emergence or reintroduction of wild or vaccine-derived type 2 poliovirus.
- Interrupt transmission in the case of outbreaks—should monovalent oral polio vaccine type 2 (mOPV2) be needed to control an outbreak of cVDPV, those primed with IPV would be expected to have a stronger immune response, thus facilitating outbreak control and interruption of polio transmission.
- Hasten polio eradication—IPV will boost immunity against poliovirus types 1 and 3 in children who have previously received OPV, which could further accelerate the eradication of these two wild viruses.

47. What are immunogenicity and vaccine efficacy of OPV in developing country like India?

In developed countries like USA, >95% seroconverted after three doses of OPV (to all types). Excellent mucosal immunity induced by OPV and invisible immunization of others due to vaccine virus spread were believed to be two factors contributing to such striking herd effect. A greater degree of vaccine virus spread and herd effect was anticipated in developing countries with poor hygiene and sanitation conditions.

When OPV was introduced in developing countries including India, suboptimal immunogenic efficacy of types 1 and 3 component was observed in several places. Studies conducted by Dr T Jacob John and his colleagues from Vellore, India have demonstrated low immunogenicity of tOPV in India as early as in 1970s and 1980s. This was further confirmed by a comprehensive review of 32 studies from developing countries, which shows low immunogenicity of tOPV for types 1 and 3 in developing countries.

Within India, when it comes to Uttar Pradesh, per dose efficacy of tOPV was calculated to be just 9% per dose. Exact cause for poor efficacy of OPV is not known, but warm climate, interference by enteroviruses, high incidence of diarrhea, and prevalence of malnutrition are some of the factors attributed for lower efficacy of OPV.

48. How can inactivated polio vaccine (IPV) be used as a complementary tool to oral polio vaccine (OPV)?

The advantages of using IPV along with OPV can be as follows:
- Excellent immunogenicity, efficacy, and safety of IPV, which guarantees individual protection.
- The risk of VAPP with this combined OPV and IPV schedule is extremely low as the child receives OPV at the time when he/she is protected against VAPP by maternal antibodies. Subsequently, he/she is protected from VAPP by IPV.
- Mucosal immunity as measured by stool excretion of virus after mOPV1 challenge is superior with combination of OPV and IPV as compared to IPV alone. IPV boosts mucosal immunity very effectively in previously OPV-vaccinated individuals.
- Switch to IPV is part of endgame strategy in postpolio eradication era in the form of at least one dose of IPV to be included in the routine EPI.

49. How many doses of oral polio vaccine (OPV) and inactivated polio vaccine (IPV) are needed to protect a child from wild polio?

There is no firm conclusion on the number of doses of OPV, mOPV, or bOPV required to ensure 100% protection, but administration of enhanced-potency vaccine in most studies has resulted in seroconversion to the three poliovirus types in 94–100% of vaccinees after two doses and high titers of serum neutralizing antibody in 99–100% of recipients after three doses. Two doses of IPV at 2 months interval produce 70–100% and three doses at 6, 10, and 14 weeks produce 63–91% seroconversion.

Various studies conducted in developed and developing countries, including India, have shown consistent immunogenicity with IPV across different geographic and environmental variabilities. IPV also protects against VAPP, e.g., Hungary has not reported any case of VAPP after introduction of one IPV dose in sequential schedule in 1992.

50. What is the duration of protection of oral polio vaccine (OPV) and inactivated polio vaccine (IPV)?

Neutralizing antibody produced by OPV (or IPV) is long lasting. Long-lasting memory responses have been demonstrated by booster doses. Low levels of neutralizing antibody can be boosted by secondary exposure to disease or by booster vaccination. Memory cells are prompted by a booster dose or secondary exposure to differentiate into plasma cells, which secrete antibody.

51. If a child has received >40 doses, does he still require further immunization during polio campaign?

Every child below 5 years of age should be given OPV in every polio campaign regardless of previous status of immunization (in routine as well as polio campaign), as gut immunity is of short duration and repeated frequent immunization with OPV is necessary to sustain gut immunity.

52. When there is no case of polio in India since January 2011 and India has received the Polio Eradication Certificate in March 2014 ("polio-free" status), should still be oral polio vaccine (OPV) recommended to be given through supplementary immunization activities (SIAs)?

Yes, because in 2019, polio remains endemic in three countries: (1) Afghanistan, (2) Nigeria, and (3) Pakistan. Until poliovirus transmission is interrupted in these countries, all countries remain at risk of importation of polio; hence, OPV is to be administered to every child till the age of 5 years during all SIAs being conducted in that area as it is necessary to sustain high level of immunity against WPV till global success in polio eradication.

53. Why oral polio vaccine (OPV) should be given despite availability of inactivated polio vaccine (IPV)?

Oral polio vaccine use should be continued due to following reasons:
- In concordance with the government policy of using OPV for polio eradication.
- Mucosal immunity as measured by stool excretion of virus after mOPV1 challenge is superior with combination of OPV and IPV as compared to IPV alone.
- By not giving OPV, we might create confusion in the minds of the parents whose children receive only IPV about the efficacy and safety of OPV and interfere with OPV uptake on the NIDs and Subnational Immunization Days (SNIDs).

54. What are the dilemmas faced by the practitioners?
- How and where to incorporate current "stand-alone" IPV in existing schedule?
- How to start "switching to IPV" without harming the national program?
- How to convince parents about need for an extra injection?
- Why should we give both OPV and IPV?
- Those who can afford the vaccine already well-protected and may not need it!

55. What are the recommendations for adult polio vaccination?

Routine adult polio vaccination or boosters are not recommended considering the epidemiology of the disease in India. Vaccination with IPV is recommended for certain adults who are at greater risk of exposure to poliovirus like laboratory workers who handle specimens that might contain polioviruses, etc.

For unvaccinated adults, two successive injections of 0.5 mL can be given at intervals of preferably 2 months. A third dose (booster) may be administered 8–12 months after the second injection.

56. What is mucosal immunity?

Mucosal immunity in polio refers to the resistance to mucosal infection by WPVs due to prior infection with WPV or immunizing experience with polio vaccines. Mucosal immunity decreases the replication and excretion (shedding) of the virus and, thus, provides a potential barrier to its transmission.

57. Which vaccine oral polio vaccine (OPV) or inactivated polio vaccine (IPV) induces better mucosal immunity? If OPV induces good mucosal immunity, then why highly vaccinated children with OPV participate in wild polio transmission?

Mucosal immunity refers to the resistance to mucosal infection by WPVs due to prior infection or immunizing experience. OPV induces a high nasopharyngeal and duodenal immunoglobulin A (IgA) response. Some more facts about mucosal immunity are:
- Immunoglobulin A response is induced more readily by infection than by stimulation by nonreplicating antigen. Thus, IgA is a marker of gut infection not necessarily mucosal immunity. Moreover, IgA is not the only medium of local mucosal immunity.
- It is not necessary that an OPV dose will cause infection every time if there is no uptake. This finding offers an explanation why repeated doses of OPV have to be given to the same children, with virtually 100% coverage, before wild virus transmission could be stopped in developing countries.
- Inactivated polio vaccine induces only low levels of IgA antibody thus, suggesting that there are other mechanisms of local immunity. So, there is more to mucosal immunity than the IgA antibody production and transport. IPV induces a very strong humoral immunity.
- There is evidence that resistance to reinfection wanes with time and high force of transmission of WPV in the area allows fully immunized children to participate in poliovirus transmission.

58. What do you mean by "endgame" strategy?

Polio endgame refers to management of the "posteradication" risks due to OPV. In 2015, WPV type 2 was declared eradicated (last case reported in 1999); WPV type 3 was declared eradicated in October 2019 (last case reported in November 2012); and while WPV type 1 has yet to be interrupted, its incidence has been reduced by over 90% since 2014. No WPV detection outside Afghanistan/Pakistan since 2016.

The Polio Eradication and Endgame Strategic Plan 2019–2023 (the Plan) developed by GPEI and spearheaded by the WHO, Rotary International, the US Centers for Disease Control and Prevention, and the United Nations Children's Fund (UNICEF), with support from the Bill and Melinda Gates Foundation, to capitalize on this new opportunity to end all polio disease. It accounts for the parallel pursuit of WPV eradication and cVDPV elimination.

59. What are the objectives of endgame strategy 2019–2023?

The strategic plan involves four objectives:
1. *Eradication*—stopping transmission
2. *Integration*—systemically collaborating with other public health sectors, capacities, and contributions beyond GPEI to help achieve and sustain eradication
3. *Certification and containment*—certify eradication and containment of all WPVs and ensure long-term polio security
4. *Enabling areas*—gender equality and equity, governance and management, research, and financial resources.

60. What will be postpolio eradication strategy?

After eradication of polio, expected by 2023, the key areas will be:
2023–2024 (Polio Postcertification Strategy)
—contain polioviruses
—protect populations
—detect and respond.

61. Should polio vaccination be continued after eradication of wild polio?

Once eradication of WPV has been confirmed, the public health benefits of RI with OPV may no longer outweigh the burden of disease due to VAPP and cVDPVs. Each OPV using country must decide whether to stop all RI against polio after OPV cessation (after OPV cessation, IPV will be the only option for those countries which decide to continue RI).

62. Is there any plan for cessation of oral polio vaccine (OPV) use after the global eradication of polio?

Yes, because as per the definition of polio eradication, it accounts for parallel pursuit of WPV eradication and cVDPV elimination. Once WPV transmission is eliminated, any polio thereafter would be exclusively vaccine caused (VAPP or VDPV). To overcome the risk of cVDPV due to OPV in posteradication era, GPEI has recommended for cessation of OPV use globally in posteradication era.

Full OPV withdrawal will take place approximately 1 year after WPV eradication is certified. Planning for OPV withdrawal will start 2 years in advance, building on the lessons learned from the switch from tOPV to bOPV. Precessation SIAs may also be considered for high-risk areas in the year prior to withdrawal.

63. What are the risks associated with oral polio vaccine (OPV) cessation?

There are two main risks associated with OPV cessation: (1) immediate risk of cVDPV emergence and (2) medium- and long-term risk of poliovirus reintroduction from a vaccine manufacturing site, research facility, or diagnostic laboratory.

64. What are the priorities for national policymakers in oral polio vaccine (OPV) using countries during preparatory phase of OPV cessation?

In the countries where OPV is being used, before its cessation, certain preparations need to be ensured. These are:
- Strengthen polio (AFP) surveillance to guide interruption of WPV transmission, certify eradication, and detect potential importations and cVDPVs.
- Fully implement and verify appropriate containment of all wild and VDPVs and prepare for Sabin virus containment.
- Raise RI coverage (>90%) to minimize the risk of spread of an imported WPV and risk of cVDPVs emergence.
- Based on analysis of risks, benefits, and opportunity costs, decide whether to stop all RI against polio after OPV cessation or continue with IPV which will be the only option.
- Conduct an iVDPV risk assessment and establish a case management plan, if needed.
- Establish national plans and mechanisms for the eventual cessation of all OPV use in RI programs and safe destruction of remaining OPV stocks.

65. Once wild poliovirus (WPV) is eliminated, what is the need of having a future vaccine policy?

When smallpox was declared eradicated, countries could decide independently whether or not to stop vaccination against the disease. For polio, this approach could prove disastrous. This is because of the safety problems associated with OPV use. Inadvertent escape of virulent virus from laboratories and malicious introduction of virulent polioviruses (bioterrorism) are the few other risks involved with posteradication era. Indeed, these are the main reasons why vaccination against polio cannot be stopped even after cessation of wild WPV transmission and achieving eradication.

66. What is the World Health Organization (WHO) stand on posteradication vaccination policy?

According to the WHO, after interruption of WPV, continued use of OPV would compromise the goal of a polio-free world. The stated strategy of the WHO is to stop using OPV in a single day, once eradication has been presumed to occur. This strategy involves simply observing for poliovirus circulation and for cases poliovirus-induced paralysis in the absence of vaccination.

67. What should be the ideal posteradication strategy for India?

The WHO has suggested that developed countries continue to use IPV in RI to prevent possibilities of import of cVDPV or WPV through bioterrorism. Stopping all polio immunization and continuing AFP surveillance alone although would be cheaper, but this strategy is fraught with danger.

68. Do you think a strategy shift from oral polio vaccine (OPV) to inactivated polio vaccine (IPV) can avoid inevitable problems associated with OPV such as vaccine-associated polio, risk of polio in immunocompromised children, and risk of vaccine-derived polio outbreaks that have occurred in few countries even after successful eradication of wild polio?

Yes, as far as vaccine VAPP and risk of polio in immunocompromised children are concerned, IPV is definite answer. However, to thwart the possibility of future emergence of vaccine-derived polio outbreaks, IPV still can work though not many precedents are available and experience is limited.

69. How can current inactivated polio vaccine (IPV) be made more efficacious?

To make the current IPV more efficacious and effective, following are the things that are being tried:
- Novel approaches to formulate and administer IPV that do not require trained medical personnel or hypodermic needles for administration, provide substantial dose sparing, and lower the overall cost without compromising efficacy.
- Novel ways to substantially increase the level of intestinal mucosal immunity induced by IPV in order to prevent viral shedding.
- Novel methods to produce an equally or more efficacious inactivated or subunit poliovirus vaccine that do not require wild virus for production and can be manufactured at scale in a cost-effective manner.

70. What is Sabin inactivated polio vaccine (sIPV)? Why there is a need of this new generation of IPV?

Sabin inactivated polio vaccine is a liquid trivalent vaccine produced from Sabin strain of OPV (types 1, 2, and 3) grown on Vero cells.

The global switch to bOPV was successfully implemented in April 2016, the first step in the global withdrawal of live polioviruses vaccines following global eradication, to be followed by a posteradication period when all immunizations will be based on IPV. More recently, the eradication of WPV3 has been declared making the global withdrawal of all OPV and substitution by IPV more imminent. However, there is a global shortage of IPV supply and increased demand will exacerbate this situation, creating an urgent need to expand manufacturing capacity and decrease costs of IPV in both the short- and long-term. Further, the Global Action Plan III (GAPIII) containment recommendations by the Strategic Advisory Group of Experts (SAGE), which accompanied the recommendation to withdraw type 2, also require stringent precautions be taken to eliminate the possibility of environmental contamination with the live polioviruses, limiting manufacture with Salk viruses to developed countries with established infrastructure.

This has led to the suggestion that attenuated Sabin strains used in OPV vaccines may be inherently safer for use in manufacturing IPV.

71. What is the current status of Sabin inactivated polio vaccine (sIPV)?

Several sIPV candidates are in clinical development, some previously shown to be safe and immunogenic in adults and in infants, leading to licensure and extensive use of sIPV in China and Japan. Takeda, a Japanese Biotech company, agreed a technology transfer from the BIKEN Foundation [formerly the Japan Poliomyelitis Research Institute (JPRI)] for viral seeds to develop the sIPV and investigate novel manufacturing technologies to enhance production capacity. The first use of the Takeda sIPV, in a combination with a DTaP vaccine (TAK-361S) in 3–67-month-old children, has been reported.

72. Is Sabin inactivated polio vaccine (sIPV) equally safe and efficacious as standard IPV?

Takeda has recently published results of their phase I/II study in which they assessed three dosages of a stand-alone sIPV. Two cohorts of 40 adults and 60 toddlers, respectively, were initially assessed for safety after receiving high-dosage sIPV compared with placebo (adults) or Salk IPV (toddlers). A cohort of 240 infants was then enrolled and randomized (1:1:1:1) to receive low-, medium-, or high-dosage sIPV or a reference Salk IPV in a three-dose primary schedule at 6, 10, and 14 weeks of age. The immunogenicity was measured as neutralization antibody titers at baseline and 4 weeks after vaccination.

They found that the sIPV had a comparable safety profile to the control arm in adults or the reference Salk IPV vaccine in toddlers and infants. Infants displayed dosage-dependent immune responses to sIPV when assayed using Sabin strains, which were equivalent to the reference IPV in the high-dosage sIPV group for serotypes 1 and 2, but not for Sabin and Salk serotype 3. SCRs of the low- and medium-dosage groups were significantly lower than the Salk IPV group for both Sabin and Salk serotypes 1 and type 2 ($P < 0.05$), with no significant differences for Salk or Sabin serotype 3. Responses to sIPV, particularly to Sabin types 1 and 2, were higher in initially seronegative infants, indicating possible interference by maternally-derived antibodies.

They concluded that their novel stand-alone sIPV was well-tolerated with an acceptable safety profile, but less immunogenic than reference Salk IPV at 6, 10, and 14 weeks of age for Salk serotypes 1 and 2, with apparent interference by maternal antibodies. Hence, more studies/data is needed to conclude that the new sIPV is as efficacious as standard Salk IPV.

73. What about oral polio vaccine (OPV) contact immunization and herd effect?

Based on the experience from developed countries, it was presumed that advantage of the invisible vaccine virus spread will be more pronounced in developing countries with poor hygiene and sanitation where fecal-oral transmission would occur more frequently and poliovirus transmission will be interrupted once 80% coverage will be reached with three doses of OPV, but this has never happened.

Herd effect: Herd effect is reduction of incidence of disease in unvaccinated segment due to vaccinating a section of population. The prerequisites for herd effect of a vaccine include two elements. First, immunization should reduce the transmission potential of the individual and second, sufficient proportion of individuals in a group should be immunized in order to have an effect on the transmission of the virus. The higher the vaccine coverage, the greater the potential of herd effect. When children in developing countries are given sufficient number of OPV doses and they seroconvert, they will be protected from the disease, most probably for life. On the other hand, gut immunity present in them soon after immunization is likely to decline as time progresses, until its level is insufficient to prevent an outbreak. Such waning gut immunity, particularly in the face of high force of virus transmission (dictated by inoculums size and/or repetitiveness of exposure) and the persistence or reintroduction of wild virus, would set the stage for large-scale poliomyelitis epidemics in well-immunized populations after a period of control of disease or even interruption of transmission. Now fully vaccinated children would also participate in virus transmission.

Herd effect of OPV was not visible in India on ground which was evident by the fact that repeated doses of OPV had to be given to the same group of children, with virtually 100% coverage, before wild virus transmission could be stopped and the median age of polio in India has not shifted to the right and remained stationary at 12–18 months from prior to introducing immunization till now.

74. What is pulse polio immunization?

It is strategy for eradication of poliomyelitis in which mass immunization is done. Extra dose of OPV (in the form of pulse) is given to all children <5 years of age in an area regardless of previous status of immunization at a time on a given day. The aim is to achieve 100% coverage.

75. Do you need to give regular polio immunization when pulse oral polio vaccine (OPV) is taken?

Yes, OPV given in SIA (pulse immunization program) is an extra dose and RI for polio should be continued as per schedule.

76. Why the polio [acute flaccid paralysis (AFP)] surveillance continue in India even after certification of polio eradication in March, 2014?

Even after certification, the polio (AFP) surveillance will continue and need to be sensitive enough to pick any importation of WPV or emergence of VDPV.

77. Can a child with isolated facial paralysis just like the Bell's palsy should also be reported as a case of acute flaccid paralysis (AFP)?

Rarely, poliomyelitis can manifest as isolated asymmetrical paralysis of face, a presentation quite indistinguishable from idiopathic "Bell's palsy". During a 16-month study period in South India, three out of five children presenting as "Bell's palsy" were in fact found suffering from poliomyelitis. This is also supported by AFP surveillance data of India. Hence, in polio-endemic countries, poliomyelitis should be considered when children present as "Bell's palsy".

78. What is polio-like syndrome?

In the past decade, newly identified strains of enterovirus have been linked to polio-like paralytic cases among children in Asia and Australia. Enterovirus infections, especially coxsackieviruses A9 and A23 (echovirus 9) and group B coxsackieviruses, frequently caused meningoencephalitis often associated with transient paralysis. Coxsackievirus A7 infection occasionally resulted in permanent paralysis.

79. What is acute flaccid myelitis?

Acute flaccid myelitis (AFM), defined as acute flaccid limb weakness, is classified using the Council of State and Territorial Epidemiologists (CSTE) case definitions of "confirmed" [magnetic resonance imaging (MRI) with spinal cord lesion largely restricted to gray matter and spanning ≥1 spinal segments], "probable" [cerebrospinal fluid (CSF) pleocytosis (>5 white blood cells/mm^3], or "not a case".

Acute flaccid myelitis is a serious neurologic condition that affects mostly children. It is characterized by rapid onset of flaccid weakness in one or more limbs and distinct abnormalities of the spinal cord gray matter as seen on MRI. AFM is one of several conditions resulting in AFP, which is the sudden onset of flaccid weakness without features typical of an upper motor neuron disorder.
- Most cases of AFM occur among children in late summer or early fall
- Acute flaccid myelitis can progress rapidly and require urgent medical intervention
- A diagnosis of AFM is made on the basis of a thorough physical and neurologic examination and MRI of the spinal cord
- There is currently no proven treatment for AFM
- Prompt recognition and reporting of AFM are critical for providing patient care and understanding the condition.

80. What is polio outbreak simulation exercise (POSE)?

The POSE is polio outbreak simulation exercise. Simulation exercise is primarily designed for health organizations to run as a discussion-based simulation exercise over 1 day. The exercise is intended to be facilitated by emergency planners with specialist assistance as required. Multiagency participation is beneficial and is enabled through the scenario and discussion points. The exercise has been designed to test a series of objectives for preparing for a possible poliovirus event or polio outbreak. Additional local objectives may be incorporated, if required. To enable the delivery of each exercise, guidance notes are provided for facilitators in addition to explanatory material for participants.

81. What is polio transition?

Polio transition is the process of transferring the necessary functions and funding from the GPEI to maintain a polio-free world and where feasible and appropriate to help achieve other health priorities. Closure of the initiative must be planned carefully, so that core functions and capacities can be sustained after certification.

- Sustaining a polio-free world after poliovirus eradication
- Strengthening immunization systems, including surveillance for vaccine preventable diseases, in order to achieve the goals of WHOs Global Vaccine Action Plan
- Strengthening emergency preparedness, detection, and response capacity in countries to fully implement the International Health Regulations (2005).

82. What is novel oral polio vaccine type 2 (nOPV2)?

The novel oral polio vaccine type 2 (nOPV2) is a new tool developed to better address the risk of circulating vaccine-derived poliovirus type 2 (cVDPV2) and VAPP. nOPV2 is a modification of the existing mOPV2 that clinical trials have shown provide comparable protection against poliovirus while being more genetically stable and less likely to revert to a form that can cause paralysis. The increased genetic stability means that there is a reduced risk of seeding new cVDPV2 outbreaks compared to the existing mOPV2. nOPV2 could eventually be used as a replacement for mOPV2.

83. Does it work? Is it indeed free from the side effects of conventional Sabin monovalent oral polio vaccine type 2 (mOPV2)?

A dedicated group of global agencies and vaccine experts has been engaged in developing candidates for nOPV2 for the past 9 years, with the first clinical study with nOPV2 implemented in 2017. In trials, the nOPV2 demonstrated noninferior immunogenicity to the historical mOPV2 control groups among infants. Assessment of viral excretion indicates that nOPV2 is unlikely to be shed in a greater rate or quantity as compared to mOPV2 and the cessation of intestinal mucosal viral replication and shedding may be earlier in infants. No direct way to quantitatively extrapolate to reduced risk of paralysis in humans, the available data support significantly improved genetic and phenotypic stability of shed nOPV2 compared to shed Sabin 2. Hence, the novel OPV2 could be an effective tool in reducing risk of vaccine-derived transmission. Phase I and phase II study results supportive of promising safety, immunogenicity, and genetic stability.

84. What are oral polio vaccine (OPV) stockpiles?

Oral polio vaccine remains the most effective tool for responding to polio outbreaks, even after certification. To prepare for full OPV withdrawal and ensure rapid and effective response after OPV cessation, the GPEI has initiated the establishment of mOPV stockpiles for types 1 and 3 as done for type 2.

SUGGESTED READING

1. Balasubramanian S, Shah A, Pemde HK, Chatterjee P, Shivananda S, Guduru VK, et al. (2018). Indian Academy of Pediatrics (IAP) Advisory Committee on Vaccines and Immunization Practices (ACVIP) Recommended Immunization Schedule (2018-19) and Update on Immunization for Children Aged 0 Through 18 Years. [online] Available from: https://www.indianpediatrics.net/dec2018/1066.pdf. [Last accessed July, 2020].
2. Centers for Disease Control and Prevention (CDC). (2013). Poliomyelitis. [online] Available from: http://www.cdc.gov/vaccines/pubs/pinkbook/downloads/polio.pdf. [Last accessed July, 2020].
3. Centers for Disease Control and Prevention (CDC). Updated recommendations of the Advisory Committee on Immunization Practices (ACIP) regarding routine poliovirus vaccination. Morb Mortal Wkly Rep. 2009;58:829-30.
4. Centers for Disease Control and Prevention (CDC). Update on vaccine-derived polioviruses—worldwide, January 2006-August 2007. Morb Mortal Wkly Rep. 2007;56:996-1001.
5. Combined Immunization of Infants with Oral and Inactivated Poliovirus Vaccines: Results of a Randomized Trial in The Gambia, Oman, and Thailand. WHO Collaborative Study Group on Oral and Inactivated Poliovirus Vaccines. J Infect Dis. 1997;175:S215-27.
6. Cramer JP, Jimeno J, Han HH, Lin S, Hartmann K, Borkwski A, et al. Safety and immunogenicity of experimental stand-alone trivalent, inactivated Sabin-strain polio vaccine formulations in healthy infants: a randomized, observer-blind, controlled phase 1/2 trial. Vaccine. 2020;38:5313-23.
7. Global Polio Eradication Initiative (GPEI). (2013). Polio Eradication and Endgame Strategic Plan 2013-2018. [online] Available from: http://polioeradication.org/wp-content/uploads/2016/07/2.8_8IMB.pdf. [Last accessed July, 2020].
8. Global Polio Eradication Initiative (GPEI). (2013). Polio Eradication and Endgame Strategic Plan 2013-2018: Working Draft. [online] Available from: http://polioeradication.org/wp-content/uploads/2013/01/EndGameStratPlan_20130123_ENG.pdf. [Last accessed July, 2020].
9. Global Polio Eradication Initiative (GPEI). (2015). Vaccine-associated paralytic polio (VAPP) and vaccine-derived poliovirus (VDPV): Factsheet. [online] Available from: https://www.who.int/immunization/diseases/poliomyelitis/endgame_objective2/oral_polio_vaccine/VAPPandcVDPVFactSheet-Feb2015.pdf. [Last accessed July, 2020].
10. Global Polio Eradication Initiative (GPEI). (2019). Polio Endgame Strategy 2019-2023: Eradication, Integration, Certification, and Containment. [online] Available from: http://polioeradication.org/wp-content/uploads/2019/06/english-polio-endgame-strategy.pdf. [Last accessed July, 2020].

11. Indian Academy of Pediatrics (IAP). (2013). IAP Guidebook on Immunization. [online] Available from: http://www.iapcoi.com/hp/iap_guidebook.php. [Last accessed July, 2020].
12. John TJ, Vashishtha VM. Eradication of vaccine polioviruses: why, when & how? Indian J Med Res. 2009;130:491-4.
13. John TJ. Vaccine-associated paralytic polio in India. Bull World Health Organ. 2002;80:917.
14. Khan M. Economics of polio vaccination in the post-eradication era: should OPV-using countries adopt IPV? Vaccine. 2008;26:2034-40.
15. Kohler KA, Banerjee K, Hlady WG, Andrus JK, Sutter RW. Vaccine-associated paralytic poliomyelitis in India during 1999: decreased risk despite massive use of oral polio vaccine. Bull World Health Organ. 2002;80:210-6.
16. Mittal SK, Mathew JL. Polio eradication in India: the way forward. Indian J Pediatr. 2007;74:153-60.
17. Peterson C, Stone DM, Marsh SM, Schumacher PK, Tiesman HM, McIntosh WL, et al. Suicide rates by major occupational group—17 states, 2012 and 2015. Morb Mortal Wkly Rep. 2018;67:1273-75.
18. Sutter RW, Bahl S, Deshpande JM, Verma H, Ahmad M, Venugopal P, et al. Immunogenicity of a new routine vaccination schedule for global poliomyelitis prevention: an open-label, randomised controlled trial. Lancet. 2015;386: 2413-21.
19. Thacker N. Critical evaluation of OPV. In: Thacker N (Ed). Polio Eradication: Challenges and Opportunities. Proceedings of Round Table Conference Series No. 24. New Delhi: Jaypee Brothers Medical Publishers (P) Ltd., 2010.
20. Vashishtha VM, Thacker N. Global Polio Eradication Initiative (GPEI): future perspectives and need for a new generation of inactivated poliovirus vaccine. J Pediatr Sci. 2010;5:e46.
21. Vashishtha VM. Proceedings of 24th Round Table Conference on Polio Eradication. New Delhi: Ranbaxy Science Foundation; 2010.
22. World Health Organization (WHO). (2005). Framework for national policy makers in OPV-using countries: Cessation of routine oral polio vaccine (OPV) use after global polio eradication. [online] Available from: https://apps.who.int/iris/bitstream/handle/10665/69083/WHO_POLIO_05.02.pdf?sequence=1&isAllowed=y. [Last accessed July, 2020].
23. World Health Organization (WHO). (2013). Meeting of the Strategic Advisory Group of Experts on immunization, November 2012—conclusions and recommendations. [online] Available from: https://www.who.int/wer/2013/wer8801.pdf?ua=1. [Last accessed July, 2020].
24. World Health Organization (WHO). (2013). Polio vaccines grading tables: Table V: Sequential administration IPV-OPV. [online] Available from: http://www.who.int/immunization/polio_sequential_administration_IPV_OPV.pdf. [Last accessed July, 2020].
25. World Health Organization (WHO). (2014). Polio vaccines: WHO position paper, January 2014. [online] Available from: https://www.who.int/wer/2014/wer8909.pdf?ua=1. [Last accessed July, 2020].
26. World Health Organization (WHO). (2015). Polio Outbreak Simulation Exercise: How to test national preparedness plans using the POSE model. [online] Available from: http://www.euro.who.int/__data/assets/pdf_file/0004/290407/Polio-Outbreak-Simulation-Exercise.pdf?ua=1. [Last accessed July, 2020].
27. World Health Organization (WHO). (2016). Fractional dose IPV. [online] Available from: https://www.who.int/immunization/diseases/poliomyelitis/endgame_

28. World Health Organization (WHO). (2016). IPV introduction and RI strengthening. [online] Available from: https://www.who.int/immunization/diseases/poliomyelitis/endgame_objective2/inactivated_polio_vaccine/en/. [Last accessed July, 2020].
29. World Health Organization (WHO). (2016). Polio vaccines: WHO position paper—March 2016. [online] Available from: https://www.who.int/wer/2016/wer9112.pdf?ua=1. [Last accessed July, 2020].
30. World Health Organization (WHO). Polio vaccines and polio immunization in the pre-eradication era: WHO position paper. Wkly Epidemiol Rec. 2010;85: 213-28.
31. Yeh MT, Bujaki E, Dolan PT, Smith M, Wahid R, Konz J, et al. Engineering the live-attenuated polio vaccine to prevent reversion to virulence. Cell Host Microbe. 2020;27:736-51.e8.

(Note: entry begins on previous page) objective2/inactivated_polio_vaccine/fractional_dose/en/. [Last accessed July, 2020].

CHAPTER 17

Diphtheria, Tetanus and Pertussis Vaccines

Vipin M Vashishtha, Unmesh A Upadhyay

PERTUSSIS EPIDEMIOLOGY AND COVERAGE ISSUES

1. What is the epidemiology of pertussis in India?

In India, the incidence of pertussis declined sharply after launch of Universal Immunization Programme (UIP). Prior to UIP, India reported 200,932 cases and 106 deaths in the year 1970 with a mortality rate of <0.001%. During the year 1987, the reported incidence was about 163,000 cases which came down to 39,091 in 2011 to 11, 875 in 2019 **(Fig. 1)** reflecting a decline of >75%. However, many cases go unreported, and many non-pertussis cases are reported and clubbed under the head of "whooping cough" cases. The actual number may be high considering the low coverage with primary and booster doses of diphtheria, tetanus, and pertussis (DTP) vaccine in the country. The data on pertussis disease and infection in adolescents and adults is lacking. There is no data on *Bordetella pertussis* infection rates in the community that may be responsible for appearance of typical pertussis disease in infants and children.

2. What is the coverage of DTP vaccine in India?

As per the data from National Family Health Survey (NFHS-4; 2015–16), the coverage of children age 12–23 months who have received three doses of diphtheria, pertussis, and tetanus (DPT) vaccine was 78.4% (urban: 80.2% and rural: 77.7%). According to the World Health Organization (WHO) data, the coverage with three doses of DPT was 91% for the year 2019 **(Fig. 2)**. However, there is marked inter-state and intra-state disparity in the coverage. The diphtheria, tetanus, and whole-cell pertussis (DTwP) vaccine is widely used in both public and private sectors since 1978. Millions of doses have been used since then, and there are no published data on the poor acceptance of the vaccine or resistance. There are not many reported incidences of serious adverse events following immunization (AEFIs) in the vaccines.

3. Can you summarize key features of pertussis disease in India?

Pertussis is still a significant problem in India. Though the disease is fairly controlled and incidence has declined sharply after the launch of UIP in India, still the surveillance quality is poor, and periodic outbreaks in different parts of country are reported. India is mainly relying of DTwP vaccine though

CHAPTER 17 Diphtheria, Tetanus and Pertussis Vaccines

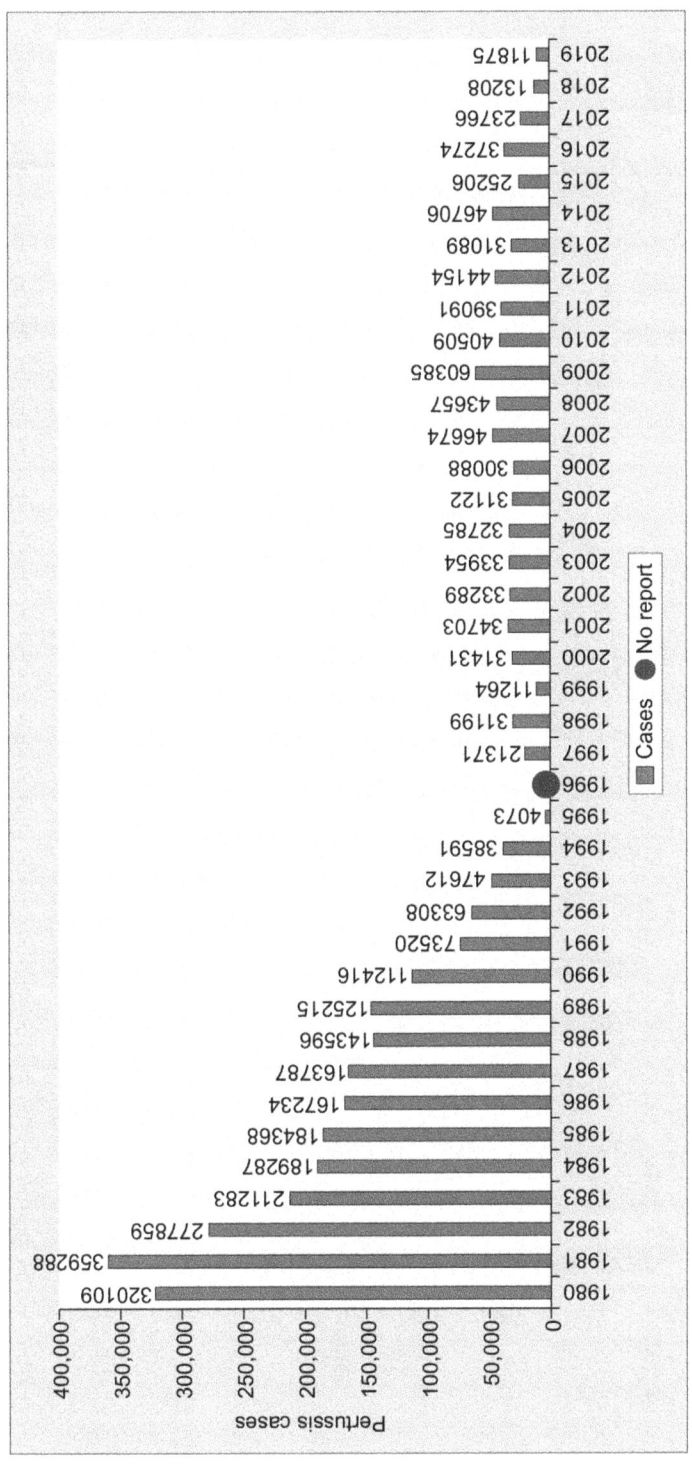

Fig. 1: Number of reported cases of pertussis to WHO from India, 1980–2019.

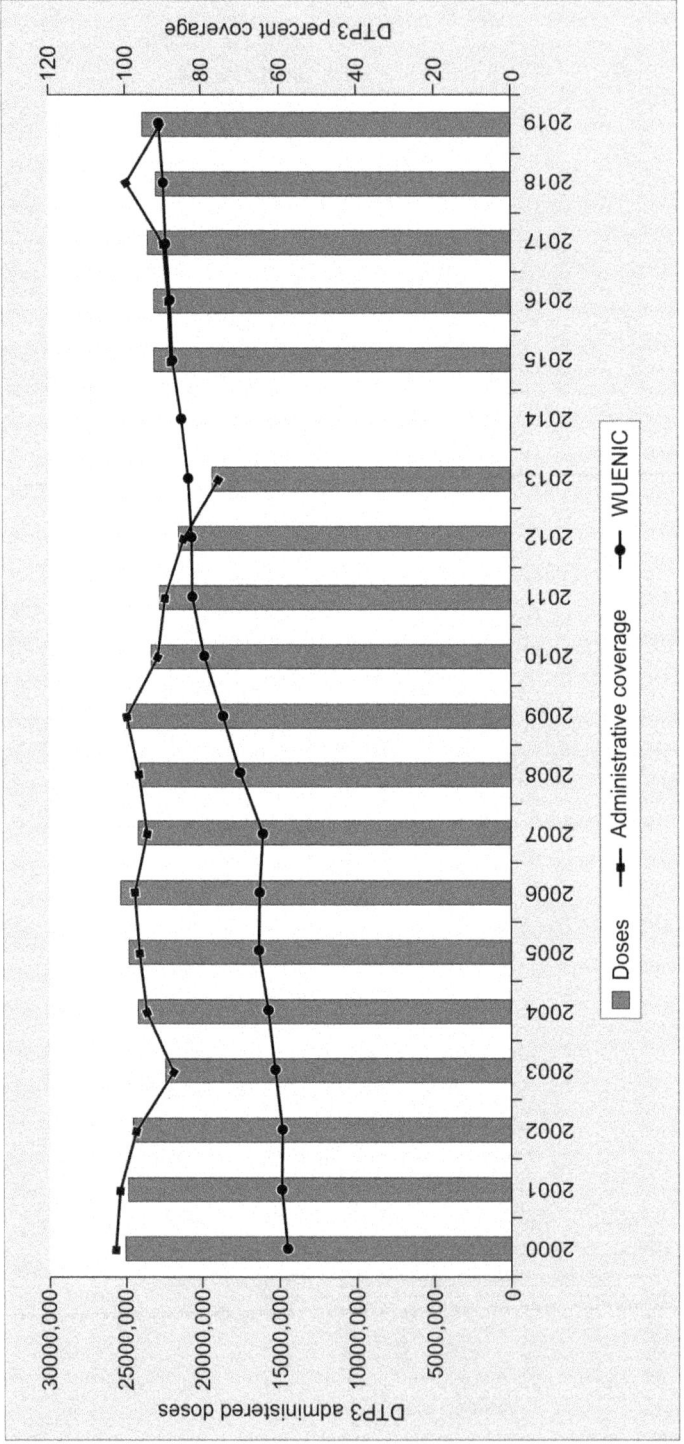

Fig. 2: Reported coverage of three doses of DTP vaccine in India from 2000 to 2019.

Source: World Health Organization. WHO data. [online] available from https://apps.who.int/immunization_monitoring/globalsummary/countries?countrycriteria%5Bcountry%5D%5B%5D=IND&commit=OK [Last accessed September, 2020].

in urban areas, particularly in private sector acellular pertussis (aP) vaccine-based penta- and hexavalent products are also used. However, there is no data on the coverage of aP vaccine use in India which seems quite miniscule in comparison to whole-cell pertussis (wP) vaccine use in large public sector. The coverage with DPT boosters is still very low. Pertussis is still a disease of young children (1–3 years) in India and burden in adolescents and adults is not specified.

PERTUSSIS VACCINES, BIOLOGY, IMMUNITY, AND CAUSES OF RESURGENCE

4. I am confused about the various vaccines that contain diphtheria, tetanus, and pertussis. Can you explain?

There are three basic products that can be used in children younger than age 7 years [DTwP, diphtheria, tetanus and acellular pertussis (DTaP), and diphtheria and tetanus (DT)] and two that can be used in older children and adults [tetanus-diphtheria (Td) and tetanus-diphtheria-pertussis (Tdap)]. Some people get confused between DTaP and Tdap and others get confused between DT and Td. Here is a hint to help you remember. The pediatric formulations usually have three to five times as much of the diphtheria component than what is in the adult formulation. This is indicated by an uppercase "D" for the pediatric formulation (i.e., DTaP, DT) and a lower case "d" for the adult formulation (Tdap, Td). The amount of tetanus toxoid in each of the products is equivalent, so it remains an uppercase "T".

5. What do the acronyms DTwP, DTaP, DT, Tdap, etc. denote?

- wP: whole-cell killed vaccine
- aP:
  - No cells, but its constituent components
  - Pertussis toxin (PT), filamentous hemagglutinin (FHA), pertactin (PRN), agglutinogens 2 and 3
  - ap—contains lower dose of acellular pertussis components (PT, FHA, PRN)
- D: diphtheria toxoid 25 limit of flocculation (Lf)
- d: lower dose with 2 Lf
- T: tetanus toxoid 5 Lf.

6. What is the maximum age of a child to receive DTwP vaccine?

Diphtheria, tetanus and whole-cell pertussis, DTaP, and DT are not given beyond 7 years of age because of high reactogenicity.

7. Can we interchange the different brands of DTaP vaccines?

The components of *pertussis bacilli* used for preparation of the acellular vaccines include PT as the essential component with or without FHA, PRN, and fimbrial protein (FIM)-type 2 and 3. Commercially available vaccines vary in number of components, quantity of components, and method of inactivation of the components. Till quite recently, following aP vaccines were available in India:

- Five-component vaccines (Tripacel™—PT, PRN, FHA, FIM 2, and 3) (not available now in India)
- Three-component vaccines (Infanrix™—PT, FHA, PRN) (not available now in India)
- A two-component combination vaccine [Pentaxim™—PT and FHA, inactivated poliovirus vaccine (IPV), *Haemophilus influenzae* type b (Hib) and Tetraxim™—IPV along with PT and FHA].

However, the five- and two-component aP vaccines are not available now. Most of the aP vaccines are now available in combination forms pentavalent (Pentaxim™) and hexavalent (Hexaxim™ and Infanrix-Hexa™). A new combination vaccine-containing two-component DTaP and IPV (Tetraxim™) has recently launched in Indian market.

CDC's Advisory Committee on Immunization Practices (ACIP) and IAP's Advisory Committee on Vaccines and Immunization Practices (ACVIP) have recommended that, whenever feasible, health care providers should use the same brand of DTaP vaccine for all doses in the vaccination series. However, if we do not know the previously used brand, use whatever DTaP/DTwP vaccine is available for all subsequent doses.

8. What are the problems with acellular pertussis (aP) vaccines?

There is no consensus about the antigenic composition of an ideal aP vaccine. The exact contribution of the different aP antigens to protection is not clear. They are derived from different sources of pertussis. They are purified with different processes and through different compounds like hydrogen peroxide, formaldehyde, and glutaraldehyde. Adjuvants used in a product are also different and adsorbed in a different way to adjuvants. According to WHO, the current generation of aP vaccines available from different manufacturers should be considered as different and unique products because of the presence of one or more different components in different concentrations, and with different degree of adsorption to different adjuvant. There is no known correlate of protection (CoP) for pertussis disease, wP and aP vaccines. Furthermore, there is no consistent, uniform performance of aP-containing products from industrialized and other countries wherever they have been employed. Different types of aP-containing products (i.e., monocomponents, bicomponents, and tricomponents) have fared differently in different regions and countries. For example, these products are found efficacious with fair to good control of the disease in few countries like Japan, Sweden, Denmark, etc. whereas documented outbreaks and resurgence have been reported from the United States of America, Australia, the United Kingdom, Spain, and many other Western countries.

In the absence of efficacy/effectiveness data, it would be hazardous to extrapolate data from one country or one geographic region to other.

Unfortunately, there is no evidence of efficacy/effectiveness of available aP vaccines from India, and most of the aP-containing products are licensed here based on bridging immunogenicity data despite knowing that there is no known CoP for aP vaccines exists.

9. **Which is the most efficacious DTaP vaccine? Does number of components of aP indeed matter?**

According to a systematic review involving 49 randomized clinical trials concluded that one- to two-component aP vaccine had lower absolute efficacy (67–70%) than vaccine with three or more components (80–84%). A recent concurrent review summarized six aP vaccine efficacy trials, including a total of 46,283 participants and 52 safety trials. The review concluded that the efficacy of multicomponent (three or more) aP vaccine varied from 84 to 85% in preventing typical whooping cough and from 71 to 78% in preventing mild pertussis disease. In contrast, the efficacy of one- and two-component vaccine varied from 59 to 75% against typical whooping cough and from 13 to 54% against mild pertussis disease. Therefore, aP vaccine having three or more components is more efficacious than the one having lesser number of components.

However, the WHO does not give much importance to the number of components present in an aP vaccine, and treat all the available aP vaccines at par.

10. **Denmark is successfully using monocomponent aP vaccine in their national immunization program for more than a decade and no resurgence of pertussis was noted. Is there any explanation to this observation?**

Combination vaccines containing a monocomponent aP vaccine, manufactured at Statens Serum Institut (SSI), Denmark, have successfully controlled *B. pertussis* infections in Denmark since 1997. The effectiveness of this aP vaccine was 93% against severe and 73% against mild pertussis in 500,000 Danish children (Thierry-Carstensen B et al., 2013) **(Fig. 3)**.

Immunoglobulin G (IgG) antibodies against PT (IgG-anti-PT) response rates after booster vaccination of adults with TdaP were considerably higher for this monocomponent aP vaccine-containing 20 μg pertussis toxoid, inactivated by hydrogen peroxide (92.0%), than for two multicomponent aP vaccines inactivated by formaldehyde and/or glutaraldehyde: three-component aP with 8 μg pertussis toxoid (77.2%) and five-component aP with 2.5 μg pertussis toxoid (47.1%). In Denmark where this monocomponent aP vaccine has been the only pertussis vaccine in use for 15 years, there has been no pertussis epidemic since 2002 (population incidence 36/100,000), in contrast to neighboring countries, where epidemics have occurred.

However, there were specific differences in the policy adopted by the Denmark's health establishment to employ pertussis vaccine in the field. They include:

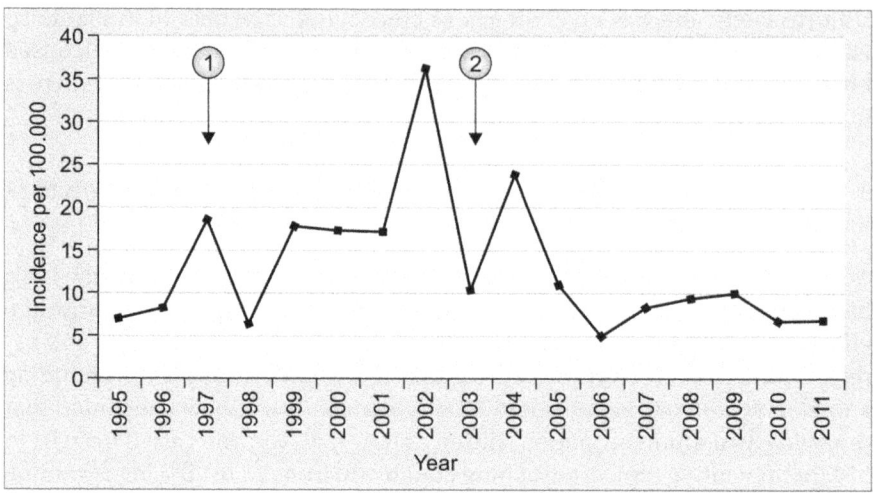

Fig. 3: Total incidence of laboratory confirmed pertussis per 100,000 (population) in Denmark, 1995–2011. (The arrows mark changes to the vaccination program: (1) Substitution of the wP vaccine with the monocomponent aP vaccine; (2) Introduction of the preschool monocomponent aP booster.)

- Higher content (40 µg instead of 20 µg) of PT was used in primary immunization schedule.
- The primary schedule was different than in the United States and some other countries: 3, 5, and 12 months.
- Extremely high coverage was achieved.
- The PT was inactivated by hydrogen peroxide than conventionally used formaldehyde or glutaraldehyde.

Furthermore, the pertussis control was better with wP before aP was introduced there in 1997 even with a moderate coverage of 80%.

11. In 2013, the ACVIP of the Indian Academy of Pediatrics (IAP) had revised their recommendations on pertussis vaccination and advised use of whole-cell pertussis (wP) vaccine instead of acellular pertussis (aP) vaccine in primary immunization. What was the rationale and evidence behind this change?

The recommendation on the exclusive use of wP vaccine in primary immunization series was based on the following reasons:
1. There was no data on the efficacy/effectiveness of aP vaccines in India and almost all the recommendations were based on the performance of these vaccines in industrialized countries. However, all these countries reported upsurge and frequent outbreaks of the disease despite using highest quality aP vaccines with an extremely high coverage (close to 100%) since mid-1990s **(Fig. 4)**. Hence, there was no evidence of effectiveness of aP vaccines from the industrialized countries also.

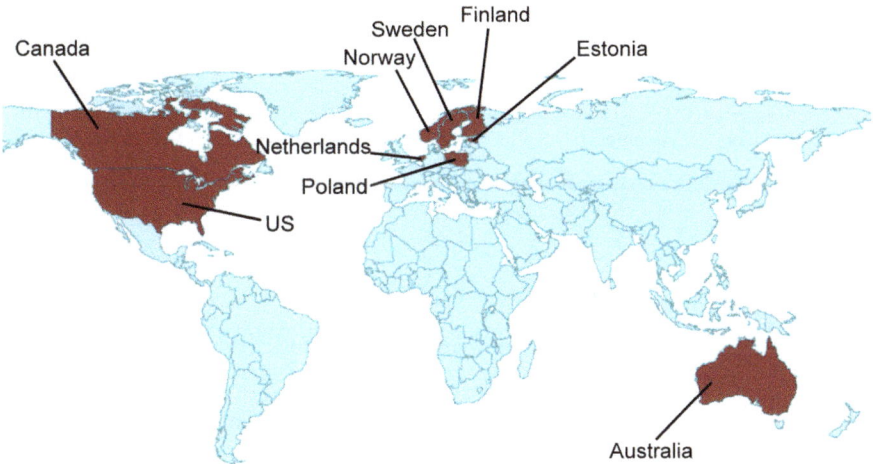

Fig. 4: Global pertussis outbreaks in vaccinated populations: pertussis re-emerged in countries highly vaccinated with DTaP vaccines.

2. The aP-containing combinations were licensed in India on the basis of immunogenicity studies only. However, in the absence of any known CoP for aP vaccines, mere presence of antibodies cannot be relied as a surrogate for efficacy or protection.
3. The studies from the United States of America, Australia, and other industrialized countries post-2009 outbreaks had demonstrated superior priming with wP vaccines and more durability of immunity following wP vaccination than aP vaccines.
4. There was strong evidence of effectiveness, real-life performance of wP vaccines from India where the widespread use of them have markedly reduced the incidence of pertussis after the launch of UIP. We had achieved a good control of pertussis (high effectiveness, not merely the efficacy) with whatever type of wP was available in the country despite with a modest coverage of around 70%.
5. World over, the widespread use of wP vaccines had almost eliminated pertussis from almost all the countries that had employed them.
6. India was, and still is, a wP vaccine using country and more than 95% of children are still vaccinated with wP vaccines. There is still no data on the efficacy or effectiveness of aP vaccines in India and almost all the recommendations are based on the performance of these vaccines in industrialized countries, mainly the United States of America. On the contrary, we have strong evidence of effectiveness, real-life performance of wP vaccines from India where the widespread use of them have markedly reduced the incidence of pertussis. On the other hand, the epidemiology of pertussis and performance of wP and aP vaccines in the United States clearly showed that early use of wP vaccines had almost eliminated pertussis, which was resurged after use of aP vaccines despite a very high coverage (close to 100%) since mid-1990s.

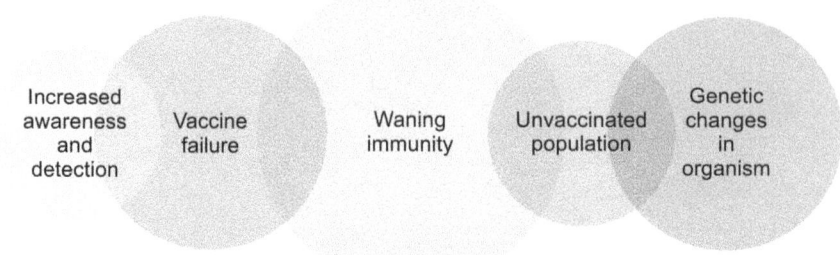

Fig. 5: Global pertussis resurgence: a combination of factors.

12. Why is the pertussis incidence rising in almost every country where aP vaccines have been introduced?

While several known factors such as waning of immunity, detection bias due to more sensitive tests [like polymerase chain reaction (PCR)] and higher awareness of the disease among practitioners, and evolutionary shifts among *B. pertussis* all likely contribute, collectively, these do not adequately explain the existing epidemiologic data, suggesting that additional factors also contribute **(Fig. 5)**. Key among these is recent data indicating that the immune responses induced by aP vaccines differ fundamentally from those induced by the wP vaccines, and do not lead to mucosal immunity. The initial aP vaccine studies were conducted in mice which were later found not a perfect animal model to study immunological changes associated with the pertussis disease.

13. Despite the poor efficacy and no effectiveness of aP vaccines, why Western countries have not reverted to wP vaccines?

Post-2012 outbreaks of pertussis in the United States, the United Kingdom, and Australia have shifted the focus back on effectiveness of the pertussis vaccines from the safety. The ACIP and many US experts on pertussis have also discussed the option of going back to wP vaccines. But the problem with them and with the entire Western world is that they cannot now revert to wP vaccines owing to "poor public acceptance" of these products. Fortunately, this is not a big issue yet in India. There is no report of poor acceptance or widespread rejection of wP vaccines both from the public or private sector.

14. In the 2018–2019 pertussis recommendations, the IAP has reverted to its past recommendations and accorded equal status to both wP and aP vaccines in the primary schedule. Do you think that equating wP and aP for the primary immunization is an appropriate decision?

No, the recommendations are usually changed when any new data emerge in the intervening period. No new study/data have emerged in last 6–7 years warranting any change of the recommendations. Most of the new publications have favored wP over aP vaccines like immunological superiority, better priming of wP, higher durability, etc.

Post-2013, after publication of many animal studies particularly in Baboons by Merkel et al., our understanding of pertussis immunity has improved to a great extent. It became clear that there is a fundamental difference in the immunology of wP and aP vaccines. The wP vaccines induce mainly T-helper cell type 17 (Th17)/Th1 type immune responses that lead to "proinflammatory" cytokine responses whereas the aP vaccines induce primarily a Th2 biased immune response that evokes an "anti-inflammatory" type of cytokines. The Th17/Th1 response prevents infection as well as disease and provides longer protection than a Th1/Th2 response. And this polarization persists throughout the life despite administration of several aP boosters.

Although aP vaccines do protect the first few years of life, the change in T-cell priming results in waning effectiveness of aP as early as 2–3 years post-boosters. Baboon models show that aP is less able to prevent nasopharyngeal colonization of *B. pertussis* than wP or natural infection. Almost all the research on aP was initially done on murine/mouse models which are probably not a perfect animal model to study/reproduce immunological changes. The use of animal model systems led to many mistakes that led the way to our present aP problems. Even a single dose of wP vaccine as a first dose of primary series is found to be more protective than using aP-containing vaccine. Switching to a wP-priming vaccination strategy could reduce pertussis incidence by up to 95%, including 96% fewer infections in neonates.

Before changing recommendations, the committee must answer the following queries:
1. Is there any new efficacy/effectiveness study on aP vaccines from India in the last 5–6 years that demonstrate better efficacy of aP over wP?
2. Is there any spurt in the incidence of serious AEFIs due to wP vaccines?
3. Are there higher incidences vaccine refusals by the parents in the last 5–6 years? On the contrary, there is a greater acceptance of wP vaccines by the parents of even affluent section.

One should not forget that India is still a largely wP vaccine using country. To change recommendations without any new evidence is not only unwarranted (no demand/no documentation of higher adverse events), and unscientific (no study proving superiority of aP over wP since last publication) but unethical (depriving a child an opportunity of getting a better and longer protection against a potentially serious disease) too. The committee is advised against revising evidence-based recommendations arbitrarily.

15. What is wrong with aP vaccine-induced immunity?

Immunologic studies show that, whereas wP vaccines orient the immune system toward Th1/Th17 responses, aP vaccines orient toward Th1/Th2 responses. Although aP vaccines do provide protection during the first years of life, the change in T-cell priming results in waning effectiveness of aP as early as 2–3 years post-boosters. In baboon models, requiring confirmation in humans, show that aP is less able to prevent nasopharyngeal colonization of *B. pertussis* than wP or natural infection. Hence, the current generation of aP vaccines fails to prevent colonization and transmission. The recent mathematical modeling has indicated that asymptomatic transmission of *B. pertussis* may be the main reason for the current resurgence of pertussis.

Although, aP vaccines prevent severe disease and death, they are inferior to wP vaccines because of following reasons:
- The type of T cell responses
- Suboptimal balance of antigens in DTaP vaccines
- Linked-epitope suppression. In DTaP vaccines, there are 3–5 antigens; in DTwP vaccines, there are >3,000 antigens
- Genetic change in *B. pertussis*. The aP vaccines are more susceptible to this than wP vaccines.

16. Tell us more about Th1/Th2 and Th17 immune responses in context with pertussis disease and vaccines immunity.

There are two main subsets of T lymphocytes, distinguished by the presence of cell surface molecules known as CD4 and CD8. T lymphocytes expressing CD4 are also known as helper T cells, and these are regarded as being the most prolific cytokine producers. This subset can be further subdivided into Th1 and Th2, and the cytokines they produce are known as "Th1-type cytokines" and "Th2-type cytokines".

Th1-type cytokines tend to produce the **proinflammatory responses** responsible for killing intracellular parasites and for perpetuating autoimmune responses. Interferon-gamma (IFN-γ) is the main Th1 cytokine. Excessive proinflammatory responses can lead to uncontrolled tissue damage, so there needs to be a mechanism to counteract this.

The Th2type cytokines include interleukin (IL)-4, IL-5, and IL-13, which are associated with the promotion of IgE and eosinophilic responses in atopy, and also IL10, which has more of an **anti-inflammatory response**. In excess, Th2 responses will counteract the Th1-mediated microbicidal action. The optimal scenario would therefore seem to be that humans should produce a well-balanced Th1 and Th2 response, suited to the immune challenge.

More recently, a third pathway was discovered of an independent lineage of cells, called the Th17 cells (so named due to dominant cytokine that drives cells down this pathway, IL-17). Of relevance, Th17 cells are found in the lungs, the gut mucosa, the skin, and play a critical role in mucosal immunity and host defense against extracellular pathogens.

It has been recently shown that infection with *B. pertussis* induces a pure Th17 response, and these cells are found to play a distinct role in the pathogenesis of *B. pertussis* infection. Hence, the Th17 and Th1 immune responses contribute to the immunity conferred by natural pertussis infection. Similarly, wP vaccines also induce a Th17 dominant responses (with a lesser Th1 contribution). By contrast aP vaccines only produced a Th2 response.

In the Merkel's Baboon animal studies, previously infected animals and wP-vaccinated animals possess strong *B. pertussis*-specific Th17 and Th1 memory, whereas aP vaccination induced a Th1/Th2 response instead.

The Th17/Th1 response prevents infection as well as disease and gives longer protection than a Th1/Th2 response **(Table 1)**.

TABLE 1: Some of the key differences between wP vaccine and aP vaccine based on animal studies data in baboons.

Whole-cell pertussis (wP) vaccine	Acellular pertussis (aP) vaccine
• Blocked disease and infection to a much higher extent than aP • Probably did this by blocking carriage (though studies were never done to prove that hypothesis)	• Blocked disease but did not block infection • Experimentally do not block carriage and permit transmission from asymptomatic to vaccine naïve animals. This observation closely mimics the cocooning strategy, and suggests a reason why it had failed to perform as anticipated
• Epidemiologically appears to offer herd effect (though not to a level sufficient to halt transmission entirely)	• Epidemiologically offers minimal or no herd effect
• Induces robust mucosal immunity	• Seemingly absent of mucosal immunity induction
• Induces robust Th17 responses	• Induces Th2 response

17. In aP-containing hexavalent combination vaccines, do you think that presence of IPV polarizes the immune responses elicited by the vaccine toward Th1 and Th17 rather than Th2-like wP-based products.

Animal studies using the baboon model suggest that wP-containing vaccines predominantly elicit a Th17/Th1 response which may provide a longer lasting protection than the Th1/Th2 response elicited by aP-containing vaccines. Furthermore, the predominant Th2 (but lower Th1 and Th17) responses seen with aP-containing vaccines may be less effective in clearing *B. pertussis* and preventing transmission.

In a recent review on hexavalent vaccines in India published in Indian Pediatrics (*Indian Pediatr. 2019;56(11):939-50*), the authors have suggested that the presence of single-stranded RNA (ssRNA) of the IPV in hexavalent products provides an adjuvant effect via toll-like receptor 7 (TLR7) and TLR8. They refer to an animal study conducted in mice (*Vaccine. 2017;35(39):5256-63*) wherein addition of a TLR7 agonist to an alum-adjuvanted aP vaccine converts it from a Th2-inducing vaccine to a more Th1/Th17-inducing vaccine with higher protective capacity, equivalent to or greater than that of a wP vaccine in a murine model.

However, before accepting the authors' perspective, one should keep the following facts in mind:
1. Both the above cited papers are published by the manufacturer of one of the hexavalent products; hence, there is a strong conflict of interest.
2. The suggested probable explanation is mere conjuncture, not even a hypothesis to be tested in clinical studies.
3. Mouse model is not a perfect animal model to study pertussis and pertussis vaccines.

4. The cited reference paper on animal study (*Vaccine. 2017*) has employed an alum-TLR7a as an adjuvant in mice study, not IPV.

The manufacturers have acknowledged the superiority of wP vaccines over aP vaccines based on elicited immune responses favoring Th1/Th17 polarization. Previously, they ascribed the resurgence of pertussis in developed countries due to the other factors such as antigenic variation in the circulating strains of *B. pertussis*, changes in surveillance and diagnostic tools, etc.

18. What do you mean by "linked-epitope suppression"?

The finding of initial priming by DTwP leading to greater efficacy than priming by DTaP can be explained by linked-epitope suppression caused by preferential responses of memory B cells following secondary exposure to vaccine components. The wP vaccines may contain > 3,000 proteins. Antibody to many of these proteins contributes to protection. Whereas the aP vaccines contain up to 5 proteins only.

Memory B cells "out-compete" naïve B cells for access to the *Bordetella* epitopes as they are more numerous, and their receptors exhibit a higher antigen affinity. Linked-epitope suppression applies as the immune response to novel epitopes is suppressed by the strong response to initial components if they are introduced together.

The lesser protection provided by DTaP, both as the initial vaccine or full primary course, may be due to linked-epitope suppression, when the initial exposure locks in the immune response to certain epitopes and inhibits response to other linked epitopes on subsequent exposures.

19. How do genetic changes in the circulating strains of *Bordetella pertussis* influence efficacy of aP vaccines?

The "vaccine pressure" has resulted in changes in PT, PRN, and FIM antigens of circulating organism. Since wP vaccines contain multiple antigens, these genetic changes are unlikely to lead to vaccine failure. Since aP vaccines contain fewer antigens, it seems clear that genetic changes are contributing to vaccine failure.

It has been suggested that an increase in the correlation of *B. pertussis* strains containing the *ptx* P3 allele rather than the *ptx* P1 allele has led to vaccine failures and more severe illness. However, there is no convincing evidence supporting this suggestion. Quite recently, the circulation of PRN-deficient mutants has been reported. Since it was noticed in earlier immunological studies that antibody to PRN correlated with protection ~70% of the time, it would seem possible that this deficiency could lead to increased vaccine failures if the deficient mutants became widespread.

There is also a dramatic increase in strains with *fim* 3B in some countries using exclusively aP vaccines. This could lead to a decrease in efficacy of the aP vaccines containing FIM 2/3 as well as PRN. However, demonstrating increased vaccine failure with either the PT, FHA, PRN, or the PT, FHA, PRN,

FIM 2/3 vaccines will be difficult because antibody to the B subunit of PT provides considerable efficacy against typical pertussis as demonstrated in Denmark, where a PT toxoid vaccine has been used for >15 years.

20. Do pertussis vaccines protect for a lifetime?

No, the pertussis vaccines are effective, but do not provide a lifelong immunity. They typically offer good levels of protection within the first few years after getting the vaccine, but then protection wanes over time. In general, aP vaccines are around 80% effective. Children who get all five doses of DTaP on schedule, effectiveness is quite high within the year following the 5th dose, but thereafter there is a significant decrease in effectiveness in each following year.

21. Now, most researchers/experts agree that aP vaccines have lower duration of protection against pertussis than wP vaccines. What is the evidence base for this notion?

There are many recent publications post-2012 that observed high effectiveness of the pertussis vaccine within 3 years of vaccination, but with clear evidence of waning of immunity beyond 4 years and little-to-no protection beyond 7 years from last vaccination. The odds of pertussis increased by 27% each year that passed after receipt of an aP vaccine. Individuals primed with aP vaccine had 2.2 times higher odds of disease than those primed with the wP vaccine. **Table 2** provides a synopsis of the observed duration of protection in different trials of wP and aP vaccines.

TDAP VACCINE, MATERNAL IMMUNIZATION, AND ITS EFFECTIVENESS

22. How effective is Tdap vaccine in adolescents and adults?

Tetanus-diphtheria-pertussis provides moderate protection 1 year after vaccination and then protection wanes rapidly. In a recent study, the vaccine effectiveness was 68.8% during the 1st year of Tdap vaccination, which decreased to 56.9% after 2 years, 25.2% after 3 years, and 8.9% after 4 years.

Wei et al. evaluated effectiveness of Tdap booster among adolescents in the Virgin Islands in 2007 and found effectiveness of 61.3% and 68.3% against probable and laboratory-confirmed pertussis, respectively. A recent unpublished trial reported that Tdap was modestly effective [vaccine effectiveness: 55.2% at preventing PCR-confirmed pertussis among Kaiser Permanente Northern California (KPNC)—adolescents and adults]. According to CDC-ACIP data, the Tdap effectiveness was noticed ranging from 66 to 78% in field observational studies. The preliminary data suggest that effectiveness wanes within 3–4 years among aP vaccine recipients and there was no evidence of herd immunity.

With the recent incidents of recurrent outbreaks of pertussis in vaccinated adolescents have raised doubts about the utility of Tdap against pertussis.

TABLE 2: Duration of protection with pertussis vaccines: A. Whole-cell pertussis vaccines; B. Acellular pertussis vaccines.

A. Whole-cell pertussis vaccines

Author	Lambert	Jenkinson	CDC	Ramsay et al.	Nielson et al.	He et al.	van Buynder et al.	Torvaldsen et al.
Year	1965	1988	1993	1993	1999	1996	1999	2003
Data source	Outbreak	Clinic patients	Outbreak	Surveillance	Surveillance	Surveillance	Surveillance	Surveillance
Country	USA	UK	USA	UK	Denmark	Finland/Switzerland	UK	Australia
Estimate of protection	12 years	4 years	4–5 years	8 years	10 years	5–10 years	5–14 years	6–9 years

B. Acellular pertussis vaccines

Publication	Simondon et al.	Tindberg et al.	Salmaso et al.	Lugauer et al.	Gustaffson et al.
Year	1997	1999	2001	2002	2006
Antigens in vaccine	PT, FHA	PT, FHA	PT, FHA, PRN	PT, FHA	PT, FHA, PRN or PT, FHA, PRN, FIM
N	4181	207	8432	10,271	Surveillance
Study type	Case control in RCT	Follow-up of RCT	RCT	Cohort study	Active surveillance
Follow-up	Up to 4.25 years	10 years	3 years	6 years	9–10 years
Country	Senegal	Sweden	Italy	Germany	Sweden
Unchanged protection	wp>aP	5.5 years	6 years	6 years	6 years

World over, the experts are now opining to adopt an alternate strategy to use Tdap in anticipation of a local pertussis outbreak rather than on a routine basis in adolescents since it provides only a short-term protection against pertussis.

23. Is there any maternal protection against pertussis to a newborn?

There is no natural maternal protection against pertussis to the newborn.

24. Why Tdap is recommended during pregnancy?

In June 2011, CDC-ACIP recommended that pregnant women who had never received the Tdap vaccine in the past should receive a single dose of the vaccine to optimize the concentration of maternal antibodies transferred to the fetus. The objective behind this recommendation was to protect newborns with maternal antibodies and decreasing the risk of transmission of pertussis to infants shortly after birth.

In October 2016, the ACIP suggested that the Tdap should be administered early in the 27- through 36-week "window" to maximize passive antibody transfer to the infant. Women who have never received Tdap and who do not receive it during pregnancy should receive it immediately postpartum. However, studies documented the superiority of Tdap given during pregnancy than at postpartum period. The Tdap must be administered in every pregnancy. This recommendation is to take care of waning of immunity following Tdap.

25. What is the scientific logic behind this recommendation?

When a woman gets Tdap during pregnancy, maternal pertussis antibodies transfer to the newborn, protecting the baby against pertussis in early life, before the baby is old enough to have received at least three doses of pertussis vaccine. Tdap also protects the mother, making it less likely that she will get infected with pertussis during or after pregnancy and thus less likely that she will transmit it to her infant.

26. What is the best time to administer Tdap vaccine?

Immunization of pregnant women with Tdap between 27 and 30 weeks is associated with highest umbilical cord geometric mean concentrations (GMCs) of IgG to PT and FHA compared with immunization beyond 31 weeks **(Fig. 6)**. However, there are some reports that favor Tdap even during second trimester. Early second-trimester maternal Tdap immunization significantly increased neonatal antibodies. Recommending immunization from the second trimester onward would widen the immunization opportunity window and could improve seroprotection (Eberhardt CS et al., 2016) **(Table 3)**.

27. Some women have closely spaced pregnancies. Should we give Tdap during each pregnancy, even if it means such women would get two doses within 12 months?

Yes. However, it is quite rare to find this occurrence, i.e., to have more than one pregnancy at an interval of 12 months or less between births. The majority

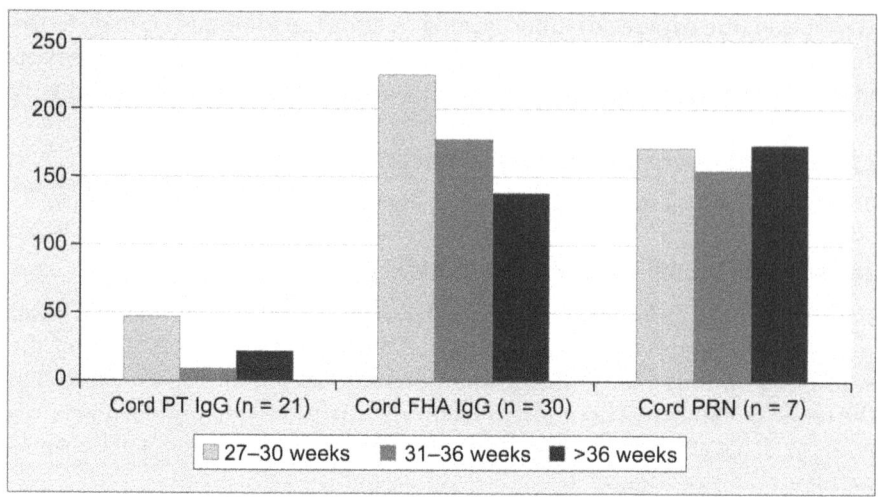

Fig. 6: Timing of maternal Tdap and cord antibodies levels.

Gestational week at maternal vaccination	No. (%)	Anti-PT GMC (95% CI)	Anti-FHA GMC (95% CI)	Infant seropositivity No. (%)
39–41	21 (6)	9.0 (5.0–16.2)	31.0 (16.9–56.6	4 (19)
37–38	74 (22)	25.1 (17.9–35.3)	92.7 (69.0–124.7	37 (50)
34–36	72 (22)	32.7 (24.1–44.3	173.0 (126.5–236.6)	40 (56)
30–33	16 (5)	74.9 (38.3–146.4)	417.3 (232.7–748.4	12 (75)
26–29	30 (9)	70.3 (49.0–100.8)	376.8 (257.0–552.7	23 (77)
22–25	54 (16)	68.3 (52.8–88.3)	291.8 (222.8–382.2	45 (83)
17–21	42 (13)	53.1 (37.2–75.7)	267.3 (205.4–347.9	32 (76)
13–16	26 (8)	44.2 (32.2–60.7)	297.9 (206.7–429.4	20 (77)

TABLE 3: Timing of maternal Tdap and anti-PT and anti-FHA GMC levels. Early second-trimester maternal Tdap immunization significantly increased neonatal antibodies.

Source: Eberhardt CS, Blanchard-Rohner G, Lemaître B, Boukrid M, Combescure C, Othenin-Girard V, et al. Maternal immunization earlier in pregnancy maximizes antibody transfer and expected infant seropositivity against pertussis. Clin Infect Dis. 2016;62(7):829-36.

of women who have two pregnancies have an interval of 13 months or more between births.

28. What could be the probable side effects of having Tdap in every pregnancy?

A theoretical risk exists for severe local reactions (e.g., Arthus reactions, whole-limb swelling) for pregnant women who have multiple, closely spaced pregnancies. However, the frequency of side effects depends on the vaccine's antigen content and product formulation, as well as on preexisting maternal antibody levels related to the interval since the last dose and the number of doses received. The risk for severe adverse events has likely been reduced with current vaccine formulations (including Tdap), which contain lower doses of tetanus toxoid than did older vaccine formulations. Most authorities believe the potential benefit of preventing pertussis disease burden in infancy outweighs the theoretical concerns of possible severe adverse events in mothers.

29. If a woman received Tdap in early pregnancy, should she get it again in the third trimester?

No, it is not recommended to give another dose of Tdap in such cases. Optimal timing for Tdap administration is between 27 and 36 weeks of gestation because of transplacental antibody kinetics. According to ACIP recommendations, "Tdap may be administered any time during pregnancy, but vaccination during the third trimester would provide the highest concentration of maternal antibodies to be transferred closer to birth".

30. How effective is giving Tdap during pregnancy at preventing pertussis in early infancy?

In one study, there was 90-93% effectiveness against pertussis infection in infants under the age of 2 months (Gkentzi D et al., 2017). In Argentina, there was a 51% relative reduction of pertussis cases in young infants whose mothers immunized against pertussis in pregnancy and who lived in states with high Tdap coverage (>50%) compared to young infants who lived in states with low coverage (<50%) of maternal pertussis immunization during pregnancy (Vizzotti C et al., 2016). There are many other recent studies that have documented effectiveness of maternal Tdap against infantile pertussis (Winter K et al., 2017; Becker-Dreps S et al., 2018)

As per the recent Centers for Disease Control and Prevention (CDC) report, the Tdap vaccination during the third trimester of pregnancy prevents 78% of pertussis cases in infants younger than 2 months of age. When infants do get pertussis, their infection is less severe if their mother received Tdap during pregnancy. A CDC evaluation found maternal vaccination is 90% effective at preventing infant hospitalization from pertussis. Another US study showed that infants whose mothers got Tdap during pregnancy had a significantly lower risk of hospitalization and shorter hospital stays. That same study showed that no infants born to vaccinated mothers required intubation or died of pertussis.

31. The American Academy of Pediatrics (AAP) has come out with some new recommendations regarding repeat doses of Tdap. Can you elaborate?

In January 2020 meeting of ACIP, a revision in the previous recommendation of Tdap use was made. According to new recommendation, people aged 11-18 years should receive a single dose of Tdap as well as a booster dose of *either Td or Tdap* every 10 years throughout life. Individuals aged 19 years or older who have not received a dose of Tdap should receive one dose of Tdap. For continued protection, either Td or Tdap can then be administered every 10 years throughout life. Earlier, only a single lifetime dose of Tdap was recommended except for pregnant mothers.

32. Tdap boosters every 10 years: how useful or relevant is it?

The Tdap has got limited use beyond employing in pregnancy to provide protection to young infant since the vaccine-induced protection wanes very fast. So, it would not be a cost-effective intervention. This is the reason why CDC-ACIP has not recommended this earlier.

33. As a pediatrician, I am concerned about protecting my newborn patients from pertussis, especially given the recent outbreaks in my community where infants have died. How many doses of pediatric DTaP vaccine do an infant need before she or he is protected from pertussis?

Vaccine efficacy is 80–85% following three doses of DTaP vaccine. Efficacy data following just one or two doses are lacking but are likely lower. Therefore, it is especially important that you advice parents of infants and all people who live with the infant or who provide care to him or her be protected against pertussis.

ACELLULAR PERTUSSIS VACCINE AT BIRTH AND OTHER RECENT DEVELOPMENTS

34. What are the new/evolving approaches to provide protection to a young infant prior routine infant pertussis immunization?

The two approaches to provide immunity to very young infants against pertussis include a dose of Tdap during pregnancy (maternal Tdap) and a dose of aP vaccine at birth. Maternal Tdap has now become standard practice to provide protection to neonates. Pregnant women should receive one dose of Tdap during each pregnancy, irrespective of their history of receiving the vaccine. Tdap should be administered at 27–36 weeks of gestation, preferably during the earlier part of this period, although it may be administered at any time during pregnancy.

35. Is the aP vaccine immunogenic and safe when given at birth?

A new study has demonstrated that monovalent aP vaccine is immunogenic and safe in neonates (Wood N et al., 2018). It may prove valuable for newborns whose mothers did not receive the Tdap vaccine during pregnancy. A birth dose of aP vaccine would significantly narrow the immunity gap between birth and 3 months of age, marking the critical period when infants are most vulnerable to severe pertussis infection. However, the monovalent aP vaccine is not yet widely available for clinical use.

36. Are there some undesirable effects of both the above strategies, i.e., maternal Tdap and monovalent aP at birth?

Both the options have undesirable impact on future infant immunization. The blunting effect of maternal Tdap on infant pertussis vaccination schedule even after booster dose, and the significantly reduced GMCs of the concomitantly administered antigens at 32 weeks with birth aP, are two main concerns.

In the above study (Wood N et al., 2018), at age 32 weeks, all infants who received the aP vaccine at birth had detectable PT IgG, but significantly lower IgG GMCs for Hib, hepatitis B, diphtheria, and tetanus antibodies. Furthermore, there is some evidence of a lower pertussis antibody level after completion of the primary vaccine series in infants with birth dose of aP born to mothers who had received Tdap within the 5 years prior to delivery.

37. Are there some ways to address the above shortcomings?

Recently, some experts have suggested a combined maternal-infant vaccination schedule with delayed infant vaccination at the start of life. In a study (Barug D et al., 2019), pregnant women received Tdap either at 30–32 weeks of pregnancy (maternal Tdap group) or within 48 hours after delivery (control group). The researchers recommended a delayed routine pertussis vaccination at the age of 3 months instead of 2 months in case of timely administration of maternal Tdap vaccination and when infants were born after term. This arrangement is applicable to developed countries using aP vaccines. Hence, in this approach, the maternal Tdap is considered equivalent to first dose of infant pertussis vaccination and the remaining two doses of the infant series are started late to avoid "blunting effect" of maternal Tdap on infant pertussis vaccination. A later age at the start of vaccination might also allow reduction of the number of doses in the primary series.

38. What is the evidence base for delaying the infant pertussis vaccination?

Pregnant women from Netherlands received Tdap either at 30–32 weeks of pregnancy (maternal Tdap group, n = 58) or within 48 hours after delivery (control group, n = 60). All term infants vaccinated with the hexavalent and 10-valent pneumococcal conjugate vaccine (PCV10) at 3, 5, and 11 months (Barug D et al., 2019). The GMCs of PT antibodies were significantly higher in infants in the maternal Tdap group than in the control group infants at age of 3 months and 2 months. However, after primary vaccination, antibody concentrations for PT, FHA, and PRN were significantly lower at all-time points in infants of the maternal Tdap group than in infants in the control group, suggesting maternal antibody interference in infant after primary and booster vaccinations with DTaP.

This trial explores the possibility of adding maternal pertussis immunization to the vaccination schedule as a first infant dose to reduce the possibility of infection before the first dose administered to the infant. However, it also suggests that the infant vaccination needs to be delayed beyond 3 months of age, in order to minimize interference with maternal antibodies.

39. Can the above-mentioned strategy be adopted here in India too?

Introduction of a delayed infant pertussis immunization schedule would place neonates of unvaccinated women in a more vulnerable situation, and maternal coverage needs to be higher to protect all babies from pertussis from the first day of their life. Moreover, the study only addresses vaccination schedules using aP vaccines in industrialized countries. The situation is completely different in low- and middle-income countries (LMICs) including India where wP vaccines are used in primary vaccination schedule and maternal immunization is still not well established. The blunting effect of maternal Tdap on wP-containing primary vaccine series may be different from the findings in the above study.

40. Why is it necessary to give at least first dose of wP-containing vaccine of the primary pertussis vaccination series?

As discussed above in details, there is a fundamental difference in the type of immune responses induced by the wP and aP vaccines. While the former elicits mainly the Th17/Th1-type cytokines, the latter induces Th2/Th1-type immunity. It is recently demonstrated that this "immune polarization" persists following wP vaccination despite repeated aP boosters later in the life.

Researchers, *da Silva Antunes R et al.* (J Clin Invest. 2018), compared the immune responses to aP boosters in individuals who received their initial doses with either wP or aP vaccines. They particularly examined pertussis-specific memory CD4+ T cell responses ex vivo, highlighting a type 2/Th2 versus type 1/Th1 and Th17 differential polarization as a function of childhood vaccination. Significantly, after a contemporary aP booster, cells from donors originally primed with aP were (1) associated with increased IL-4, IL-5, IL-13, IL-9, and transforming growth factor-β (TGF-β) and decreased IFN-γ and IL-17 production, (2) defective in their ex vivo capacity to expand memory cells, and (3) less capable of proliferating in vitro **(Fig. 7)**. These differences appeared to be T cell specific, since equivalent increases of antibody titers and plasmablasts after aP boost were seen in both groups. They conclude that there are long-lasting effects and differences in polarization and proliferation of T cell responses in adults originally vaccinated with aP compared with those that initially received wP, despite repeated acellular boosters.

41. How does priming with wP or aP affect the later immune responses to Tdap booster?

In a study by van der Lee S et al. (Front Immunol. 2018) aimed to determine whether memory immune responses to aP, diphtheria, and tetanus vaccine antigens following booster vaccinations at 4 and 9 years of age differ between wP- versus aP-primed children, it was noticed that after the preschool booster

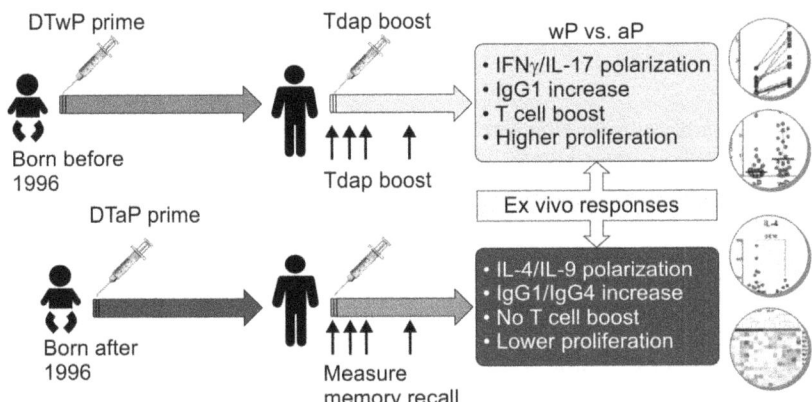

Fig. 7: Th1/Th17 polarization persists following wP vaccination despite repeated aP boosters (A contemporary Tdap booster was administered more than 15 years later and memory recall response measured using ex vivo analysis of T cell or B cell reactivity, proliferation assays, and transcriptomic profiling. The major immunological differences for each cohort (wP vs. aP) are depicted in the boxes.

vaccination, IgG levels were significantly higher in aP-primed as compared with wP-primed children until 6 years of age. Before the Tdap booster, humoral and cellular immune responses were similar in aP- and wP-primed children. However, the Tdap booster induced lower vaccine antigen-specific humoral, B-cell, and T-helper 1 (Th1) cell responses resulting in significantly lower Th1/Th2 ratios in aP-primed compared with wP-primed children. The memory immune profiles at preadolescent age to all DTaP vaccine antigens are already determined by the wP or aP combination vaccines given in infancy, showing a beneficial Th1-dominated response after wP-priming. These immunological data corroborate epidemiological data showing that DTaP-primed adolescents are less protected against clinical pertussis than DTwP-primed children.

Another study concludes that *B. pertussis* infection is processed differently between individuals immunized with wP or aP vaccines in childhood leading to a distinct infection-induced antibody response.

42. What are the new developments related to Tdap vaccine?

Recently a new TdaP (PTgen/FHA) that contains a genetically inactivated PT along with FHA as two-component pertussis vaccine with tetanus toxoid and reduced dose of diphtheria toxoid is licensed in Thailand. This new Tdap is found to induce higher pertussis responses 28 days after vaccination than does the available licensed Tdap vaccine. Further, after 1 year, persistent seroconversion for PT neutralizing antibodies was seen in significantly higher number of participants than in conventional Tdap group (41% vs. 8%) (Sricharoenchai S et al., 2018). Results of this trial led to the licensure of new aP vaccines containing genetically inactivated PT in Thailand. Hence, the novel TdaP, not only induced a higher antibody response but these responses sustained for longer duration than those achieved with the Tdap comparator vaccine.

43. Is there any study on monovalent aP vaccine dose administered in place of Tdap dose to pregnant mothers?

During the above trial (Sricharoenchai S et al., 2018), a monovalent aP vaccine with genetically inactivated PT and FHA without Td toxoid was also tried. It was also found superior to conventional Tdap in relation to pertussis protection.

Recently, in a baboon animal study, maternal vaccination with a PT-only vaccine was found sufficient to protect newborn baboons from disease following exposure to pertussis. The avoidance of the other antigens in Tdap would ameliorate issues related to suppression of infant responses to routine vaccination.

44. There is a theoretical risk of severe local reactions following too frequent administration of TT- and DT-containing vaccines. What could be other disadvantages of using maternal Tdap vaccine?

A recent report using a large database of infant vaccine studies conducted by one manufacturer indicated that preexisting maternal antibody affected immune responses to 20 of 21 antigens administered to infants. In the study, for aP antigens, twofold higher maternal antibody was associated with 11% lower post-vaccination antibody for PT and FHA and 22% lower PRN antibody. The influence of maternal antibody was still evident in reduced responses to booster doses of aP at 12–24 months of age (Voysey M et al., 2017).

Maternal antibody concentrations and infant age at first vaccination both influence infant vaccine responses. These effects are seen for almost all vaccines contained in global immunization programs and influence immune response for some vaccines even at the age of 24 months. These data highlight the potential for maternal immunization strategies to influence established infant programs.

Hence, one must be aware that all of the antigens included in the maternal immunization cocktail have the potential to suppress infant immune responses to primary immunization and that only antigens absolutely needed for maternal protection or infant protection in the 6–8 weeks before onset of the infant primary vaccination series should be administered.

PERTUSSIS RESURGENCE IN ACELLULAR PERTUSSIS USING COUNTRIES: THE WAY OUT

45. Following resurgence of pertussis in many developed, industrialized countries in last few years, it is now believed that aP vaccines are having certain limitations. How are these countries going to address this issue?

Following new options are being explored by researchers to address the poor efficacy and short duration of protection offered by aP vaccines **(Table 4)**:

TABLE 4: Possible strategies to control pertussis resurgence.

Strategy	Remarks
1. Return to the use of wP	Not practical and unacceptable
2. Develop less reactogenic wP	Not yet complete
3. Maternal vaccination to protect newborn	Now recommended
4. Vaccination of newborn contacts (cocoon strategy)	Difficult to obtain complete coverage
5. More frequent boosters with aP	Costly and difficult to put in place
6. Use antigens from currently circulating strains	Uncertain effect
7. Increase quantities of current antigens	Would require large trials
8. Inactivate PT by genetic mutation or mild	Advisable to increase immunogenicity
9. Add new virulence factors	Would require large trials
10. Use stronger adjuvants	Would require large trials
11. Use live attenuated B. pertussis vaccine intranasally	In clinical trial stage

1. Vaccines containing only aP components
2. Modification of antigens in current vaccines—novel DTaP formulations
3. Addition of antigens to current vaccines—aP with additional antigens
4. Modification of adjuvant in current vaccines
5. Change in delivery system
6. Whole-cell pertussis vaccines with low endotoxin content
7. Newer techniques using outer membrane vesicles
8. aP vaccines with new adjuvants
9. Development of new pertussis vaccines like live attenuated pertussis vaccine

46. What are the challenges to developing a new pertussis vaccine?

There are several challenges to develop new pertussis vaccines. Some of them are enumerated here:
- Costly: huge amount of finances is needed.
- Better understanding of the disease, transmission, and immunity are needed.
- Most advances over last 20 years have been with bridging to efficacy studies from the 1990s; new field efficacy studies will be difficult!
- Vaccines that produce protection through different immune mechanisms would not be able to be bridged.
- Regulatory pathway is complex.
- May take several years before licensure.

47. What is the current status of development of new pertussis vaccines?

Recent studies in nonhuman primates have shown that neither wP nor aP vaccines prevent infection and transmission of *B. pertussis,* in contrast to prior exposure. There are several candidates in early preclinical development. The most advanced is the live attenuated nasal vaccine BPZE1.

48. Tell us more about this live attenuated nasal vaccine, called as "BPZE1".

This vaccine candidate has successfully completed a phase I clinical trial and has shown to be safe in young male volunteers, able to transiently colonize the nasopharynx and to induce antibody responses to *B. pertussis* antigens in all colonized individuals. Whether BPZE1 will indeed be useful to ultimately control pertussis obviously needs to be assessed by carefully conducted human efficacy trials. Following are the key attributes of this vaccine:
- Genetic modifications made to remove/or inactivate three major toxins, pertussis toxin (PTX), tracheal cytotoxin (TCT), and dermonecrotic toxin (DNT).
- This vaccine has successfully completed a phase I clinical trial in humans.
- The vaccine was given in each nostril as a 100 μL nasal drop suspension.
- A single intranasal administration led to strong and prolonged B cell and Th1 T cell responses, inducing protection against challenge infection.
- A single nasal administration of BPZE1 in infant mice was associated with stronger protection than that induced by two inoculations of aP vaccine and was lasting substantially longer.
- In addition to mice, juvenile baboons were protected by a single nasal administration of BPZE1 against infection and whooping cough disease upon challenge with a highly virulent *B. pertussis*.

49. Does live attenuated pertussis vaccine, BPZE1 also have heterologous, nonspecific effects (NSEs) like bacillus Calmette–Guérin (BCG)?

Yes, in experimental animal studies, this vaccine is also found having NSEs. In mice, BPZE1 was found to protect against inflammation resulting from heterologous airway infections, including those caused by other *Bordetella* species, influenza virus, and respiratory syncytial virus. Furthermore, the nonspecific protection conferred by BPZE1 was also observed for noninfectious inflammatory diseases, such as allergic asthma, as well as for inflammatory disorders outside of the respiratory tract, such as contact dermatitis. It is speculated to offer some nonspecific protection against severe acute respiratory syndrome-associated coronavirus 2 (SARS-CoV-2) also.

SAFETY ISSUES, PRECAUTIONS, AND CONTRAINDICATIONS

50. Can we give assurance to parents about full safety of the DTaP vaccine?

In real life, no vaccine is truly "painless". It is true that minor local and systemic adverse events like pain, induration, fever, etc., are much more following wP vaccines than aP vaccines. However, as far as serious adverse effects are concerned, the frequency of these effects are rare even with wP vaccines. Adverse events that had occurred following previous pertussis vaccination may still occur with DTaP though less likely as compared to DTwP. So, use precautions while using the vaccine. Do not assure there will be no side effects as incidence of minor and major adverse effects are reduced by two third only.

51. There is lot of confusion about contraindications for administering DTP vaccines. Can you clarify?

"Absolute contraindications" to any pertussis vaccination (DTwP/DTaP/Tdap):
- Severe allergic reaction to vaccine component or following a prior dose;
- Encephalopathy within 7 days following previous DTwP vaccination (not due to another identifiable cause)

In case of anaphylaxis further immunization with any diphtheria/tetanus/pertussis vaccine is contraindicated as it is uncertain which component caused the event.

For patients with history of encephalopathy following vaccination any pertussis vaccine is contraindicated and only DT vaccines may be used.

52. What are the "precautions" for DTP vaccines?

Following events are considered as precautions for DTP vaccines:
- Moderate or severe acute illness
- Persistent inconsolable crying of more than 3 hours duration
- Hyperpyrexia (fever > 40.50°C)
- Hypotonic hyporesponsive episode (HHE) within 48 hours of DTwP administration
- Seizures with or without fever within 72 hours of administration.

The above events are considered as precautions but not contraindications to future doses of DTwP/DTaP vaccines because these events generally do not recur with the next dose and they have not been proven to cause permanent sequelae.

Progressive/evolving neurological illnesses is a relative contraindication to first dose of DTwP immunization. However, DTwP can be safely given to children with stable neurologic disorders.

53. What precautions are needed with Tdap vaccination?

Tdap precautions:
- Guillain–Barré syndrome (GBS) within 6 weeks after a previous dose of TT-containing vaccine
- Progressive neurologic disorder until the condition is stabilized.
- Severe local reaction (Arthus reaction) following a prior dose of tetanus/diphtheria toxoid-containing vaccine
- Moderate or severe acute illness.

54. If a baby had inconsolable crying for greater than 3 hours after the first DTwP vaccine, should we give second dose of DTaP?

Inconsolable crying for more than 3 hours is a contraindication to use it further. Here DTaP can be used with a precaution or warning and after discussing with the parents.

55. If a child shows reactions like high fever, convulsion, and "inconsolable crying, can we give DTwP in subsequent doses? Is it preferable to switch to DTaP as the next doses?

Events such as persistent inconsolable crying of more than 3 hours duration/hyperpyrexia (fever > 40.50°C)/HHE within 48 hours of DTwP administration and seizures with or without fever within 72 hours of administration of DTwP are considered as precautions but not contraindications to future doses of DTwP because these events generally do not recur with the next dose and they have not been proven to cause permanent sequelae. Wise option, but parents must be explained that such side effects can also occur with DTaP, though much less frequently. Severe local/systemic reactions to DTP are two-thirds less with DTaP.

56. Do the same precautions that apply to DTaP also apply to Tdap?

No. Many of the precautions to DTaP (e.g., temperature of 105°F or higher, collapse or shock-like state, persistent crying lasting 3 hours or longer, seizure with or without fever) do not apply to Tdap.

57. Can an adult receive Tdap if they had a contraindication or precaution to DTP as a child?

Tdap has two contraindications and four precautions. The contraindications are:
1. Anaphylactic reaction to a prior dose of the vaccine or any of its components and
2. Encephalopathy within 7 days of a previous dose of DTaP or DTP; in this case, give Td instead of Tdap.
The precautions have already been enumerated above.

58. Can we give further doses of DTaP to an infant who had an afebrile seizure within 3 hours of a previous dose?

An infant who experiences an afebrile seizure following a dose of DTaP requires further evaluation. An infant with a recent seizure or an evolving neurologic condition should not receive further doses of DTaP, or DT until the condition has been evaluated and stabilized. Other indicated vaccines may be administered on schedule. To assure that the child is at least protected against Td, the decision to give either DTaP or DT should be made no later than the first birthday.

59. What are the safety profiles of wP and aP vaccines?

There is a very wide range among various aP with varying frequencies for individual side effects. Impossible to identify an aP with the most (or least) favorable adverse event profile.

The wP vaccines often cause minor (but troublesome) side effects and rarely more serious adverse events. Relatively high incidence of the former is sometimes unacceptable to care-givers and care-providers; this is what prompted the development of aP. The incidence of frequent side effects (fever, erythema, swelling, fretfulness, drowsiness) is reported to be significantly less with aP as compared to wP **(Table 5)**.

Relative risk for some events is less with aP, the absolute risk difference is comparable to wP because such events are very rare with both. Meta-analysis of data from large randomized controlled trials (RCTs) on serious adverse events shows that although the relative risk (RR) for some events is less with aP, the absolute risk difference is comparable to wP because such events are very rare with both **(Table 6)**.

TABLE 5: Frequency of common side effects with pertussis vaccines.

Event	Whole-cell pertussis vaccine	Acellular pertussis vaccine	
	Average	Average	Range
Fever < 38.3°C	44.5%	20.8%	16–29.2%
Fever > 38.3°C	15.9%	3.7%	1.6–5.9%
Erythema	56.3%	31.4%	15–44%
> 2.0 cm	16.4%	3.3%	1.4–5.9%
Swelling	38.5%	20.1%	7.5–24.2%
Drowsiness	62.0%	42.7%	29.4–52.2%

Source: Adapted from Mathew JL. Acellular pertussis vaccines: pertinent issues. Indian Pediatrics. 2008;45:727-9.

TABLE 6: Meta-analysis of serious adverse events with pertussis vaccines.

Event	Frequency with aP	Frequency with wP	Pooled RR (95% CI)	Interpretation
High fever (>40°C)	227/99,323 (0.23%)	996/96,879 (1.03%)	0.18 (0.08–0.44)	RR is about 80% less with aP than with wP, but the absolute difference is 2%
Seizures (within 48 hours)	58/106,204 (0.05%)	224/103,474 (0.22%)	0.28 (0.13–0.61)	RR is about 72% less with aP than with wP, but the absolute difference is negligible
Hypotensive-hyporesponsive episode	20/106,204 (0.02%)	491/103,474 (0.47%)	0.04 (0.01–0.19)	RR is about 96% less with aP than with wP, but the absolute difference is negligible

Source: Adapted from Mathew JL. Acellular pertussis vaccines: pertinent issues. Indian Pediatrics. 2008;45:727-9.

GENERAL ADMINISTRATION AND SCHEDULING ISSUES

60. A child is brought for vaccination at 45 days with a background of prematurity with a birth weight of 1.8 kg and hypocalcemic seizures in the nursery. The mother is concerned about safety of DTP vaccines. How will you counsel?

Diphtheria, tetanus, and pertussis vaccination should be given since prematurity, low birth weight (LBW) and an identifiable nonprogressive neurologic disease (hypocalcemic seizures) are all not contraindications for DTP vaccination.

61. We are routinely scheduling the fourth dose of DTaP in children at 15–18 months, but occasionally would like to give it earlier. Is that okay?

The fourth dose of DTaP may be given as early as age 12 months if at least 6 months have passed since the third dose, and if, in the provider's opinion, the child might not return for another visit at 15–18 months of age.

62. Should further doses of pertussis vaccine be given to an infant or child who has had culture-proven pertussis?

After the recent resurgence of pertussis in many developed countries, it has become clear that there is gradual waning of immunity following vaccination and even after natural infection, and it is not lifelong. Hence, individuals with a history of pertussis should continue to receive vaccination with pertussis-containing vaccine as per the recommended schedule.

63. Can a child or an adult who has had pertussis get the disease again?

Reinfection appears to be uncommon but does occur. Reinfection may present as a persistent cough rather than typical pertussis. Hence, it is essential to immunize even those children recovering from pertussis as natural disease may not offer complete protection.

64. When a child comes in for his vaccinations at age 4–6 years and presents with an incomplete history of 0–2 doses of DTwP/DTaP vaccine, how do we determine how many more doses are needed?

You should try to achieve at least four total doses. Give additional doses of DTwP/DTaP with 4-week intervals until you achieve three total doses. Then, give the last (third or fourth) dose at least 6 months after the previous dose.

65. What is the minimum interval between DTwP/DTaP number 4 and DTwP/DTaP number 5?

The minimum interval between DTwP/DTaP number 4 and DTwP/DTaP number 5 is 6 months. Remember that the minimum age for DTwP/DTaP number 5 is 4 years.

CHAPTER 17 Diphtheria, Tetanus and Pertussis Vaccines

66. Is there a recommendation about how many doses of DTwP/DTaP a child can receive by a certain age?

According to CDC-ACIP, children should not receive more than six doses of diphtheria and tetanus toxoids (TT) (e.g., DT, DTwP/DTaP) before the seventh birthday because of concern about adverse reactions, primarily local reactions.

67. We now know that wP vaccines have better priming and longer duration of protection than aP vaccines. In which circumstances, DTaP vaccine be preferred over DTwP?

DTaP vaccine may be preferred to DTwP vaccine in those children who have history of severe adverse effects with DTwP vaccine or children with neurological disorders.

68. Can DT be used as second booster?

No, it should not be used as second childhood booster. Pertussis vaccine is still required to protect against childhood pertussis.

69. Can Tdap vaccine be used as a second booster dose in place of DTwP/DTaP vaccine?

No. Tdap not only contains about one-third or even less amount of aP vaccine content but even diphtheria toxoid content is also less than what is recommended for 2nd booster **(Table 7)**. Further, both CDC-ACIP and IAP recommend this vaccine for use in those above 7 years of age.

TABLE 7: A comparative analysis of available DTaP-containing and Tdap products in India.

Product	Infanrix-hexa (+IPV+Hib+HB)	Hexaxim (+IPV+Hib +HB)	Pentaxim (+IPV+Hib)	Tetraxim (+IPV)	Adacel (Tdap)	Boostrix (Tdap)
Tetanus toxoid	5 Lf	5 Lf	5 Lf	5 Lf	5 Lf	5 Lf
Diphtheria toxoid	≥15 Lf	≥15 Lf	15 Lf	15 Lf	2 Lf	2.5 Lf
Acellular pertussis						
Pertussis toxoid (PT)	25 µg	25 µg	25 µg	25 µg	2.5 µg	8 µg
FHA	25 µg	25 µg	25 µg	25 µg	5 µg	8 µg
Pertactin (PRN)	8 µg		---		3 µg	2.5 µg
Fimbriae (FIM) types 2 and 3	---		---		5 µg	---

70. When can one use Td?

Used in children above 7 years of age as replacement to TT.

71. The Government of India (GoI) has recently replaced TT with Td. Should IAP write to GoI to replace even Td with Tdap?

No. This strategy may not be a cost-effective since there is fast waning of pertussis protection in the recipients of Tdap.

72. How will you immune a child who has not received complete primary immunization against diphtheria/tetanus and pertussis and is more than 7 years?

One dose of Tdap + two doses Td at 0, 1, 6 months followed by Td/Tdap every 10 years.

73. Should a teenage be given Tdap dose even if the child has received a dose of Td at age 11.5 years?

Yes, all adolescents should receive dose of Tdap vaccine to protect them from pertussis, even if they have already received Td. It is important to do this right away if they are in contact with an infant younger than age 12 months, working in a health care center or live in a community where cases of pertussis are occurring.

74. What is the difference between the two Tdap products—Boostrix™ and Adacel™?

Both vaccines provide protection against DTP. Boostrix™ (GlaxoSmithKline) is licensed for people ages 10-64 years, and Adacel™ (Sanofi Pasteur) is licensed for people ages 11-64 years. Both are approved for one dose only, not multiple doses in a series. The two vaccines also contain a different number of pertussis antigens and different concentrations of pertussis antigen and diphtheria toxoid **(Table 7)**.

75. If an adolescent or adult who has never received their one-time dose of Tdap is either infected with or exposed to pertussis, is vaccination with Tdap still necessary, and if so when?

Yes. Adolescents or adults who have a history of pertussis disease generally should receive Tdap according to the routine recommendation. In the United States, two Tdap products are licensed for use. Adacel (Sanofi Pasteur) is licensed for use in people age 11-64 years, and Boostrix (GSK), is licensed for people age 10-64 years. This practice is recommended because the duration of protection induced by pertussis disease is unknown (waning might begin as early as 7 years after infection) and because diagnosis of pertussis can be difficult to confirm, particularly with tests other than culture for *B. pertussis*. Administering pertussis vaccine to people with a history of pertussis presents no theoretical risk.

76. Someone gave Tdap to an infant instead of DTaP. Now what should be done?

If Tdap was inadvertently administered to a child, it should not be counted as either the first, second, or third dose of DTaP. The dose should be repeated with DTaP. Continue vaccinating on schedule. According to CDC-ACIP, if the dose of Tdap was administered for the fourth or fifth DTaP dose, the Tdap dose can be counted as valid.

77. If a dose of DTaP or Tdap is inadvertently given to a patient for whom the product is not indicated (e.g., wrong age group), how do we rectify the situation?

The first step is to inform the parent/patient that you have administered the wrong vaccine. Next, follow these guidelines:
- Tdap given to a child younger than age 7 years as either dose one, two or three is not valid. Repeat with DTaP as soon as feasible.
- Tdap given to a child younger than age 7 years as either dose four or five can be counted as valid for DTaP dose four or five.
- Tdap given to a child age 7 through 9 years can be counted as valid for the one-time Tdap dose.
- DTaP given to patients age 7 or older can be counted as valid for the one-time Tdap dose.

78. When a patient with a recent injury has come to you for a tetanus shot, which vaccine should be given TT/Td or Tdap?

Adolescents and adults ages 10–64 years who require a tetanus toxoid-containing vaccine as part of wound management should receive a single dose of age appropriate Tdap instead of Td, if they have not previously received Tdap if Tdap is not available or was previously administered these people should receive Td.

79. I have a patient who received single-antigen tetanus (TT) in the emergency room for wound management rather than Td or Tdap. Should he be revaccinated?

The CDC-ACIP recommends that patients always be given Td or, if appropriate, Tdap rather than TT, as long as there is no contraindication to the other vaccine components. However, since it is already been given, you can wait until the next scheduled booster dose is due and administer Td (or Tdap) at that time. There are exceptions (e.g., the patient plans to travel internationally, is a contact of an infant younger than age 12 months) in which case you should administer Td (or Tdap).

80. When should tetanus immune globulin (TIG) be administered as part of wound management?

Tetanus immune globulin is recommended for any wound other than a clean minor wound if the person's vaccination history is either unknown, or she/he has had less than a full series of three doses of Td vaccine. TIG should be given as soon as possible after the injury.

81. How long after a wound occurs is tetanus immune globulin no longer recommended?

According to CDC-ACIP, for a person who has been vaccinated but is not up to date, there is probably little benefit in giving TIG more than a week or so after the injury. For a person believed to be completely unvaccinated, we would suggest increasing this interval to 3 weeks (i.e., up to day 21 post-injury). Td or Tdap should be given concurrently.

82. Can a booster dose of Tdap be given to people age 65 years and older?

No brand of Tdap is approved for people age 65 years or older. CDC-ACIP does not recommend off-label use of Tdap for this age group. However, a clinician may choose to administer Tdap to a person age 65 years or older if both patient and clinician agree that the benefit of Tdap outweighs the risk of a local adverse event.

83. Why the Tdap vaccine is not licensed for people older than 64 years? And why this vaccine was not recommended or at least suggested for health care workers age 65 years and older who are in contact with young children.

There are no safety and efficacy data for this age group; FDA did not approve the vaccine for anyone older than age 64 years, and ACIP has not recommended off-label use of Tdap for this age group. However, there is no reason to believe that Tdap is any less safe for people age 65 years and older than it is for younger adults. Clinicians may decide that the benefit of Tdap exceeds the hypothetical risk in these situations.

SUGGESTED READING

1. Acosta AM, DeBolt C, Tasslimi A, Lewis M, Stewart LK, Misegades LK, et al. Tdap vaccine effectiveness in adolescents during the 2012 Washington State pertussis epidemic. Pediatrics. 2015;135:981-9.
2. Barug D, Pronk I, van Houten MA, Knol MJ, van de Kassteele J, Berbers GA, et al. Maternal pertussis vaccination and its effects on the immune response of infants aged up to 12 months in the Netherlands: an open-label, parallel, randomised controlled trial. Lancet Infect Dis. 2019;19(4):392-401.
3. Briere EC, Pondo T, Schmidt M, Skoff T, Shang N, Naleway A, et al. Assessment of Tdap vaccination effectiveness in adolescents in integrated health-care systems. J Adolesc Health. 2018;62:661-6.
4. Cauchi S, Locht C. Non-specific effects of live attenuated pertussis vaccine against heterologous infectious and inflammatory diseases. Front Immunol. 2018;9:2872.
5. Cherry JD. Pertussis: challenges today and for the future. PLoS Pathog. 2013;9(7):e1003418.
6. Cherry JD. Why do pertussis vaccines fail? Pediatrics. 2012;129(5):968-70.
7. Choudhury J. Vaccines at doorstep: Tdap. In: Ghosh TK (Ed). Vaccines at Doorstep and in Pipeline. Kolkata: Indian Academy of Pediatrics; 2008. pp. 82-7.
8. da Silva Antunes R, Babor M, Carpenter C, Khalil N, Cortese M, Mentzer AJ, et al. Th1/Th17 polarization persists following whole-cell pertussis vaccination despite repeated acellular boosters. J Clin Invest. 2018;128(9):3853-65.
9. Edwards KM. How can we best protect infants from pertussis? J Infect Dis. 2018;217(8):1177-9.

10. Gabutti G, Rota MC. Pertussis: a review of disease epidemiology worldwide and in Italy. Int J Environ Res Public Health. 2012;9(12):4626-38.
11. Gkentzi D, Katsakiori P, Marangos M, Hsia Y, Amirthalingam G, Heath PT, et al. Maternal vaccination against pertussis: a systematic review of the recent literature. Arch Dis Child Fetal Neonatal Ed. 2017;102:F456-63.
12. Immunization Action Coalition. (2020). Ask the experts: diphtheria, tetanus, pertussis. [online] Available from https://www.immunize.org/askexperts/experts_per.asp [Last accessed September, 2020].
13. Indian Academy of Pediatrics. (2019). IAP Guidebook on Immunization, 2018-2019. [online] Available from http://acvip.org/files/iap-guidebook-2019.pdf [Last accessed September, 2020].
14. Klein NP, Bartlett J, Fireman B, Baxter R. Waning Tdap effectiveness in adolescents. Pediatrics. 2016;137:e20153326.
15. Klein NP, Bartlett J, Fireman B, Rowhani-Rahbar A, Baxter R. Comparative effectiveness of acellular versus whole-cell pertussis vaccines in teenagers. Pediatrics. 2013;131(6):e1716-22.
16. Klein NP, Bartlett J, Rowhani-Rahbar A, Fireman B, Baxter R. Waning protection after fifth dose of acellular pertussis vaccine in children. N Engl J Med. 2012;367(11):1012-9.
17. Koepke R, Eickhoff JC, Ayele RA, Petit AB, Schauer SL, Hopfensperger DJ, et al. Estimating the effectiveness of tetanus-diphtheria-acellular pertussis vaccine (Tdap) for preventing pertussis: evidence of rapidly waning immunity and difference in effectiveness by Tdap brand. J Infect Dis. 2014;210:942-53.
18. Lapidot R, Gill CJ. The Pertussis resurgence: putting together the pieces of the puzzle. Trop Dis Travel Med Vaccines. 2016;2:26.
19. Liko J, Robison SG, Cieslak PR. Priming with whole-cell versus acellular pertussis vaccine. N Engl J Med. 2013;368(6):581-2.
20. Locht C. Will we have new pertussis vaccines? Vaccine. 2018;36(36):5460-9.
21. Meade BD, Plotkin SA, Locht C. Possible options for new pertussis vaccines. J Infect Dis. 2014;209 Suppl 1:S24-7.
22. Pitisuttithum P, Chokephaibulkit K, Sirivichayakul C, Sricharoenchai S, Dhitavat J, Pitisuthitham A, et al. Antibody persistence after vaccination of adolescents with monovalent and combined acellular pertussis vaccines containing genetically inactivated pertussis toxin: a phase 2/3 randomised, controlled, non-inferiority trial. Lancet Infect Dis. 2018;18(11):1260-8.
23. Raeven RH, van der Maas L, Pennings JL, Fuursted K, Jørgensen CS, van Riet E, et al. Antibody specificity following a recent Bordetella pertussis infection in adolescence is correlated with the pertussis vaccine received in childhood. Front Immunol. 2019;10:1364.
24. Sheridan SL, Ware RS, Grimwood K, Lambert SB. Number and order of whole cell pertussis vaccines in infancy and disease protection. JAMA. 2012;308(5):454-6.
25. Sricharoenchai S, Sirivichayakul C, Chokephaibulkit K, Pitisuttithum P, Dhitavat J, Pitisuthitham A, et al. A genetically inactivated two-component acellular pertussis vaccine, alone or combined with tetanus and reduced-dose diphtheria vaccines, in adolescents: a phase 2/3, randomised controlled non-inferiority trial. Lancet Infect Dis. 2018;18:58-67.
26. Thierry-Carstensen B, Dalby T, Stevner MA, Robbins JB, Schneerson R, Trollfors B. Experience with monocomponent acellular pertussis combination vaccines for infants, children, adolescents and adults—A review of safety, immunogenicity, efficacy and effectiveness studies and 15 years of field experience. Vaccine. 2013;31:5178-91.

27. van der Lee S, Hendrikx LH, Sanders EA, Berbers GA, Buisman AM. Whole-cell or acellular pertussis primary immunizations in infancy determines adolescent cellular immune profiles. Front Immunol. 2018;9:51.
28. Voysey M, Kelly DF, Fanshawe TR, Sadarangani M, O'Brien KL, Perera R, et al. The influence of maternally derived antibody and infant age at vaccination on infant vaccine responses: an individual participant meta-analysis. JAMA Pediatr. 2017;171(7):637-46.
29. Warfel JM, Merkel TJ. Bordetella pertussis infection induces a mucosal IL-17 response and long-lived Th17 and Th1 immune memory cells in nonhuman primates. Mucosal Immunol. 2013;6(4):787-96.
30. Warfel JM, Zimmerman LI, Merkel TJ. Acellular pertussis vaccines protect against disease but fail to prevent infection and transmission in a nonhuman primate model. Proc Natl Acad Sci U S A. 2014;111(2):787-92.
31. Witt MA, Arias L, Katz PH, Truong ET, Witt DJ. Reduced risk of pertussis among persons ever vaccinated with whole cell pertussis vaccine compared to recipients of acellular pertussis vaccines in a large US cohort. Clin Infect Dis. 2013;56(9):1248-54.
32. Witt MA, Katz PH, Witt DJ. Unexpectedly limited durability of immunity following acellular pertussis vaccination in preadolescents in a North American outbreak. Clin Infect Dis. 2012;54(12):1730-5.
33. Wood N, Nolan T, Marshall H, Richmond P, Gibbs E, Perrett K, et al. Immunogenicity and safety of monovalent acellular pertussis vaccine at birth: a randomized clinical trial. JAMA Pediatr. 2018;172(11):1045-52.

CHAPTER 18

Measles Vaccines

Baldev S Prajapati, Arun Wadhwa

1. What is measles and how can you differentiate from rubella and roseola?

Measles, also called as morbilli, rubeola, red measles, and English measles, is a highly contagious infectious disease caused by measles virus. Incubation period is usually 10–12 days and the disease lasts for 7–10 days. It is an extremely contagious disease—nine out of 10 people who are not immune and share living space with an infected person will be infected. Initial symptoms typically include fever, often greater than 104°F, cough, runny nose, and inflamed eyes. Small white spots known as Koplik's spots may form inside the mouth 2 or 3 days after the start of symptoms. A red, flat rash, which usually starts on the face and then spreads to the rest of the body typically begins 4 days after the start of symptoms. Common complications include diarrhea (8%), middle ear infection (7%), and pneumonia (6%). Less commonly, seizures, blindness, or encephalitis may occur. Rubella, also known as German measles, fifth disease (erythema infectiosum), and roseola infantum are different diseases caused by unrelated viruses. They are milder and the fever typically vanishes on 4–5th day as soon as the rash appears.

2. What is modified (incomplete) measles?

Modified measles is an attenuated form of infection that may occur in individuals who have received immunoglobulin as prophylaxis after exposure to measles. It may occur in individuals with passively acquired antibodies, such as recipients of blood products or intravenous immunoglobulins few days before the exposure. The clinical manifestations of modified or incomplete measles are milder than those of typical infection and the incubation period is prolonged (15–20 days). The rash may be indistinct, brief, or rarely entirely absent. Complications are rarely observed following modified measles.

3. What is atypical measles?

Atypical measles occurs in adults infected with natural virus who had previously received killed measles vaccine between 1963 and 1968. These persons have a sudden onset of fever accompanied by abdominal pain, cough, vomiting, and pleuritic chest pain. Koplik's spots are rarely present and rash begins distally and progresses in a cephalad direction, with less involvement of face and upper part of trunk. The rash is not generalized and confluent as in typical measles. Although rash is erythematous and maculopapular, it often has a vesicular component. Cough and conjunctivitis are not prominent features of atypical measles. Pulmonary symptoms accompanied by radiographic evidence of pneumonia, hilar adenopathy, and pleural effusions are common. Recovery from atypical measles may take 2 weeks or longer.

4. What is the disease burden of measles?

Measles is now rare in many industrialized developed countries, but it still prevails as a common illness in many developing countries, particularly in parts of Africa and Asia. Measles is a highly contagious disease; in prevaccination era, >90% of the individuals were infected by 10 years of age. In the early part of 20th century, major epidemics occurred every 2–3 years leading to an estimated 2.6 million deaths each year. Now >95% of measles deaths occur in countries with low per capita incomes and weak health infrastructures.

5. What is the situation in India?

While India has made significant progress in reducing child mortality, measles still remains a leading cause of death and disability among young children. India stood fourth among 194 countries in the number of measles cases registered between July 2018 and June 2019, according to the latest measles surveillance data released by the World Health Organization (WHO). With 39,299 cases, India bagged the fourth spot after Madagascar (150,976), Ukraine (84,394), and Philippines (45,847). However, India had the lowest measles incidence rate per million in the top 10 countries—29.68.

6. Has regular measles vaccination made a significant impact on the disease incidence?

Accelerated immunization activities have had a major impact on reducing measles deaths. In 2007, measles vaccine coverage of at least one dose reached around 82% worldwide. During the 2000–2018 period, measles vaccination prevented an estimated 23.2 million deaths. Global measles deaths decreased by 73% from an estimated 536,000 in 2000 to 142,000 in 2018. In India, after the introduction of measles vaccination in Universal Immunization Program (UIP) in 1985, measles deaths have been reduced from 106,000 in 2005 to 65,000 in 2010 and to 29,336 in 2012. While India has increased its measles vaccination coverage, it is still far from achieving the WHOs deadline of 95% coverage till 2020.

7. What are the efficacy and effectiveness of the measles vaccine?

In controlled studies, it has been found that measles vaccine efficacy is 89% when given at 9 months of age and approximately 99% when given above 12 months of age. As expected, vaccine effectiveness, however, is lower. It is around 85% when given at 9 months and 95% when given after 1 year of age.

8. Which strains of measles virus are used for preparing measles vaccines at present?

All currently used measles vaccines are live attenuated vaccines and the strains originate from the original Edmonston strain. They are Schwarz, Edmonston-Zagreb, Moraten, and Edmonston B strains. Indian vaccines are usually formulated from the Edmonston-Zagreb strain grown on human diploid cells or purified chick embryo cells.

9. Being live viral vaccine, measles vaccine is more labile. What precautions should be taken to maintain its potency?

Measles vaccine is supplied as freeze-dried in single dose or multidose vials with distilled water as a diluent. The vaccine may be stored frozen or at 2–8°C (shelf-life 2 years). Reconstituted vaccine is destroyed by light and is very heat labile. It loses 50% potency at 20°C and 100% potency at 37°C after 1 hour. Therefore, it should be protected from light, kept at 2–8°C, and used within 4–6 hours of reconstitution. This is particularly applicable to multidose vials.

10. What are the contraindications of measles vaccination?

- Severely immunocompromised child—congenital or acquired
- History of severe allergic reaction to any of the constituents
- Pregnancy.

Human immunodeficiency virus (HIV)-infected individuals and history of egg allergy are not contraindications for measles vaccination.

11. What is the schedule of measles vaccination in an outbreak?

The immunogenicity and efficacy of the measles vaccine depends on the age of administration due to interference by preexisting maternal antibodies. Seroconversion rates are around 60% at the age of 6 months, 80–85% at the age of 9 months, and >95% at the age of 12–15 months. Therefore, the best time for the measles vaccination is 12–15 months of age. However, in India, a significant proportion of measles cases occur below the age of 12 months. Hence, in order to achieve the best balance between these competing demands of early protection and high seroconversion, completed 9 months of age have been recommended as the appropriate age for measles vaccination in India. In case of an outbreak, however, the vaccine can be given to infants as young as 6 months (scientifically feasible and epidemiologically relevant). An additional dose of measles vaccine preferably as measles, mumps, and rubella (MMR) vaccine at the age of 15 months is required for durable and possibly lifelong protection against measles.

12. What are adverse reactions of measles vaccination?

Measles vaccine is remarkably safe vaccine and side effects are few and generally mild. Measles-like illness may develop 7–10 days after measles vaccination in 2–5% of the vaccinees. Thrombocytopenic purpura may occur in some vaccinees. The depression of cell-mediated immunity (CMI) may occur, it is harmless, and recovers within 4–6 weeks. It does not create any problem with early HIV or unrecognized tuberculosis. Subacute sclerosing panencephalitis (SSPE) is rare complication following measles vaccination. It may occur 7–8 years after the vaccination in one out of 1 million vaccinees.

13. What is toxic shock syndrome following measles vaccination? How can it be prevented?

Toxic shock syndrome following measles vaccination is due to contamination of measles vaccine with *Staphylococcus aureus* bacteria due to use of unsterile syringes, needles, and using a vaccine vial beyond 4 hours after reconstitution. It happens more often when multidose vials are used. Reconstituted measles vaccine is susceptible to contamination, as it does not have any preservative or antibiotics. It can occur after 30 minutes to few hours after vaccination presenting with fever, vomiting, diarrhea, and shock.

Use of sterile syringes, needles, aseptic precautions, and prevention of contamination of reconstituted measles vaccine can prevent toxic shock syndrome. Hence, once reconstituted, the measles vaccine should be used within 4 hours.

14. Is it true that measles vaccine may be given along with all childhood vaccines, except Bacillus Calmette-Guérin (BCG) vaccine?

Earlier it was postulated that depression of CMI following measles vaccination may cause disseminated tuberculosis due to vaccine strain of Bacillus Calmette-Guérin (BCG) vaccine, if both the vaccines are given on the same day. The recommended minimum interval between two vaccines was 4 weeks. Now, it is known that depression of CMI takes at least 2 weeks. Therefore, even BCG vaccine can be given along with the measles vaccine on the same day. In fact, in many African countries, simultaneous campaign of both BCG and measles vaccines are undertaken by the WHO.

15. Can measles vaccine be given in a human immunodeficiency virus (HIV)-infected child? At what age? How many doses?

Children infected by HIV are vulnerable to develop severe measles disease with high mortality rate. In early life, most vaccines in this group are safe and efficacious including measles vaccine as the immune system is relatively well-preserved. It is noted that in HIV-infected infants following measles vaccination, seroconversion rates are superior at 6 months of age compared to 9 months due to progressive immunodeficiency with the age. Hence, the Indian Academy of Pediatrics Committee on Immunization (IAPCOI) recommends two doses of measles vaccine in HIV-infected infants at 6 and 9 months of age. The measles vaccine should be administered to those with

HIV infection, irrespective of degree of immunocompromise as here the benefits outweigh the risks.

16. If the mother gives the history of fever and measles-like rashes to the child in the past, what decision should be taken to administer measles vaccine?

The measles vaccine should be given irrespective of prior history of measles as any exanthematous illness is often considered as measles.

17. Is there any role of measles vaccine as postexposure prophylaxis?

Available data suggest that live measles virus vaccine, if given within 72 hours of measles exposure, will prevent or modify the disease. Exposure to measles is not a contraindication to measles immunization.

18. What is the risk of epidemiological shift of measles cases?

Infants are protected from measles up to 6–9 months of age by maternal antibodies. Thereafter, measles and MMR vaccines protect them. If measles vaccination coverage is persistently >85%, children will be well-protected from the disease. But the older children and adults who are not protected will be more susceptible to measles disease. Thus, the measles epidemiology may shift to older group and the disease severity is likely more in this group.

19. Before launching the measles and rubella (MR) vaccination program, the Government of India had earlier launched a Mass Measles Vaccination Program. Was this scientifically strong? Why should a child already vaccinated with measles and then measles, mumps, and rubella (MMR) that suffer unnecessary pricks?

The country needs 95% vaccination coverage to control measles. The first time that the measles vaccine is given at 9 months. We know that giving measles at 9 months is an epidemiological compulsion; there is a 15–20% primary vaccination failure due to maternal antibodies. Therefore, at least two to three doses of measles-containing vaccines are required for protection. Even then, 5–8% remain susceptible. Therefore, giving a measles vaccine/measles-containing vaccine for more than two times is scientifically sound. So, even if the child has already received a measles-containing vaccine, the extra dose offered under the Government of India (GOI) Measles-rubella Immunization Program does not do any harm, but is also scientifically valid. The Mass Measles Vaccination Program is like the supplementary immunization activity that was carried out for polio eradication.

20. What are the new recommendations of National Technical Advisory Group on Immunization (NTAGI)/Government of India (GOI) on measles-rubella immunization?

Recently, following the National Technical Advisory Group on Immunization (NTAGI) Standing Technical Subcommittee recommendation of two doses of measles and rubella (MR) vaccines in UIP at 9 months and 16–24 months at the time of first booster of diphtheria, tetanus, and pertussis (DTP) vaccine, the GOI has decided to implement this policy. Further, India has now joined the global initiative of elimination of MR and control of congenital rubella syndrome (CRS).

21. What is the Indian Academy of Pediatrics-Advisory Committee on Vaccines and Immunization Practices (IAP-ACVIPs) stand on the Government new policy of rescheduling the measles and rubella (MR) vaccine at 9 months and 16–24 months?

The academy has argued very strongly in favor of MMR instead of MR vaccine in UIP schedule because of various reasons. Mumps carries as much significance as rubella in terms of morbidity and complications. Moreover, the MMR vaccine has been in use since decades and therefore, its acceptance by doctors and parents would be much easier than of MR vaccine with which no one has been so far acquainted. Also, it is more sensible in terms of logistics as it will require the same effort, money, and manpower to eliminate three illnesses instead of two.

22. Does it mean stand-alone measles vaccine will become obsolete?

Yes, it is highly unethical to use stand-alone measles vaccine when effective MR and MMR vaccines are available in the country.

23. Why the Government of India is not willing to include measles, mumps, and rubella (MMR) in place of measles and rubella (MR) in its Universal Immunization Program (UIP)?

Probably, they are still not convinced about the burden of mumps in the country. Lack of large-scale studies has also hampered the moves to include mumps in National Immunization Program/UIP. Cost also could be a consideration.

24. What is the cause of so many measles outbreaks across the world?

Measles outbreaks refer to a substantial global increase in the number of measles cases reported, relative to previous year (**Box 1 and Fig. 1**). As of April 2019, the number of measles cases reported worldwide represented a 300% increase from the number of cases seen in 2018. In the first half of 2019, the WHO received reports of 364,808 measles cases from 182 countries, up 182% from the same time period of 2018 when 129,239 confirmed cases were reported by 181 countries. Countries reporting maximum cases were USA (New York and California), France, Brazil, Nigeria, Israel, Democratic Republic of the Congo (DRC), and Philippines. The outbreaks happened due to nonavailability of vaccine in some places or more often due to opposition to vaccination (vaccine hesitancy). Outbreaks might increase if there is a break in routine immunizations or if mass vaccine campaigns stop because of prolonged lockdown due to coronavirus disease 2019 (COVID-19).

BOX 1: Global measles outbreaks in top 10 countries in 2019.

Top 10 countries by case counts (2019)
1. *Democratic Republic of the Congo (DRC)*: 19,166
2. *Nigeria*: 6,371
3. *Brazil*: 6,069
4. *Kazakhstan*: 4,755
5. *India*: 4,516
6. *Uzbekistan*: 4,508
7. *Philippines*: 4,424
8. *Central African Republic*: 4,194
9. *Bangladesh*: 3,627
10. *Ethiopia*: 2,434

Source: Centers for Disease Control and Prevention (CDC).

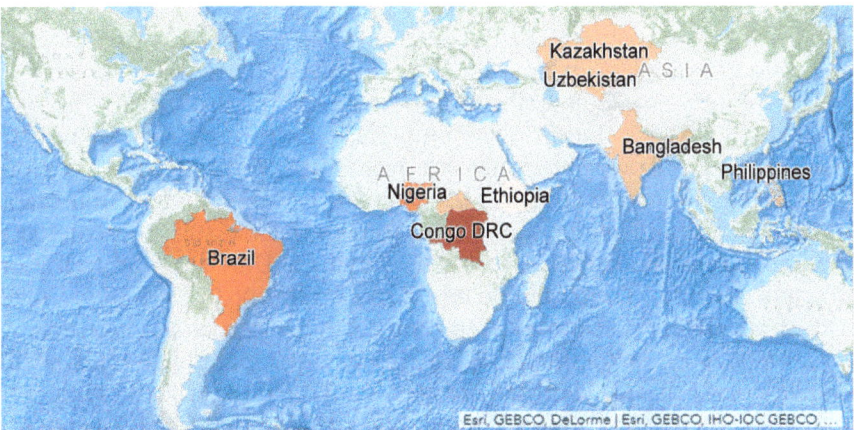

Fig. 1: Top 10 countries with measles outbreaks in 2019.
Source: Centers for Disease Control and Prevention (CDC).

SUGGESTED READING

1. Centers for Disease Control and Prevention (CDC). (2020). Global Measles Outbreaks. [online] Available from: https://www.cdc.gov/globalhealth/measles/globalmeaslesoutbreaks.htm. [Last accessed July, 2020].
2. Ghosh TK, Kundu R, Ganguly N. Controversies Answered: A Monograph on Vaccinology. New Delhi: Jaypee Brothers Medical Publishers (P) Ltd; 2007.
3. Kliegman RM, Behrman RE, Jenson HJ, Stanton BF. Nelson Textbook of Pediatrics, 18th edition. New York: Elsevier; 2008.
4. Plotkin S, Orenstein W, Offit P. Vaccines, 5th edition. New Delhi: Jaypee Brothers Medical Publishers (P) Ltd; 2008.
5. Singhal T, Amdekar YK, Agarval RK. IAP Guidebook on Immunization, 4th edition. New Delhi: Jaypee Brothers Medical Publishers (P) Ltd; 2007.
6. Thacker N, Shah NK. Immunization in Clinical Practice. New Delhi: Jaypee Brothers Medical Publishers (P) Ltd; 2005.
7. Vashishtha VM, Choudhury P, Kalra A, Bose A, Thacker N, Yewale VN, et al. Indian Academy of Pediatrics (IAP) recommended immunization schedule for children aged 0 through 18 years—India, 2014 and updates on immunization. Indian Pediatr. 2014;51:785-800.

CHAPTER 19

Measles, Mumps and Rubella Vaccines

Arun Wadhwa, Baldev S Prajapati, Sudhir Kumar Choudhary

1. What is the disease burden of measles, mumps, and rubella (MMR)? Why is it important to give MMR vaccine routinely?

Measles is a highly contagious disease caused by a virus of paramyxovirus family. In prevaccination era, >90% of the individuals were infected by the age of 10 years. Before the introduction of measles vaccine in 1963 vaccination, measles caused many outbreaks and an estimated 2.6 million deaths annually. Now, global measles deaths have decreased by 73% from an estimated 536,000 in 2000 to 142,000 in 2018. More than 95% of measles deaths now occur in low-income countries with weak health infrastructures. After the introduction of measles vaccination in the Universal Immunization Program (UIP) in 1985, measles deaths reduced from 106,000 in 2005 to 29,336 in 2012, but still India contributes to almost 47% of global measles deaths.

Mumps is a highly contagious virus that causes painful swelling of the parotid glands. It can lead to viral meningitis, pancreatitis, orchitis, and subsequent sterility. Mumps vaccine had been introduced in 122 countries by the end of 2018.

Rubella is a viral disease which is usually mild in children, but infection during early pregnancy may cause fetal death or congenital rubella syndrome, which can lead to defects of the brain, heart, eyes, and ears. Rubella vaccine was introduced in 168 countries by the end of 2018 and global coverage was estimated at 69%.

The exact disease burden of mumps and rubella in India is not known.

2. What are the Advisory Committee on Vaccines and Immunization Practices (ACVIP) recommendations for routine and catch-up immunization for measles, mumps, and rubella (MMR)?

The Advisory Committee on Vaccines and Immunization Practices (ACVIP) recommends three doses of measles, mumps, and rubella (MMR).

First dose as MMR at the completion of 9 months, second dose as MMR at 15–18 months, and third dose as MMR at 5 years of age.

Catch-up vaccination: All the school-aged children above 5 years of age, if not vaccinated earlier, should at least be vaccinated with MMR vaccine with minimal interval of 4 weeks between the two doses. Give second dose if the child has previously received one dose of MMR after 1 year of age.

3. What are the World Health Organization (WHO) recommendations for optimal timing of measles, mumps, and rubella (MMR) doses?

In countries where the risk of measles transmission and mortality remains high, measles-containing vaccine first dose (MCV1) should be administered at 9 months of age to ensure optimal protection during the susceptible period in infancy. These countries should administer the second dose of MCV2 at 15–18 months of age. The minimum interval between MCV1 and MCV2 is 4 weeks. In countries with low levels of measles transmission, MCV1 may be administered at 12 months of age to take advantage of the higher seroconversion rates achieved at this age. If MCV1 coverage is high (>90%) and school enrolment is high (>95%), administration of routine MCV2 at school entry is an effective strategy for achieving high coverage and preventing outbreaks in schools.

4. Why measles, mumps, and rubella (MMR) vaccine is not included in the Expanded Program on Immunization (EPI) schedule?

Measles, mumps, and rubella vaccine is not incorporated in the Expanded Program on Immunization (EPI) schedule by the Government of India (GOI) due to following reasons.

The main reason why government has not included mumps in their immunization schedule is lack of documentation of existing burden of the mumps in the community. So, the recommendation of giving MMR in place of measles vaccine should be viewed in this background.

Another reason is higher cost of MMR in comparison to measles and rubella (MR), though it was not the main reason.

The Indian Academy of Pediatrics (IAP) has been arguing for inclusion of MMR instead of MR in the UIP also. The committee considers the decision of using MR as "unethical" and a sort of "missed opportunity" when three instead of two vaccine-preventable diseases (VPDs) can be targeted simultaneously with almost similar logistics and efforts.

As of June 2020, 122 countries have introduced MMR or mumps-containing vaccine in their National Immunization Programs (NIPs) globally **(Fig. 1)**.

5. Why the Indian Academy of Pediatrics (IAP) has changed its recommendations pertaining to measles, mumps, and rubella (MMR) vaccine?

The relook becomes unavoidable following the National Technical Advisory Group on Immunization (NTAGI) Standing Technical Subcommittee (STSC) recommendation of two doses of MR vaccines in the UIP at 9 months and 16–24 months at the time of first booster of diphtheria, tetanus, and pertussis (DTP) vaccine. Since the Academy has argued very strongly in favor of MMR instead of MR vaccine in the UIP schedule, the revised recommendations will facilitate inclusion of mumps vaccine in the NIP in near future. Furthermore, it will be more sync with the upcoming UIP schedule.

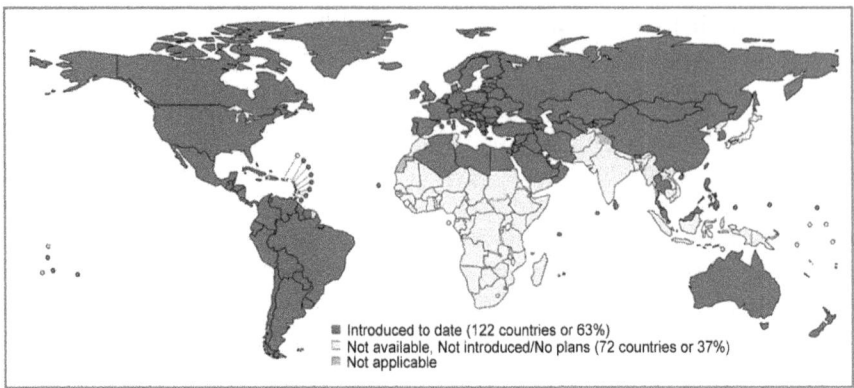

Fig. 1: Countries with mumps-containing vaccine in the National Immunization Program (NIP).

6. **Initially in the Universal Immunization Program (UIP), the recommendation was for one dose of measles, then it was changed to two doses, and then from stand-alone measles to measles and rubella (MR). Why?**

One dose of measles was included in 1985 in the UIP, but the dropouts, poor coverage, vaccine failures, and waning immunity, >40% of the cohort remained unimmunized. Hence, two doses of MCV one at 9 months, as stand-alone measles, and second as MR at 15 months were initiated. Though exact rubella disease burden estimates are not known and difficult to assess but since India has committed to the elimination of measles and control of congenital rubella syndrome (CRS) by the year 2020, rubella vaccine has been introduced in the NIP, as MR vaccine replacing both doses of MCV at 9 months as 16–24 months.

7. **Why is there a variation between the Indian Academy of Pediatrics (IAP) and Government recommendations—measles and rubella (MR) in Government and measles, mumps, and rubella (MMR) in the IAP?**

The GOI recommends MR vaccine in the NIP because of lack of evidence of disease burden data, less morbidity-mortality, and probably cost factor. The IAP recommends MMR vaccine in place of MR at 9 months and 16–24 months. The IAP considers mumps morbidity as significant as much as rubella. There are complications of mumps like aseptic meningitis, encephalitis, pancreatitis, orchitis, transverse myelitis, polyradiculitis, etc., with lifelong repercussions and disabilities.

Globally, most countries use MMR vaccine instead of monovalent measles or MR and thereby the burden of mumps has reduced substantially in the developed world.

8. **What is measles-rubella initiative?**

The MR initiative is a global partnership aimed at ensuring no child dies of measles or is born with CRS. It was launched in 2001 by the American Red

Cross, the Centers for Disease Control and Prevention (CDC), the United Nations International Children's Emergency Fund (UNICEF), and the World Health Organization (WHO). Since 2001, the initiative has delivered >1 billion doses of measles vaccines to help to raise and maintain measles vaccination coverage to 85% globally and thereby reduce global measles death by 74%. These efforts have contributed significantly in reducing child mortality.

9. Are there any changes to the childhood vaccination schedule for mumps during an outbreak?

During an outbreak, vaccine schedules of all children should be checked. If any dose pending, it should be given. If the child has received one or two doses at 9 and 15 months, third dose can be given 4 weeks from the last dose. All healthcare professional and high-risk individuals should take an extra dose.

10. The Indian Academy of Pediatrics-Advisory Committee on Vaccines and Immunization Practices (IAP-ACVIP) recommends first dose of measles, mumps, and rubella (MMR) at 9 months. Do you think MMR will be effective before 12 months of age? Is there adequate data to support this recommendation?

There are many studies both from India and from other countries demonstrating efficacy and safety of MMR vaccine given at 9 months of age **(Table 1)**.

11. Why is a second dose of measles, mumps, and rubella (MMR) necessary?

Between 2 and 5% of persons do not develop measles immunity after the first dose of vaccine. This occurs for a variety of reasons and especially so if first dose was given before 1 year of age. The second dose is to provide another chance to develop measles immunity for persons who did not respond to the first dose.

12. What is the rationale for measles, mumps, and rubella (MMR) third dose?

For lifelong immunity against mumps, you need three doses of mumps or two doses given after 1 year of age. In view of the outbreaks of mumps in older age groups, another dose at 5 years has been recommended.

13. How long does it take to develop immunity to mumps after vaccination with measles, mumps, and rubella (MMR)?

In one study, 86.6% of vaccinees had evidence of mumps seroconversion at 4 weeks after immunization and 93.3% had evidence of seroconversion after 5 weeks. However, seroconversion may not result in immunity. About 80% of persons who have received one dose can be considered protected and 90% after two doses.

TABLE 1: Summary of studies evaluating seroconversion after measles, mumps, and rubella vaccines administered at different ages.

Authors	Place	Year	Ages/age groups compared	Seroconversions at different age groups		
				Measles	Mumps	Rubella
Schoub BD et al.	South Africa	1990	9 and 15 months	Better at 9 months	Similar in both groups	Similar in both groups
Giammanco G et al.	Italy	1993	10–12 and 15–24 months	Similar, but lower geometric mean titers (GMTs) at 9–12 months	Similar, but lower GMTs at 9–12 months	Similar, same GMTs
Singh R et al.	Vellore, India	1994	9, 12, and 15 months	Lower at 9 months (80%) than at 12 and 15 months (95%)	Lower at 9 months (75%) than at 12 and 15 months (92%)	Similar (92%) at all the three age groups
Forleo-Neto E et al.	Brazil	1997	9 and 15 months	Similar in both groups	Similar in both groups	GMTs higher in 15 months age group
Klinge J et al.	Germany	2000	9–11, 12–14, or 15–17 months	Lower seroconversion in one and three groups only (84.8% vs. 100%)	Similar in all the groups	Similar in all the groups
Yadav S et al.	New Delhi, India	2003	9–10 and 15–18 months	Similar (92% in each group)	Similar (100% vs. 96%)	Similar (98% vs. 94%)
Goh P et al.*	Singapore	2007	9 and 12 months	Similar (>92% in each group)	Similar	Similar

*Seroconversion of varicella along with measles, mumps, and rubella was also studied.

Source: Adapted from Vashishtha VM, Yewale VN, Bansal CP, Mehta PJ, Indian Academy of Pediatrics, Advisory Committee on Vaccines and Immunization Practices (ACVIP). IAP perspectives on measles and rubella elimination strategies. Indian Pediatr. 2014;51:719-22.

14. If you can give the third dose of measles, mumps, and rubella (MMR) as early as 28 days after the first dose, why do we routinely wait until school entry to give the third dose?

The third dose of MMR may be given as early as a month after the first dose and be counted as a valid dose if both doses were given after the first birthday. It is convenient to give the third dose at school entry, since the child will have an immunization visit for other school entry vaccines. The third dose is not a "booster"; it is intended to produce immunity in the small number of persons who fail to respond to the first dose.

15. What about postexposure prophylaxis?

For preventing measles, MCV vaccine has to be administered within 72 hours of exposure and immunoglobulin (IG) administered within 6 days of exposure. People who are at risk for severe illness and complications from measles, such as infants younger than 12 months of age, pregnant women without evidence of measles immunity, and people with severely compromised immune systems, should receive IG. If MMR vaccine is not administered within 72 hours of exposures as postexposure prophylaxis (PEP), MMR should still be offered in order to offer protection from future exposures. In case of exposure to mumps or rubella, MMR can be given till 10 days after exposure because of the long incubation period of the disease (around 15–17 days).

16. What is the recommended length of time a woman should wait after receiving rubella [or measles, mumps, and rubella (MMR)] vaccine before becoming pregnant?

Four weeks. In October 2001, the Advisory Committee on Immunization Practices (ACIP) voted to change its recommendation for the waiting interval following the administration of rubella vaccine. The interval was reduced from 3 months to 4 weeks. The waiting period for measles and mumps vaccine was already 1 month.

17. What should be done if inadvertent immunization with measles, mumps, and rubella (MMR) takes place in early pregnancy?

The rubella component of MMR vaccine can cause teratogenic effect on the fetus and it may result in CRS as this is the period of organogenesis. Therefore, a female should avoid pregnancy for the 4 weeks after the MMR vaccination. Still inadvertent MMR vaccination in early pregnancy is not an indication for termination of pregnancy. The babies born to women inadvertently vaccinated in pregnancy have been followed up and development of any malformation of CRS has not observed. Close contact with a pregnant woman is not a contraindication to MMR vaccination of the contact. Breastfeeding is not a contraindication to vaccination of either the woman or the breastfeeding child.

18. **Would you consider a person with two documented doses of measles, mumps, and rubella (MMR) vaccine after the first birthday to be immune even if their serology for one or more of the antigens comes back negative?**

There is no ACIP recommendation for this situation. A negative serology would more likely be the result of an insensitive test than of a true vaccine failure. No more doses are necessary.

19. **If a pregnant woman had a positive rubella titer in the past and now has a negative rubella titer, she would not need another measles, mumps, and rubella (MMR) vaccination. Does not the negative rubella titer mean her immunity has waned and she needs a booster dose?**

Rubella antibody levels may decline with time and may even fall below the level of detection of standard screening tests. However, data from surveillance of rubella and CRS suggest that waning immunity with increased susceptibility to rubella disease does not occur (https://www.cdc.gov/mmwr/preview/mmwrhtml/rr6204a1.htm). Studies of persons who have "lost" detectable rubella antibody indicate that almost all had antibody detectable by more sensitive tests or demonstrated a booster-type response [absence of immunoglobulin M (IgM) antibody and a rapid rise in immunoglobulin G (IgG) antibody] after revaccination.

20. **If a woman has a negative rubella titer during her first pregnancy, should she be given measles, mumps, and rubella (MMR) vaccine or only rubella vaccine alone prior to hospital discharge?**

She should be given MMR, unless she has documentation of immunity to measles and mumps (birth before 1957, documented vaccination, or serologic evidence of immunity).

21. **Is pregnancy test required before giving measles, mumps, and rubella (MMR) to a lady of childbearing age group?**

No. The ACIP recommends that women of childbearing age be asked if they are currently pregnant or attempting to become pregnant. Vaccination should be deferred for those who answer "yes." Those who answer "no" should be advised to avoid pregnancy for 4 weeks following vaccination.

22. **Should we give a measles, mumps, and rubella (MMR) to a 15-month-old whose mother is 2 months pregnant?**

Yes. MMR vaccine viruses are not transmitted from the vaccinated person, so MMR does not pose a risk to a pregnant household member.

23. **What are the contraindications of measles, mumps, and rubella (MMR) vaccination?**

Measles, mumps, and rubella is contraindicated in patients with severe immunodeficiency, pregnancy, and those with history of serious allergic reaction to vaccine or its components. Pregnancy is considered as an absolute contraindication to MMR vaccination. Egg allergy is not a contraindication.

24. Which component of measles, mumps, and rubella (MMR) vaccine can cause aseptic meningitis? What are its sequelae?

Aseptic meningitis can rarely occur 2–3 weeks following MMR vaccination due to mumps. The peak incidence is in the 3–4 years of age. It is usually mild and fortunately death or long-term sequelae is very rare.

25. Can measles, mumps, and rubella (MMR) be given on the same day as other live virus vaccines (e.g., varicella)?

Yes. However, if two live vaccines (e.g., MMR and varicella) are not administered on the same day, they should be separated by an interval of at least 28 days.

26. If exposed, will the measles, mumps, and rubella (MMR) vaccine prevent mumps infection?

Mumps vaccine has not been shown to be effective in preventing mumps in already infected persons.

27. Should an immunoglobulin G (IgG) be drawn after two doses of measles, mumps, and rubella (MMR)?

No. After vaccination, it is not necessary to test patients for IgG to confirm immunity.

28. A box of measles, mumps, and rubella (MMR) vaccine (undiluted) was left at room temperature for 3 hours. Is it okay to use?

Ideally, vaccine vial monitor (VVM) should be used in all live vaccines. By the WHO guidelines, MMR is stable at 37°C for 2 days so should be safe to use it. However, if you suspect that this vaccine or any vaccine has been mishandled, you should contact the manufacturer for guidance on its use. This is particularly important for labile live virus vaccines like MMR and varicella. Unfortunately, errors in vaccine storage and handling are common.

29. Once measles, mumps, and rubella (MMR) vaccine has been reconstituted with diluent, how soon must it be used?

It is preferable to administer MMR immediately after reconstitution. If not used immediately, it should be stored in a refrigerator and used within 6 hours (PIL Tresivac).

30. I misplaced the diluent for the measles, mumps, and rubella (MMR) dose, so I used sterile water instead. Is there any problem with doing this?

Only the diluent supplied with the vaccine should be used to reconstitute any vaccine.

31. Can single antigen preparations for measles and rubella vaccines be mixed together? We have measles, mumps, and rubella (MMR) vaccine and single antigen vaccines for those who only need one.

Absolutely not. Vaccines should *never* be mixed except when specifically approved by the Food and Drug Administration (FDA). Also, the ACIP recommends use of combined MMR whenever one or more of the antigens are indicated, so there is little need to stock single antigen vaccines.

32. Our clinic has given measles, mumps, and rubella (MMR) by the wrong route [intramuscular (IM) rather than subcutaneous (SC)] for years. Should these doses be repeated?

All live injected vaccines (MMR, varicella, and yellow fever) are recommended to be given subcutaneously. However, intramuscular (IM) administration is not likely to decrease immunogenicity and doses given IM do not need to be repeated.

33. We often need to give measles, mumps, and rubella (MMR) vaccine to large adults. Is a 25-gauge needle with a length of 5/8" sufficient for a subcutaneous injection?

Yes. A 5/8" needle is recommended for SC injections for people of all sizes.

34. As far as mumps antigen is concerned, there are different strains used to produce different vaccine product. Which strain is the best to use?

Recently, with introduction of a new strain of mumps vaccine—Jeryl-Lynn (J-L) strain [Priorix, GlaxoSmithKline (GSK)] which is almost four times costlier than available vaccines in Indian market raised a controversy on safety and efficacy of different mumps vaccine virus strains used in MMR vaccines over the years. The other mumps vaccine (Tresivac, marketed by Serum Institute of India) available and widely used in India contains L-Zagreb strain of the virus. The concern raised in the Indian vaccine market is on tendency of L-Zagreb strain to cause higher incidence of aseptic meningitis in the recipients. Before passing any judgment on the safety and efficacy of different strains, lets analyze the various facts associated with different strains **(Table 2)**.

- All the strains used in monovalent, bivalent (MM), or trivalent (MMR) vaccines are live, attenuated, and contain >1,000 cell culture infective doses of mumps virus per dose.
- The following strains are used for the development of live vaccines:

TABLE 2: Comparative efficacy and rates or aseptic meningitis of different strains used in mumps vaccines.

Name of strain	Developed by	Efficacy (after single dose)	Risk of aseptic meningitis (cases per 1 lac doses)
Urabe	Japan	92–100%	100
Jeryl-Lynn	USA	75–91%	0.1–1.0
L-Zagreb	Croatia	92–99%	2–90
Leningrad-3	Soviet Union	92–99%	20–100
Rubini	Switzerland	6.3–12.4%	Not known

- Jeryl-Lynn strain
- Leningrad-3 strain
- L-Zagreb strain
- Urabe strain
- Rubini strain.

This is clear from above **Table 2** that all the available mumps virus antigens (except Rubini) are highly efficacious against protecting the disease. The manufacturers of Rubini strain have now recommended two doses of the vaccine instead of one dose (WHO).

The risk of aseptic meningitis is negligible with all the strains, though it is highest with Urabe strain and lowest with J-L strain. Urabe strain though associated with highest incidence of aseptic meningitis, but is found to be the most potent of all available strains. In most comparative studies involving with J-L strain, the Urabe strain was shown to provide more sustained protection. On the other hand, waning of protective immunity was noticed with J-L strain over the passing years.

Hence, all the available mumps vaccines (apart from those containing Rubini strain, not available in India) are highly effective and safe. The controversy over association of aseptic meningitis as adverse effect of mumps vaccination is quite inconsequential and unwarranted. So far, the world over >500 million doses of the vaccine have been administered and the adverse events are found to be extremely rare and mild. The fears about aseptic meningitis are quite unfounded and unjustified. The aseptic meningitis associated with mumps vaccination is quite benign—asymptomatic, self-limiting, and resolves without sequelae within a week. On the other hand, the incidence of aseptic meningitis following natural mumps infection is quite high and even entails some degree of morbidity. The more pertinent issue would be how to increase coverage of MMR vaccine. Right now, the usage in pediatric population is not sufficient to make any impact at the epidemiology of the diseases protected by the vaccine.

35. Are there special vaccination recommendations for colleges and other post-high school educational institutions?

Risks for transmission of MMR at post-high school educational institutions can be high because these institutions bring together large concentrations of persons who may be susceptible to these diseases. Therefore, colleges, universities, technical and vocational schools, and other institutions for post-high school education should require that all undergraduate and graduate students have received two doses of MMR vaccine after 1 year of age or have other acceptable evidence of MMR immunity before enrollment.

Students who do not have documentation of MMR vaccination or other acceptable evidence of immunity at the time of enrollment should be admitted to classes only after receiving the first dose of MMR vaccine. These students should be administered a second dose of MMR vaccine 1 month later (but no sooner than 28 days after the first dose).

36. An 18-year-old college student says he had measles and mumps at ages 4 and 5, but never had measles, mumps, and rubella (MMR) vaccine. Is rubella vaccine recommended in such a situation?

Actually, this student should receive two doses of MMR, separated by at least 28 days (it is recommended that all persons attending school receive two doses of MMR vaccine). A personal history of measles and mumps is not acceptable as proof of immunity. Acceptable evidence of measles and mumps immunity includes a positive serologic test for antibody, physician diagnosis of diseases, birth before 1957, or written documentation of vaccination. For rubella, only serologic evidence or documented vaccination should be accepted as proof of immunity. Additionally, persons born prior to 1957 may be considered immune to rubella unless they are women who have the potential to become pregnant.

37. My patient has had two documented doses of measles, mumps, and rubella (MMR). Her rubella titer was nonreactive at a prenatal visit. What should I do?

It is possible that she failed to respond to both doses. It is also possible that she did respond, but has a low level of antibody. Failure to respond to two properly timed doses of MMR vaccine would be expected to occur in one or two persons per 1,000 vaccinees, at most. A small number of people appear to develop a relatively small amount of antibody following vaccination with rubella and other vaccines. This level of antibody may not be detectable on relatively insensitive commercial screening tests. Controlled trials with sensitive tests indicate a response rate of >99% following two doses of rubella-containing vaccine. Ideal way would be to make a note of her documented vaccination and stop testing. Another approach would be to administer one additional dose of MMR. However, there are no data on the administration of additional doses of rubella-containing vaccine in this situation.

38. Can I give measles, mumps, and rubella (MMR) to a child whose sibling is receiving chemotherapy for leukemia?

Yes. MMR and varicella vaccines should be given to the healthy household contacts of immunosuppressed children. Oral polio is the only vaccine that should not be given to a healthy child if an immunosuppressed person resides in the household.

39. Is it true that egg allergy is no longer considered a contraindication to measles, mumps, and rubella (MMR) vaccine?

Several studies have documented the safety of measles and mumps vaccine (which are grown in chick embryo tissue culture) in children with severe egg allergy. The American Academy of Pediatrics (AAP) "Red Book" Committee no longer considers egg allergy a contraindication to MMR vaccination. The new ACIP statement on MMR also recommends routine vaccination of egg-allergic children without the use of special protocols or desensitization procedures.

40. Is it contraindicated to give measles, mumps, and rubella (MMR) to a breastfeeding mother or to a breastfed infant?

No. Breastfeeding does not interfere with the response to MMR vaccine. Vaccination of a woman who is breastfeeding her infant poses no risk to the infant being breastfed. Although, it is believed that rubella vaccine virus, in rare instances, may be transmitted via breast milk, the infection in the infant is asymptomatic.

41. How soon after delivery can measles, mumps, and rubella (MMR) be given?

Measles, mumps, and rubella can be administered any time after delivery. The vaccine should be administered to a woman who is susceptible to either MMR before hospital discharge, even if she has received RhoGAM during the hospital stay, leaves in <24 hours, or is breastfeeding.

42. Can a purified protein derivative (PPD) (tuberculin skin test) test be given on the same day as a dose of measles, mumps, and rubella (MMR) vaccine?

A purified protein derivative (PPD) can be applied 2 days before or on the same day that MMR vaccine is given. However, if MMR vaccine is given on the previous day or earlier, the PPD should be delayed for at least 1 month. Live measles vaccine given prior to the application of a PPD can reduce the reactivity of the skin test because of mild suppression of the immune system.

43. Is there anything that can be done for unvaccinated people who have already been exposed to measles?

Measles vaccine may be effective if given within the first 3 days (72 hours) after exposure to measles. Immune globulin may be effective for as long as 6 days after exposure.

44. A story on measles, mumps, and rubella (MMR) vaccine suggested administering each component of MMR in separate injections to decrease the risk of autism. Is there any reason to do this?

There is no scientific reason for or benefit to separating the antigens. There is no credible evidence that measles vaccine or MMR increases the risk of autism. Separating the doses put children (and pregnant women who may be exposed to them) at increased risk for these diseases by extending the amount of time children remain unvaccinated. Studies have shown that if parents have to schedule additional appointments for vaccinations, there is an increased risk that their children may not receive all the vaccines they need.

45. Is there any evidence that measles, mumps, and rubella (MMR) or thimerosal causes autism?

No. This issue has been studied extensively in recent years, including a thorough review by the independent Institute of Medicine (IOM). The IOM issued a report in 2004 that concluded there is no evidence supporting an association between MMR vaccine or thimerosal-containing vaccines and the development of autism.

46. How likely is it for a person to develop arthritis from rubella vaccine?

Arthralgia (joint pain) and transient arthritis (joint redness or swelling) following rubella vaccination occur only in persons who were susceptible to rubella at the time of vaccination. Joint symptoms are uncommon in children and in adult males. About 25% of postpubertal women report joint pain after receiving rubella vaccine and about 10% report arthritis-like signs and symptoms. When joint symptoms occur, they generally begin 1–3 weeks after vaccination, persist for 1 day to 3 weeks, and rarely recur. Chronic joint symptoms attributable to rubella vaccine are very rare, if they occur at all.

47. If a healthcare worker develops a rash and low-grade fever after measles, mumps, and rubella (MMR) vaccine, is she/he infectious?

Approximately 5–15% of susceptible persons who receive MMR vaccine will develop a low-grade fever and/or mild rash 7–12 days after vaccination. However, the person is not infectious and no special precautions (e.g., exclusion from work) need to be taken.

48. What is measles, mumps, rubella, and varicella (MMRV)? What age can it be used?

The MMRV vaccine is a combination of MMR and varicella vaccine. The advantage is that it reduces one additional prick to the recipient as both these are usually given together. World over, it is available as Priorix-Tetra™ (GSK) and ProQuad™ [Merck Sharp & Dohme (MSD)]. Measles, mumps, rubella, and varicella (MMRV) can be used at 15 months of age and again at 5 years of age. It is licensed for use from through 12 years of age. GSK MMRV was available in India for a couple of years but now withdrawn.

49. What are the main safety issues with the measles, mumps, rubella, and varicella (MMRV) vaccines?

For children aging <2 years, the MMRV vaccine is associated with more adverse events compared to separate administration of MMR and varicella vaccinations on the same day. In prelicensure studies, incidence of fever was reported at a significantly higher rate (0–42 days postvaccination) in children aged 12–23 months who received a first dose of MMRV vaccine than in children who received first doses of MMR and varicella vaccine as separate injections. Further, the MMRV vaccines (Priorix-Tetra™ and ProQuad™) are also found to be associated with a higher risk of febrile seizures after vaccination among children aged 12–23 months, compared with children receiving separate MMR and varicella vaccinations. The incidence rate of febrile seizures was twice as high in children receiving a first dose of MMRV compared to those receiving monovalent varicella vaccination and MMR at the same time, either 5–12 or 7–10 days postvaccination, amounting to one extra febrile seizure for every 2,300–2,700 children vaccinated.

SUGGESTED READING

1. Balasubramanian S, Shah A, Pemde HK, Chatterjee P, Shivananda S, Guduru VK, et al. Indian Academy of Pediatrics (IAP) Advisory Committee on Vaccines and Immunization Practices (ACVIP) Recommended Immunization Schedule (2018-19) and Update on Immunization for Children Aged 0 Through 18 Years. Indian Pediatr. 2018;55:1066-74.
2. Centers for Disease Control and Prevention (CDC). (2019). Mumps: Outbreak-Related Questions and Answers for Patients. [online] Available from: https://www.cdc.gov/mumps/outbreaks/outbreak-patient-qa.html. [Last accessed July, 2020].
3. Centers for Disease Control and Prevention (CDC). (2019). Q&As About Vaccination Options for Preventing Measles, Mumps, Rubella, and Varicella: Questions and Answers for Healthcare Providers. [online] Available from: https://www.cdc.gov/vaccines/vpd/mmr/hcp/vacopt-faqs-hcp.html. [Last accessed July, 2020].
4. Forleo-Neto E, Carvalho ES, Fuentes IC, Precivale MS, Forleo LH, Farhat CK. Seroconversion of a trivalent measles, mumps, and rubella vaccine in children aged 9, 12 and 15 months. Vaccine. 1997;15:1898-901.
5. Giammanco G, Li Volti S, Salemi I, Giammanco Bilancia G, Mauro L. Immune response to simultaneous administration of a combined measles, mumps and rubella vaccine with booster doses of diphtheria-tetanus and poliovirus vaccine. Eur J Epidemiol. 1993; 9:199-202.
6. Goh P, Lim FS, Han HH, Willems P. Safety and immunogenicity of early vaccination with two doses of tetravalent measles-mumps-rubella-varicella (MMRV) vaccine in healthy children from 9 months of age. Infection. 2007;35:326-33.
7. Immunization Action Coalition (IAC). (2020). Ask the Experts: Measles, Mumps, and Rubella. [online] Available from: http://www.immunize.org/askexperts/experts_mmr.asp. [Last accessed July, 2020].
8. Klinge J, Lugauer S, Korn K, Heininger U, Stehr K. Comparison of immunogenicity and reactogenicity of a measles, mumps and rubella (MMR) vaccine in German children vaccinated at 9-11, 12-14 or 15-17 months of age. Vaccine. 2000;18:3134-40.

9. Schoub BD, Johnson S, McAnerney JM, Wagstaff LA, Matsie W, Reinach SG, et al. Measles, mumps, and rubella immunization at nine months in a developing country. Pediatr Infect Dis J. 1990; 9:263-7.
10. Singhal T, Amdekar YK, Agarwal RK. IAP Guidebook on Immunization. New Delhi: Jaypee Brothers Medical Publishers (P) Ltd; 2019.
11. Singh R, John TJ, Cherian T, Raghupathy P. Immune response to measles, mumps and rubella vaccine at 9, 12 and 15 months of age. Indian J Med Res. 1994; 100:155-9.
12. Vashishtha VM, Choudhury P, Kalra A, Bose A, Thacker N, Yewale VN, et al. Indian Academy of Pediatrics (IAP) recommended immunization schedule for children aged 0 through 18 years—India, 2014 and updates on immunization. Indian Pediatr. 2014;51:785-800.
13. Vashishtha VM, Yewale VN, Bansal CP, Mehta PJ, Indian Academy of Pediatrics, Advisory Committee on Vaccines and Immunization Practices (ACVIP). IAP perspectives on measles and rubella elimination strategies. Indian Pediatr. 2014;51:719-22.
14. Yadav S, Thukral R, Chakarvarti A. Comparative evaluation of measles, mumps & rubella vaccine at 9 & 15 months of age. Indian J Med Res. 2003;118:183-6.

CHAPTER 20

Hepatitis B Vaccines

Ajay Kalra, Sanjay Verma

1. What is the magnitude of problem of hepatitis B in the world?

Hepatitis B is one of the most common viral infections in the world. In 2015, the global prevalence of hepatitis B virus (HBV) infection was estimated at 3.5% with about 257 million persons living with chronic HBV infection. An estimated 887,220 persons died due to HBV infection—337,454 due to hepatocellular carcinoma, 462,690 due to cirrhosis, and 87,076 due to acute hepatitis. A substantial burden of chronic HBV infection persists because birth-dose coverage is still low, estimated at 39% globally. Most of the burden results from infection acquired in infancy through perinatal or early childhood exposure, as infection acquired in early age is more likely to become chronic than infection acquired later in life.

2. What is its prevalence in different countries of the world?

Australia, North America, and countries in Northern Europe have low prevalence rates. Countries of West and South Asia, South America, Eastern Europe, and those in the Mediterranean belt have intermediate prevalence. China, countries of tropical Africa and Pacific region, and the Southeast Asian countries have carrier rates ranging from 7% to 20% and have, therefore, high prevalence rates.

3. Which zone does India belongs to?

With the average carrier rate being estimated as 3.8–4.2%, India belongs to the group of countries with intermediate prevalence rates.

4. What are the features of hepatitis B virus (HBV)?

Hepatitis B virus is a deoxyribonucleic acid (DNA) virus belonging to the family Hepadnaviridae. The virion of hepatitis B consists of surface and core components. The core contains DNA polymerase, core antigen, and e-antigen. The DNA structure of the virus is double-stranded and circular. Hepatitis B surface antigen (HBsAg) (Australia antigen) is an antigen determinant found on the surface of virus. HBsAg is a marker of infectivity and its presence indicates either acute or chronic HBV infection. Anti-HBs antibody to HBsAg is a marker of immunity. Its presence indicates immune response to HBV infection or vaccination or presence of passively acquired antibody. Hepatitis B e-antigen (HBeAg) is a marker of high degree of HBV infectivity and it correlates with high level of HBV replication.

5. What are the modes of transmission of hepatitis B virus (HBV) infection?

The following are known modes of transmission:
- *Vertical transmission*: From pregnant mother to her fetus and baby during the perinatal period. Perinatal transmission is mostly acquired during birth. In utero transmission is rare.
- *Parenteral transmission*: Transmission through blood and blood products is the major contributor for parenteral transmission. Needlestick injuries, unsterile needles, tattooing, ear piercing, and acupuncture can also transmit infection.
- *Sexual transmission*: It is a major mode of transmission in developed countries. It is mainly seen among male homosexual individuals and those with promiscuous heterosexual behavior. Transmission can also occur during artificial insemination.
- *Horizontal transmission*: Virus transmission is known to occur unrelated to sexual, vertical, and parenteral modes of transmission. This transmission is probably due to close contact. In 50% of cases, no definite history of contact can be elicited.

Fifty percent of the carrier pool is contributed by vertical transmission while other modes of transmission account for the rest. Risk of developing HBV infection varies inversely with age.

6. Which categories of individuals are most susceptible of hepatitis B virus (HBV) infection?

The following individuals are at high risk to suffer from HBV infection:
- Infants born to HBsAg-positive mothers
- Homosexual men, heterosexuals individuals with multiple sex partners or with sexually transmitted diseases (STDs)
- Parenteral drug users who share needles
- Patients on hemodialysis therapy, healthcare professionals coming in contact with blood and secretions
- Patients receiving blood or blood products (especially on multiple occasions)
- Household contacts of HBsAg-positive individuals
- Sexual partners of persons with acute HBV infection or carriers
- Inmates of institution for developmentally disabled children
- Prison inmates and staff.

7. When does vertical transmission of hepatitis B virus (HBV) occur?

Vertical transmission is because of contact between secretions of mother and the baby. This most commonly occurs in late perinatal period or at the time of delivery. It is known to occur via breastfeeding and handling by mother in the postnatal period. Hence, there is the importance of timely vaccination in the neonatal period.

8. What is the efficacy of vertical transmission and what does it depend on?

The overall efficacy of vertical transmission is 30–40%. This increases to 70–90% if mother is also HBeAg positive, but drops to >30% if she has anti-HBe antibodies. In India, about 10% of carrier mothers are also HBeAg positive as many as 90% of these newborns infected at birth have potential to become chronic carriers.

9. What happens to newborns infected through vertical transmission?

Newborns infected through vertical transmission usually do not develop acute symptoms, but have a high risk of developing chronic carrier state. Approximately, 90% of newborns infected at birth become chronic carriers and over 25% of these will die from cirrhosis or hepatocellular carcinoma in later life. Thus, perinatally acquired infection has serious consequences for the infant.

10. Is horizontal transmission known to occur with hepatitis B virus (HBV)?

Yes, familial clustering of hepatitis B is known. Children attending daycare centers can also possibly transmit HBV infection to each other. Whenever close- and long-term contact exists, HBV may become widely disseminated through horizontal transmission. The 25% of HBV infections are known to follow familial clustering. Almost 50% of carrier pool is estimated to be due to horizontal transmission.

11. Can hepatitis B virus (HBV) be transmitted in daycare centers via saliva, e.g., drooling infants?

Though HBV has been found in saliva, there are no data to suggest that saliva alone transmits HBV infection. There have been reports of HBV transmission when an HBV-infected person bites another person. In these reports, bloody saliva was usually present in the infected person's mouth and the blood was more likely the vehicle of transmission. HBV is not spread by kissing, hugging, sneezing, coughing, food or water, sharing eating in utensils or drinking glasses, or casual contact.

12. Can hepatitis B virus (HBV) be transmitted by sharing cups or straws?

There are no data to suggest that sharing drinking cups, straws, or other eating in utensils have been associated with HBV transmission.

13. More of my patients are getting tattoos and body piercing. Should they be concerned about contracting a blood-borne infection like hepatitis B virus (HBV)?

Yes, tattooing and body piercing have the potential to transmit blood-borne infections, including HBV, hepatitis C virus (HCV), and human immunodeficiency virus (HIV), if the person doing the tattoos or body piercing does not use good infection control practices.

14. What is the risk for transmitting hepatitis B virus (HBV) by oral sex?

There are no specific data on transmission of blood-borne viruses through oral-genital sex. Saliva has not been associated with HBV transmission unless biting has taken place. HBV is not spread by kissing, hugging, sneezing, coughing, food or water, sharing eating in utensils or drinking glasses, or casual contact.

15. Can kissing transmits hepatitis B virus (HBV)?

Although HBV has been found in saliva, there is no data to suggest that kissing transmits HBV; however, there have not been studies to specifically look at kissing.

16. I tested positive for chronic hepatitis B virus (HBV) infection about 5 months ago. I know there is a vaccine to prevent transmission; however, I would like to know how long my sex partner (I do not have one now) should wait after taking this vaccine, before having sex with me without any risk of transmission?

You should use condoms (the efficacy of latex condoms in preventing infection with HBV is unknown, but their proper use might reduce transmission) until a postvaccination blood test (anti-HBs) shows that your sex partner is protected from HBV infection. For example, your sexual partner should have the three-dose series of hepatitis B vaccine and postvaccination testing 1–2 months after the last dose of vaccine. If your sexual partner's test shows adequate anti-HBs (at least 10 mIU/mL), then he/she should be protected against HBV infection.

17. What are the signs and symptoms of hepatitis B?

About 7 out of 10 adults with acute hepatitis B have signs or symptoms when infected with HBV. Children under age of 5 years, who become infected rarely, show any symptoms. Signs and symptoms of hepatitis B might include nausea, lack of appetite, vomiting, malaise, pain in joints and muscles, headache, photophobia, jaundice, dark urine, clay colored or light stool, and abdominal pain. People who have such signs or symptoms generally feel quite ill and might need to be hospitalized. The case fatality rate among persons with reported cases of acute hepatitis B is approximately 1.5%, with the highest rates occurring in adults who are over 60 years of age.

18. How long does it take to show signs of illness after a person becomes infected with hepatitis B virus (HBV)?

The incubation period ranges from 45 to 160 days (average 120 days).

19. If a patient is diagnosed with acute hepatitis B and then resolves the infection, can the patient ever get hepatitis B again?

Generally speaking, no. However, it is possible for a person to have two different HBV infections, the second due to an HBV variant or a different HBV subtype.

20. How stable is hepatitis B virus (HBV) in the environment and what types of equipment cleaners are virucidal against HBV?

Any high level disinfectant that is tuberculocidal will kill HBV. It is important to note that HBV is quite stable in the environment and remains viable for 7 or more days on environmental surfaces at room temperature. So, the virus is capable of transmitting HBV despite the absence of visible blood.

21. What are hepatitis B virus (HBV) mutants?

Table 1 describes HBV mutants that are known to occur.

TABLE 1: Hepatitis B virus (HBV) mutants and their biological significance.

Mutant form	Mutation	Biological significance
Precore	Single or multiple mutations in the precore region, at codon 28 or 29; preventing synthesis of HBeAg	Most common mutation, association with severe disease and fulminant hepatitis
Core	Clustering mutations in core gene, often associated with precore mutations	Progressive liver disease
Envelope vaccine escape mutant	Does not synthesize HBsAg, HBV-DNA is positive	Responsible for vaccine failure, sometimes associated with chronic liver disease
X-gene	Mutations in X-gene	Not known
Pre-S gene	Mutation in Pre-S region	Not known

Incidence of mutants in India varies from 5% to 14% of total HBV infections.
(DNA: deoxyribonucleic acid; HBeAg: hepatitis B e-antigen; HBsAg: hepatitis B surface antigen)

22. How do mutants matter?

The significance of mutants is that:
- Some mutants can escape recognition by routine HBV serology.
- Hepatitis B virus serology being negative, these persons may be accepted as blood donors and hence transmission of infection can occur.
- Vaccination may not be able to offer protection against some of the mutants.
- Some mutants do not have HBeAg and hence do not induce formation of anti-HBe antibodies. The virus replication continues in spite of HBeAg being negative leading to a false sense of security.

23. I understand that if a person is hepatitis B e-antigen (HBeAg) negative and hepatitis B surface antigen (HBsAg) positive, he/she is not infectious. Am I correct?

No, HBsAg-positive people are infectious independent of their HBeAg status. HbeAg positivity indicates higher levels of HBV in the blood compared to an HBeAg-negative person. A person who is HBsAg positive and HBeAg negative is still infectious, but has lower levels of HBV in their blood.

24. Can hepatitis B virus (HBV) infection be in a remission? Would you please comment on the appropriateness of this terminology?

"Remission" is not a good term to be used for a persistent infection such as HBV. HBV infection should be described in terms of virologic markers, infectivity, and evidence of liver disease. Some persons might resolve their infection (i.e., become HBsAg negative and hence are not infectious) spontaneously or from antiviral therapy. Other persons might remain HBsAg positive and hence infectious, but have no evidence of chronic liver disease (i.e., the often used term "healthy carriers"). We assume that the use of "remission" in the question might refer to either of these scenarios.

25. What are possible risk factors for developing liver disease among persons with chronic hepatitis B virus (HBV) infection?

Risk factors include older age, male gender, presence of HBeAg, mutations in the precore and core promoter regions of the viral genome, and coinfection with hepatitis D (delta) virus. An association between alcohol use and progression to hepatocellular carcinoma in persons with chronic hepatitis B has been reported in some studies, but not in others; these discrepancies might be related to accuracy of the alcohol history.

26. What are the various serologic tests for hepatitis B?

Various serologic tests for hepatitis B are listed in **Table 2**.

27. How do I interpret some of the common hepatitis B panel results?

Interpretation of some of the common hepatitis B tests and results are given in **Table 3**.

28. Is it safe for a hepatitis B surface antigen (HBsAg)-positive mother to breastfeed her infant?

Yes. An HBsAg-positive mother, who wishes to breastfeed, should be encouraged to do so, including immediately following delivery. However, the infant should receive hepatitis B immunoglobulin (HBIG) and hepatitis B vaccine within 12 hours of birth. Although HBsAg can be detected in breast

TABLE 2: Hepatitis B laboratory nomenclature.

HBsAg	HBsAg is a marker of infectivity. Its presence indicates either acute or chronic HBV infection. Anti-HBs antibody to HBsAg is a marker of immunity. Its presence indicates an immune response to HBV infection, an immune response to vaccination, or the presence of passively acquired antibody (it is also known as HBsAb, but this abbreviation is best avoided since it is often confused with abbreviations such as HbsAg)
Anti-HBc (total)	Antibody to HBcAg is a nonspecific marker of acute, chronic, or resolved HBV infection. It is not a marker of vaccine-induced immunity. It may be used in prevaccination testing to determine previous exposure to HBV infection (it is also known as HBcAb, but this abbreviation is best avoided since it is often confused with other abbreviations)
Anti-HBc IgM	IgM antibody subclass of anti-HBc positivity indicates recent infection with HBV (within the past 6 months)
HBeAg	HBeAg is a marker of a high degree of HBV infectivity and it correlates with a high level of HBV replication. It is primarily used to assess and monitor the treatment of patients with chronic HBV infection
Anti-HBe	Antibody to HBeAg may be present in an infected or immune person or in persons with chronic HBV infection. Its presence suggests a low viral titer and a low degree of infectivity. HBV-DNA is a marker of viral replication and it correlates well with infectivity. It is used to assess and monitor the treatment of patients with chronic HBV infection

(DNA: deoxyribonucleic acid; HBc: hepatitis B core; HBV: hepatitis B virus; HBs: hepatitis B surface; HBcAb: hepatitis B core antibody; HBcAg: hepatitis B core antigen; HBeAg: hepatitis B e-antigen; HBsAb: hepatitis B surface antibody; HBsAg: hepatitis B surface antigen; IgM: immunoglobulin M)

TABLE 3: Interpretation of some common hepatitis B tests and results.

Tests	Results	Interpretation	Vaccinate
HBsAg Anti-HBc Anti-HBs	Negative Negative Negative	Susceptible	Vaccinate, if indicated
HBsAg Anti-HBc Anti-HBs	Negative Negative Positive with ≥10 mIU/mL*	Immune due to necessary vaccination	No vaccination necessary
HBsAg Anti-HBc Anti-HBs	Negative Negative Positive	Immune due to natural infection	No vaccination necessary
HbsAg Anti-HBc IgM anti-HBc Anti-HBs	Positive Positive Negative Negative	Actually infected	No vaccination necessary
HbsAg Anti-HBc IgM anti-HBc Anti-HBs	Positive Positive Negative Negative	Chronically infected	No vaccination necessary (may need treatment)

Contd...

Contd...

Tests	Results	Interpretation	Vaccinate
HbsAg	Negative	Four interpretations possible**	Use clinical judgment
Anti-HBc	Positive		
Anti-HBs positive	Negative		

*Postvaccination testing, when it is recommended, should be performed 1–2 months after the last dose of vaccine. Infants born to HbsAg-positive mothers should be tested for HbsAg and anti-HBs after completion of at least three doses of a licensed hepatitis B vaccination series, at age 9–18 months (generally at the next well child visit)

**(1) May be recovering from acute HBV infection; (2) May be distantly immune, but the test may not be sensitive enough to detect a very low level of anti-HBs in serum; (3) May be susceptible with a false-positive anti-HBc; and (4) May be chronically infected and have an undetectable level of HBsAg present in the serum.(HBsAg: hepatitis B surface antigen; HBc: hepatitis B core; HBs: hepatitis B surface; IgM: immunoglobulin M)

milk, studies done before hepatitis B vaccine was available showed that breastfed infants born to HBsAg-positive mothers did not demonstrate an increased rate of perinatal or early childhood HBV infection. More recent studies have shown that, among infants receiving postexposure prophylaxis to prevent perinatal HBV infection, there is no increased risk of infection among breastfed infants.

29. What is possibility of maternal hepatitis B virus (HBV) transmission when breastfeeding an infant if the mother is hepatitis B surface antigen (HBsAg) positive and has cracked or bleeding nipples?

As stated before, although HBsAg can be detected in breast milk, there is no evidence that HBV is transmitted by breastfeeding. Babies born to HBsAg-positive mothers should be immunized with hepatitis B vaccine and HBIG, which will substantially reduce the risk of perinatal transmission and protect the infant from modes of postnatal HBV transmission, including the theoretical exposure to HBV from cracked or bleeding nipples during breastfeeding. To prevent cracked and bleeding nipples, all mothers who breastfeed should be instructed on proper nipple care.

30. What types of hepatitis B vaccines are available?

Earlier, two types of vaccines against hepatitis B were available:
1. Plasma-derived vaccine
2. Deoxyribonucleic acid recombinant vaccine.

The plasma-derived vaccine consisted of purified inactivated HBsAg particles obtained from the plasma of chronic carriers.

Now only the DNA recombinant vaccine is available. In the DNA recombinant vaccine, the antigen particles are obtained from the yeast *Saccharomyces cerevisiae* through recombinant DNA technology. These are adjuvanted with aluminum salts and lipid A. Both thimerosal-preserved and thimerosal-free vaccines are available. The vaccines are available as single and multidose vials. They need to be stored at 2–8°C. Single pediatric dose vial of vaccine contains 10 µg of antigen and that for adult use contains 20 µg of antigen. Multidose vials are available containing 20 µg/mL.

31. Is there any new brand of hepatitis B vaccine available elsewhere?

Heplisav-B is a new hepatitis B vaccine approved by the United States Food and Drug Administration (USFDA) in November 2017 for persons 18 years of age and older. Heplisav-B contains a novel immunostimulatory adjuvant (CpG 1018) that binds to toll-like receptor 9 to stimulate a directed immune response to HBsAg. It is provided in a single dose 0.5 mL vial and given as a two-dose series with doses separated by 1 month.

Heplisav-B was approved based on clinical trials that compared seroprotection rates (SPR, defined as anti-HBs of 10 mIU or higher) following two doses of Heplisav-B to rates following three doses of Engerix-B (GlaxoSmithKline). Among persons 18 through 70 years of age, SPRs were 90–95% following two doses of Heplisav-B and 65–81% following three doses of Engerix-B. Local reactions were most commonly reported (injection site pain, redness, and swelling) and were similar in frequency to those following Engerix-B.

32. Can Heplisav-B be used to complete a vaccination series started with Engerix-B?

Yes. However, data are limited on the safety and immunogenicity effects when Heplisav-B is interchanged with hepatitis B vaccines from other manufacturers. When feasible, the same manufacturer's vaccines should be used to complete the series. However, vaccination should not be deferred when the manufacturer of the previously administered vaccine is unknown or when the vaccine from the same manufacturer is unavailable.

The two-dose hepatitis B vaccine series for adults only applies when both doses in the series consist of Heplisav-B. Series consisting of a combination of one dose of Heplisav-B and a vaccine from a different manufacturer should consist of three total vaccine doses and should adhere to the three-dose schedule minimum intervals of 4 weeks between doses 1 and 2, 8 weeks between doses 2 and 3, and 16 weeks between doses 1 and 3. Doses administered at less than the minimum interval should be repeated. However, a series containing two doses of Heplisav-B administered at least 4 weeks apart is valid, even if the patient received a single earlier dose from another manufacturer.

33. What is the dose and schedule of routine vaccination?

The dose of vaccine is age dependent. It is 10 µg for children <10 years and 20 µg for children above 10 years or adults. There are a number of schedules. In all schedules, at least three doses are recommended. The classic schedule is 0, 1, and 6 months. A four-dose schedule, where monovalent birth dose is followed by three (combination vaccine) doses, usually given with other routine infant vaccination, is also appropriate. It is preferable to start vaccination as early as possible. The World Health Organization (WHO) recommends that all national programs should include a monovalent hepatitis B vaccine birth dose, ideally within 24 hours. Importance of birth dose should be emphasized in preventing vertical transmission, which is important for our country. Although effectiveness declines progressively in the days after birth, after 7 days, a late birth dose can still be effective in preventing horizontal transmission and therefore remains beneficial. Therefore, the WHO recommends that all infants receive the late birth dose during the first contact with healthcare providers at any time up to the time of the next dose of the primary schedule. The route of vaccination is intramuscular (IM). The site of vaccination is anterolateral thigh in neonates and infants and deltoid in children and adults. Vaccination given by any other route than IM or any other site than anterolateral part of thigh or deltoid should not be considered as valid.

34. What if the child comes late for subsequent doses?

If there is a gap of up to 6 months between the first and second dose or a gap of up to 1 year between second and third dose, there is no need to restart vaccination. Complete the remaining doses as per the original schedule. However, such delays are not desirable, as the person remains unprotected till the schedule is completed. The Centers for Disease Control and Prevention (CDC) recommendations state:
- When the hepatitis B vaccine schedule is interrupted, the vaccine series does not need to be restarted
- If the series is interrupted after the first dose, the second dose should be separated by an interval of at least 8 weeks
- If only the third dose is delayed, it should be administered as soon as possible, after age of 24 weeks (168 days)
- It is not necessary to restart the vaccine series for infants switched from one vaccine brand to another, including combination vaccines.

35. What is the efficacy of hepatitis B vaccine?

Protective serum titers of anti-HBs (>10 mIU/mL) develop in 95–98% of healthy infants and children who receive a series of three IM doses. In carefully conducted field trials, efficacy has been estimated to be up to 95%. Vaccine has been shown to induce long-term protection for 20 or more years due to immunologic memory. Therefore, booster doses are not routinely recommended.

36. What are the reasons for vaccine failure?

Improper storage of vaccine and failure to maintain cold chain are the most important causes of vaccine failure. Immunocompromised individuals (those on chemotherapy, etc.) may also fail to respond. Surface mutants of HBV may be able to cause infection even in vaccinated children. In addition, there are individuals who do not respond to the vaccine for no apparent reason. However, half of these people who do not develop anti-HBs antibodies after a three-dose series will do so after additional dose(s).

37. What are other factors that can affect the extent of immunogenicity?

The recommended series of three IM doses of hepatitis B vaccine induces a protective antibody response in >90% of healthy adults younger than 40 years of age. After the age of 40 years, the cumulative age-specific decline in immunogenicity drops to <90% and by age of 60 years, only 65–70% vaccines develop protective antibody level. Therefore, the earlier the vaccination starts, the better it is. Besides age, other factors, which decrease immunogenicity to hepatitis B vaccination, include obesity, smoking, presence of chronic disease and human immunodeficiency virus (HIV) infection, and malignancy like leukemia in whom the response has been seen to be as poor as 20–40% with the vaccines and these cases need to be protected by HBIG prophylaxis. Genetic nonresponders and injection given in the gluteal region also elicit decreased immune response. Whenever doubtful about uptake of vaccine, anti-HBs antibody titer should be done 2–3 weeks after last dose of vaccine to ensure vaccine uptake.

38. For how long is hepatitis B vaccine protective?

Studies indicate that immunologic memory remains intact for at least 30 years and confers protection against clinical illness and chronic HBV infection, even though anti-HBs levels that once measured adequate might become low or decline below detectable levels. If exposed to HBV, people whose immune systems are competent will mount an anamnestic response and develop protective anti-HBs. Studies are ongoing to assess whether booster doses of hepatitis B vaccine will be needed in the future.

39. What are the adverse effects of hepatitis B vaccination?

Adverse effects of hepatitis B vaccine are very few. They consist primarily of local reactions or low-grade fever. Serious reactions like anaphylaxis are very rare, but can occur as with any other vaccine.

40. Who should not receive the vaccine?

Persons with a history of serious adverse events, including anaphylaxis, after receipt of hepatitis B vaccine, should not receive additional doses. Persons allergic to yeast should not be vaccinated with vaccines containing yeast. As with other vaccines, vaccination of persons with moderate or severe acute illness, with or without fever, should be deferred until the illness improves. Vaccination is not contraindicated in persons with a history of multiple sclerosis, Guillain-Barré syndrome, or autoimmune diseases such as systemic lupus erythematosus or rheumatoid arthritis.

41. What schedule is used for immunocompromised children or children on hemodialysis?

These include primarily those with advanced HIV infection, chronic renal failure, chronic liver disease, and diabetes. It is estimated that 10% of the 40 million people infected with HIV infection worldwide are coinfected with

HBV; the presence of HIV markedly increases the risk of developing HBV-associated liver cirrhosis and hepatocellular carcinoma.

In immunocompromised hosts, one should use double the recommended dose for that age. They may also require additional doses in case they do not show seroconversion following three doses. In situations where early seroconversion is required, one may use accelerated schedule of doses at 0, 1, 2, and 12 months. Despite this, it has been shown that not >30% of children with leukemia undergoing chemotherapy show seroconversion. In such cases, it may be better to use regular passive prophylaxis with HBIG. For hemodialysis patients, the need for booster doses should be assessed by annual testing for antibody levels and booster doses should be provided when antibody levels decline below 10 mIU/mL.

42. Can we give the vaccine by intradermal route?

Intradermal administration of hepatitis B vaccine reduces the cost tremendously as the dose consists of 0.1 mL, but it has not been found to result in protective antibody titers in all recipients. Hence, testing for antibody response becomes mandatory in these persons. Also, antibody titers may not persist for long in these patients. Thus, this route has not been routinely advocated.

As a matter of fact, hepatitis B vaccine administered by any route or site other than intramuscularly in the anterolateral thigh or deltoid muscle should not be counted as valid.

43. If you want to test and vaccinate your patient for hepatitis B on the same day, does it matter if you test or vaccinate first?

Yes, you should draw the blood first and then administer the first dose of vaccine, as transient HBsAg positivity has been found to occur after a dose of hepatitis B vaccine.

44. How long should a person wait to donate blood after a dose of hepatitis B vaccine?

It is advisable to wait for 1 month. Studies published in the last several years have found that transient HBsAg positivity (lasting <21 days) can be detected in certain persons after vaccination.

45. Which schedule is recommended for immunizing a neonate born to a hepatitis B surface antigen (HBsAg)-positive mother?

In infants born to HbsAg-positive mothers, the first dose of HBV should be given at birth (within 12 hours). This should be given along with HBIG in the dose of 0.5 mL. Both vaccine and HBIG can be given at the same time, but they should be administered intramuscularly at separate sites; the second dose of vaccine should be given at the age of 1 month and the third dose at 6 months of age. One can also use accelerated schedule of four doses given at 0, 1, 2, and 12 months.

46. What about vaccination in preterm and low birth weight infants?

Preterm infants born to HBsAg-positive women and women with unknown status must receive immunoprophylaxis with hepatitis B vaccine and HBIG beginning at shortly after birth. Preterm infants having low birth weight have a decreased response to hepatitis B vaccine administered before 1 month of age; however, by chronological age of 1 month. Preterm infants, regardless of initial birth weight or gestational age, are likely to respond as adequately as full-term infants. Since the HBsAg status of most mothers is usually not known in our country, it is advisable to give the vaccine as recommended above within 12 hours. The next dose given at 1 month of age will take care of the immunological incompetence if any of the preterm baby.

For preterm infants weighing <2 kg at birth:

- *If maternal HBsAg status is positive*: Give HBIG plus hepatitis B vaccine within 12 hours of birth. Give three additional doses (with single-antigen vaccine at ages 1, 2, 3, and 6 months or 2, 4, and 12–15 months). Test for HBsAg and antibody to HBsAg 1–2 months after completion of at least three doses of a licensed hepatitis B vaccine series (i.e., at age of 9–18 months, generally at the next well-child visit). Testing should not be performed before age of 9 months nor within 4 weeks of the most recent vaccine dose.
    - *If maternal HBsAg status is unknown*: Give HBIG plus hepatitis B vaccine within 12 hours of birth. Be sure to test the mother's blood for HBsAg. Give three additional hepatitis B vaccine doses (with single-antigen vaccine at ages 1, 2, 3, and 6 months or hepatitis B containing combination vaccine at ages 2, 4, and 6 months or 2, 4, and 12–15 months).
    - *If the maternal HBsAg status is negative*: If you are certain that appropriate maternal testing was done and a copy of the mother's original laboratory report indicating that she was HBsAg negative during this pregnancy is placed on the infant's chart, delay the first dose of hepatitis B vaccine until age 1 month or hospital discharge, whichever comes first. Administer vaccine as per the recommended schedule.

For preterm infants weighing 2 kg or more at birth, follow the recommendations for full-term infants, including the birth dose for all, keeping in mind the special needs of newborns whose mother's HBsAg status is positive or unknown.

47. An infant was given monovalent hepatitis B vaccine at birth. Later, we gave her monovalent vaccine at age of 1 month and age of 4 months. Did we give her the third dose too early?

Yes. Poorer immune response rates are seen in infants who complete the vaccination schedule prior to age of 6 months. Do not count dose number three, which you gave at age of 4 months. Repeat dose number three when the infant is at least 6 months old (not earlier than age 24 weeks).

48. **What is the recommended time to do hepatitis B testing for evidence of success or failure of immunoprophylaxis given at birth to an infant born to a hepatitis B surface antigen (HBsAg)-positive mother?**

For infants born to HBsAg-positive mothers, postvaccination testing is recommended 1–2 months after completion of at least three doses of a licensed hepatitis B vaccine series (i.e., at age of 9–18 months, generally at the next well-child visit). Testing should not be performed before age 9 months, as HBIG might still be present for 6–8 months nor should testing be performed within 4 weeks of the most recent vaccine dose, as a false positive HBsAg might occur. Anti-HBc testing of infants or children is not recommended because passively acquired maternal anti-HBc might be detected up to age 24 months in children of HBV-infected mothers.

Hepatitis B surface antigen-negative infants with anti-HBs levels of at least 10 mIU/mL are protected and need no further medical management. HBsAg-negative infants with anti-HBs levels <10 mIU/mL should be revaccinated with a second three-dose series and retested 1–2 months after the final dose of vaccine. Children who are HBsAg positive should receive medical evaluation and ongoing follow-up.

49. **An infant of a hepatitis B surface antigen (HBsAg)-positive mother received appropriate postexposure prophylaxis and tested negative for anti-HBs and HBsAg at 12 months of age. How many more doses of hepatitis B vaccine do I need to give before I retest?**

The recommended approach is to complete a second three-dose schedule of vaccine and retest for both HBsAg and anti-HBs 1–2 months after the third dose of vaccine. If anti-HBs and HBsAg are still negative after revaccination, the child is considered a nonresponder to hepatitis B vaccine.

50. **When screening an adopted infant for hepatitis B, at what age would you expect the infant to not show anti-HBs or anti-HBc if it were passively transferred antibody from the mother?**

Passively acquired maternal anti-HBs might be detected until age 6–8 months and passively acquired maternal anti-HBc might be detected until age 24 months.

All foreign-born persons (including immigrants, refugees, asylum seekers, and internationally adopted children) born in Asia, the Pacific Islands, Africa, and other regions with high endemicity of HBV infection that should be tested for HBsAg, regardless of vaccination status. Persons testing HBsAg positive should be referred for medical evaluation and ongoing follow-up.

51. **Can adolescents be immunized on a 0-, 2-, and 4-month schedule for hepatitis B?**

Yes. There are data that show adequate seroprotection using this schedule in young adults. If this schedule is used, you should be aware that the studies were in young adults and might not translate to older adults (≥40 years). There are other schedules that offer flexibility in vaccination as well.

52. Three years ago at a middle school, my patient received the first dose of the hepatitis B vaccine series. Should I give her the second dose now or do I need to start over again with the first dose?

There is no need to restart the series. Give the second dose now and be sure there are at least 8 weeks between that dose and the third dose. No apparent effect on immunogenicity has been documented when minimum spacing of doses is not achieved precisely. Increasing the interval between the first two doses has little effect on immunogenicity or final antibody concentration.

The third dose confers the maximum level of seroprotection, but acts primarily as a booster and appears to provide optimal long-term protection. Longer intervals between the last two doses result in higher final antibody levels, but might increase the risk for acquisition of HBV infection among persons who have a delayed response to vaccination. No differences in immunogenicity have been observed when one or two doses of hepatitis B vaccine produced by one manufacturer are followed by doses from a different manufacturer.

53. At what anatomic site should hepatitis B vaccine be administered to adults? What needle size should be used?

The deltoid muscle is recommended for routine IM vaccination among adults. The gluteus muscle should not be used as a site for administering hepatitis B vaccine. The suggested needle size is 1-2 inch depending on the recipient's gender and weight (1 inch for females weighing <70 kg; 1.5 inch for females weighing 70-100 kg; 1-1.5 inch for males weighing <120 kg; and 2 inch for males weighing 120 kg or more and females weighing >100 kg). A 22-25 gauge needle should be used. For optimal protection, it is crucial that the vaccine can be administered IM and not subcutaneously.

54. I would like more information about Twinrix®, the combination of hepatitis A and B vaccine.

Twinrix® [GlaxoSmithKline (GSK)] is an inactivated combination vaccine containing both hepatitis A virus (HAV) and HBV antigens. The vaccine contains 720 enzyme-linked immunosorbent assay units (ELU) of hepatitis A antigen (half of the Havrix® adult dose) and 20 µg of hepatitis B antigen (the full Engerix-B adult dose). In the US, Twinrix® is licensed for use in people who are aged 18 years or older. It can be administered to persons who are at risk for both hepatitis A and hepatitis B such as certain international travelers, men who have sex with men, illegal drug users, or to persons who simply want to be immune to both diseases. Primary immunization consists of three doses given intramuscularly on a 0-, 1-, and 6-month schedule. For those who need rapid protection like travelers, earlier three-dose schedule of Twinrix® was advised (0, 7, and 21 days). In March 2007, the USFDA also approved a four-dose schedule. Now, it consists of three doses given within 3 weeks, followed by a booster dose at 12 months (0, 7, 21-30 days, and 12 months). The four-dose schedule could benefit individuals needing rapid protection from hepatitis A and hepatitis B such as persons traveling to high-prevalence areas imminently and emergency responders, especially those being deployed to disaster areas overseas. Twinrix® cannot be used for postexposure prophylaxis.

55. I have seen adults who had one or two doses of Twinrix®, but we only carry single-antigen vaccine in our practice. How should we complete their vaccination series with single-antigen vaccines?

Twinrix® is licensed as a three-dose series for persons of age 18 years and older. If Twinrix® is not available or if you choose not to use Twinrix® to complete the Twinrix® series, you should do the following: If one dose of Twinrix® was given, complete the series with two adult doses of hepatitis B vaccine and two adult doses of hepatitis A vaccine. If two doses of Twinrix® were given, complete the schedule with one adult dose of hepatitis A vaccine and one adult dose of hepatitis B vaccine. Another way to consider this is as follows:
- Any combination of three doses of adult hepatitis B or three doses of Twinrix® is equal to a complete series of hepatitis B vaccine
- One dose of Twinrix® with two doses of adult hepatitis A is equal to a complete series of hepatitis A vaccine
- Two doses of Twinrix® plus one dose of adult hepatitis A are equal to a complete series of hepatitis A vaccine.

56. We are thinking of using Twinrix® and we are wondering whether we can use it for doses number 1 and number 3 only and use single antigen hepatitis B vaccine for dose number 2?

No. Twinrix® contains 50% less hepatitis A antigen component than Havrix®, GSK's monovalent hepatitis A vaccine (720 vs. 1,440 ELU), so the patient would not receive the recommended dose of hepatitis A vaccine antigen. For this reason, three doses of Twinrix® must comprise the series.

57. What blood test should be used to screen a pregnant woman to prevent perinatal hepatitis B virus (HBV) infection?

Screening should be done with the HBsAg test only. This blood test will tell whether a woman has current HBV infection that can be transmitted to her infant. Ordering other blood tests such as total antibody to hepatitis B core antigen (total anti-HBc) and/or antibody to HBsAg (anti-HBs) are not useful when screening to prevent perinatal HBV infections and should not be included in screening pregnant women for perinatal HBV infection. Total anti-HBc will be positive in all HBsAg-positive persons and anti-HBs are rarely positive in an HBsAg-positive person. Women who are found to be HBsAg positive should then be referred for counseling and medical evaluation that will include further testing. If there is a reason to suspect recently acquired HBV infection in a pregnant woman, immunoglobulin M (IgM) class anti-HBc (IgM anti-HBc) could be tested to differentiate recently acquired HBV infection from chronic HBV infection. IgM anti-HBc is the blood test that is positive in recently acquired HBV infection.

58. A female patient was immunized against hepatitis B about 4 years ago. She was recently found to be "hepatitis B positive" by her gynecologist. Is this possible? Could it be a false positive?

It is possible, but unlikely. The HBsAg test has high sensitivity and specificity and is quite trustworthy. She might have already been HBsAg positive when she was vaccinated; therefore, the vaccine would not have been effective. You should make sure that the positive test was actually HBsAg and not another hepatitis B test such as anti-HBs (sometimes confusingly referred to as HBsAb) or anti-HBc. A positive anti-HBs test is expected after vaccination with hepatitis B vaccine, but not a positive anti-HBc or HBsAg. If you are certain after careful checking that the test and reported result are correct, you should then make sure the laboratory result was correct. If she is ultimately determined to be truly HBsAg positive, she should be referred to a liver disease specialist for counseling and medical evaluation.

59. Do women who have been vaccinated previously against hepatitis B virus (HBV) infection still need to be screened during pregnancy?

Yes. Women who have received hepatitis B vaccine should still be screened for HBsAg early in each pregnancy. Just because a woman has been vaccinated does not mean she is HBsAg negative. Since postvaccination testing is not performed for most vaccinated persons, she could have been vaccinated even though she was already HBsAg positive.

60. Is it safe to give hepatitis B vaccine to a pregnant woman?

Yes, limited data indicate no apparent risk for adverse events to developing fetus. Current vaccines contain noninfectious HBsAg and should cause no risk to the fetus. If the mother is being vaccinated because she is at risk for HBV infection [e.g., a healthcare worker (HCW), a person with an STD, an injection drug user (IDU), and multiple sex partners], vaccination should be initiated as soon as her risk factor is identified during the pregnancy. In contrast, HBV infection affecting a pregnant woman might result in severe disease for the mother and chronic infection for the newborn.

61. Should a pregnant lady who is hepatitis B surface antigen (HBsAg) positive for liver disease should be evaluated during her pregnancy only or should the evaluation wait until the postpartum period? What should I recommend for her husband and her children? How urgent is the time frame?

An HBsAg positive pregnant lady should be evaluated during her pregnancy, at the earliest possible opportunity. Consultation with a liver disease specialist (i.e., hepatologist, gastroenterologist, and infectious disease specialist) should be done. The consulting/referral physician should be completely aware of the patient's obstetrical status. In addition, the patient's sex partner and children or other household contacts should be tested for HBV infection (total anti-HBc and HBsAg) as soon as possible. If any of them are susceptible to HBV infection (anti-HBc and HBsAg negative), they should be vaccinated; if any are HBsAg positive, they should be referred to or have consultation with a liver disease specialist.

62. What advances have occurred with regard to the hepatitis B vaccine?

Over the years, the following advances have occurred:
- Improvement in antigenicity by including the pre-S component
- Combining hepatitis B antigen with other antigens like diphtheria, pertussis, and tetanus (DPT) or diphtheria, tetanus, and acellular pertussis (DTaP), killed polio vaccines, hepatitis A vaccine, *Haemophilus influenzae* type b (Hib) vaccine, etc. For example:
    - Hepatitis A + Hepatitis B (Twinrix®)
    - Diphtheria, tetanus, and acellular pertussis + Killed polio vaccine + Hepatitis B (pentavalent vaccine)
    - Diphtheria, tetanus, and acellular pertussis + Killed polio vaccine + Hepatitis A + Hepatitis B + Hib (septavalent vaccine)
    - A new Hepatitis-B vaccine with a nolvel adjuvant (CpG 1018) (Heplisav-B).

63. What is the role of hepatitis B virus (HBV) vaccine containing pre-S component?

This vaccine has better immunogenicity, especially protection against HBV surface mutant as well.

64. Till what age can the hepatitis B virus (HBV) vaccination be given?

Vaccination against HBV can be started at any age. The earlier one starts, the better it is.

After three IM doses of hepatitis B vaccine, >90% of healthy adults and >95% of infants, children, and adolescents (from birth to 19 years of age) develop adequate antibody response. However, there is an age-specific decline in immunogenicity. After age 40 years, approximately 90% of recipients respond to three-dose series and by 60 years, only 75% of vaccines develop protective antibody titers.

65. What is the role of hepatitis B immunoglobulin (HBIG)?

Postexposure prophylaxis with HBIG is recommended for newborn babies born to HBsAg-positive mothers. Postexposure prophylaxis with HBIG is also recommended for health personnel who suffer from accidental needlestick injury and for patients who receive HBsAg-positive blood inadvertently. Pre-exposure passive prophylaxis with HBIG is needed for individuals failing to respond to vaccine (e.g., immunocompromised children) or in children with disorders that preclude a response (e.g., agammaglobulinemia), when they are likely to be exposed to the risk of acquiring HBV infection.

66. What are the Centers for Disease Control and Prevention (CDC) recommendations for postexposure prophylaxis after exposure to hepatitis B virus in occupational setting?

Table 4 summarizes course of actions in this situation as recommended by the CDC.

TABLE 4: Recommendations for postexposure prophylaxis after percutaneous or mucosal exposure to hepatitis B virus (HBV) in an occupational setting.

Vaccination and antibody response status of exposed persons	Treatment			
	Source is HBsAg positive	Source is HBsAg negative	Source is unknown or not tested	
			High risk	Low risk
Unvaccinated	HBIG† (one dose) and begin a hepatitis B vaccine series	Begin a hepatitis B vaccine series	Begin a hepatitis B vaccine series	Begin a hepatitis B vaccine series
Known responder	No treatment	No treatment	No treatment	No treatment
Nonresponder				
Not revaccinated*	HBIG (one dose) and begin a revaccination series	Begin a revaccination series	HBIG (one dose) and begin a revaccination series	Begin a revaccination series
After revaccination	HBIG (two doses)†	No treatment	HBIG (two doses)†	No treatment
Antibody response unknown	Treat for anti-HBs if adequate§, no treatment if inadequate, HBIG × 1, and vaccine booster	No treatment	Test for anti-HBs†† if adequate§, no treatment if inadequate, give vaccine booster, and check anti-HBs in 1–2 months	–

*Person known to have HBV infection in the past or who are chronically infected do not require HBIG or vaccine.
†HBIG (0.06 mL/kg) administered intramuscular (IM).
§Adequate response is anti-HBs of at least 10 mIU/mL after vaccination.
¶Revaccination: Additional three-dose series of hepatitis B vaccine administered after the primary series.
**First dose as soon as possible after exposure; add the second dose 1 month later.
††Testing should be done as soon as possible after exposure.
(HBs: hepatitis B surface; HBsAg: hepatitis B surface antigen; HBIG: hepatitis B immunoglobulin)
Source: Adapted from Updated U.S. Public Health Service Guidelines for the Management of Occupational Exposures to HBV, HCV, and HIV and Recommendations for Postexposure Prophylaxis. MMWR Recomm Rep. 2001;50:1-42.

Pool may take decades to manifest. However, effects on carrier pool are already evident in countries that took to universal immunization earlier. Now the cost of vaccine has also come down drastically. The Indian Academy of Pediatrics recommends that universal immunization of all children should be followed.

67. A nurse who received the hepatitis B vaccine series >10 years ago and had a positive follow-up titer (at least 10 mIU/mL) at present, her titer is negative (<10 mIU/mL). What should be done now?

Nothing. Data show that vaccine-induced anti-HBs levels might decline overtime; however, immune memory (anamnestic anti-HBs response) remains intact indefinitely following immunization. Persons with anti-HBs concentrations that decline to <10 mIU/mL are still protected against HBV infection. For HCWs with normal immune status who have demonstrated adequate anti-HBs (at least 10 mIU/mL) following vaccination, booster doses of vaccine or periodic anti-HBs testing is not recommended.

68. A person who is a known nonresponder to hepatitis B vaccine has a percutaneous exposure to hepatitis B surface antigen (HBsAg)-positive blood. According to older Advisory Committee on Immunization Practices (ACIP) recommendations, I have the option to give hepatitis B immunoglobulin (HBIG) × 2 or HBIG × 1 and initiate revaccination. How do I decide which to do?

Current recommendations have been revised. The recommended postexposure prophylaxis for persons who are nonresponders to hepatitis B vaccine (i.e., have not responded to an initial three-dose series and revaccination with a three-dose series) is to give HBIG as soon as possible after exposure and a second dose of HBIG 1 month later. Exposed persons, who are known not to have responded to a primary vaccine series, but have not been revaccinated with a second three-dose series, should receive a single dose of HBIG and reinitiate the hepatitis B vaccine series with the first dose of hepatitis B vaccine as soon as possible after exposure.

69. Does giving hepatitis B vaccine to a chronically infected person cause any harm?

No, it will neither harm nor help the person.

70. For prevention of hepatitis B virus (HBV) infection, which is preferred high-risk approach or universal immunization approach?

Considering the high cost of vaccination, initially high-risk approach was followed, wherein individuals at added risk for acquiring infection (such as intravenous drug abusers, patients on chronic hemodialysis therapy, individuals requiring blood and blood products, spouse of an infected or carrier person, infants born to HBsAg-positive mothers, laboratory and healthcare personnel likely to come to contact with blood and body fluids, sex workers, etc.) were targeted. However, these failed to have any impact on the size of carrier pool in the population.

Universal immunization targets every newborn, child, and adult, thereby eliminating all modes of transmission. It also raises the possibility of ultimate eradication of this dreaded virus, as humans are its only reservoirs. Universal immunization may be expensive in the short-term and reduction in carrier.

71. Are there any countries where vaccination against hepatitis B is included as universal immunization?

Yes, USA and most of the European countries have advised universal immunization against hepatitis B.

72. What is the future for hepatitis B vaccination?

The available vaccines are quite efficacious. However, any research on developing better vaccines would focus on bringing down the number of doses, making vaccines for nonresponders, therapeutic vaccines for chronic cases, and exploring the possibility of oral vaccines.

73. Whether hepatitis B birth dose should be given at birth to low birth weight/premature babies?

A birth dose of hepatitis B vaccine can be given to low birth weight and premature infants. For these infants, the birth dose should not count as part of primary three-dose series; the three dose of the standard primary serious should be given according to the national vaccination schedule.

SUGGESTED READING

1. Centers for Disease Control and Prevention (CDC). Epidemiology and Prevention of Vaccine Preventable Diseases, 10th edition. Washington DC: Department of Health and Human Services; 2007. pp. 222-3.
2. Damme PV, Ward J, Daniel SD. Hepatitis B vaccines. In: Plotkin SA, Orenstein WA, Offit PA (Eds). Vaccines, 6th edition. Philadelphia: Saunders Elsevier; 2013. pp. 205-34.
3. Dutta AK. Immunization against hepatitis B. In: Thacker N, Shah NK (Eds). Immunization in Clinical Practice. New Delhi: Jaypee Brothers Medical Publishers (P) Ltd.; 2005. pp. 109-18.
4. Immunization Action Coalition (IAC). (2013). Ask the Experts: Hepatitis B. [online] Available from: http://immunize.org/askexperts/experts_hepb.asp. [Last accessed June, 2020].
5. Ray G. Current scenario of hepatitis B and its treatment in India. J Clin Transl Hepatol. 2017;5(3):277-96.
6. World Health Organization (WHO). (2017). Summary of WHO Position Paper on Hepatitis B Vaccines. [online] Available from: https://www.who.int/immunization/policy/position_papers/who_pp_hepb_2017_summary.pdf?ua=1. [Last accessed June, 2020].
7. Yewale V, Choudhury P, Thacker N. IAP Guidebook on Immunization. Mumbai: Indian Academy of Pediatrics; 2011. pp. 78-85.

CHAPTER 21

Hepatitis A Vaccines

Arun Wadhwa, Nigam P Narain

1. What is hepatitis A? How is it transmitted?

Hepatitis A is the most common infection of the liver caused by hepatitis A virus (HAV), which is a ribonucleic acid (RNA) virus belonging to Picornavirus family. HAV spreads mainly through direct person-to-person contact. Transmission often occurs through food and water contamination or, rarely, through blood.

Persons from developed countries who travel to underdeveloped parts of the world are at risk of HAV infections. Among those who travel to countries with high or intermediate endemicity, the risk is approximately three cases per 1,000 people per month of stay.

Common source outbreaks and sporadic cases can occur from exposure to fecally-contaminated food or water. Uncooked HAV-contaminated foods have been recognized as a source of outbreaks. Cooked foods also can transmit HAV if the temperature during food preparation is inadequate to kill the virus or if food is contaminated after cooking, as it occurs commonly in outbreaks associated with infected food handlers.

2. What is the epidemiological significance of hepatitis A?

The epidemiology varies according to socioeconomic and sanitary level of the country or area concerned. In some industrialized countries, HAV transmission has practically ceased. In developing countries, HAV infections usually occur early in life, resulting in high levels of asymptomatic disease. Once infection occurs, it gives lifelong immunity.

Countries are classified as low/medium or highly endemic for hepatitis A. In countries with high endemicity like India, most individuals acquire natural infection in childhood and burden of disease including incidence of outbreaks is low. As a shift occurs toward medium endemicity due to improvements in hygiene and sanitation, a certain proportion of children remain susceptible till adulthood. Thus, burden of symptomatic disease and incidence of outbreaks paradoxically increase. Epidemiologic data from India, though limited, suggests an upward shift in epidemiology of disease and HAV susceptibility in 30–40% of adolescents and adults belonging to the high socioeconomic class.

Hepatitis A epidemic occurs in two different forms—(1) common source outbreaks (polluted water, hotels, and restaurants) and (2) community-wide outbreaks. Community-wide outbreaks are of two different types. In the most common community-wide outbreak, the highest clinical infection rate occurs in those of age 5–14 years, but the main transmitters of HAV are assumed to be asymptomatic infected toddlers. These outbreaks tend to occur periodically. In the other type of community-wide outbreaks, the epidemics are not usually periodic.

3. How serious is hepatitis A?

Hepatitis A virus infection is a relatively benign infection in young children. As many as 85% of children below 2 years and 50% of those between 2 and 5 years infected with HAV are anicteric and may just have nonspecific symptoms like any other viral infection. On the contrary, hepatitis A in adults is symptomatic in 70–95% with a mortality of 1%. The disease severity increases in those with underlying chronic liver disease.

Rarely, hepatitis A can be serious. Studies show that only a few children with hepatitis A are hospitalized, with people age 60 years and older are more likely to be hospitalized. Many days of work are missed due to hepatitis A as well. Certain people, such as people with chronic hepatitis C, can get very sick and die from hepatitis A. Death from hepatitis A is rare in healthy young people, but more common in people aged 60 years and older.

Hepatitis A cannot be differentiated from other types of viral hepatitis on the basis of clinical or epidemiological features alone. Appropriate blood tests must be used.

- *Anti-HAV*: Total antibody to HAV. This diagnostic test detects total antibody of both immunoglobulin G (IgG) and immunoglobulin M (IgM) subclasses of HAV. Its presence indicates either acute or resolved infection.
- *Immunoglobulin M anti-HAV*: IgM antibody is a subclass of anti-HAV. Its presence indicates a recent infection with HAV (6 months or less). It is used to diagnose acute (recently acquired) hepatitis A.

Total anti-HAV, which appears early in the course of infection, remains detectable for the person's lifetime and provides lifelong protection against the infection/disease. To confirm a diagnosis of acute HAV infection, serologic testing for IgM anti-HAV is required. In the majority of persons, serum IgM anti-HAV becomes detectable 5–10 days before onset of symptoms and lasts about 6 months. However, there have been reports of persons who test positive for IgM anti-HAV for up to a year or more following infection.

4. Can hepatitis A virus (HAV) cause chronic infection?

No, it causes only acute infection. A condition of prolonged cholestatic syndrome has been described that waxes and wanes over several months. Pruritus and fat malabsorption are problematic symptoms, but need only supportive care. The syndrome occurs in the absence of any liver synthetic dysfunction and resolves without sequelae.

5. How long can a person with hepatitis A infection spread hepatitis A virus (HAV)?

Generally, duration of spread is 2 weeks before the appearance of symptoms and 1 week after the onset of symptoms.

6. Can a person get infected with hepatitis virus more than once?

No. Once a person recovers from infection, he develops antibody called anti-HAV that provides lifelong protection in immunocompetent person.

7. How can it be prevented?

It can be prevented by scrupulous good general hygiene, proper environmental sanitation, and immunization by vaccine.

8. Which type of vaccine is used for immunization?

Two types of vaccines are used for immunization. First type is inactivated virus vaccine and second type is live attenuated vaccine made up of H2 strain.

9. What are the different types of inactivated vaccines available in India?

Most of the currently available inactivated vaccines are derived from HM175/GBM strains and grown on MRC-5 human diploid cell lines. The virus is formalin inactivated and adjuvanted with aluminum hydroxide. The vaccine is stored at 2–8°C.

Another inactivated vaccine is a liposomal adjuvanted vaccine derived from the RG-SB strain, harvested from disrupted MRC-5 cells, and inactivated by formalin (HAVpur). The liposome adjuvant is immunopotentiating reconstituted influenza virosomes (IRIV) composed from an H1N1 strain of influenza virus another vaccine is the CR326F strain vaccine which uses the aluminium hydroxyphosphate adjuvant **(Table 1)**. However, the last two vaccines are not available in India.

10. What is the vaccine schedule for inactivated hepatitis A vaccine? Is there any difference in efficacy of these vaccines?

The vaccines are given in a two-dose schedule, 6 months apart intramuscularly. Two doses are recommended for primary immunization. First dose is given at the age of 12–18 months. Second dose is given after 6–12 months after the first dose.

The adult formulation should be used after the recommended cutoff age of 15 years (Avaxim™) and 18 years (Havrix™). Protective antibodies are seen in 95–100% 1 month after the first dose and almost 100% after the second dose. Serologic correlate of protection has been fixed at 20 mIU/mL. The protective efficacy is around 90–100% and onset of protection is 2 weeks to 1 month after the first dose of the vaccine. The vaccine efficacy is lower in the elderly, immunocompromised, those with chronic liver disease, in transplant recipients, and those with preexisting maternal antibodies. The vaccine may

TABLE 1: Different inactivated hepatitis A virus (HAV) vaccines available currently.				
Vaccine	Havrix	Vaqta*	Avaxim	Epaxal*
Manufacturer	GSK	MSD	Sanofi	Crucell
Strain	HM175	CR326F	GBM	RG-SB
Antigen	Elisa units (EIU)	Units (U)	Antigen units (AU)	International units (IU)
Adult dose (cutoff age)	1,440 EIU/1.0 mL (>18 years)	50 U/1.0 mL (>18 years)	160 AU/0.5 mL (> 15 years)	24 IU/0.5 mL (>1 year)
Pediatric dose (cutoff age)	740 EIU/0.5 mL (<18 years)	25 U/0.5 mL (<18 years)	80 AU/0.5 mL (1–15 years)	12 IU/0.5 mL (>1 year)
Adjuvant	Aluminum hydroxide	Aluminum hydroxyphosphate	Aluminum + formaldehyde	Virosome (IRIV)
Preservative	Phenoxyethanol	Nil	Phenoxyethanol	Nil
Schedule	0 month, 6–12 months	0 month, 6–18 months	0 month, 6–12 months	0 month, 6–12 months

*These vaccines are not available in India.
(GSK: GlaxoSmithKline; IRIV: immunopotentiating reconstituted influenza virosomes; MSD: Merck Sharp & Dohme)

be safely given with other childhood vaccines and interchange of brands is permitted, though not routinely recommended. Immunity is lifelong due to anamnestic response and no boosters are recommended at present in the immunocompetent. Adverse reactions are minor and usually include local pain and swelling. Both the vaccines have the same efficacy.

11. Can this vaccine be given in second or third year? If yes, then which year is the best?

Yes. It can be given at this age, of which second year is the best because:
- It will protect those who do not have maternal antibody.
- It is easier to integrate with existing immunization schedule.
- By the third year, many children get immunized by natural subclinical infection.

12. How is hepatitis A vaccine given?

The vaccine is given by an injection into the muscle of anterolateral part of thigh in toddlers and upper part of arm in adults and older children. In patients with bleeding disorders like hemophilia, it has found to be safe and immunogenic when given by subcutaneous route.

13. What are the characteristics of live attenuated hepatitis A vaccine?

This vaccine is derived from the H2 strain of the virus attenuated after serial passage in human diploid cell (KMB17 cell line). It has been in use in China since the 1990s in mass vaccination programs. The vaccine meets requirements of the Chinese drug authority and the World Health Organization (WHO). It is also now licensed and available in India (Biovac A).

14. What is the dose and schedule of live hepatitis A vaccine? Is a single dose of live vaccine adequate to protect an individual?

The recommended dose is 0.5 mL subcutaneous (SC) (106.5 CCID50/mL) in children aged 1–15 years and in adults also. Immunogenicity studies with single dose show seroconversion rate of >98% 2 months after vaccination and persistence of protective antibodies in >80% of vaccines at 10 years follow-up. Uncontrolled studies show an efficacy of almost 100% sustained over 10 years, despite decline in seroprotection rate and antibody titers. Recent immunogenicity studies from India have shown 97.3% seroconversion 5 years following single dose of the vaccine in a multicentric study and 79.3% up to 6 years in another study. Therefore, a single dose of live vaccine is adequate to protect an individual.

15. What are the Indian Academy of Pediatrics-Advisory Committee on Vaccines and Immunization Practices (IAP-ACVIP) recommendations for use of live hepatitis A vaccine?

When introduced 12 years ago, it was advised to be given as two doses 6 months apart. Later, the committee then revised its recommendations based on the above studies. Now, a single dose of this vaccine is recommended at 12 months of age overriding the previous recommendation of two doses.

16. Why has the Indian Academy of Pediatrics (IAP) changed its earlier recommendation? Do we have adequate data from Indian studies or the committee has relied on old Chinese data?

There were studies (unicentric and multicentric) from India on the long-term persistence of antibodies against HAV among children vaccinated with a single dose of live attenuated hepatitis A vaccine. The data showed 79.3% of 121 children were seroprotected (considering >20 mIU/mL of anti-HAV antibody titer as seroprotection levels) up to 6 years follow-up in the pivotal single-center study whereas 97.3% of 111 children had shown seroprotection after 5 years of follow-up period of multicentric group. In the multicentric study, the test subjects maintained good geometric mean titer (GMT) levels even after 5 years of follow-up. The committee had earlier shown its concern on waning of seroprotection in a subgroup of individuals of original single-center study cohort. However, it was later disclosed that only a handful subjects had shown this phenomenon and most of these subjects were of comparatively higher age groups than other study subjects. The decision was also facilitated by the Strategic Advisory Group of Experts (SAGE)/WHO recommendations of single dose of live attenuated hepatitis A vaccine. Hence, the committee is now convinced on the long-term immunogenicity and safety of a single dose of live attenuated H2-strain hepatitis A vaccine in healthy Indian children after reviewing the long-term follow-up data **(Table 2)**.

TABLE 2: Long-term immunogenicity results following one dose of live attenuated hepatitis A (H2-strain) vaccine in 1–3-year-old children.

Follow-up time	Subjects	% seroprotected (>20 mIU/mL)	Geometric mean titer (GMT) (mIU/mL)
Baseline	220	0%	–
2 months	220	98.6%	287
12 months	219	93.6%	226
6 years	176	83.3%	173
10 years	155	80.2%	145
15 years	134	81.3%	128

17. Which vaccine should be used and what schedule is recommended by the Indian Academy of Pediatrics-Advisory Committee on Vaccines and Immunization Practices (IAP-ACVIP)?

If a decision to administer the vaccine is taken, any of the licensed vaccines may be used as all have nearly similar efficacy and safety [exception for postexposure prophylaxis (PEP)/immunocompromised patients where only inactivated vaccines may be used]. Two doses 6 months apart are recommended for all inactivated vaccines. A single dose of live attenuated vaccine is sufficient for long-term protection. All hepatitis A vaccines are licensed for use in children aged 1 year or older. Prevaccination screening for hepatitis A antibody is likely to be cost-effective in children older than 10 years at which age the estimated seropositive rates exceed 50%.

18. For how long does a hepatitis A vaccine protect?

Protection after primary immunization ranges from 15 to 20 years in children and longer in adults.

19. How long after first dose we get protection to hepatitis A infection?

It takes 2–4 weeks after first dose. Anti-HAV antibody forms in this duration and helps in protection to HAV infection.

20. Is hepatitis A vaccine safe?

Yes. It has excellent safety profile. No serious side effects have been attributed definitively to HAV vaccine.

21. What are the side effects of hepatitis A vaccine?

Most common side effect is soreness at injection site. Other side effects are—headache, loss of appetite, low-grade fever, or tiredness.

22. Can hepatitis A vaccine be administered concurrently with other vaccine?

Yes, it can be safely given with hepatitis B, diphtheria, polio, tetanus, oral typhoid, Japanese encephalitis, rabies vaccines, and even immunoglobulins can be given at the same time but at different sites.

23. Can a different brand of inactivated hepatitis A vaccine be used to complete a primary course?

Yes. Any current brand of hepatitis A vaccine can be used to boost another. Both the doses must be inactivated vaccine. For live vaccine, one dose is sufficient.

24. Does a course of inactivated hepatitis A vaccine need to be repeated if there has been a long interval between the first and the second dose?

No. An excellent immune response is obtained after a single dose of hepatitis A vaccine and second dose (if missed) may be given as soon as possible, but there is no need to repeat the first dose.

25. Is there a need for a booster dose inactivated hepatitis A vaccine after a two-dose schedule has been completed?

Not at present. A long-term immunity (25 years) is obtained after two doses of vaccine, so there is no need for extra dose of vaccine. Boosting also occurs by natural infections.

26. Is there a vaccine that protects against both hepatitis A virus (HAV) and hepatitis B virus (HBV) infection?

Yes. Twinrix™ is a combination of both vaccines, but it is recommended only for persons of above 18 years age. This vaccine is given by a schedule of 0, 1, and 6 months **(Table 3)**.

27. Who should not receive hepatitis A vaccine?

This vaccine should not be given to the following:

TABLE 3: Dosage schedule of Twinrix™ vaccine.

Vaccine	Age group	Antigens used	Volume	Doses#	Schedule
Combination vaccine using hepatitis A and hepatitis B vaccines					
Twinrix™ [GlaxoSmithKline (GSK)]	18 years and older	Havrix (720 EIU) combined with Engerix-B (20 µg)	1.0 mL	3	0, 1, and 6 months
				4	0, 7, 21–30 days, 12 months

Number of doses.

- Persons who have hepatitis A infection in past and have recovered from disease
- Persons who are allergic to any component of vaccine
- Children < 1 year
- Pregnant and nursing mothers as data regarding safety profile is not available
- Those who are sick or have exanthema (can be delayed).

28. What is the importance of screening before giving this vaccine?

The cost-effectiveness of this approach will depend on the likelihood of being anti-HAV positive before getting this vaccination. The general rule is that if 50% of the target population are anti-HAV positive, then screening is cost-effective.

29. What is the role of this vaccine in cases of chronic liver disease (CLD)? Why is hepatitis A vaccination recommended for people with CLD?

Although not at increased risk for HAV infection, people with chronic liver disease (CLD) are at increased risk for fulminant hepatitis A if they should become infected with HAV. For this reason, hepatitis A vaccination is recommended for them.

30. What is the role of this vaccine in hepatitis B carriers?

Few studies indicate that if hepatitis B carriers get infected by HAV, their disease (hepatitis A) becomes more severe. However, the Centers for Disease Control and Prevention (CDC) does not agree with this due to lack of sufficient evidence.

31. What are the recommendations for postexposure prophylaxis (PEP) for hepatitis A?

Healthy persons who have completed the two-dose hepatitis A vaccination series at any time do not need additional PEP if they are exposed to HAV. Persons who have recently been exposed to HAV and who have not received hepatitis A vaccine previously should receive PEP as soon as possible within 2 weeks of exposure.

Persons age 12 months and older exposed to HAV within the past 14 days and who have not previously completed the two-dose hepatitis A vaccine series should receive a single dose of hepatitis A vaccine as soon as possible. In addition to vaccine, immune globulin (IG, 0.1 mL/kg) may be administered to persons older than 40 years of age depending on the providers' risk assessment. For long-term immunity, the hepatitis A vaccine series should be completed with a second dose at least 6 months after the first dose. However, the second dose is not necessary for PEP. A second dose should not be administered sooner than 6 calendar months after the first dose, regardless of HAV exposure risk.

Twinrix™ should not be used for PEP but may be used to confer protection to at-risk, but not yet exposed persons during an outbreak.

Infants younger than 12 months of age and persons for whom vaccine is contraindicated should receive IG (0.1 mL/kg) instead of hepatitis A vaccine as soon as possible and within 2 weeks of exposure. Measles, mumps, and rubella (MMR) and varicella vaccines should not be administered sooner than 3 months after IG administration.

32. Are the postexposure prophylaxis (PEP) recommendations same for immunocompromised individuals?

No, there are some differences. People age 1 year or older who are immunocompromised or have CLD and who have been exposed to HAV within the past 14 days and have not previously completed the two-dose hepatitis A vaccination series should receive both IG (0.1 mL/kg) and hepatitis A vaccine at the same visit in a different anatomic site (for example, separate limbs) as soon as possible after exposure. For long-term immunity, the hepatitis A vaccination series should be completed with a second dose at least 6 months after the first dose. However, the second dose is not necessary for PEP. A second dose should not be administered sooner than 6 calendar months after the first dose, regardless of HAV exposure risk.

33. How does immune globulin (IG) work?

Immune globulin provides protection against HAV infection through passive transfer of antibody. Depending on the IG dosage, protection lasts from 1 to 2 months. When administered for pre-exposure prophylaxis, a dose of 0.1 mL/kg will provide protection for up to 1 month and a dose of 0.2 mL/kg will provide protection for up to 2 months. A dose of 0.2 mL/kg can be repeated every 2 months. For PEP, the recommended dosage is 0.1 mL/kg. There is no maximum dosage of IG for hepatitis A prophylaxis.

SUGGESTED READING

1. Averhoff F, Shapiro CN, Bell BP, Hyams I, Burd L, Deladisma A, et al. Control of hepatitis A through routine vaccination of children. JAMA. 2001;286:2968-73.
2. de Febres OC, de Petrola MC, de Escalona LC, Naveda O, Naveda M, Estopinan M, et al. Safety, immunogenicity and antibody persistence of an inactivated hepatitis A vaccine in 4 to 15 year old children. Vaccine. 1999;18:656-64.
3. Immunization Action Coalition (IAC). (2019). Ask the Experts. [online] Available from: https://www.immunize.org/askexperts/experts_hepa.asp. [Last accessed June, 2020].
4. Immunization Action Coalition (IAC). (2016). Hepatitis A: Questions and answers: Information about the disease and vaccines. [online] Available from: http://www.immunize.org/catg.d/p4204.pdf. [Last accessed June, 2020].
5. Koff RD. Vaccine recommendations challenges and controversies hepatitis vaccine. Infect Dis Clin North Am. 2001;15:83-95.
6. Linglöf T, van Hattum J, Kaplan KM, Corrigan J, Duval I, Jensen E, et al. An open study of subcutaneous administration of inactivated hepatitis A vaccine (VAQTA) in adults: Safety, tolerability, and immunogenicity. Vaccine. 2001;19:3968-71.

7. López EL, Del Carmen Xifró M, Torrado LE, De Rosa MF, Gómez R, Dumas R, et al. Safety and immunogenicity of a pediatric formulation of inactivated hepatitis A Vaccine in Argentinean Children. Pediatr Infect Dis J. 2001;20:48-52.
8. Ragni MV, Lusher JM, Koerper MA, Manco-Johnson M, Krause DS. Safety and immunogenicity of subcutaneous hepatitis A vaccine in children with haemophilia. Hemophilia. 2000;6:98-103.
9. Singhal T, Amdekar YK, Agarwal RK. IAP Guidebook on Immunization, 4th edition. New Delhi: Jaypee Brothers Medical Publishers (P) Ltd.; 2009.
10. Vashishtha VM, Choudhury P, Kalra A, Bose A, Thacker N, Yewale VN, et al. Indian Academy of Pediatrics (IAP) recommended immunization schedule for children aged 0 through 18 years—India, 2014 and updates on immunization. Indian Pediatr. 2014;51:785-800.
11. Vashishtha VM, Kalra AK, Shah NK. IAP Textbook of Vaccines, 2nd edition. New Delhi: Jaypee Brothers Medical Publishers (P) Ltd.; 2009.

CHAPTER 22

Varicella Vaccines

Vijay N Yewale, Dhanya Dharmapalan

1. How significant is varicella disease in India?

Varicella, caused by the varicella zoster virus (VZV), is a highly contagious disease which in the absence of a vaccination program affects nearly every person by mid-adulthood in most populations. It is usually a self-limiting and benign illness in children. The mean age of infection is higher in tropical climates as compared to that in the temperate climates, leading to higher number of cases occurring in adolescents and young adults. This could be one of the reasons for a higher morbidity and mortality in the tropical developing countries as compared to the west. The exact burden of varicella in India is not known, but outbreaks are reported. One study from India suggests that 15% of adults are seronegative and susceptible to varicella. The susceptibility of the unimmunized adults, pregnant women and their infants, and of immunocompromised people from close contacts suffering from varicella is a cause for concern.

2. What is the content of a varicella vaccine?

Varicella vaccine is a live-attenuated vaccine derived from the original Oka strain, grown in human diploid cells. Oka is the main strain in use throughout the world for manufacture of single antigen and combination vaccines. The minimum infectious virus content should be 1,000 plaque units. Clinical studies suggest that the ratio of total viral antigen to total infectious viral particles is important to elicit appropriate immune response to vaccination. Vaccine medium may vary according to the manufacturer, but generally contains sucrose and buffering salts. The vaccine is marketed in lyophilized form to improve the stability during prolonged storage. It is reconstituted with sterile distilled water (0.5 mL) according to the instructions provided by the manufacturer. It should be used within 30 minutes of reconstitution.

3. How is the vaccine administered?

The recommended dose is 0.5 mL to be administered subcutaneously. Presently, in India, it is recommended in all healthy children who can afford the vaccine after one-to-one discussion with the parents.

4. What happens if the vaccine is administered intramuscularly?

The vaccine is to be administered subcutaneously and the seroconversion and efficacy data are based on data from individuals administered the vaccine subcutaneously. However, inadvertent intramuscular (IM) administration does not led to a significant reduction in immunogenicity and seroconversion.

5. What is the efficacy of varicella vaccine and how is it determined?

Primary antibody response to the vaccine at 6 weeks postvaccination is correlated with protection against disease. A titer of >5 glycoprotein enzyme-linked immunosorbent assay (gpELISA) units/mL or fluorescent-antibody-to-membrane-antigen (FAMA) titer > 1:4 at 16 weeks postvaccination correlates with protection against disease, though does not guarantee protection.

A meta-analysis of postlicensure varicella vaccine effectiveness (VE) concluded that one dose of varicella vaccine was moderately effective in preventing all varicella and very effective in preventing severe varicella. The second dose provides added protection against all varicella.

6. What are the side effects of the vaccine?

It is a very safe vaccine. Local side effects are: pain, redness, and swelling in <5% of vaccines. Systemic side effects like fever are rare. About 3–7% of vaccines can develop varicella-like rash, which is very mild with rapid recovery. It can occur up to 6 weeks after vaccination.

7. What is breakthrough varicella?

Varicella, which occurs in children vaccinated >6 weeks before rash onset, is called breakthrough varicella and is generally mild and atypical, predominantly maculopapular with little or no fever. But these children should be considered as potentially infectious and isolated like the typical varicella-infected children.

8. Why is occurrence of breakthrough varicella a matter of concern?

Approximately 15% of vaccine recipients remain at increased risk of breakthrough disease. These susceptible children may be at risk of severe varicella associated with VZV infection in adolescence and adulthood.
- Studies done in school outbreaks show that schoolchildren with breakthrough disease can serve as the index case for an outbreak
- Because vaccinated cases are mild, recognition or exclusion may be difficult, resulting in more opportunities to infect others. Education of physicians, school officials, and parents about the appearance of varicella in vaccinated persons are important for early recognition of outbreaks
- Varicella infection in immunized population may raise concern regarding vaccine efficacy and a misunderstanding by physicians or parents who may conclude that vaccine efficacy is declining. This misperception can lead to frustration among both parents and physicians and they may

lose faith in the varicella vaccine program, especially among people who perceive varicella as a mild illness of childhood
- Because immunized children who experience breakthrough diseases, are coinfected with both wild and vaccine strains of varicella virus, they may be at increased risk of zoster from the reactivated wild-type strain later in life, compared with vaccine recipients who do not experience breakthrough disease.

9. What are the causes of vaccine failure?

Primary vaccine failure is defined as failure to mount a protective immune response after a dose of vaccine and secondary vaccine failure is defined as a gradual loss of immunity after an initial immune response over a period of years after vaccination (waning immunity). The observed vaccine failure after one dose of vaccine may be explained in most probability as that immunized children either:
- Do not develop humoral immunity to VZV at all, or
- There is an initial immune "burst" of immunity that is enough to generate a positive gpELISA result, but is inadequate to generate a sustained memory T-cell response leading to waning of immunity over a period of time.

10. Does breakthrough varicella occur due to primary vaccine failure or due to waning immunity?

It is still controversial whether the breakthrough varicella occurs due to primary vaccine failure or due to waning immunity.

One study done to estimate primary vaccine failure in 148 healthy child vaccines found that 113 (76%) seroconverted and 24% had no detectable VZV FAMA antibodies at 4 months after vaccination. Their data suggested that many cases of varicella in immunized children are due to primary vaccine failure.

The risk of breakthrough varicella and severity of the disease are directly proportionate to the time lapsed from the date of immunization suggesting waning of the immunity acquired by immunization rendering these individual susceptible.

A study involving 11,356 children in California found that breakthrough varicella was twice as likely to be severe (defined as manifesting over 50 skin lesions) in children who became ill >5 years after vaccination compared with those who developed breakthrough disease after a short interval. Also, it was found that the annual breakthrough rate of disease was six times higher in children vaccinated 9 years before compared with those vaccinated 5 years previously. Though this study suggests a waning immunity, the possibility of primary vaccine failure being the causative factor cannot be ruled out.

Studies in Japan indicate persistence of antibodies for at least 20 years; however, these studies were conducted during a period when a substantial amount of wild-type VZV was present in the community with many opportunities for natural boosting of immunity by subclinical infection.

Thus, the available data are inconclusive regarding waning of immunity after one dose of varicella vaccine.

11. Why are the other concerns regarding primary vaccine failure in countries with a good coverage with vaccine?

Primary vaccine failure in just 10% of vaccinees after a single dose could result in progressive accumulation of susceptible individuals over time and lead to an increased incidence of varicella in young adults. Such an increment is potentially dangerous and therefore strongly supports the use of a second dose of vaccine for all children without a history of disease. The unacceptably high rate of primary vaccine failure suggests that the interval between the first and second doses of vaccine should be a matter of months rather than years. Correction of the problem of primary vaccine failure is thus urgent; if done, it will probably prevent not only the current phenomenon of isolated outbreaks of breakthrough disease, but a subsequent epidemic of serious varicella in vaccinated but unprotected adults.

12. If breakthrough varicella occurs due to primary vaccine failure, why is it milder compared to varicella occurring in unimmunized persons?

It is postulated that an insufficient number of virus-specific memory T-cells are generated after one-dose vaccination. According to the hypothesis, the immune memory response is less intense after a moderate initial stimulus than after a strong one because the virus-specific effector cell populations are downregulated within weeks or months after the primary contact with the antigen. In this view, the generally moderate course of breakthrough disease indicates that priming has indeed taken place after the single dose of vaccine, but that the initial stimulus did not suffice for complete protection. The fact that a second dose of vaccine brings about a stronger immune memory response supports this hypothesis, as a stronger response would not be expected if a robust primary immune response had already occurred.

13. What are the risk factors for breakthrough varicella?

They include:
- Vaccinating a child <16 months of age
- Not observing a gap of 28 days between measles, mumps, and rubella (MMR) and varicella vaccination
- Time elapsed since vaccination.

14. Does increasing the virus content in the vaccine help in reducing the risk of breakthrough varicella?

No, because, as the quantity of antigen increases, a plateau effect comes about, so that the immune response probably cannot be made any stronger.

15. If breakthrough varicella occurs due to waning immunity, will the immunity wane after second dose of vaccine?

Quite possible. Waning might also be an issue with the newly recommended two-dose vaccination schedule. Sustained surveillance for varicella outbreaks in populations with varicella immunization programs, therefore, is mandatory.

16. What are the current recommendations of the Indian Academy of Pediatrics-Advisory Committee on Vaccines and Immunization Practices (IAP-ACVIP) on varicella vaccine?

Current guidelines recommend two doses of 0.5 mL subcutaneously administered varicella vaccines in all children above 12 months, adolescents and adults with no prior history of varicella. The first dose of varicella vaccine can be given between 15 and 18 months and second dose just before school entry, i.e., between 4 and 6 years.

However, during an outbreak, the 1st dose may be administered at 12 months of age if it is ensured that the 2-dose schedule will be completed by the individual child. The second dose may be administered any time 3 months after the first dose.

It also recommends vaccine to children belonging to certain high-risk groups as enumerated below:
- Children with humoral immunodeficiencies
- Children with human immunodeficiency virus (HIV) infection, but with CD4+ counts 15% and above the age-related cutoff
- Leukemia but in remission and off chemotherapy for at least 3–6 months
- Children on long-term salicylates. Salicylates should be avoided for at least 6 weeks after vaccination
- Children likely to be on long-term steroid therapy. The vaccine may be given at any time if the children are on low-dose steroids/alternate day steroids, but only 4 weeks after stopping steroids if the patients have received high-dose steroids (2 mg/kg) for 14 days or more
- In household contacts of immunocompromised children
- Adolescents who have not had varicella in past and are known to be varicella immunoglobulin G (IgG) negative, especially if they are leaving home for studies in a residential school/college
- Children with chronic lung/heart disease
- Seronegative adolescents and adults, if they are inmates of or working in the institutional setup, e.g., school teachers, day care center workers, military personnel, and healthcare professionals.

For postexposure prophylaxis in susceptible healthy nonpregnant contacts, preferably within 3 days of exposure (efficacy 90%) and potentially up to 5 days of exposure (efficacy 70% against severe disease 100%).

17. What are the latest recommendations of varicella vaccine by the Advisory Committee on Immunization Practices (ACIP)?

The Advisory Committee on Immunization Practices (ACIP) recommends two doses of varicella vaccine.

For children aged >12 months, adolescents and adults are without evidence of immunity. For routine vaccination, the first dose can be administered between 15 and 18 months and second dose between 4 and 6 years.

For children aged 12 months to 12 years, the recommended minimum interval between the two doses is 3 months. However, if the second dose was administered ≥28 days after the first dose, the second dose is considered valid and needs not to be repeated.

For persons aged ≥13 years, the recommended minimum interval between two doses is 4–8 weeks. If >8 weeks elapse after the first dose, the second dose may be administered without restarting the schedule. Only single-antigen varicella vaccine may be used for vaccination of persons in this age group. Measles, mumps, rubella, and varicella (MMRV) is not licensed for use among persons aged ≥13 years.

18. What is the rationale behind the Advisory Committee on Immunization Practices (ACIP) recommending the two-dose schedule for children?

Despite the successes of the one-dose vaccination program in children in US, vaccine effectiveness of 85% has not been sufficient to prevent breakthrough varicella outbreaks which are contagious.

Studies of the immune response after one and two doses of varicella vaccine demonstrate a greater than ten-fold boost in geometric mean titers (GMTs) when measured 6 weeks after the second varicella vaccine dose. A higher proportion (>99%) of children achieve an antibody response of >5 gpELISA units after the second dose compared with 76–85% of children after a single dose of varicella vaccine.

The efficacy of a single dose versus two doses of vaccine was tested in a randomized clinical study involving 2,216 children who were vaccinated in the USA from 1991 to 1993. Over 10 years of follow-up, the cumulative rate of breakthrough disease in children who had been vaccinated twice was lower by a factor of 3.3 than that of children who had been vaccinated once (2.2% compared to 7.3%; $p < 0.001$). Breakthrough disease was most commonly occurred 2–5 years after vaccination in both groups. Among the children who had been vaccinated twice, no breakthrough disease at all arose during the interval from 7 to 10 years after vaccination. Hence, in June 2006, US implemented a routine two-dose varicella vaccination program for children, with the first dose administered at age 12–15 months and the second dose at age 4–6 years.

19. When implementing a two-dose schedule below 13 years, what should be the ideal gap between the two doses?

A study where the second dose was given 4–6 years after the first dose found a large increase in the antibody levels during the 7–10 days after the second dose, indicating an anamnestic response (GMT on the day of second dose:

25.7 and on days 7–10 after second dose: 143.6). However, the antibody levels after two doses administered 4–6 years apart were comparable to those levels seen when two doses were administered 3 months apart.

The timing of the second dose recommended in US at 4–6 years was partially for compatibility with the MMR dose schedule. But since breakthrough varicella has been observed to have occurred commonly as early as 2 years, the second dose of varicella can be administered early, i.e., at any time 8 weeks after first dose.

20. What are the current Indian Academy of Pediatrics-Advisory Committee on Vaccines and Immunization Practices (IAP-ACVIP) recommendations on varicella vaccination?

The Advisory Committee on Vaccines and Immunization Practices (ACVIP) recommendations are almost same as advised by the Centers for Disease Control and Prevention (CDC)-ACIP. They are as follows for the routine vaccination:
- *Minimum age*: 12 months
- Administer the first dose at age 15 through 18 months and the second dose 3 months after the first dose or at age 4 through 6 years
- If the second dose was administered at least 4 weeks after the first dose, it can be accepted as valid
- The risk of breakthrough varicella is lower if given 15 months onward.

21. What are the Indian Academy of Pediatrics-Advisory Committee on Vaccines and Immunization Practices (IAP-ACVIP) recommendations for catch-up immunization?

Catch-up vaccination:
- Ensure that all persons aged 7 through 18 years without "evidence of immunity" have two doses of the vaccine.
- "Evidence of immunity" to varicella includes any of the following:
  - Documentation of age-appropriate vaccination with a varicella vaccine
  - Laboratory evidence of immunity or laboratory confirmation of disease
  - Diagnosis or verification of a history of varicella disease by a healthcare provider
  - Diagnosis or verification of a history of herpes zoster (HZ) by a healthcare provider
- For children aged 12 months through 12 years, the recommended minimum interval between doses is 3 months. However, if the second dose was administered at least 4 weeks after the first dose, it can be accepted as valid
- For persons aged 13 years and older, the minimum interval between doses is 4 weeks

- For persons without evidence of immunity, administer two doses if not previously vaccinated or the second dose if only one dose has been administered.

22. What do you mean by "evidence of immunity"?

"Evidence of immunity" to varicella includes any of the following:
- Documentation of age-appropriate vaccination with a varicella vaccine
- Laboratory evidence of immunity or laboratory confirmation of disease
- Diagnosis or verification of a history of varicella disease by a healthcare provider
- Diagnosis or verification of a history of HZ by a healthcare provider.

23. Why the second dose at 4–6 years of age? Is there any advantage of delaying the second dose to 4–6 years of age?

Though technically, the second dose can be administered after 3 months of first dose and there are many trials to support that, but why the CDC-ACIP is insisting for 4-6 years is because of following reasons:
- The recommended ages for routine first (at age 12-15 months) and second (at age 4-6 years) doses of varicella vaccine are harmonized with the recommendations for MMR vaccine use and intended to limit the period when children have no varicella antibody. The recommended age for the second dose is supported by the current epidemiology of varicella, with low incidence and few outbreaks among preschool-aged children and higher incidence and more outbreaks among elementary school-aged children.
- Although, the most studies are done when second dose is given after 3 months of the first, there are few trials where the two schedules were compared and it was concluded that among children, VZV antibody levels and GMTs after two doses administered 4-6 years apart were comparable to those obtained when the two doses were administered 3 months apart (seroconversion: 99.2% vs. 99.6%; GMTs: 212.4 vs. 142.6, respectively).
- However, the cell-mediated immunity (CMI) responses were measured by mean stimulation index (SI), a marker of CMI was 36.9 for second dose after 3 months of primary dose and 58.6 when second dose was given at 4-6 years of age.

But, the main reasons why 4-6 years were preferred for second dose in primary schedule are contained in first dose. Probably, the only benefit of providing second dose after 3 months of first dose (given at 15 months) could be insignificant, miniscule reduction in cases of breakthrough varicella occurring in the window period of 15 months to 4 years.

24. There are many chickenpox vaccine brands available in Indian market. Are all the same? What are the key differentiating features of them?

Different brands of monovalent varicella vaccine are available in India now for over the last 2 decades. There are currently five different brands of monovalent varicella vaccine available in Indian market. Besides the two multinational brands, VARIPED® and VARILRIX®, there are three other brands manufactured by three Chinese manufacturers and imported in India by different Indian vaccine companies. Another Japanese product, OKAVAX® by Biken marketed by M/s Sanofi Pasteur, is not available in Indian market. All vaccines are freeze dried, lyophilized products, and licensed for use in persons aged ≥12 months.

Table 1A summarizes the key attributes like composition, process of development, and stability of available varicella vaccine brands in India whereas **Table 1B** enlists the comparative study of the various brands available in India. The Indian Academy of Pediatrics-Advisory Committee on Vaccines and Immunization Practices (IAP-ACVIP) approves all the available monovalent varicella vaccine brands in the Indian market for use in pediatric population for prevention of varicella disease.

25. How is varicella vaccination related to the incidence of herpes zoster?

Some studies have suggested that the exposure of individuals with latent wild-type VZV infection (as a result of natural infection) to individuals with varicella reduces the risk for HZ, presumably by externally boosting VZV immunity. After implementation of vaccination program, there is a predicted rise in HZ cases especially for a short to medium term (up to 70 years) although in the long term, a reduction in zoster cases is expected to occur provided that the vaccine recipients have a lower risk of developing zoster than persons who acquire natural infection.

26. Is varicella vaccine recommended for adolescents and adults? What is the Indian scenario of susceptibility of adolescents and adults to varicella?

Yes, healthy adolescents and adults with no evidence of immunity should receive two doses of varicella vaccine 4–8 weeks apart. Varicella is a more severe disease in adults. Nearly 100% seropositivity to VZV has been documented by 11–13 years in USA. However, a study from India revealed that the prevalence of antibodies to varicella gradually increases through childhood, adolescence, and adulthood. An overall seropositivity rate of >70% was reached between the ages of 11 and 15 years which increased to nearly 90% at the age of 30 years demonstrating that a significant proportion of adolescents and adults are susceptible to varicella in India.

The epidemiology of VZV infection is different in tropical countries in which VZV infection is common in adolescents and adults than in temperate countries where adolescents and adults are almost immune with universal seroconversion occurring by late childhood. The varicella disease is also a far more serious ailment with greater morbidity and mortality in adolescents and adults than in early childhood. Furthermore, VZV infection during pregnancy may have serious health hazards for the fetus and newborn infant.

TABLE 1A: Key attributes such as composition, process of development, and stability of available varicella vaccine.

Brand name*	Manufacturer/ marketer	Composition (Vaccine formulation)					Process of development		Stability (Shelf-life at (2–8°C)
		Strain	Quantity of antigen	Preservative	Stabilizer	Antibiotic	Other	Adherence to GMP	Other	
VARIPED	Merck sharp and Dohme (MSD) Pharmaceuticals	Oka/ Merck varicella	Minimum of 1,350 PFU	None	MSGO 36 mg sucrose and hydrolyzed Gelatin 8.9 mg	Neo-mycin (traces)	Sodium phosphate and potassium phosphate as pH regulators; Bovine calf serum and trace residual components of MRC-5 cells	Yes	USFDA and European medicines agency approved	24 months
VARILRIX	Glaxo Smith Kline (GSK) vaccines	OKA/GSK strain	Not less than $10^{3.3}$ PFU	None	Anhydrous lactose, Sorbitol, Mannitol, Amino acids	Neo-mycin (traces)	Human serum albumin	Yes	European medicines agency approved	24 months
BIOVAC-V	Manufactured by Changchun Changsheng Life Sciences, China; marketed in India by M/s Wockhardt India Ltd	Oka strain (VR 795 varicella Oka strain)	2,511 PFU	Fucose 17.5 mg	MSG 3.0 mg, Sorbierite 2.5 mg	None	Dextran and L-arginine	–	Approved by State Food and Drugs Administration, China	24 months

Contd...

Contd...

Brand name	Manufacturer/ marketer	Composition (Vaccine formulation)						Process of development		Stability (Shelf-life at (2–8°C)
		Strain	Quantity of antigen	Preservative	Stabilizer	Antibiotic	Other	Adherence to GMP	Other	
VARIVAX	Changchun Institute of Biological Products, China marketed in India by M/s VHB Life Sciences Ltd	Oka strain	Not less than 2,000 PFU	None	MSG 0.7 mg, Gelatin 2.1 mg, Dextran, Socrose	Neo-mycin (traces)	Mannitol as a humectant, Human Albumin, Sodium Orthophosphate and Potassium phosphate	–	No information	24 months
NEXIPOX	Changchun BCHT Biotechnology (Baiko) China, marketed in India by M/s Novo Medi Sciences Pvt Ltd	Oka strain (VR 795 varicella Oka strain	≥ 2,000 PFU	Human albumin 5 mg	Trehalose 10 mg, Sucrose, Dextran	Neo-mycin (traces)	Human albumin, Bovine calf serum, Mannitol as a humectant	–	Certificate of GMP from Peoples Republic of China	36 months

(GMP: good manufacturing practice; MSG: monosodium L-glutamate; PFU: plaque forming units; USFDA: United States Food and Drug Administration)

CHAPTER 22 Varicella Vaccines 323

TABLE 1B: Comparative analysis of available varicella vaccine brands in India: Clinical data on immunogenicity, efficacy, effectiveness, and safety.

Brand name*	Immunogenicity data		Efficacy data		Effectiveness data			Safety data		Clinical experience/usage	
	Indian trial	Publication in an indexed journal	Efficacy studies	Publication in an indexed journal	Effectiveness study/impact data	Publication in an indexed journal	Population impact data	PMS trial	Publication	National	Worldwide
VARIPED	Yes	No (poster presentation only)	Yes	Yes	Yes	Yes (33 studies, 28 studies with one dose and five studies with two doses)	Yes (US, Canada, Germany, Spain, Australia, and Taiwan)	Yes	Yes	Marketing approval received in India in 2014	191 million doses used worldwide in 38 countries
VARILRIX	Yes	Yes (MMRV trial in India)	Yes	Yes	Yes	Yes (13 studies, all with one dose)	Yes (Uruguay, Australia, Germany, and Taiwan)	Yes	Yes	Marketing approval in 1998; approximately 4.98 million doses sold since launch	62.9 million doses used in over 90 countries since 1986
BIOVAC-V	Yes	Yes	No	No	Yes	Yes (two studies)	No	Yes (studies done in few districts of China)	No	Marketing approval in June 2014; approximately 1.9 million doses sold since launch	20.7 million doses used in China, Philippines, Pakistan, and Guatemala

Contd...

Contd...

Brand name®	Immunogenicity data		Efficacy data		Effectiveness data		Population impact data	Safety data		Clinical experience/usage	
	Indian trial	Publication in an indexed journal	Efficacy studies	Publication in an indexed journal	Effectiveness study/impact data	Publication in an indexed journal		PMS trial	Publication	National	Worldwide
VARIVAX	Yes	?	No	No	–	Yes (one study)	No	?	?	Marketing approval in 2004; approximately 5.0 million doses sold since launch	No information
NEXIPOX	Yes	Yes (studies published in Chinese journals)	No	No	Yes	Yes (one study)	No	Yes (studies done in few districts of China)	Yes (studies published in Chinese journals)	0.25 million doses sold since its approval in India	More than 90 million doses sold since 2008 in Philippines, Macau, and China

(MMRV: measles, mumps, rubella, and varicella; PMS: postmarketing surveillance)

27. Can a 30-year-old seronegative/susceptible lady be administered varicella vaccine?

It is not very stringent in India, unlike in countries like US, to furnish an evidence of immunity for varicella to decide whether vaccine is to be given. A history of varicella infection in the past is fairly acceptable. Documentation of age-appropriate vaccination with a varicella vaccine, diagnosis or verification of a history of varicella disease/HZ by a healthcare provider, and laboratory evidence of immunity or laboratory confirmation of disease are hardcore evidences, but not easily available. In absence of these evidences, it is better to provide the vaccine.

28. Are there some groups of adults for whom varicella vaccination is especially important?

Yes, varicella vaccination is especially important for the following groups of susceptible adults:
- Persons who have close contact with persons at high risk for serious complications from VZV infection; for example, healthcare workers and family members/close contacts of people with impaired immune systems
- Persons who live or work in environments in which VZV transmission is likely; for example, teachers of young children, childcare employees, and residents/staff in institutional settings
- Persons who live or work in places where VZV transmission can readily occur; for example, college students, inmates and staff of correctional institutions, and military personnel
- Nonpregnant women of childbearing age (women should avoid pregnancy for 1 month following each vaccine dose)
- Adolescents and adults living in households with children
- International travelers.
  However, all healthy susceptible adults should be vaccinated.

29. When is the vaccine contraindicated?

Varicella vaccine is contraindicated in the following situations:
- In persons allergic to the vaccine or its constituent
- In persons who have any malignant condition, including blood dyscrasias, leukemia, lymphomas of any type, or other malignant neoplasms affecting the bone marrow or lymphatic systems
- Varicella vaccines should not be administered to persons who have a family history of congenital or hereditary immunodeficiency in first-degree relatives (e.g., parents and siblings) unless the immune competence of the potential vaccine recipient has been clinically substantiated or verified by a laboratory
- Varicella vaccines should not be administered to persons receiving high-dose systemic immunosuppressive therapy, including persons on oral steroids >2 mg/kg of body weight or a total of >20 mg/day of prednisone

or equivalent for persons who weigh >10 kg when administered for >2 weeks
- Because the effects of the varicella virus vaccine on the fetus are unknown, pregnant women should not be vaccinated. Nonpregnant women who are vaccinated should avoid becoming pregnant for 1 month after each injection. If a pregnant woman is vaccinated or becomes pregnant within 1 month of vaccination, she should be counseled about potential effects on the fetus. A registry of such patient, however, has not reported any adverse outcome so far.

30. In which patients should the clinician takes a decision to vaccinate with precaution?

Vaccination of persons, who have acute severe illness, including untreated, active tuberculosis, should be postponed until recovery. The decision to delay vaccination depends on the severity of symptoms and on the etiology of the disease.

31. Can a child with idiopathic thrombocytopenic purpura (ITP) be given varicella vaccine?

Cases of thrombocytopenia have been reported after MMR vaccine and after varicella vaccination, but it is not a contradiction for receiving varicella vaccine.

32. Can an individual who has received antibody-containing product like whole blood or immunoglobulin be given the vaccine?

Because of the potential inhibition of the response to varicella vaccination by passively transferred antibodies, varicella vaccines should not be administered for the same intervals as measles vaccine (3–11 months, depending on the dosage) after administration of blood (except washed red blood cells, plasma, or IG).

33. Can the vaccine be given to a child receiving salicylates and is salicylate contraindicated after varicella immunization?

No adverse events associated with the use of salicylates after varicella vaccination have been reported; however, the vaccine manufacturer recommends that vaccine recipients avoid using salicylates for 6 weeks after receiving varicella vaccines because of the association between aspirin use and Reye syndrome after varicella. Vaccination with subsequent close monitoring should be considered for children who have rheumatoid arthritis or other conditions requiring therapeutic aspirin. The risk for serious complications associated with aspirin is likely to be greater in children in whom natural varicella develops than it is in children who receive the vaccine-containing attenuated VZV.

34. Can varicella vaccine be coadministered with measles, mumps, and rubella (MMR) even though both are live vaccines?

Single-antigen varicella vaccine is well-tolerated and effective in healthy children aged ≥12 months when administered simultaneously with MMR vaccine either at separate sites and with separate syringes or separately ≥4 weeks apart.

35. How does one protect a newborn who is exposed to a case of varicella?

A full-term healthy newborn is not at increased risk for complications and does not merit prophylaxis with varicella zoster immune globulin (VZIG)/intravenous immunoglobulin (IVIG) if exposed to varicella. All neonates born at <28 weeks of gestation with birth weight <1,000 g exposed in the neonatal period should be administered VZIG. All preterm neonates born at >28 weeks of gestation and exposed to varicella in the neonatal period should be administered VZIG only if their mothers are negative for anti-varicella IgG.

36. What is the risk to the newborn delivered to a mother having varicella at the time of delivery?

A maternal rash erupting 5 days before and 2 days after delivery is frequently associated with clinically severe varicella in the newborn, leading to high mortality if untreated. Then, the newborn is infectious and must be isolated till scabs are formed. In this setting, acyclovir is generally recommended (60 mg/kg divided every 8 hours). VZIG 125 units/kg IM should be given as soon as possible after delivery.

37. Who should be administered varicella zoster immune globulin (VZIG)?

The IAP-ACVIP recommends the use of VZIG for postexposure prophylaxis in the following *susceptible individuals* with *significant contact* with varicella/HZ who are at high risk for severe disease. Here, susceptible is defined as:
- All unvaccinated children who do not have a clinical history of varicella in the past
- All unvaccinated adults who are seronegative for anti-varicella IgG. Bone marrow transplant recipients are considered susceptible even if they had disease or received vaccinations prior to transplantation.

A significant contact is defined as any face-to-face contact or stays within the same room for a period >1 hour with a patient with infectious varicella (defined as 1–2 days before the rash till all lesions have crusted) or disseminated HZ.

Patients meeting these two criteria and who are at high risk of developing severe disease merit prophylaxis with VZIG.

38. What is the problem of chickenpox in immunocompromised host?

Varicella can be very severe in immunocompromised host. Chances of complications like encephalitis, pneumonitis, generalized varicella, or hemorrhagic varicella are high. 50% of them have secondary bacterial soft tissue infections, 70% develop encephalitis, and 40–50% develop pneumonitis. Mortality is 7% in children and 50% in adults. Though only 0.1% cases of all chickenpox cases occur in immunocompromised hosts, it contributes to 25% of mortality due to varicella disease. Hence, these children, except the ones with severe T-cell defects, should be immunized irrespective of age. They should receive two doses of the vaccine.

39. How does one protect an immunocompromised child with leukemia (or any other malignancy) on exposure to varicella?

All immunocompromised children especially neoplastic disease, congenital or acquired immunodeficiency, or those receiving immunosuppressive therapies should be administered VZIG. Patients who received IVIG @ 400 mg/kg in the past 3 weeks are considered protected and need not to be given VZIG.

40. How late can varicella zoster immune globulin (VZIG) be administered to a patient? What is the dose and how is it administered?

Varicella zoster immune globulin should be given as soon as possible but not later than 96 hours following exposure. VZIG reduces the risk of disease and complications and the duration of protection lasts for 3 weeks. The currently available VZIG is for intravenous use (Varitect) and is administered at a dose of 0.2–1 mL/kg diluted in normal saline over 1 hour. The efficacy against death in cases where neonatal exposure has occurred is almost 100%. Side effects include allergic reactions and anaphylaxis. Since VZIG prolongs the incubation period, all exposed should be monitored for at least 28 weeks for disease manifestations.

41. Can one use intravenous immunoglobulin (IVIG) in place of varicella zoster immune globulin (VZIG)?

The cost of VZIG is prohibitive and is not easily available. If unaffordable/not available, the options with uncertain efficacy include IVIG @ 200 mg/kg or oral acyclovir 80 mg/kg/day beginning from the 7th day of exposure and given for 7–10 days.

42. What should be the interval between administration of varicella zoster immune globulin (VZIG) and varicella vaccine?

Any patient who receives VZIG to prevent varicella should receive varicella vaccine subsequently, provided the vaccine is not contraindicated. Varicella vaccination should be delayed until 5 months after VZIG administration. Varicella vaccine is not needed if the patient has varicella after administration of VZIG.

43. What is the data on contagiousness of varicella vaccine?

Transmission of the vaccine virus from vaccinees to contacts is rare, especially in the absence of a vaccine-related rash in the vaccinees. However, vaccine recipients who develop a rash should avoid contact with persons without evidence of immunity who are at high risk for severe complications.

44. How contagious is breakthrough varicella?

A study demonstrated that vaccinated persons with varicella with <50 lesions were only one-third as contagious as unvaccinated persons with varicella. However, vaccinated persons with varicella who had >50 lesions were as contagious as unvaccinated persons with varicella. Vaccinated persons with varicella tend to have milder disease, and, although they are less contagious than unvaccinated persons with varicella, they might not receive a diagnosis and be isolated. As a result, they might have more opportunities to infect others in community settings, thereby further contributing to VZV transmission. Vaccinated persons with varicella also have been index case-patients in varicella outbreaks.

45. Can the sibling of a child undergoing chemotherapy be given the varicella vaccine?

Yes. The IAP-ACVIP, the ACIP, and the American Academy of Pediatrics (AAP) recommend that healthy household contacts of immunocompromised persons be vaccinated. This is the most effective way to protect the immunocompromised person from exposure to wild-type varicella. However, because of the small risk of household transmission of vaccine virus, vaccinees who develop a vaccine-related rash should avoid contact with immunocompromised persons while the rash is present. To date, there have been no documented cases of transmission of varicella vaccine virus to immunocompromised persons. If a susceptible immunocompromised person is inadvertently exposed to a person with a vaccine-related rash, postexposure treatment with VZIG is not needed because the disease associated with this type of transmission would be expected to be mild. On the basis of available data, the benefit of vaccinating susceptible household contacts of immunocompromised persons outweighs the low potential risk of transmission of vaccine virus to immunocompromised persons.

46. Can persons with human immunodeficiency virus (HIV)/acquired immunodeficiency syndrome (AIDS) receive the vaccine?

Screening for HIV infection is not indicated before routine varicella immunization. Vaccine is contraindicated in individuals with clinically manifest HIV. After weighing potential risks and benefits, varicella vaccine should be considered for HIV-infected children in the CDC class I with a CDC T-lymphocyte percentage of 15%.

Human immunodeficiency virus-infected children in this group should receive two doses of the single-antigen vaccine, separated by

3 months. They are encouraged to return to their healthcare provider, if they experience a postvaccination, varicella-like rash. Previously, this vaccine was recommended for children in the CDC classes N1 and A1 who have age-specific CD4+ percentages >25%.

Data on the use of varicella vaccine in HIV-infected adolescents and adults are lacking and the immunogenicity may be lower in this group of HIV-infected individuals. However, based on expert opinion in examining the risk of severe disease from wild varicella infection compared to the benefit of vaccination, vaccination (two doses administered 3 months apart) of HIV-infected persons >8 years of age who are in the CDC clinical class A or B and have CD4+ T-lymphocyte counts ≥200 cells/µL may be considered.

If inadvertent vaccination of HIV-infected person results in clinical disease, acyclovir may be used to modify the disease.

47. Can a child on budesonide, budecort metered-dose inhaler for asthma since past 6 months receive varicella vaccine?

Yes. The child on metered-dose inhaler (MDI) can be given varicella vaccine though the data are lacking on whether persons receiving inhaled, nasal, or topical steroids without evidence of immunity can be vaccinated safely. It is recommended that persons without evidence of immunity who are receiving systemic steroids for certain conditions and who are not otherwise immunocompromised can be vaccinated if they are receiving <2 mg/kg of body weight or total of <20 mg/day of prednisone or its equivalent. Some experts suggest withholding steroids for 2–3 weeks after vaccination if that can be done safely.

48. Is it safe to administer the vaccine to a child of nephrotic syndrome on daily oral steroids (>2 mg/kg/day) since past 3 weeks?

It is recommended that persons who are receiving high doses of systemic steroids (i.e., ≥2 mg/kg prednisone) for ≥2 weeks may be vaccinated once steroid therapy has been discontinued for at least 1 month. This child can be given the vaccine once the steroids have been discontinued for at least 1 month.

49. Can a postpartum lactating woman who is seronegative (susceptible) be administered the varicella vaccine?

Postpartum vaccination of women without evidence of immunity need not be delayed because of breastfeeding. Women who have received varicella vaccination postpartum may continue to breastfeed. The majority of live vaccines are not associated with virus secretion in breast milk. Therefore, single-antigen varicella vaccine may be administered to nursing mothers without evidence of immunity.

SUGGESTED READING

1. American Academy of Pediatrics Committee on Infectious Diseases. Prevention of varicella: recommendations for use of varicella vaccines in children, including a recommendation for a routine 2-dose varicella immunization schedule. Pediatrics. 2007;120:221-31.
2. Arvin A, Gershon A. Control of varicella: why is a two-dose schedule necessary? Pediatr Infect Dis J. 2006;25:475-6.
3. Auriti C, Piersigilli F, de Gasperis MR, Seganti G. Congenital varicella syndrome: still a problem? Fetal Diagn Ther. 2009;25:224-9.
4. Balasubramanian S, Shah A, Pemde HK, Chatterjee P, Shivananda S, Guduru VK, et al. Indian Academy of Pediatrics (IAP) Advisory Committee on Vaccines and Immunization Practices (ACVIP) Recommended Immunization Schedule (2018-19) and Update on Immunization for Children Aged 0 Through 18 Years. Indian Pediatr. 2018;55:1066-74.
5. Centers for Disease Control and Prevention (CDC). (2019). Varicella Vaccine-Q&A about Eligibility. [online] Available from: http://www.cdc.gov/vaccines/vpd-vac/varicella/vac-faqs-clinic-eligible.htm. [Last accessed July, 2020].
6. Centers for Disease Control and Prevention (CDC). Outbreak of varicella among vaccinated children—Michigan, 2003. MMWR Morb Mortal Wkly Rep. 2004;53:389-92.
7. Chaves SS, Gargiullo P, Zhang JX, Civen R, Guris D, Mascola L, et al. Loss of vaccine-induced immunity to varicella over time. N Engl J Med. 2007;356:1121-9.
8. Singhal T, Amdekar YK, Agarwal RK (Eds). IAP Guidebook on Immunization. New Delhi: Jaypee Brothers Medical Publishers (P) Ltd; 2009.
9. Gershon AA, Takahashi M, Seward JF. Varicella vaccines. In: Plotkin SA, Orenstein WA (Eds). Vaccines, 5th edition, Philadelphia: Saunders; 2008. pp. 467-517.
10. Kuter B, Matthews H, Shinefield H, Black S, Dennehy P, Watson B, et al. Ten year follow-up of healthy children who received one or two injections of varicella vaccine. Pediatr Infect Dis J. 2004;23:132-7.
11. Lokeshwar MR, Agrawal A, Subbarao SD, Chakraborty MS, Ram Prasad AV, Weil J, et al. Age related seroprevalence of antibodies to varicella in India. Indian Pediatr. 2000;37:714-9.
12. Lopez AS, Guris D, Zimmerman L, Gladden L, Moore T, Haselow DT, et al. One dose of varicella vaccine does not prevent school outbreaks: is it time for a second dose? Pediatrics. 2006;117:e1070-7.
13. Marin M, Güris D, Chaves SS, Schmid S, Seward JF. Prevention of Varicella: Recommendations of the Advisory Committee on Immunization Practices (ACIP). MMWR Recomm Rep. 2007;56:1-40.
14. Marin M, Marti M, Kambhampati A, Jeram SM, Seward JF. Global varicella vaccine effectiveness: a meta-analysis. Pediatrics. 2016;137:e20153741.
15. Marin M, Meissner HC, Seward JF. Varicella prevention in the United States: a review of successes and challenges. Pediatrics. 2008;122:e744-51.
16. Michalik DE, Steinberg SP, Larussa PS, Edwards KM, Wright PF, Arvin AM, et al. Primary vaccine failure after 1 dose of varicella vaccine in healthy children. J Infect Dis. 2008;197:944-9.
17. National Center for Immunization and Respiratory Diseases. General recommendations on immunization: Recommendations of the Advisory Committee on Immunization Practices (ACIP). MMWR Recomm Rep. 2011;60:1-64.

18. Pickering LK, Baker CJ. Varicella-zoster infections. In: Pickering LK, Baker CJ, Kimberlin DW (Eds). Red Book: Report of the Committee on Infectious Diseases, 28th edition. United States: American Academy of Pediatrics; 2009. pp. 714-27.
19. Prevention of varicella: Recommendations of the Advisory Committee on Immunization Practices (ACIP). Centers for Disease Control and Prevention. MMWR Recomm Rep. 1996;45:1-36.
20. Seward JF, Zhang JX, Maupin TJ, Mascola L, Jumaan AO. Contagiousness of varicella in vaccinated cases: a household contact study. JAMA. 2004;292:704-8.
21. White CJ, Kuter BJ, Hildebrand CS, Isganitis KL, Matthews H, Miller WJ, et al. Varicella vaccine (VARIVAX) in healthy children and adolescents: results from clinical trials, 1987 to 1989. Pediatrics. 1991;87:604-10.
22. Wutzler P, Knuf M, Liese J. Varicella: efficacy of two-dose vaccination in childhood. Dtsch Arztebl Int. 2008;105:567-72.

CHAPTER 23

Typhoid Vaccines

Chandra Mohan Kumar, Vipin M Vashishtha, Ajay Kalra

1. What is the global burden of typhoid?

Although with improved sanitation and access to drinking water, the disease burden has reduced globally, still typhoid fever remains a public health problem. Globally, 14.3 million cases of enteric fever (typhoid and paratyphoid fever) occurred in 2017, a 44.6% decline from 25.9 million in 1990. It accounts for over 140,000 deaths each year globally. As the disease is primarily associated with poor hygienic and sanitary conditions, mainly the developing countries bear the brunt of the disease. **Figure 1** depicts the status of typhoid and paratyphoid fevers, by country, in 2017.

2. What is the status of typhoid fever in India and neighboring countries?

As Indian subcontinent has the maximum disease burden, around 5 million cases occur annually in India. In 2016, India had 6.6 million typhoid cases (499 cases/100,000 population) and 66,439 typhoid deaths, more than half were in children below 15 year of age. Population-based studies from urban population in India suggest that the incidence of typhoid fever on decline over last 20 years. In 1990s, it was 2,730 out of per 100,000 people-years (PY) among 0-4 years old children and 1,170 per 100,000 PY every year in 5- to 19-year age group but a recent pooled data meta-analysis suggests that the current incidence is between 377 and 499 cases per 100,000 PY. Majority of cases are in children and young adults. Ten percent of cases occur in the infant age group because diagnosis is difficult and hence mortality is higher.

A major problem in the last four decades has been the emergence of plasmid-encoded multidrug resistance it ranges from 17 to 90% of isolates as reported by various studies, drug resistance is seen especially to the quinolones. Off late extensively drug-resistant (XDR) cases too have been reported where resistance to ceftriaxone and azithromycin too have made the treatment more challenging. Children constitute 40–50% cases of multidrug-resistant (MDR) typhoid fever with higher case fatality rates. India has 86% fluoroquinolone resistance and 9.4% MDR. Luckily XDR is rare in India but the fact that our neighboring country Pakistan has 34% XDR resistance is a matter of grave concern.

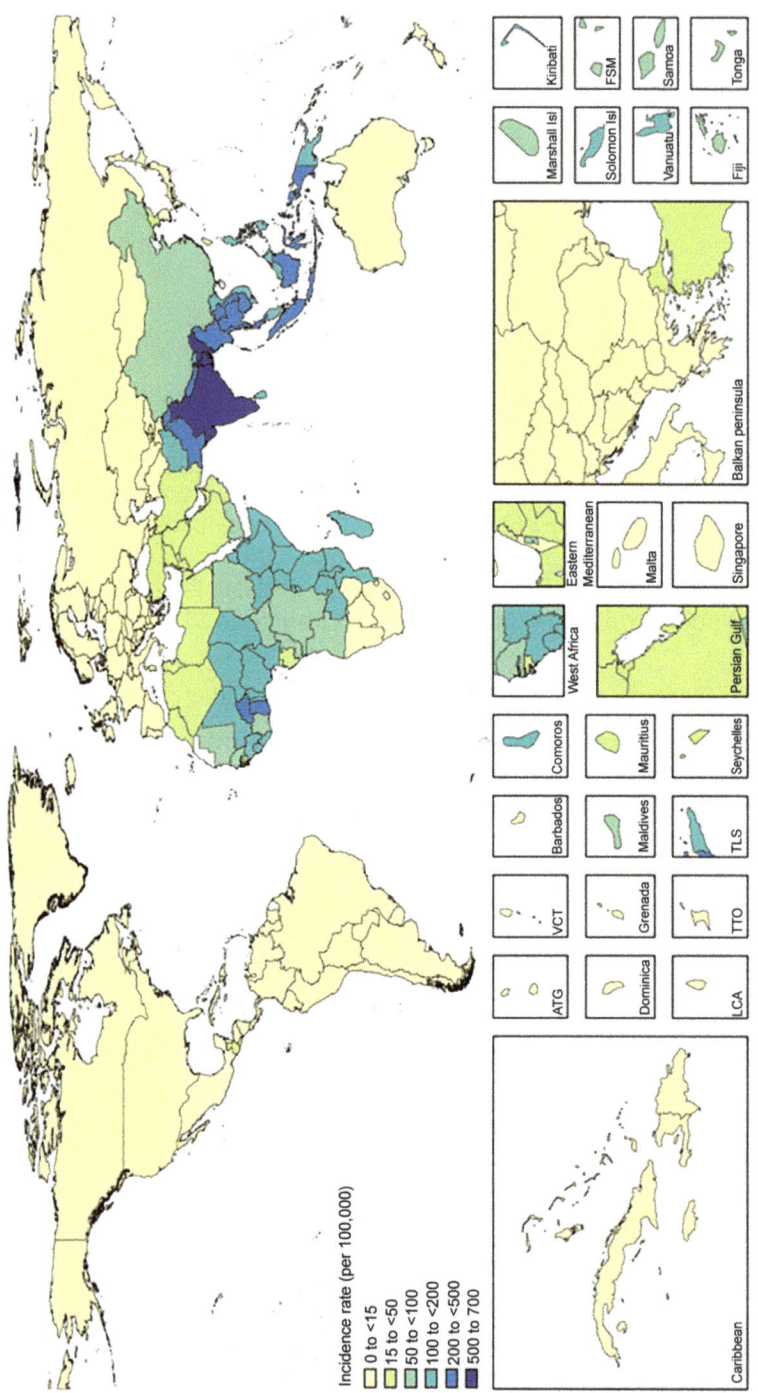

Fig. 1: Incidence rates (per 100,000) of typhoid and paratyphoid fevers, by country, in 2017.

3. How can typhoid fever be prevented?

The mode of transmission of typhoid fever is via fecal-oral route. WASH (water, sanitation, and hygiene) holds the key for prevention. Therefore, the best solution would be to provide the entire population with treated, bacteriologically monitored safe water for drinking and proper sanitation for disposal of human waste without contaminating water. Despite a great improvement in sanitation with success of *Swachh Bharat Abhiyan* leading to reduction in open defecation and some progress made in providing piped water to urban and rural masses still such principles of hygiene and public health remain at best a distant reality to be an effective preventive step and the only practical viable option is vaccination. Typhoid vaccines are on the WHO's list of essential medicines, which are the most effective and safe medicines needed within a health system.

4. What are the various types of typhoid vaccines manufactured?

Over the years, various types of typhoid vaccines have been manufactured and have been made available for vaccination from time to time. These are: parenteral vaccine and oral vaccine. There are two types of parenteral vaccine: (1) typhoid conjugate vaccine (TCV) and (2) polysaccharide vaccine **(Fig. 2 and Table 1)**.

- *Typhoid conjugate vaccine*: This is the newest type of typhoid vaccine using conjugation technique of vaccine production which increases the immunogenicity of a vaccine and makes it usable at a lower age. As the typhoid disease prevalence is higher in young children and infants, there was a need for a vaccine which can be used during infancy as the polysaccharide vaccine cannot be used in children below 2 years of age.

  In this, Vi capsular polysaccharide (Vi-CPS) has been conjugated with tetanus toxoid toxin. A major breakthrough in the field of vaccinology has been the method to conjugate polysaccharide vaccines making them T cell-dependent leading to immunogenic response even in infants and inducing long and lasting immunoglobulin G (IgG) response and T cell memory.

- Vi capsular polysaccharide vaccine: This is a subunit vaccine, first licensed in the United States in 1994 and is made from the purified

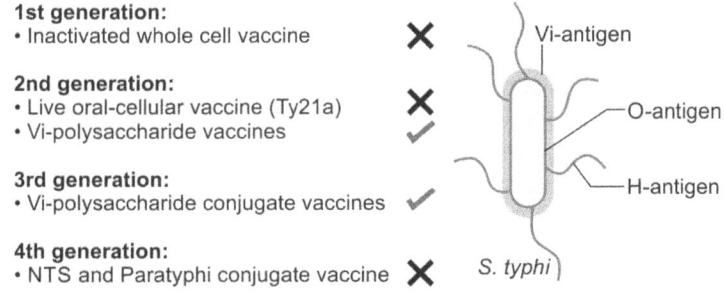

Fig. 2: Overview of typhoid vaccines.

TABLE 1: Comparative features of different types of typhoid vaccines.

Characteristics	Whole-cell killed vaccines	Ty21a	Vi-PS	TCV (Typbar-TCV™)
Type	Killed	Live	Subunit	Subunit
Route	Intramuscular (IM)/ Subcutaneous (SC)	Oral	IM/SC	IM
Doses	2	3	1	1
Revaccination	3–5 years	3–5 years	3 years	?
Immunogenicity	++	+	+	+++
Efficacy	51–79%	35–67%	55–72%	Around 80%
Duration of protection	7 years	7 years	3 years	Up to 5 years, at least
Herd immunity	?	Yes	?	?
Adverse effects	++++	+	++	++
Age group	>6 months	>6 years	>2 years	>6 months
Boostability	-	-	-	++
Mass vaccination	Unsuitable	Suitable	Suitable	Suitable
Availability	No	Not in India	Yes	Yes

Vi-CPS from the Ty2 *Salmonella typhi* strain. As for other polysaccharide vaccines, the Vi vaccine is not effective in children aged < 2 years. The vaccine is moderately immunogenic (approximately 65%) and requires repeat dosing every 3 years. Many different formulations are available, but only one, Typhim Vi™, is WHO prequalified.

The polysaccharide antigen stimulates B cells directly and T helper cells do not get stimulated. Being T cell-independent, it can induce only IgM antibody. IgM to IgG switch requires regulation by T helper cells. T-independent antigens do not induce the production of memory T cells or memory B cells, so, the serum antibody response is not boosted by administration of additional doses of Vi vaccine. As with other T cell-independent purified polysaccharide vaccine, it is not a good immunogen in children < 2 years of age and most infants fail to respond to this antigen.

– *Multivalent combination vaccines*: Combined Vi-CPS and hepatitis A vaccines (Hepatyrix™, GSK; Viatim™, Aventis Pasteur) contain 25 µg Vi polysaccharide (Vi-PS) antigen of *S. typhi* combined with either 1,440 ELU or 160 AU of inactivated hepatitis A virus grown in human diploid cells and adsorbed onto aluminum hydroxide.

• *Oral Ty21a live vaccine*: This vaccine was developed in the early 1970s, using mutagenic techniques, a mutant strain of *S. typhi* was produced which has a mutation in the galE gene and lacks enzyme uridine diphosphate galactose-4 epimerase. This enzyme is necessary for capsular polysaccharide formation as shown here.

$$\text{UDP Glucose} \xrightarrow{\text{UDP Gal-4 epimerase}} \text{UDP Galactose} \longrightarrow \text{Lipopolysaccharide (LPS) capsule}$$

Ty21a, the first live oral attenuated *Salmonella* vaccine was developed in Switzerland by chemical mutagenesis of wild-type *S. typhi* strain Ty2. This strain does not possess the functional galactose-epimerase gene and the Vi antigen and is highly attenuated.

This results incomplete lipopolysaccharide (LPS) which does not allow the bacteria to multiply beyond one or two generations making it immunogenic but not pathogenic. Ty21a is a galE mutant of *Salmonella typhi* which cannot synthesize Vi-PS capsule. This vaccine stimulates serum and mucosal antibodies to O, H, and other surface antigens and elicits strong cell-mediated immunity (CMI) but cannot stimulate Vi antibody production because the antigen is lacking.

The Ty21a also offers some protection against infection from *Salmonella* Paratyphi A and B. Ty21a is a moderately effective vaccine with an efficacy of 53–78% against culture-proven typhoid fever in large efficacy trials, conducted in Chile.

The Ty21a vaccine is available in two formulations: (1) liquid formulation for children above 2 years of age and (2) an enteric-coated capsule for administration to older children. The liquid formulation of Ty21a is licensed for use in individuals aged 2 years and above, whereas the enteric-coated capsule is available for individuals aged 5 years and above.

Limitations: Ty21a requires at least three doses for optimal protection and is supplied as gelatin capsules coated with phthalate. Each coated capsule contains $2–6 \times 10^9$ colony-forming units (CFU) of Ty21a, $5–50 \times 10^9$ nonviable Ty21a or sachets containing lyophilized Ty21a, a mutant strain of *Salmonella enterica* serovar typhi (*S. typhi*). The liquid formulation is not readily available. Another disadvantage of this vaccine is that it cannot be used in children below 6 years of age so in a country like India having a high disease burden in under-5 children, it is not very useful. The oral typhoid vaccine is not a WHO prequalified vaccine.

5. How efficacious are the Vi-CPS vaccines?

Two randomized controlled trials suggest an efficacy of this vaccine in the range of 64–72%.

Studies conducted among children above 2 years of age in Nepal, South Africa, China, India, and Pakistan demonstrated protective vaccine effectiveness/efficacy (VE) ranging from 31% in Pakistan to 72% in Nepal in different age groups. These vaccines have shown a reasonable duration of protection against typhoid fever that ranges from 2 to 3 years.

However, most of these studies have been done in children above 5 years of age and no data is available for the 2–5 years age group. There have been concerns that as this vaccine does not protect against Vi-negative *Salmonella*, widespread use might make it the dominant strain causing typhoid fever, though this concern has been largely baseless scientifically.

SECTION 2 Licensed Vaccines

Table 2 demonstrates the key features of vaccine effectiveness trial of Vi-CPS vaccine in India (Kolkata) and Pakistan (Karachi).

6. What are the limitations of Vi-CPS vaccines?

It is well known that these unconjugated Vi-PS vaccines are not effective in children below 2 years of age; however, their efficacy in the age group of 2–5 years is also not uniformly demonstrated. Two cluster-randomized effectiveness trials of Vi-PS typhoid vaccine in the low socioeconomic areas of Kolkata, India and Karachi, Pakistan were conducted. While in Kolkata, the vaccine was found highly effective [VE: 80% (95% CI, 53, 91)] in 2- to 5-year-old children with reasonably good herd protection, in Karachi, the same vaccine failed to provide any protection [VE: 38% (95% CI: –192, 35%)] in the younger age group and no herd effect was noticed **(Table 2)**.

There are several other limitations of Vi-PS vaccines **(Box 1)**. Being purely PS vaccine, these do not induce T-cell immunity; hence, there is no immune memory, and frequent revaccinations with extra doses are needed. The antibody response following the PS vaccine results in low titers of poor affinity IgG antibodies. Further, there is a possibility of hyporesponsiveness with subsequent doses of Vi-PS vaccines. The Vi-PS vaccine is also not fit

TABLE 2: A comparative analysis of the effectiveness trials of Vi-CPS vaccine in Kolkata and Karachi.

Attributes	Kolkata trial	Karachi trial
Time period	2004–2006	2002–2007
Vaccine used (Control vaccine: Havix)	Typherix®, GSK	Typherix®, GSK
Target population	2 years and above	2–16 years
Coverage (in Vi-vaccine cluster)	61%	52%
Vaccine effectiveness (VE) (among Vi-vaccine recipients)	61% (95% CI, 41, 75)	31% (95% CI:–28%, 63%)
VE 2–5 years	80% (95% CI, 53, 91)	–38% (95% CI:–192%, 35%)
VE 5–16 years	59% (95% CI, 18, 79)	57% (95% CI: 6%, 81%)
Overall VE (all residents of Vi vaccine clusters)	57% (95% CI: 37, 71)	26% (95% CI:–21%, 55%)
Herd effect VE (in vaccine clusters)	44% (95% CI: 2, 69)	–10% (95% CI:–116%, 44%)

BOX 1: Limitations of Vi-CPS vaccines.
- Short duration of protection
- Not effective in younger age groups
- Poor affinity antibodies
- T cell-independent immunity, no immune memory, frequent boosters are needed
- Hyporesponsiveness a theoretical concern
- Not fit for administration in combination with other routine childhood EPI vaccines

for coadministration with other routine childhood vaccines provided under "Expanded Program on Immunization (EPI)".

7. What is the status of first-generation, whole-cell inactivated typhoid vaccines? Are they still produced?

No, the old generation whole-cell vaccines are no longer produced now. Various types were invented depending on the process of inactivation namely heat inactivated phenol preserved, acetone inactivated, formol inactivated, and alcohol inactivated vaccines. Initially, these were a combination of typhoid and paratyphoid A and paratyphoid B vaccines. However, it was realized that paratyphoid is a less common cause of enteric fever and the vaccines have poor protection while at the same time increasing the adverse effects. Hence, from the TAB vaccine it became TA vaccine and later T vaccine, i.e., *S. typhi* vaccine. The efficacy of acetone inactivated preparation (79–88%) was better than the phenol killed (51–66%) vaccine. Now all these vaccines have been discontinued as safer vaccines have become available.

8. What are the key differences between a polysaccharide and a protein-polysaccharide conjugate vaccine?

Table 3 summarizes the key differentiating features of an unconjugate polysaccharide (PS) and a protein-polysaccharide conjugate vaccine.

9. Which was the first typhoid conjugate vaccine (TCV) developed globally?

The first typhoid conjugate polysaccharide vaccine Vi-rEPA was developed by Szu et al. in which the Vi-antigen of typhoid has been conjugated with the nontoxic recombinant exotoxin A of the *Pseudomonas aeruginosa*.

TABLE 3: Key differences between an unconjugate polysaccharide and a protein-polysaccharide conjugate vaccine.

Characteristic	Unconjugated polysaccharide vaccine	Conjugated protein-polysaccharide vaccine
Cells stimulated	B cells	B and T cells
Antibody titers, type	Low, IgM	High, IgG
Quality of antibody (Avidity)	Low	High
Cell-mediated immunity	Absent	Present
Duration of response	Short-lived	Long-lived
Immune memory	Poor	Strong
Booster response	Poor	Strong
Hyporesponsiveness (on repeated doses)	May be present	No
Effective ages	>2 years	All ages

Successful field trials in Vietnam on 13,766 children aged 2–4 years have shown the vaccine to be highly immunogenic (100% showing at least tenfold increase in Vi antibody levels). The efficacy was as high as 93% at 27 months of age when two doses were given at 6 weeks interval and 89% at 46 months postvaccination. Even with a single dose there was an efficacy of 91% and even the vaccines who developed typhoid had a milder disease. Further, trials are going on to validate these results especially in the infant age group. The side effects of fever and local reactions were seen in less than 2% vaccines making it very safe.

10. What are the different TCVs available in the market?

Currently, in Indian market, two different TCVs, Typbar-TCV™ and Zyvac-TCV™ are available. Another TCV, PedaTyph™ which was the first licensed TCV in the world and developed by M/s BioMed Ltd. is no longer freely available in the market. The TCV by M/s BBIL, India is the only WHO prequalified vaccine. **Tables 4 and 5** provide a comparative analysis and current status of all the available, previously developed, and upcoming TCVs.

11. The different TCVs displayed in Table 3 have employed different carrier proteins for conjugation with polysaccharide. Which is the best carrier protein to use for conjugation to get the best results?

Vi capsular PS is a linear homopolymer of (1→4) alpha-D-galacturonic acid with N- and O-acetylation at its O2 and O3 positions. The degree of O-acetylation, which may be variable in different Vi-PS preparations, influences the immunogenicity of a glycoconjugate the most. Therefore, it is necessary to quantify the optimal level of O-acetylation that can provide adequate antigenic stimulation. The immunodominant epitopes of Vi-PS molecule are the two hydrophobic groups, O-acetyl and N-acetyl, which overhang on both sides of the PS, whereas the carboxyl groups are less exposed; hence, they remain an insignificant determinant of Vi-PS immunogenicity. The carboxyl group is, therefore, selected as the linking site for carrier protein **(Fig. 3)**.

The most critical step in the development of a Vi-PS protein conjugate is the selection of a correct "linker scheme". In clinical settings, the two commonly employed schemes are hetero-bi-functional cross-linker N-succinimidyl-3-(2-pyridyldithio) propionate (SPDP) and homo-bi-functional linker adipic acid dihydrazide (ADH). The protein-ADH scheme consistently elicited a higher amount of anti-Vi IgG antibodies than the SPDP scheme.

Four different carrier proteins have been employed in the production of different TCVs so far. They include recombinant exoprotein A from *Pseudomonas aeruginosa* (rEPA), tetanus toxoid (TT), diphtheria toxoid (DT), and cross-reactive material 197 (CRM197), a nontoxic mutant of diphtheria toxin **(Table 4)**. The immunogenicity of a glycoconjugate is affected more by the degree of O-acetylation and conjugation scheme rather than the carrier protein used or the source of Vi-PS.

TABLE 4: Comparative analysis of few key typhoid conjugate vaccines (TCVs).

Vaccine attributes	Typbar-TCV	PedaTyph	Vi-rEPA	Vi-CRM197	Vi-DT
Developer/Manufacturer	Bharat Biotech International Ltd., India	BioMed Pvt Ltd., India	National Institutes of Health, USA	Novartis Vaccines Institute for Global Health, Italy	International Vaccine Institute, Korea
Vi-PS dose	25 µg	5 µg	25 µg	5 µg	25 µg
Carrier protein	Tetanus toxoid	Tetanus toxoid	Recombinant exoprotein A from Pseudomans	CRM197	Diphtheria toxoid
Source of Vi polysaccharide	Ty2 strain of S. typhi	S. typhi	S. typhi	Citrobacter freundii	S. typhi strain from India (C6524)
Study group	6 months–45 years	3 months–12 years	2 years to adults; infants (Unpublished)	6 weeks–45 years	2–45 years (Phase II and III trials ongoing)
Dose schedule	Single dose	Two doses	Two doses	Two to three doses (Biological E Ltd. is using 25 µg of Vi-PS in a single dose)	Two doses
Trial under 2 years of age	Yes	Yes	Yes (Unpublished)	Yes	No
Efficacy/effectiveness study	No (trials ongoing)	Yes	Yes	No	No
Long-term protection	Up to 5 years	Up to 2.5 years	Up to 4 years in 2–5 years old children	Not examined	Not examined
Booster responses: elicited	Yes	Not studied	Yes (Unpublished, NIH trials)	No, titers decreased after booster dose	Not studied
Licensure	In 2013	In 2009 in India	Not licensed	Not licensed	Not licensed
WHO prequalification	Yes	No	NA	Interest shown for WHO-PQ	Interest shown for WHO-PQ

TABLE 5: Current status of different typhoid conjugate vaccines (TCVs).				
Typbar-TCV	PedaTyph	Vi-rEPA	Vi-CRM197	Vi-DT
• Licensed in India and Nepal • M/s Cadila Healthcare Limited, India has developed a similar product Zyvac TCV™, based on Vi-TT conjugation employing 25 µg of Vi-PS; got national licensure and market authorization in 2018 in India	• Licensed in India • No interest shown in WHO-PQ • Not freely available now	• Technology transfer to Lanzhou Institute of Biological Products (LIBP), China • LIBP, China has completed phase 3 in adults, preschool and school-aged children • Submitted for licensure for use in persons >2 years old	• Technology transfer to Biological E Ltd. India • Biological E Ltd., India (in partnership with GSK) and Eubiologics, South Korea are developing this vaccine; BE with 25 µg dose of Vi-PS • Interest expressed to apply for WHO-PQ	• Technology transfer to four different manufacturers, i.e., Shantha Biotechnics (India), PT Biofarma (Indonesia), SK Chemicals (Korea), and Incepta (Bangladesh) • Phase 3 trial in progress • Davac (Vietnam) and Finlay Institute (Cuba), are also developing Vi-DT conjugate • Shantha Biotechnics (India) has stopped development • Finlay Institute (Cuba) in most advanced stage

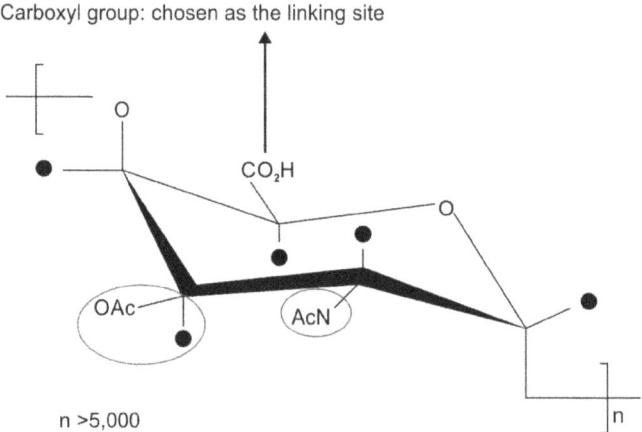

Fig. 3: Vi-PS structure at the molecular level.

12. What is "epitope suppression"?

There is a concern that a "pre-exposure" or "co-exposure" of a carrier protein containing TT or DT can adversely affect the immunogenicity of the carbohydrate moiety to which conjugation is done through a phenomenon referred to as "epitope suppression". However, as stated above, the type of carrier protein is not the sole criteria, and many other factors such as chemical linking, PS size, the degree of O-acetylation and presence of a spacer affect the final immunogenicity of glycoconjugate vaccines. It needs to be emphasized that the making of a Vi-protein conjugate is a complex process and every Vi conjugate product is distinct.

13. What should be the optimal dose of Vi-PS for an ideal TCV?

The two licensed TCVs, the Typbar-TCV™ and PedaTyph™, contain 25 and 5 µg of Vi-PS, respectively. The two experimental TCVs, the Vi-rEPA and Vi-CRM, also have a different amount of Vi-PS **(Table 4)**. The amount of PS in the currently used other conjugate vaccines ranges from 2 µg/injection for pneumococcal conjugate vaccines to 10 µg/mL for *Haemophilus influenzae* type b. The first, experimental TCV, Vi-rEPA employed 25 µg of PS. The dose of 25 µg was selected based on the amount of PS present in the licensed Vi-PS vaccine.

As per the WHO guidelines to vaccine manufacturers, it is mandatory to determine an adequate dose and schedule of a candidate TCV, and extrapolation must be avoided even if the same carrier protein is employed. The immunogenicity of the Vi-PS conjugate vaccines is found to be dose dependent.

The issue of the exact dose of Vi-PS in a TCV is still unsettled. A very low antigen dose of 1.25 µg of Vi-PS in TCV was found as immunogenic or even better than 25 µg/dose of unconjugated Vi-PS vaccine in a trial of another TCV employing CRM197 as a carrier protein. Most of the manufacturers of TCVs have adopted a high-end dose, 25 µg of Vi-PS, in their upcoming products **(Tables 4 and 5)**. However, more studies are needed, mainly, on long-term effectiveness trials, to get a final answer.

14. Tell us in detail about PedaTyph™, the first TCV licensed in India.

In India, PedaTyph™ was introduced by M/s BioMed. PedaTyph was the first TCV to be licensed in India. In this, Vi-CPS has been conjugated with tetanus toxoid toxin **(Table 4)**. There is little field efficacy data for this vaccine. A randomized comparative trial was conducted in 400 healthy Indian children aged 3 months to 5 years who received one dose of PedaTyph (n = 200) or two doses 8 weeks apart (n = 200). In 101 children aged < 2 years and 24 children aged < 1 year who were available for follow-up, a seroconversion rate (≥4-fold increase over preimmunization titer) of 83% was reported at 8 weeks postvaccination, with the highest seroconversion rate in infants (seroconversion rates of 73%, 89%, and 96% for children aged > 2 years, ≤ 2 years, and < 1 year, respectively). The vaccine in this study was found to be highly immunogenic in infants and children < 2 years of age.

A quasi-randomized, open-label trial (OLT) was conducted post-licensure in 905 Kolkata children aged 6 months to 12 years who received two doses of PedaTyph 6 weeks apart and were followed with active surveillance for 1 year, along with 860 unvaccinated controls. Incidence of culture-positive typhoid fever in the control group was 1.27% and zero in the vaccinated group. In a subgroup evaluated for immunogenicity, an antibody titer value of 1.8 EU/mL (95% CI, 1.5, 2.2), 32 EU/mL (95% CI, 27.0, 39.0), and 14 EU/mL (95% CI, 12.0, 17.0) at baseline, 6 weeks, and 12 months, respectively, was observed. Seroconversion among the subgroup was 100% after 6 weeks postvaccination and 83% after 12 months considering a fourfold rise from baseline. The efficacy of the vaccine was 100% (95% CI, 97.6, 100) in the first year of follow-up, with minimal adverse events postvaccination. PedaTyph was licensed in India in 2009 and is recommended for children aged > 3 months as a single dose of 0.5 mL followed by boosters at age 2.5–3 years.

15. What are the specific details available about the only WHO-PQ vaccine, Typbar-TCV™?

Bharat Biotech in Hyderabad, India, developed a TCV using tetanus toxoid as the carrier protein with Vi-PS. **Table 4** provides details about Typbar-TCV. This vaccine has been tested in children (aged 2–17 years) for safety, immunogenicity, and dose ranging. In a clinical trial, the immunogenicity of Vi-TT was compared to that of the polysaccharide vaccine in 981 participants (age 6 months–45 years). There were fourfold seroconversion rates in each treatment arm at 6 weeks postvaccination.

In a randomized controlled trial, Typbar-TCV recipients attained higher anti-Vi IgG geometric mean titers (GMTs) 42 days after immunization [seroconversion (SCN), 97%; GMT, 1,293 (95% confidence interval (CI), 1,153–1,449)] than recipients of Vi-PS vaccine, Typbar [SCN, 93%; GMT, 411 (95% CI, 359–471); $p < 0.001$)]. Typbar-TCV was highly immunogenic in the open-label trial [SCN, 98%; GMT, 1,937 (95% CI, 1,785–2,103)].

In a randomized controlled trial, 2 years after vaccination, anti-Vi titers remained higher in Typbar-TCV recipients [GMT, 82 (95% CI, 73–92)] and exhibited higher avidity [geometric mean avidity index (GMAI), 60%] than in Typbar recipients [GMT, 46 (95% CI, 40–53); GMAI, 46%; $p < 0.001$]. Typbar-TCV™ recipients achieved GMT of 48 (95% CI, 42–55) and GMAI of 57%. Typbar-TCV induced multiple IgG subclasses and strong booster responses in all ages. No serious vaccine-attributable adverse events were observed.

Based on the above results, the Bharat Biotech received marketing authorization for Typbar-TCV in India in 2013. Additional studies were conducted with Typbar-TCV to demonstrate noninterference of measles-containing vaccine when administered simultaneously to age-eligible recipients. Study results showed that TCV can be successfully coadministered with measles vaccine at age 9 months without interfering with the immune response to measles at 4 and 8 weeks postvaccination compared to baseline.

16. What are the key trials conducted so far with the Typbar-TCV™ vaccine?

There are five trials conducted so far with the Typbar-TCV™.
- A randomized controlled trial Typbar-TCV versus Typbar vaccine in subjects 2–45 years of age (pivotal trial)

- An open-label trial < 2 years to assess the safety and immunogenicity of Typbar-TCV in infants 6–11 months and toddlers 12–23 months (pivotal trial)
- A randomized controlled trial comparing Typbar-TCV versus Typhim Vi in 2–15 years of age
- Coadministration of Typbar-TCV with measles (at 9 months) and MMR (measles, mumps and rubella) (at 15 months)
- Human challenge trial in adults
- An efficacy trial of Typbar-TCV in Nepal, 2019.

Apart from these trials, a large, community-based effectiveness trial is underway in Navi Mumbai, India.

17. What are the key takeaways from these trials?

- The Typbar-TCV elicits significantly higher titers of Vi IgG Ab than Vi-PS (both after primary and booster immunization; boostability is demonstrated).
- Typbar-TCV produces higher amount of high avidity antibodies than Vi-PS vaccine.
- Duration of elevated Vi IgG antibody titers till 5 years after a single dose in both groups (6–23 months and 2–45 years).
- In 6–23 months old cohort, children still had elevated titers after 3 years (around 80%) and 5 years (around 75%).
- Human challenge study shows that Typbar-TCV offers better protection.
- A retrospective analysis of seroresponses calculated the efficacy of Typbar-TCV and found it around 85%.

18. What was the efficacy of Typbar-TCV vaccine in the human challenge study in adults?

The human challenge study with Typbar-TCV™ was conducted in naïve adult volunteers in a nonendemic setting. The Typbar-TCV™ was found to have an estimated efficacy of 54.6% (95% CI: 26.8–71.8%) based on the original primary endpoint of persistent fever or *S. typhi* bacteremia and 87.1% (95% CI: 47.2–96.9%) based on a *post hoc* analysis of alternative diagnostic criteria of persistent fever followed by positive blood culture. The respective figures for the comparator Vi-PS vaccine were 52.0 (23.2–70.0) and 52.3% (−4.2–78.2).

19. In a retrospective seroefficacy trial (Voysey M et al., 2018) calculated the efficacy of Typbar-TCV around 85%. What is the basis of this study?

The vaccine efficacy can be computed from immunogenicity data alone, by modeling serologically defined infections and comparing the incidence of these infections between randomized groups in a clinical trial. The detection of Vi-antibody responses to natural exposure can be used to estimate the incidence of clinical or subclinical infections if blood samples are taken from participants at appropriate times and Vi IgG antibodies are serially measured. These spikes in anti-Vi IgG antibodies may serve as a marker of typhoid infection. Antibody decay was analyzed using a Gaussian mixture model during two-time periods (6 weeks–18 months; and 18–24 months). That a single Vi immunization would lead to a decay of antibody in the first period and that anyone with higher levels of antibody at 18 months than at 6 weeks postimmunization, had had an additional exposure to Vi antigen.

However, since the timing of an infection is unpredictable, infection events may be missed if the antibody response to exposure is small or if the antibody has waned by the time a blood sample is taken.

Voysey M et al. (Clin Infect Dis. 2018) obtained data from a previously published phase 3 randomized controlled trial comparing Typbar-TCV with Vi-PS vaccine in participants aged 2–45 years. An additional open-label arm administered Typbar-TCV to children aged 6–23 months. The proportion of participants with presumed clinical or subclinical infection ("seroincidence") was determined using mixture models and compared using relative risks (RRs). They studied 387 participants, 21% were classified as having presumed typhoid infection during the 2-year postvaccination period. The seroincidence was lower in participants randomized to Typbar-TCV rather than Vi-PS.

There was no difference in seroincidence for Typbar-TCV between those aged 2–45 years and those aged 6–23 months. The researchers calculated the vaccine seroefficacy as 85% (95% CI, 80–88%).

20. Does measurement of anti-Vi IgG antibodies sufficient? What more is required?

No. Antibodies, produced in response to both typhoid infection and vaccination, are generally used as the gold standard for measuring vaccine immunogenicity even though their role in clearance of *S. typhi* infections is undefined, and not properly understood. The protection is primarily conferred by higher level of anti-Vi antibodies as suggested by both the earlier trials of Vi-PS vaccine.

However, serum IgG titers were found to be poor correlates of protection for Vi-PS vaccines in some communities. In the recent human challenge study of Typbar-TCV™, no significant difference in titers of anti-Vi IgG antibodies was found between individuals who were diagnosed with typhoid fever and those who did not in the Typbar-TCV™ group. This observation suggests that antibody functionality is equally important for protection as total antibody quantity. Role of subclasses of IgG antibodies (IgG1–IgG4) is emerging, and functional Vi-antibodies such as those involved with neutralization, opsonization and/or antibody-dependent cellular-cytotoxicity activity, etc., may be more important determinant of protection. In the trials of Vi-PS vaccine, IgG2 titers were found to be main determinant of protection. Similarly, antibody avidity is also considered as a main factor responsible for the strength of the anamnestic response.

21. It means that functional antibodies are more significant determinant of protection against typhoid fever. What is the current thinking and knowledge about typhoid immunity?

Immunity to *S. typhi* is complex and involves both systemic antibodies (against O, H, Vi, and other *S. typhi* antigens) and local (IgA) antibodies along with CMI. Because *S. typhi* can persist intracellularly in the human host, CMI is expected to be essential in eliminating *S. typhi* infection thus preventing carrier stage. Both CD4+ helper T cells and CD8+ cytotoxic T cells might play key roles in defense against *S. typhi*, and recent reports suggest a more dominant role of CMI in protection against typhoid. Evidences gathered through trials of live attenuated, oral Ty21a vaccine reveal that CMI responses consist of both Th1-type [cytokine production such as interferon-gamma (IFN-γ), tumor necrosis factor-alpha (TNF-α), etc.] and cytotoxic T cell responses (elimination of cells infected with intracellular organisms) along with lymphoproliferation. However, in these trials, no correlations were observed between CMI and serum antibody responses.

The role of gut homing, circulating IgA antibody-secreting cells (ASCs) in providing protection against the typhoid was studied in Ty21a trials. The magnitude of the IgA ASC responses against O antigen after immunization with Ty21a correlated with efficacy. However, boost in IgA ASC responses did not correlate with serum anti-*S. typhi* lipopolysaccharide O responses.

Hence, human immunity to *S. typhi* elicited by immunization is quite wide and complex. However, the immunologic "correlate of protection" (CoP) remains mostly indeterminate. It is critical to identify which immune responses, if any, correlate with the protection. This information will be of utmost significance to select a consistent CoP for evaluation of next-generation typhoid vaccines. Further, this would greatly facilitate the licensing and availability of the new TCVs and should obviate the needs of costly and time-consuming efficacy trials.

22. In some earlier trials, attempts were made to determine a reliable immune correlate of protection (CoP) for typhoid vaccines. Is there any CoP for typhoid conjugate vaccines known?

In the past, several attempts were made to decide a reliable CoP for TCV. However, these attempts were limited by the lack of efficacy trials with TCV because only one large efficacy trial of any TCV has been conducted so far. During the Vi-rEPA efficacy trial, the CoP was first proposed to be 8.7 µg/mL of anti-Vi IgG level based on the 27 months of active surveillance and subsequently lowered to 4.3 µg/mL (equal to 3.52 EUs) at 46 months. Later, in a reanalysis of the anti-Vi IgG levels in different age groups of children in the Vietnam efficacy trial, a much lower estimate (in the range of 1.4–2.0 µg/mL) was described. The WHO has also analyzed the clinical data of Vi-rEPA and concluded that it is not possible to identify a cutoff based on the old National Institutes of Health (NIH)-sponsored trial data. So, currently, no exact CoP is known.

23. Different vaccine manufacturers are using different enzyme-linked immunosorbent assay (ELISA) kits to study anti-Vi antibodies levels. Is there a need for a standardized international reference and validation of ELISA kits?

Yes, there is an urgent need of having validation of different ELISA kits used in immunogenicity trials. Before any cutoff based on protective antibody level is applied to a new candidate TCV, it is of paramount importance to calibrate ELISA kits used by different vaccine manufacturers in their trials. To evaluate new TCVs, it is essential to quantify anti-Vi IgG antibodies in serum accurately. Currently, the antibody levels are expressed in EUs assigned arbitrarily by different laboratories. However, the assignment of EU varies extensively among different developers with no common reference to calibrate. This shortcoming rendered the comparison of clinical results of different trials nearly impossible. A standardized human reference is essential to estimate and compare the immune responses of a candidate TCV with the existing known levels.

24. How effective was the Typbar-TCV vaccine in efficacy trial conducted in Nepal?

According to early, interim analysis after 12 months, the Typbar-TCV has around 80% efficacy against culture-proven typhoid fever in children.

Following is the detail of the trial:
In this phase III, participant- and observer-blinded randomized controlled trial in Lalitpur, Nepal, children aged 9 months to <16 years of age, were randomized 1:1 to receive either TCV or a group A meningococcal conjugate vaccine (Men A) as control. Here the interim analysis after 12 months of follow-up, for safety, immunogenicity and efficacy are presented.

About 10,005 participants received TCV and 10,014 received Men A. Blood culture-confirmed typhoid fever occurred in 7 participants who received TCV and 38 receiving Men A; vaccine efficacy: 81.6% (95% CI, 58.8%, 91.8%, $p < 0.001$).

Overall, 132 SAEs occurred in the first 6 months with one (pyrexia) identified as vaccine-related. The participant remains blinded. Seroconversion (≥4-fold rise in Vi IgG 28 days after vaccination) was 99% in the TCV group (N = 677/683) and 2% in the control group (N = 8/380). This is the first large-scale, individually randomized controlled trial of Vi-TCV in children in an endemic setting.

25. Apart from PedaTyph™ and Typbar-TCV™, one more TCV with the brand name of Zyvac-TCV™ is available in Indian market. Is it the same vaccine as Typbar-TCV™?

No, this is another TCV developed by M/s Zydus Cadila, using tetanus toxoid as the carrier protein. Phase 2 and 3 clinical trials were conducted at seven sites in India for immune noninferiority with Typbar-TCV (238 participants in all age groups). After this noninferiority study, a dossier was submitted to Indian National Regulatory Authority for marketing authorization in India.

This vaccine is now licensed in India as a single dose of 25 µg from age 6 months onward.

26. What is the status of another TCV, being developed by the International Vaccine Institute (IVI) South Korea? How does it differ from the existing TCV?

With initial know-how from the US NIH, IVI scientists at Manila developed the TCV, which consists of the Vi-PS purified from *S. typhi* chemically conjugated to diphtheria toxoid. IVI transferred the technology for production and quality control of Vi-DT to three manufacturing partners (SK Chemicals, South Korea; Biofarma, Indonesia; and Incepta, Bangladesh) and is working with them to complete the clinical development with the aim of local licensure and later on WHO prequalification. Two partner manufacturers (SK Chemicals, South Korea and Biofarma, Indonesia) have completed phase 1 clinical trials. Following the successful completion of a Phase II trial among children aged between 6–23 months, large-scale Phase III studies with a single-dose of Vi-DT have started in the Philippines and Nepal in 2020. So, more options of TCVs vaccines are in the pipeline. The current status of different typhoid conjugate vaccines (TCVs) is given in **Table 5**.

27. There are many reports of vaccinated children developing culture-proven typhoid fever despite having received even two doses of TCV. How will you explain this phenomenon?

One should remember that no vaccine is 100% effective and breakthrough cases may surface. The same is true even for the current generation of TCVs. At best, they provide moderate protection against typhoid fever, in the range of 60–70%. Hence, it is not unusual to find few cases of vaccine failure.

28. What is the administration schedule of TCV in India? What is the WHO and Indian Academy of Pediatrics (IAP), Advisory Committee on Vaccines and Immunization Practices (ACVIP) guidelines?

In the March 2018 position paper on typhoid vaccines, the WHO recommended the administration of TCV as a 0.5 mL single dose for infants and children from 6 months of age and in adults up to 45 years in typhoid endemic regions. The WHO recommended the introduction of TCV in the National Immunization Program (NIP) at the same time as other vaccine visits at 9 months of age (MR/MMR), or in the second year of life. The WHO also recommended catch-up vaccination with TCV up to 15 years of age. The need for a second dose or a booster was not recommended as per available data.

These recommendations were based on the background paper to the Strategic Advisory Group of Experts (SAGE) on typhoid vaccine policy recommendations prepared by the SAGE Working Group on Typhoid Vaccines and the WHO Secretariat in its version dated 24 September 2017. At that time, the 5-year follow-up data of Typbar-TCV was available, which showed persistence of high GMTs and seroconversion rates (SCRs) till the end of 5 years. In its 2018–2019 recommendations, the IAP ACVIP endorsed these recommendations in toto.

29. Current recommendations on Typbar-TCV suggest no indication for booster doses for children or adults in typhoid endemic regions. Do you concur with the above schedule? Do you think there is no need of a booster dose of TCV?

Deciding the need and the appropriate timing of a booster dose of TCV is somewhat problematic. The schedule may differ among different age groups and populations. The older children may get considerable natural boosting especially in a highly endemic setting. On the other hand, regular boosters may be required in certain low endemic regions so that a minimum concentration of antibodies is maintained to confer protection.

For young children, particularly those under 2 years of age, some key issues need to be considered before recommending a "single-dose, no-booster" policy.

- First, as a rule, immune responses elicited during infancy and young age lack certain key "immunological edifices" needed for providing a long-lasting immunity owing to immaturity of immune system.
- In some of the trials with candidate TCVs, there is a perceptible drop in the anti-Vi IgG titers at 6–12 months after vaccination following an initial rise in the antibody levels after the first dose. Whether this observation warrants consideration of a booster dose, is difficult to determine in the absence of reliable knowledge about the protective antibody levels in different age groups.
- In the last, due to comparatively lower burden of typhoid infection below 2 years of age than in 2–5 years age group, there is limited opportunity to get natural boosting secondary to subclinical infections.

30. So, what should be the ideal schedule of TCV in different age groups?

It is difficult to sketch out an administration schedule for a vaccine where you do not have any known CoP, no long-term immunogenicity data, a heterogeneous population in terms of susceptibility, and most importantly, no long-term efficacy data. Nevertheless, based on the available data, following schedule can be practiced till more information becomes available:

Under 2 years of age (<2 years)
- *Primary dose:* At 9 months along with MMR.
- *Booster:* Booster at 2 years of age.
- *Catch-up schedule (<2 years):* Single dose between 9 and 23 months followed by a booster dose either at 2 years of age or after 2 years of first dose. However, a minimum 6 months gap should be there between the two doses.

Giving the booster at 2 years will have additional advantages also:
- Maturation of immune system.

TABLE 6: Typbar-TCV™ long-term immunogenicity data—unboosted cohort [open-label trial (OLT) and randomized controlled trial (RCT) cohorts].

Parameter	42 days	2 years	3 years	5 years	7 years
Cohor 2 (RCT) 2–45 years					
GMTs	1301.44	81.7	81.9	106.9	61.57
SC (>4 folds)	97.3%	74.1%	83.6%	69.2%	59.3%
Cohort 1 (OLT) 6 months–2 years					
GMTs	1937	48.7	58.4	80.16	54.3
SC (>4 folds)	98.05%	59.5%	72.7%	76.6	45.34

TABLE 7: Typbar-TCV™ long-term immunogenicity data—boosted cohort [open-label trial (OLT) and randomized controlled trial (RCT) cohorts].

Parameter	Day 0	Day 42	2 years (720D)	42 days after booster (762D)	3 years	5 years	7 years
Cohort 2 (RCT) 2–45 years							
GMTs	10.4	1292.5	81.7	1685.3	287.09	179.2	130.5
SC		97.3%	74.1%		90.2%	86.2%	80.3%
Cohort 1 (OLT) 6 months–2 years							
GMTs	9.5	1937.4	48.7	1721.9	302.68	132.29	101.7
SC		98.05%	59.5%		92.4%	83.78	66.06

- Documentation of immune kinetics since the parent company of Typbar-TCV had also given a booster at 2 years of age.
- Taking into consideration the impact of natural boosting.

Above 2 years of age (>2 years)
- *Primary schedule:* Single dose of TCV.
- *Booster dose/s:* Single booster dose after 5 years of primary dose.

There is definite waning of seroconversion (**SCR:** Seroconversion rate—Those vaccinated and still having more than fourfold rise in Vi IgG antibodies) at 5 years in unboosted cohort after an initial, smaller boost (probably, secondary to subclinical infections). However, this fall is not visible in the GMTs levels. In one study titres based on the titers in the **boosted cohort**, there is gradual waning starting from 6 weeks after the boosting till 7 years **(Tables 6 and 7)**. Similar gradual waning is visible in **"Avidity Index"** also.

Further, one should remember the fact that unconjugate Vi-PS typhoid vaccines do provide protection up to 3 years postprimary immunization (based on data in the large efficacy trials).

Since there is no known CoP and no efficacy trial with long-term follow-ups, it is difficult to predict the future needs of further booster doses of the vaccine.

Ideally, this issue should be settled with either a known CoP or through long-term follow-ups of subjects in large, prospective, efficacy/effectiveness studies. One can also have an assessment of CoP based on the efficacy data if immune responses are measured serially as happened with Vi-rEPA trial. It may be hazardous to extrapolate data from Vi-rEPA to Vi-TT TCV vaccine.

31. With the ready availability of TCVs, is there any role of unconjugated Vi-PS typhoid vaccines?

Though both conjugate and unconjugated Vi-PS vaccines can be used in the age group of >2 years. However, available data and WHO Position Paper on Typhoid Vaccines published in 2018 favors conjugate vaccine since it has higher seroprotection and GMCs than polysaccharide vaccine and longer protection which obliviates the need to administer boosters at regular intervals. Furthermore, the quality of antibodies induced by TCVs is superior than those elicited by Vi-PS vaccines as evident by the higher avidity index of TCVs. The only justification of still using Vi-PS vaccines could be their lower cost than TCVs.

32. What are the limitations of the existing TCVs?

- The current TCVs are only "moderately" efficacious.
- There are no large scale, long-term field efficacy data available for the licensed products.
- The Human Challenge study with Typbar-TCV˚ was conducted in naïve adult and in a nonendemic setting.
- Do not provide protection against Paratyphi A and nontyphoidal *Salmonella* (NTS).
- Ineffective against Vi-negative *S. typhi* strains.
- Do not produce broad immune responses including CMI.
- Fail to induce intestinal secretory IgA (sIgA) response.
- Expensive to develop.

33. What are the options to deal with limitations of the existing TCVs? What are the new developments in the field of typhoid vaccines?

Considering the above-mentioned limitations of the TCVs, there is a need for new typhoid vaccines which are more efficacious and have serotype-independent coverage against all *Salmonella* strains. There are new advanced technologies underway to develop more effective and broadly protective typhoid vaccines. A few such novel approaches include the use of single or multiprotein subunit vaccines, use of novel linking methods and exploration of the dual role of proteins as a carrier and protective antigen. Although protein subunit vaccines may overcome some of the limitations of TCVs, yet the challenge is to recognize suitable antigens that can be developed into effective human vaccines. One such protein antigen could be the outer membrane vesicles (OMVs) which are secreted naturally from

> **BOX 2:** Future perspectives on new generation of typhoid vaccines.
> - Need of new typhoid vaccines having higher efficacy and serotype-independent coverage
> - Single or multiprotein subunit vaccines
> - Novel linking methods in which covalent bonding may not be required, and protein carriers can be directly coupled to activated glycans
> - Use of novel carrier systems like nanoparticles
> - Use of antigens universally present in all *S. typhi* such as O-specific polysaccharides
> - Exploration of dual role of proteins as carrier and protective antigen.

several gram-negative bacteria including *Salmonella* and have already been used in some vaccine development studies. The OMVs contain LPS and other membrane proteins that act as a natural adjuvant and are found protective against both *S. typhi* and Paratyphi A.

Another exciting development is the exploration of new ways to present carbohydrate antigens to the immune system. Conventionally, PS antigens are covalently attached to carrier proteins to convert T-independent antigens into T-dependent ones. The evidence is now emerging that the covalent bonding may not be required, and protein carriers can be directly coupled to activated glycans to introduce functional groups for subsequent conjugation. Genetically modified proteins can also be employed to predetermine the site of linking with PS for *in vivo* expression. These new advancements along with the use of novel carrier systems such as nanoparticles have been projected as alternative methods to develop new glycoconjugates.

With the looming threat of Vi-negative strains, there is a greater focus on antigens universally present in all *S. typhi* such as O-specific PSs. These new typhoid vaccines will be considerably cost-effective than the TCVs at present. Unlike Vi-based vaccines, these would be effective against Vi-negative strains as well as *Salmonella* Paratyphi A infection **(Box 2)**.

34. A new generation typhoid vaccine using a new technology has recently undergone phase 1 trial. Write the details of this vaccine and the trial.

The vaccine is named Typhax™, being developed by M/s Matrivax as an alternative to conjugate vaccines. The manufacturer has applied a novel "virtual conjugation" Protein Capsular Matrix Vaccine (PCMV) technology to manufacture, which is composed of Vi-PS entrapped in a cross-linked CRM197 matrix.

A randomized, double-blinded, dose escalating phase 1 study was performed to compare the safety and immunogenicity of three dose levels of aluminum phosphate adjuvanted Typhax (0.5 µg, 2.5 µg, or 10 µg of Vi antigen) to the comparator vaccine, Typhim Vi.

Following one dose of Typhax™, seroconversion rates at day 28 were 12.5%, 77.8%, and 66.7% at the 0.5 µg, 2.5 µg, and 10 µg dose levels, respectively, compared to 55.6% and 0% in the Typhim Vi and placebo groups, respectively.

The results from this phase 1 clinical trial indicate that Typhax™ is safe, well tolerated, and immunogenic. After a single dose, Typhax™ at the 2.5 µg and 10 µg dose levels elicited comparable anti-Vi IgG titers and seroconversion rates as a single dose of Typhim Vi (25 µg dose). A second dose of Typhax™ at day 28 did not elicit a booster response. All Typhax™ vaccine regimens were well tolerated, and adverse events were low in number and primarily characterized as mild in intensity and similar in incidence across the treatment groups.

SUGGESTED READING

1. Browne AJ, Kashef Hamadani BH, Kumaran E, Rao P, Longbottom J, Harriss E, et al. Drug-resistant enteric fever worldwide, 1990 to 2018: a systematic review and meta-analysis. BMC Med. 2020;18:1.
2. Cartee RT, Thanawastien A, Griffin IV TJ, Mekalanos JJ, Bart S, Killeen KP. A phase 1 randomized safety, reactogenicity, and immunogenicity study of Typhax: a novel protein capsular matrix vaccine candidate for the prevention of typhoid fever. PLoS Negl Trop Dis. 2020;14(1):e0007912.
3. Coalition Against Typhoid. (2018). Typhoid vaccines. [online] Available from: https://www.coalitionagainsttyphoid.org/the-issues/typhoid-vaccines/ [Last accessed September, 2020].
4. GBD 2017 Typhoid and Paratyphoid Collaborators. The global burden of typhoid and paratyphoid fevers: a systematic analysis for the Global Burden of Disease Study 2017. Lancet Infect Dis. 2019;19(4):369-81.
5. John J, Van Aart CJ, Grassly NC. The burden of typhoid and paratyphoid in India: systematic review and meta-analysis. PLoS Negl Trop Dis. 2016;10:e0004616.
6. Khan MI, Soofi SB, Ochiai RL, Habib MA, Sahito SM, Nizami SQ, et al. Effectiveness of Vi capsular polysaccharide typhoid vaccine among children: a cluster randomized trial in Karachi, Pakistan. Vaccine. 2012;30:5389-95.
7. Klugman KP, Koornhof HJ, Robbins JB, Le Cam NN. Immunogenicity, efficacy and serological correlate of protection of Salmonella typhi Vi capsular polysaccharide vaccine three years after immunization. Vaccine. 1996;14:435-8.
8. Levine MM. Typhoid fever vaccines. Plotkin SA, Orenstein WA (Eds). Vaccines. USA: Saunders; 2004. pp. 1057-95.
9. Lin FY, Ho VA, Khiem HB, Trach DD, Bay PV, Thanh TC, et al. The efficacy of a Salmonella typhi Vi conjugate vaccine in two-to-five-year-old children. N Engl J Med. 2001;344:1263-9.
10. Ochiai RL, Khan MI, Soofi SB, Sur D, Kanungo S, You YA, et al. Immune responses to Vi capsular polysaccharide typhoid vaccine in children 2 to 16 years old in Karachi, Pakistan, and Kolkata, India. Clin Vaccine Immunol. 2014;21(5):661-6.
11. Shakya M, Colin-Jones R, Theiss-Nyland K, Voysey M, Pant D, Smith N, et al. Phase 3 efficacy analysis of a typhoid conjugate vaccine trial in Nepal. N Engl J Med. 2019;381(23):2209-18.
12. Steele AD, Hay Burgess DC, Diaz Z, Carey ME, Zaidi AK. Challenges and opportunities for typhoid fever control: a call for coordinated action. Clin Infect Dis. 2016;62(Suppl 1):S4-8.
13. Sur D, Ochiai RL, Bhattacharya SK, Ganguly NK, Ali M, Manna B, et al. A cluster-randomized effectiveness trial of Vi typhoid vaccine in India. N Engl J Med. 2009;361(4):335-44.
14. Szu SC, Lin KF, Hunt S, Chu C, Thinh ND. Phase I clinical trial of O-acetylated pectin conjugate, a plant polysaccharide based typhoid vaccine. Vaccine. 2014;32:2618-22.

15. Szu SC. Development of Vi conjugate—a new generation of typhoid vaccine. Expert Rev Vaccines. 2013;12:1273-86.
16. Vashishtha VM, Choudhury P, Kalra A, Bose A, Thacker N, Yewale VN, et al. Indian Academy of Pediatrics (IAP) recommended immunization schedule for children aged 0 through 18 years—India, 2014 and updates on immunization. Indian Pediatr. 2014;51(10):785-800.
17. Vashishtha VM, Kalra A. The need and the issues related to new-generation typhoid conjugate vaccines in India. Indian J Med Res. 2020;151(1):22-34.
18. Voysey M, Pollard AJ. Seroefficacy of Vi polysaccharide-tetanus toxoid typhoid conjugate vaccine (Typbar TCV). Clin Infect Dis. 2018;67:18-24.
19. Wahdan MH, Serie CH, Germainer R, Lackany A, Cerisier Y, Guerin N, et al. A controlled field trial of live oral typhoid vaccine Ty21a. Bull World Health Organ. 1980;58:469-74.
20. World Health Organization. Typhoid vaccines: WHO position paper—March 2018. Wkly Epidemiol Rec. 2018;93:153-72.

CHAPTER 24

Haemophilus influenzae Type B Vaccines

Jaydeep Choudhury

1. What is the *Haemophilus influenzae* type b disease burden in India?

In India, the estimated *Haemophilus influenzae* type b (Hib) incidence is 50–60/100,000 children <5 years of age. Invasive Bacterial Infections Surveillance (IBIS) study done in India has shown that 76% of Hib occurs before age of 1 year with peak incidence at 6–9 months. From hospital-based data in India, 30–45% of cases of pyogenic meningitis and 8–12% of cases of pneumonia in children are due to Hib infection, but the burden of Hib infection and disease is often underestimated in our country. The various factors are that many cases of community-acquired pneumonia are nonbacteremic, there is widespread prior use of antibiotics, cultures are often not sent, and poor yield as Hib is difficult to culture.

2. What is the current status of *Haemophilus influenzae* type b (Hib) vaccine use globally?

Haemophilus influenzae type b vaccine had been introduced in almost all the countries of the world. As of June 2020, 192 countries have introduced Hib vaccine in their National Immunization Program **(Fig. 1)**. Global coverage with three doses of Hib vaccine is estimated at 72%. There is great variation between regions. The World Health Organization (WHO) regions of the

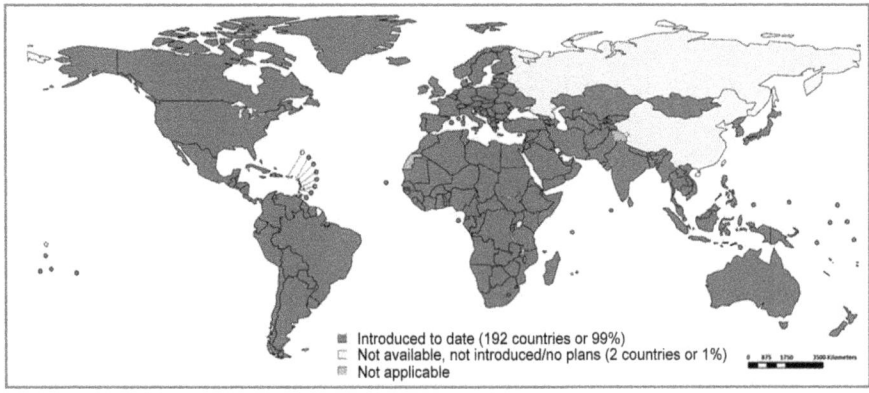

Fig. 1: Countries with *Haemophilus influenzae* type b (Hib) vaccine in the National Immunization Program.

Americas and Southeast Asia are estimated to have 87% coverage while it is only 23% in the WHO Western Pacific Region.

3. **What is the profile of clinical presentation of invasive *Haemophilus influenzae* type b (Hib) disease?**

Capsulated *Haemophilus influenzae* has six serotypes, of which type b is the most important. Hib infection is a common cause of invasive and noninvasive severe bacterial infections in children. Meningitis accounts for over 50% of all recognized cases of invasive Hib disease in infants and children under the age of 5 years. Pneumonia is another serious condition with a high morbidity and mortality in children below 5 years of age. Despite early diagnosis and effective antibiotic therapy, mortality figures are high, about 50% in Hib meningitis and about 20% in Hib pneumonia. Invasive Hib infections may also manifest as bacteremia, septicemia, epiglottitis, cellulitis, pericarditis, osteomyelitis, septic arthritis, and peritonitis. Hib may also cause peripartum septicemia in mothers. Noncapsulated Hib disease including bronchitis, otitis media, sinusitis, and some types of pneumonia are not amenable to prevention at present and can occur at all ages.

4. **Why cannot *Haemophilus influenzae* type b (Hib) infection be treated with antibiotics alone?**

Haemophilus influenzae type b infection is often serious and needs prolonged hospitalization and sometimes intensive care management. Since 1970, drug-resistant Hib strains have emerged. In India, the initial cases were reported in 1990 from Chandigarh. Subsequently, Vellore has reported 42.5% MDR strains in 1992. IBIS reported 56% Hib resistance to chloramphenicol and 40% resistance to ampicillin in 1999. With increasing spectrum of resistance, Hib infection is better prevented than cured.

5. **What are the various formulations of *Haemophilus influenzae* type b (Hib) vaccine?**

Various formulations of Hib vaccine are depicted in **Table 1**.

TABLE 1: Different formulations of Hib vaccine displaying carrier protein and immunogenicity.

Hib vaccine	Carrier protein	Immunogenicity	Formulation
PRP-D	Diphtheria toxoid	Poor, effective only above 12 months age	Lyophilized
HbOC	CRM197	Late response with good booster effect	Liquid
PRP-OMP	OMP	High for short-term protection, modest booster effect	Not available
PRP-T	Tetanus toxoid	Late response with good booster effect	Lyophilized

[CRM197: nontoxic mutant of *Corynebacterium diphtheriae* toxin protein; HbOC: *Haemophilus* b conjugate; OMP: outer membrane protein complex of *Neisseria meningitidis*; PRP-D or T: polyribosyl-ribitol phosphate (capsular polysaccharide) covalently bound to either diphtheria or tetanus toxoid]

6. Why polyribosylribitol phosphate-outer membrane protein (PRP-OMP) *Haemophilus influenzae* type b (Hib) vaccine is not available?

The polyribosylribitol phosphate-outer membrane protein (PRP-OMP) Hib vaccine is unique in producing a dramatic antibody response to the very first dose, even in infants below 6 months of age. Majority of infants achieve anti-PRP antibody levels of >1.0 µg/mL, but it produces minimal further increase in antibody concentration to subsequent doses. After the initial rise, antibody titers decrease significantly over time. Consequently, the final antibody levels are about 30% of those obtained with *Haemophilus* b conjugate (HbOC) or PRP-T. Hence, PRP-OMP was withdrawn.

7. Why is it ideal to use conjugated *Haemophilus influenzae* type b (Hib) vaccine?

Majority of Hib infections occur in children <18 months of age, with peak incidence of invasive disease at around 6–7 months of age. All Hib vaccines are conjugated vaccines where the Hib capsular polysaccharide (polyribosylribitol phosphate or PRP) is conjugated with a protein carrier, so as to provide protection in the early years of life when it is most needed.

8. Can we use the *Haemophilus influenzae* type b (Hib) vaccines interchangeably?

The Hib vaccines HbOC, PRP-T, and PRP-OMP can be used interchangeably even in the primary immunization schedule with good immune response.

9. What is the vaccination schedule of *Haemophilus influenzae* type b (Hib) vaccine?

The vaccination schedule for Hib consists of three doses when initiated in children below 6 months of age; two doses between 6 and 12 months and one dose between 12 and 15 months. In every schedule, a booster is given at 18 months. The interval between two doses of Hib vaccine should be at least 4 weeks. For children aged >15 months, a single dose may suffice. As Hib disease is essentially confined to infants and young children, catch-up vaccination is not recommended for healthy children above 5 years. However, the vaccine should be administered to all individuals with functional/anatomic hyposplenia irrespective of age.

10. Why three doses of *Haemophilus influenzae* type b (Hib) vaccines are required in infants below 6 months?

The first dose of the Hib vaccines, HbOC and PRP-T, stimulates an exceptionally low antibody response in infants below 6 months of age. The infants show a late response and three doses are required to achieve seroprotective antibody levels in infants below 6 months of age. The vaccine may not protect the infants until after the third dose.

11. Why is booster dose necessary for *Haemophilus influenzae* type b (Hib) vaccine?

There is demonstrable waning immunity in general for all types of Hib vaccine formulations available. After the three primary doses of Hib vaccination, >90% vaccines achieve an antibody titer >1.0 µg/mL which gives protection till 15–18 months of age. In >50% of them, the protective level falls. Being a vaccine intended for boosting the natural immunity and as the prevalence of Hib disease is mainly in children below 5 years, if a booster is given at 18 months of age, the titer rises and protects till the age of 5 years.

12. Being a conjugate vaccine (i.e., T-dependent antigen), memory cells are formed during induction phase. Then, why are they not being able to provide protection at the time of natural infection during 2nd year of life and booster is needed?

This is to be noted that presence of memory B cells does not mean protection against a disease, which requires reactivation of memory B cells into antibodies secreting plasma cells. This transition usually takes around 4–7 days. However, invasive Hib diseases are characterized by short incubation period, hence by the time, memory B cell transforms into plasma cells, the disease already advances, and causes morbidity and mortality. This is the reason, why boosters are needed for organisms having short incubation period like pneumococcal, influenza, meningococcal, etc., whereas diseases like hepatitis B and A, which have long incubation period, boosters are not required and memory is sufficient to accord in protection.

13. Does the tetanus protein in polyribosylribitol phosphate-tetanus toxoid (PRP-T) *Haemophilus influenzae* type b (Hib) immunize against tetanus?

No. Here, the tetanus protein is conjugated to bring the PRP component into contact with the immunologically competent T lymphocytes. This does not replace the routine dose of tetanus vaccine.

14. What are the available combination *Haemophilus influenzae* type b (Hib) vaccines?

Combination Hib vaccines available in India are:
- Diphtheria, tetanus, and whole-cell pertussis (DTwP)/Hib
- Diphtheria, tetanus, and whole-cell pertussis/hepatitis B/Hib
- Diphtheria, tetanus, and whole-cell pertussis/Hib/inactivated polio vaccine (IPV)
- Diphtheria, tetanus, and whole-cell pertussis/hepatitis B/Hib/IPV
- Diphtheria, tetanus, and acellular pertussis (DTaP)/IPV/Hib
- Diphtheria, tetanus, and acellular pertussis/hepatitis B/Hib/IPV.

15. Is it true that when the combination formulation of diphtheria, tetanus, and acellular pertussis (DTaP)/*Haemophilus influenzae* type b (Hib) is used, the antibody level of the Hib component is decreased?

Some studies have shown that administering DTP and Hib combination results in reduced mean PRP Hib antibody levels compared to giving the same components separately. The reduction in PRP Hib antibody is more significant in DTaP than DTwP. However, even in these studies, the antibody levels are well above the protective titers. Thus, reduced immunogenicity of Hib when given in combination with DTP appears to be of no clinical significance. Hence, the DTaP/Hib vaccine formulation can safely be used.

16. Is there any difference between lyophilized and liquid *Haemophilus influenzae* type b (Hib) combination vaccines?

Lyophilized or dry powder Hib vaccine has to be mixed with the liquid DTP vaccine, which acts as the diluent. Here, PRP-T Hib vaccine is used whereas in liquid combination Hib vaccine HbOC is used where CRM197 is the carrier protein and the vaccine is in dissolved state. Immunologically, both the forms are equally effective.

17. If a healthy infant received one dose of *Haemophilus influenzae* type b (Hib) at 5 months and another at 15 months, does he/she need any more doses?

No. If a healthy child receives a dose of Hib vaccine at 15 months of age or older, he or she does not need any further doses regardless of the number of doses received before 15 months of age.

18. Is it feasible to combine *Haemophilus influenzae* type b (Hib) vaccines ad hoc?

Providers should not create their own ad hoc combinations by mixing separate vaccines in the same syringe unless there is an evidence establishing the stability, safety, and immunogenicity of the resultant combinations as reflected in the package inserts.

19. A 4-year-old girl received third dose of *Haemophilus influenzae* type b (Hib) vaccine at 6 months of age. She is now brought to complete her vaccination schedule. Does she need fourth dose of Hib vaccine also?

Yes. All children <5-year-old need at least one dose of Hib vaccine on or after the first birthday. The last dose should be separated from the previous dose by at least 8 weeks.

20. A 7-year-old boy is brought to my outpatient department (OPD) for completion of his vaccination schedule. The parents do not have any past record of *Haemophilus influenzae* type b (Hib) vaccination. Should he receive a dose of Hib vaccine now?

No, the routine Hib vaccination of healthy children aging 5 years or more is not recommended, even if they have no prior history of Hib vaccination.

21. *Haemophilus influenzae* type b (Hib) vaccine is usually not recommended above 5 years of age for healthy children, even if the person did not receive Hib vaccine as a child nor it is recommended for adults. But in certain conditions, older children and even adults are required to get vaccinated against Hib. What are these conditions?

In the following conditions, the Centers for Disease Control and Prevention-Advisory Committee on Immunization Practices (CDC-ACIP) recommends a dose of Hib vaccine:
- A dose of Hib vaccine to persons who have anatomical or functional asplenia or sickle cell disease or are undergoing elective splenectomy if they have not previously received Hib vaccine.
- *Haemophilus influenzae* type b vaccine should be administered 14 or more days before splenectomy, along with pneumococcal conjugate vaccine (PCV) and meningococcal vaccines if possible.
- If vaccines are not administered before surgery, they should be administered as soon as the person's condition stabilizes after surgery.
- Recipients of a hematopoietic stem cell transplantation (HSCT) should be vaccinated with a three-dose series of Hib vaccine 6–12 months after a successful transplant, regardless of vaccination history; at least 4 weeks, it should separate doses.

However, the Hib vaccine is not recommended for adults with human immunodeficiency virus (HIV) infection since their risk for Hib disease is low.

22. A 5-month-old unimmunized boy developed *Haemophilus influenzae* type b (Hib) meningitis. Should he be vaccinated with Hib vaccine following recovery?

Haemophilus influenzae type b invasive disease does not always result in development of protective antibody levels. Children younger than 2 years of age who develop invasive Hib disease should be considered susceptible and should receive Hib vaccine. Vaccination of these children should start as soon as possible during the convalescent phase of the illness. A complete series as recommended for the child's age should be administered.

SUGGESTED READING

1. American Academy of Pediatrics. *Haemophilus influenzae* infections. In: Pickering L, Baker C, Long S, McMillan J (Eds). Red Book: 2006. Report of the Committee on Infectious Diseases, 27th edition. Elk Grove Village: American Academy of Pediatrics; 2006. pp. 310-8.
2. Atkinson W, Hamborsky J, McIntyre L, Wolfe S. Epidemiology and Prevention of Vaccine-preventable Disease, 10th edition. Washington DC: Public Health Foundation; 2007. pp. 115-27.
3. Centers for Disease Control and Prevention (CDC). Progress toward elimination of *Haemophilus influenzae* type b disease among infants and children—United States, 1998-2000. Morb Mortal Wkly Rep. 2002;51:234-7.

4. Immunization Action Coalition (IAC). (2018). Ask the expert: *Haemophilus influenzae* type b (Hib). [online] Available from: https://www.immunize.org/askexperts/experts_hib.asp. [Last accessed July, 2020].
5. Mehta P, Choudhury J. Immunization against *Haemophilus influenzae* type b. In: Thacker N, Shah NK (Eds). Immunization in Clinical Practice, 2nd edition. New Delhi: Jaypee Brothers Medical Publishers (P) Ltd; 2016. pp. 148-52.
6. National Family Health Survey (NFHS). (2019). National Family Health Survey of India-3 (NFHS-3). [online] Available from: http://rchiips.org/NFHS/nfhs3.shtml. [Last accessed July, 2020].
7. Prospective multicentre hospital surveillance of *Streptococcus pneumoniae* disease in India. Invasive Bacterial Infection Surveillance (IBIS) Group, International Clinical Epidemiology Network (INCLEN). Lancet. 1999;353: 1216-21.

CHAPTER 25

Pneumococcal Diseases Vaccines

Shobha Sharma, Neha Goel

1. What is the disease spectrum of pneumococcal disease in children?

Pneumococcal diseases are a global healthcare concern caused by the pathogen, *Streptococcus pneumoniae* (*S. pneumoniae*) (Pneumococcus); however, these diseases are preventable. Pneumococcal diseases are broadly classified into invasive and noninvasive forms. Invasive pneumococcal disease (IPD) is diagnosed when the pathogen is identified in normally sterile body fluids (cerebrospinal fluid, blood, and pericardial fluid) of an affected individual, e.g., bacteremia, meningitis, etc. Non-IPD includes sinusitis, acute otitis media (AOM), and community-acquired pneumonia. It can spread from nasopharynx, locally to middle ear, leading to AOM, or to sinuses leading to sinusitis. It can spread focally to lungs leading to nonbacteremic pneumonia. Lastly, it can also spread via bloodstream leading to IPD like bacteremia, sepsis, meningitis, or bacteremic pneumonia. Besides, it can also lead to uncommon noninvasive infections like cellulitis, peritonitis, joint infections, etc. The peak incidence of pneumococcal disease in children occurs at 6–24 months of age. IPD is a notable cause of morbidity and mortality in the US, despite the availability of 7-valent pneumococcal conjugate vaccine (PCV7) and 13-valent pneumococcal conjugate vaccine (PCV13). After introduction of PCV7 in 2000, rates were reduced by 64–77% among adults and older children and down to less than one case per 100,000 among children under-five for the included serotypes. In 2010, PCV13 further lowered rates. Pneumonia is one of the most common causes of morbidity and mortality in children younger than 5 years in India. The Millennium Development Goal (MDG) 4, which focuses on reduction of under-five mortality, has generated significant momentum for accurate assessment of cause-specific under-five morbidity and mortality. In 2004, incidence of clinical pneumonia in children younger than 5 years was 0.28 episodes per child-year globally, with an interquartile range of 0.21–0.71 episodes per child-year in developing countries (**Fig. 1**). In 2008, the Child Health Epidemiology Reference Group (CHERG) established by the World Health Organization (WHO) identified lack of exclusive breastfeeding, undernutrition, indoor air pollution, low birth weight, crowding, and lack of measles immunization as leading risk factors contributing to pneumonia incidence. In addition, they mentioned that five countries where 44% of the world's children aged <5 years live (India, China, Pakistan, Bangladesh, Indonesia, and Nigeria) contribute more than

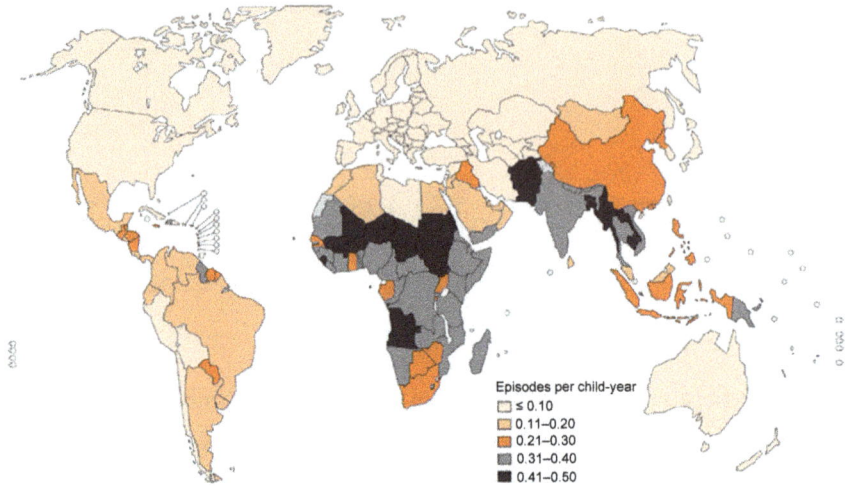

Fig. 1: Incidence of childhood clinical pneumonia at the country level.

half of the new pneumonia cases annually. For India, they predicted around 43 million pneumonia cases (23% of the world's total) and estimated an incidence of 0.37 episodes per child-year for clinical pneumonia.

2. What is the pneumococcal disease burden in children?

Incidence of IPD varies from 25–50/100,000 children under 5 years in Europe to 90/100,000 under 5 years in the United States of America (USA) to 500/100,000 under 5 years in the Gambia and Apache Indians. 90% of bacteremia, 30–50% of severe community-acquired pneumonia, 30–45% of pyogenic meningitis, and 30–60% of all bacterial AOM are caused by Pneumococcus. The mortality rate of invasive disease is 6–20% and there are long-term sequels like central nervous system (CNS) squeal who survive meningitis and deafness with recurrent AOM. *S. pneumoniae* is responsible for 15–50% of all episodes of community-acquired pneumonia, 30–50% of all cases of AOM, and a significant proportion of bacterial meningitis and bacteremia. *S. pneumoniae* kills at least 1 million children under the age of 5 every year, which is more than malaria, acquired immunodeficiency syndrome (AIDS), and measles combined. For a large country like India, pneumonia burden estimates level are still not available accurately. India accounts for 23% of the global pneumonia burden and 36% of the WHO regional burden. A large nationally representative survey has reported that in 2005, pneumonia contributed 13.5% of deaths in children age 1–59 months with girls in central India having a five times higher mortality rate (per 1,000 live births) from pneumonia than boys in south India. The estimated annual severe pneumonia incidence varied greatly from one state to another: 7.2 episodes [95% confidence interval (CI): 6.6–7.8%] per 1,000 children in Manipur to 50.3 episodes (95% CI: 46.2–54.9%) per 1,000 children in Jharkhand. Southern states (Kerala, Tamil Nadu) and Northeastern states

(Sikkim, Manipur) have significantly lower incidence and mortality from severe pneumonia as compared to rest of the India. In age-stratified analysis, severe pneumonia-related morbidity was highest morbidity in the 0–1 year age group (51%) followed by the 1–2 years age group (22%). Jharkhand had the highest incidence of severe pneumonia, but Uttar Pradesh (UP) had the highest number of cases because of a large population of children younger than 5 years (**Figs. 2A and B**).

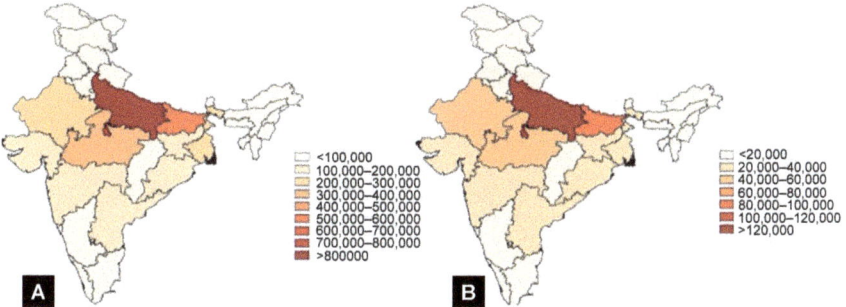

Figs. 2A and B: Distribution of severe pneumonia episodes and pneumonia deaths in children younger than 5 years in India. (A) Number of severe pneumonia cases in India in age 0–59 months; (B) Number of pneumonia-related deaths in India in age 0–59 months.

Source: Adapted from Farooqui H, Jit M, Heymann DL, Zodpey S. Burden of severe pneumonia, pneumococcal pneumonia and pneumonia deaths in Indian states: modelling based estimates. PLoS One. 2015;10(6):e0129191.

3. What is the burden of pneumococcal pneumonia and mortality?

Despite the difficulties of producing estimates with available evidence, pneumonia has consistently been estimated as the leading single cause of childhood mortality. Factors contributing to difficulty in estimating the burden and death include large differences in case definition of pneumonia between studies, low specificity of verbal autopsies in community-based studies, the fact that similar symptoms from both pneumonia and malaria lead to death, difficulties in distinguishing pneumonia from sepsis in neonates, and the synergy between several disorders leading to a single death. The African region has, in general, the highest burden of global child mortality. Although it comprises about 20% of the world's population of children aged <5 years, it has about 45% of global under-five deaths and 50% of worldwide deaths from pneumonia in this age group. More than 90% of all deaths due to pneumonia in children aged <5 years take place in 40 countries and according to the official estimates from the WHO for the year 2000, two-thirds of all these deaths are concentrated in 10 countries with maximum numbers in India (408,000 deaths) (**Fig. 3**). In India, it was estimated that of 1.4 million under-five deaths every year, 20.3% were caused by pneumonia, i.e., 0.29 million deaths, contributing 23.5% of all pneumonia deaths in the world. India also contributes 40 million episodes of clinical pneumonia. As bacteriological diagnosis of pneumococcal infection is difficult, exact

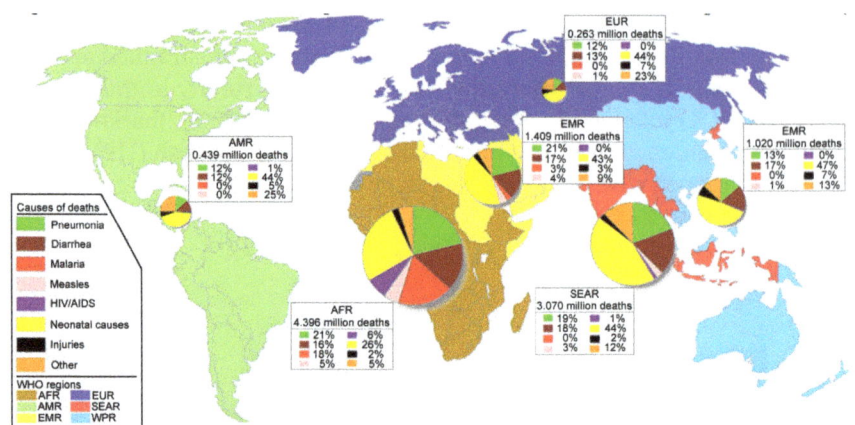

Fig. 3: Distribution of deaths from pneumonia and other causes in children aged <5 years by the WHO region.

(AFR: Africa; AIDS: acquired immunodeficiency syndrome; AMR: America; EMR: Eastern Mediterranean; EUR: Europe; HIV: human immunodeficiency virus; SEAR: Southeast Asia; WHO: World Health Organization; WPR: Western Pacific)

Source: Adapted from Rudan I, Boschi-Pinto C, Biloglav Z, Mulholland K, Campbell H. (2008). Epidemiology and etiology of childhood pneumonia. [online] Available from: who.int/bulletin/volumes/86/5/07-048769/en/. [Last accessed August, 2020].

magnitude of its burden is not known. *S. pneumoniae* is estimated to constitute for 30% of all bacterial pneumonias. For pneumonia, between 8.7% and 52.4% of cases occur in infants aged <6 months. In 2010, 3.6 million episodes of severe pneumonia and 0.35 million all-cause pneumonia deaths occurred in children under the age of 5 years in India. Among those, 0.56 million episodes of severe pneumonia (16%) and 0.10 million deaths (30%), respectively, were caused by pneumococcal pneumonia.

4. What are the prevalent serotypes of Pneumococcus in children in India and how many of them are covered by the pneumococcal conjugate vaccine (PCV)?

Out of >90 serotypes of *S. pneumoniae*, serotypes 1, 2, 3, 4, 5, 6A, 6B, 7F, 8, 9A, 9N, 9V, 10A, 12F, 14, 15B, 18C, 19A, 19F, and 23F are responsible for 85% of IPD. Children under the age of 2 years are at greatest risk for IPD. Results of the Invasive Bacterial Infection Surveillance (IBIS) study in patients with IPD showed that serotypes 1, 2, 3, 4, 5, 6A, 6B, 7F, 8, 9A, 9N, 9V, 10A, 12F, 14, 15B, 18C, 19A, 19F, and 23F are the most prevalent, with serotypes 1 and 5 accounting for 30% of IPD. It is also known that the serotypes causing pneumonia and otitis media differ from those causing IPD and usually reflect those serotypes present in nasopharyngeal carriage. In India, 6, 14, 18, 5, 19, and 1 serotypes were the most frequent. In a study from Bengaluru, serotypes 6A, 14, 6B, 1, 18C, 19A, 9V, 4, 10C, and 18A showed antibiotic resistance. In another Indian study, most common pneumococcal serotypes causing invasive infections in children <5 years of age were 14, 19F, 5, 6A, and 6B

(13, 24, and 25). The Asian Network for Surveillance of Resistant Pathogens (ANSORP) data of 2008 shows that 19A is on rise in most Asian countries, as also in India. 19A is covered by PCV13 but not by PCV10. Two recent studies from India have looked at serotype distribution in IPD in children <5 years of age. PCV7 covers 55% of serotypes seen in children under 5 years and PCV10 and PCV13 covers around 75%. The Pneumonet study showed that PCV10 covers 63.8% of prevalent serotypes and PCV13 covers 91.6% of prevalent serotypes. The Alliance for Surveillance of Invasive Pneumococci (ASIP) study which was a multicentric study sponsored by GlaxoSmithKline (GSK) India showed that PCV10 covers 64.1% of prevalent serotypes and PCV13 covers around 74.3% of prevalent serotypes.

5. **Which different pneumococcal conjugate vaccine (PCV) is available in market? How do they differ?**

There are two types of pneumococcal vaccine—(1) pneumococcal polysaccharide vaccine (PPSV) and (2) pneumococcal conjugate vaccine (PCV). The PPSV is unconjugated 23-valent vaccine (PPSV23) containing 23 serotypes, i.e., 1, 2, 3, 4, 5, 6B, 7F, 8, 9N, 9V, 10A, 11A, 12F, 14, 15B, 17F, 18C, 19F, 19A, 20, 22F, 23F, and 33F. But the disadvantage is that being a T-cell independent vaccine, it is poorly immunogenic below the age of 2 years, has low immune memory, does not reduce nasopharyngeal carriage, and also does not provide any herd immunity. It is given as 0.5 mL intramuscular (IM) or subcutaneous (SC) dose with maximum recommended three doses. It mounts serotype-specific immunoglobulin G (IgG), immunoglobulin A (IgA), and immunoglobulin M (IgM) antibodies. Although efficacy is shown in healthy adults against IPD, evidence of efficacy against invasive disease or pneumonia in other high-risk populations with underlying diseases or immunosuppressed individuals is lacking.

Pneumococcal conjugate vaccines were developed primarily to address the problem of low immunogenicity of the polysaccharide vaccine in children below the age of 2 years by conjugating them with carrier proteins like cross-reactive material 197 (CRM197), a nontoxic mutant diphtheria toxin, diphtheria toxoid, tetanus toxoid, or a meningococcal outer membrane protein (OMP) complex (**Table 1**).

Three of these vaccines containing 7, 10, or 13 serotypes of Pneumococcus, respectively (PCV7, PCV10, and PCV13) were licensed globally. The only PCV licensed to date in India is CRM197 PnC-7v (henceforth referred to as PCV7, Pfizer) containing polysaccharide antigen of serotypes 4, 6B, 9V, 14, 18C, 19F, and 23F linked to CRM197. Till recently, only PCV7 and unconjugated 23-valent PPSV (PPSV23) were available in India. However, in mid-2010, a new PCV13 was launched in India. PCV13 has replaced PCV7 world over, including India. PCV13 contains six additional strains (i.e., 1, 3, 5, 6A, 19A, and 7F), which protect against the majority of the remaining pneumococcal infections. Another PCV, a 10-valent pneumococcal conjugate vaccine (PCV10) from GlaxoSmithKline (GSK) is now available internationally

TABLE 1: WHO prequalified/submitted for the WHO prequalification pneumococcal conjugate vaccines (PCVs) along with serotypes included in each product.

Product	Formulation specifications	Type of carrier protein(s)	Conjugation method	Serotypes												
				1	3	4	5	6A	6B	7F	9V	14	18C	19A	19F	23F
Currently WHO prequalified																
Synflorix™ (GSK)	10-valent Preservative: 1-dose vial - none 2-dose vial - none 4-dose vial - 2-phenoxyethanol	Protein D (PD), tetanus toxoid (TT), diphtheria toxoid (DT)	CDAP**	1 μg PD		3 μg PD	1 μg PD		1 μg PD	1 μg PD	1 μg PD	1 μg PD	3 μg TT		3 μg DT	1 μg PD
Prevenar 13® (pfizer)	13-valent Preservative: 1-dose vial* - none 4-dose vial - 2-phenoxyethanol	CRM$_{197}$	Reductive amination	2.2 μg CRM$_{197}$	2.2 μg CRM$_{197}$	2.2 μg CRM$_{197}$	2.2 μg CRM$_{197}$	2.2 μg CRM$_{197}$	4.4 μg CRM$_{197}$	2.2 μg CRM$_{197}$	2.2 μg CRM$_{197}$	2.2 μg CRM$_{197}$	2.2 μg CRM$_{197}$	2.2 μg CRM$_{197}$	2.2 μg CRM$_{197}$	2.2 μg CRM$_{197}$
Submitted for WHO prqualification																
Pneumosil® (SII)	10-valent Preservative: 1-dose vial* - none 5-dose vial - thimerosal	CRM$_{197}$	CDAP**	2 μg CRM$_{197}$			2 μg CRM$_{197}$	2 μg CRM$_{197}$	4 μg CRM$_{197}$	2 μg CRM$_{197}$	2 μg CRM$_{197}$	2 μg CRM$_{197}$		2 μg CRM$_{197}$	2 μg CRM$_{197}$	2 μg CRM$_{197}$
No longer available																
Prevenar 7® (wyeth/pfizer)	7-valent Preservative: 1-dose vial* - none	CRM$_{197}$	Reductive amination			2 μg CRM$_{197}$			4 μg CRM$_{197}$		2 μg CRM$_{197}$	2 μg CRM$_{197}$	2 μg CRM$_{197}$		2 μg CRM$_{197}$	2 μg CRM$_{197}$

* Other formulations/presentations (e.g. pre-filled syringe) may be available in some countries but are not currently WHO-prequalified
** CDAP: 1-cyano-4-dimethylaminopyridinium tetrafluoroborate

and soon will be available in India too developed by the Serum Institute of India as the Serum Institute of India Pvt. Ltd. (SIIPL)-PCV. PCV13 contains polysaccharides of the capsular antigens of *S. pneumoniae* serotypes 1, 5, 7F, 3, 6A, and 19A, in addition to the seven polysaccharides of the capsular antigens of 4, 6B, 9V, 14, 18C, 19F, and 23F present in the PCV7, individually conjugated to a nontoxic diphtheria CRM carrier protein (CRM197). PCV10 covers three additional serotypes besides PCV7, i.e., 1, 5, and 7F. Three different carrier proteins are used in this formulation (**Table 2**). It contains aluminum phosphate as an adjuvant.

TABLE 2: Antigen concentration of different serotypes and carrier proteins used in the development of 10-valent pneumococcal conjugate vaccine (PCV10).

Serotypes	1, 5, 6B, 7F, 9V, 14, and, 23F	4	18C	19F
Antigen concentration	1 µg	3 µg	3 µg	3 µg
Carrier proteins	Nontypeable *Haemophilus influenzae* (NTHi) protein D		Tetanus toxoid	Diphtheria toxoid

Pfizer's PCV13 has been used in India's Universal Immunization Program (UIP). The vaccine is being introduced in a phased manner; it has been introduced in Himachal Pradesh and parts of Bihar, Uttar Pradesh, Madhya Pradesh, and Rajasthan. From August 2020, the PCV13 has been introduced in all the districts of Uttar Pradesh.

6. **What are the strains used in Serum Insititute of India Pvt. Ltd.-pneumococcal conjugate vaccine (SIIPL-PCV) (Pneumosil™)? What will be its impact on economy?**

The 10-valent candidate PCV has been developed by the SIIPL, SIIPL-PCV containing most prevalent IPD-causing serotypes 1, 5, 6A, 6B, 7F, 9V, 14, 19A, 19F, and 23F. One of the major advantages of this vaccine is its low cost by optimizing three critical components of the manufacturing process: (1) carrier protein production, (2) polysaccharide production, and (3) conjugation efficiency. It can thus be provided at a considerably lower price than currently licensed PCVs, provided it is found to be safe and immunogenic. The company has submitted the reports of phase III trial to the Drug Controller General of India (DCGI). The vaccine has got approval from the DCGI, the Union Health Ministry said on 14th July 2020. With the help of Special Expert Committee (SEC) for vaccines, the drug regulator reviewed the phase I, II, and III clinical trial data submitted by the Serum Institute of India and then granted the market approval for pneumococcal polysaccharide conjugate vaccine.

So, now there are three PCVs are licensed in India. The vaccine will be available to low- and middle-income countries for just $2 a dose, which is 30% cheaper than the Global Alliance for Vaccines and Immunization (GAVI) price. Countries that get the vaccine through GAVI shell out nearly $3 per dose, while GAVI puts in an equal amount. Hence, the $2 per dose will be far cheaper for countries that do not get the vaccines through GAVI.

7. What is the schedule of pneumococcal conjugate vaccine (PCV)?

Considering the burden of pneumococcal disease among underprivileged children in India, the PCVs are thus of public health importance and ideally should be available to all children. However, the high cost of PCVs and the limited coverage of the currently available vaccine are impediments. The risk of IPD is significantly lower in healthy children above the age of 2 years and thus benefit achieved with vaccination of these children is likely to be lower. Vaccination with single dose of PCV vaccine may be considered in children aged 2–5 years. Pneumococcal vaccination is not recommended in children aged 5 years and above. The recommended dosage for PCV13 is 0.5 mL and the vaccination route is IM.

Infants and children who have not previously received PCV7 or PCV13: The Indian Academy of Pediatrics (IAP) recommends three doses at 6, 10, and 14 weeks with a booster at 15 months. Infants receiving their first dose at age <11 months should receive three doses of PCV13 at intervals of approximately 4 weeks with a booster at 15 months. Children aged 12–23 months should receive two doses with an interval of at least 8 weeks between doses. Unvaccinated healthy children aged 24–59 months should receive a single dose of PCV13.

Children incompletely vaccinated with PCV7 or PCV13: Infants <24 months should receive one or more doses based on the number of doses of PCV7 received to date and the age of the child.

Children who have received four doses of PCV7: A single dose of PCV13 is recommended for all children 14–59 months of age.

Children 6–18 years of age with high-risk conditions: A single dose of PCV13 may be administered for who are at increased risk for IPD in age 2 years and older with chronic heart disease (particularly cyanotic congenital heart disease and cardiac failure); chronic lung disease (including asthma treated with high-dose oral corticosteroids); diabetes mellitus, with cerebrospinal fluid leak; candidate for or recipient of cochlear implant, with sickle cell disease and other hemoglobinopathies; anatomic or functional asplenia; congenital or acquired immunodeficiency; human immunodeficiency virus (HIV) infection; chronic renal failure; nephrotic syndrome; malignant neoplasms, leukemias, lymphomas, Hodgkin disease, and other diseases associated with treatment with immunosuppressive drugs or radiation therapy; and solid organ transplantation, multiple myeloma regardless of whether they have previously received PCV7 or PPSV23.

Contraindications: Do not give PCV13 to a child who has experienced a serious reaction (e.g., anaphylaxis) to a prior dose of the vaccine or to any of its components (including to any diphtheria toxoid-containing vaccine).

8. What is the efficacy of pneumococcal conjugate vaccine (PCV) on invasive pneumococcal disease (IPD)?

Significant effectiveness against vaccine-type (VT) IPD in children ≤5 years was reported for ≥1 dose of PCV13 in the 3 + 1 (86–96%) and 2 + 1 schedules (67.2–86%) and for PCV10 for the 3 + 1 (72.8–100%) and 2 + 1 schedules (92–97%). In children <12 months of age, PCV13 vaccine efficacy (VE) against serotype 19A postprimary series was significant for the 3 + 1 but not the 2 + 1 schedule. PCV10 cross-protection against 19A was significant in children ≤5 years with ≥1 dose (82.2% and 71%). Neither PCVs were found effective against serotype 3.

9. What is the efficacy of pneumococcal conjugate vaccine (PCV) on nasopharyngeal (NP) carriage and otitis media?

With the introduction of PCV7, reduction in the colonization of VT strains has been observed in vaccinated subjects but with increase of non-VT (NVT) colonization, resulting in no significant changes in the overall carriage rates. Decrease in VT carriage was shown not only in vaccinated subjects, but also in nonvaccinated siblings if they lived in a household or community of PCV7-vaccinated infants and children showing that PCV7 reduces VT colonization and colonization density with an increase in NVT colonization in both vaccines and household contacts. Similar results were found in a study in Atlanta, US, comparing nasopharyngeal (NP) carriage serotype distribution between 1995 and 2009 before the introduction of PCV7 and PCV13, respectively. PCV7 serotypes decreased substantially, with an increase in non-PCV7 serotypes, with serotype 19A as the leading serotype. After introduction of PCV13, a reduction in PCV13 serotypes was reported. NP carriage rates for serotypes 19A and 7F, two of six additional serotypes, were significantly lower in PCV13-vaccinated subjects than that in PCV7-vaccinated subjects. The reduction of serotype 6C, which is not included in PCV13, suggests cross-protection against pneumococcal disease by serotype 6C. The effect of PCV10 on NP carriage is of interest in two aspects: (1) the impact on carriage of nontypeable *Haemophilus influenzae* (NTHi) and (2) the impact on *S. pneumoniae*. VT serotype carriage was reduced by 22–35% in those vaccinated with PCV10. For carriage of any *H. influenzae*, subjects vaccinated with PCV10 showed a nonsignificant increase during the first year after booster vaccination (VE: 3.5%; 95% CI: 30.7–18.0%) and a nonsignificant decrease for NTHi carriage (VE: 1.7%; 95% CI: 25.5–23.0%).

Acute otitis media: Since it is not ethically permissible and practically feasible to do middle ear tap and middle fluid culture for every suspected case of AOM to establish the etiology, therefore, it is difficult to prove the efficacy of PCV against AOM. Only few studies were designed where middle ear tap and culture were routinely done as a standard of care in management of AOM, as was done in Finnish study. PCV7 showed 57% efficacy against vaccine serotype AOM and 34% against all serotype AOM with simultaneous increase in AOM due to nonvaccine serotype pneumococci and AOM due to other pathogens like *H. influenzae* and *Moraxella catarrhalis (M. catarrhalis)*. Overall, there was 8% decrease in all-cause AOM, 50% decrease in all-cause

AOM with effusion, 18% decrease in all-cause recurrent AOM, and 39% decrease in all-cause AOM needing positron emission tomography (PET) insertion on long-term follow-up.

Experimental PCV11 (a different vaccine than the current PCV10 in its contents) was tried in one study for otitis media. The efficacy against vaccine serotype AOM was 57% and against all-cause AOM was 33.6%. There was decrease of 35% in NTHi AOM and increase in AOM due to *M. catarrhalis*.

The 13-valent pneumococcal conjugate vaccine has shown significant effectiveness against AOM in various studies. A prospective study on AOM in Israel after use of PCV13 showed that the incidence of AOM per 1,000 children decreased significantly from 12.2 to 6 and that caused by NTHi from 5.7 to 3.8. In Greece, PCV13 use led to 47.4% reduction in AOM caused by six additional serotypes present in PCV13 compared to PCV7, including AOM caused by serotypes 19A, 6A, and 3.

10. What is the efficacy of pneumococcal conjugate vaccine (PCV) against pneumonia?

Streptococcus pneumoniae is a leading cause of bacterial pneumonia, but the definition differs between the physicians and it is difficult to determine the causative agent of pneumonia in children since blood culture is positive in only 10% of cases and lung tap, though is positive in 50% of cases, is unethical and hazardous. Owing to these difficulties, the WHO developed a standardized definition based on evidence of alveolar consolidation on chest radiography. The efficacy of PCV against pneumonia has been studied in clinical trials evaluating a 9-valent pneumococcal conjugate vaccine (PCV9) and an 11-valent pneumococcal conjugate vaccine (PCV11) as well as PCV7. An initial study conducted in the Northern California Kaiser Permanente (NCKP) district showed a VE of 27% based on the WHO definition of pneumonia. Based on the studies of PCV7, PCV9, and PCV11, according to a Cochrane systematic review, the VE was 27% (95% CI: 15–36%) for the WHO radiologically defined pneumonia. An extensive analysis on the serotype changes of pneumococcal pneumonia from 2000 to 2004 in Uruguay showed that serotype 14 (30.5%) was the most prevalent, followed by serotypes 1 (19.9%), 5 (17.8%), and 3 (6.5%). According to this study, PCV7 covers 60%, PCV10 covers 83.8%, and PCV13 covers 93.9% of the serotypes. Subsequently in Uruguay, PCV7 was introduced in the routine vaccination program (2 + 1 schedule) in 2008 and PCV7 was replaced by PCV13 in April 2010. The incidence of pneumococcal empyema in children <14 years of age decreases by 77% in 2012, compared with the prevaccination period, 2005–2007. After the introduction of PCV7 in the US by 2004, hospitalizations for pneumococcal pneumonia in children <2 years of age decreased by 65% and those for all-cause pneumonia decreased by 39%. Within 30 months of PCV7 introduction in Australia, all-cause pneumonia decreased by 36% in children <2 years of age. Study in Uruguay showed 79% reduction in consolidated pneumonia hospitalization in children after second primary dose and 85% reduction after the booster dose after PVC13 introduction with a significant reduction of 69.2% in hospitalizations for empyema and complicated pneumonia. There was also significant 19% reduction in pneumonia hospitalization rates in 5-14 years of age suggesting her defect against CAP of PCV13 in this age group for the first time ever.

11. Will use of pneumococcal conjugate vaccine (PCV) leads to replacement disease with nonvaccine serotypes?

It was earlier observed that with reduction of NP carriers with vaccine serotypes, there was increase in nonvaccine serotypes. Almost 100% replacement of vaccine serotypes with nonvaccine serotypes in NP carriage and partial increase in AOM due to nonvaccine serotype pneumococci and other pathogens like *H. influenzae* and *M. catarrhalis* have been noted after use of PCV7. Hence, such replacement disease in IPD remains a potential risk.

Study done on Alaskan region in children under 2 years of age observed the incidence of vaccine serotype IPD fell by 265,100,000 population in 6 years after introduction of PCV7 with simultaneous increase in incidence of nonvaccine serotype IPD by 133,100,000 population during same period nullifying the benefits of vaccine on IPD by 50%. There was only small increase in nonvaccine serotype in other age groups of native Alaskan population. No significant increase in nonvaccine serotype IPD was noted in any age group of nonnative Alaskan population. Study done by Active Bacterial Core Surveillance (ABCS) group in USA did not show significant increase in nonvaccine serotype IPD as compared to massive decrease in vaccine serotype IPD in all the age groups. Serotype 19A contributes to 50% of the replacement disease in US. Increase in 19A disease may be due to secular trends, misuse of antimicrobials, and reduction in the vaccine serotype colonization due to PCV7 use. The predominant serotypes causing replacement disease were those found in the higher valency formulations of PCV. Fortunately, no replacement is seen following use of PCV10 or PCV13 in vaccinated children in countries using these vaccines in the National Immunization Program (NIP) since last 4 years. The WHO recommends that surveillance for replacement disease should continue especially in developing countries where the potential for replacement may be different from that in industrialized countries.

12. What is the herd effect with pneumococcal conjugate vaccine (PCV) against invasive pneumococcal disease (IPD)?

A surveillance program done by ABCS system in USA considered data from 1998 to 1999 as a pre-PCV7 launch and 2003 data as a post-PCV7 era. PCV7 was successfully included in 2000 in the NIP for use in children <2 years of age with catch-up program for children up to the age of 5 years. Vaccine uptake rapidly reached national average of 70%. It was found that IPD rates in children under 2 years fell by 96% for vaccine serotypes and 80% for all serotypes and for children under 5 years fell by 94% for vaccine serotypes and 75% for all serotypes. The IPD rates fell by 41% in 20–39 years age group, by

20% in 40–64 years age group, and by 31% in elderly >65 years of age who were not even the target for the vaccination. Even in babies <60-day-old, who have not received their first dose of the vaccine, the IPD rates fell by 42.5% and in <90-day-old (before the first dose can offer any protection) by 39%.

The Finnish Invasive Pneumococcal disease (FinIP) study showed reductions in hospital-diagnosed suspected nonconfirmed IPD and/or culture-confirmed VT IPD in older unvaccinated children following PCV10 introduction in the NIP.

Herd effects with PCV13 were shown in ABCS, USA data after the introduction of PCV13 in 2010. The incidence of five extra serotypes in PCV13 reduced significantly in 2011–2012 as compared to pre-PCV13 era by 88% in children <5 years, by 59% in 5–17-year-old, by 65% in 18–49-year-old, by 54% in 50–64-year-old, and by 47% in >65-year-old.

13. What about herd effect against noninvasive pneumococcal disease?

Since the incidence of non-IPD is 10–100 times more than the even little herd effect on these episodes will be significant. In a study done in the US by Grijalva et al. comparing the incidence of hospitalization due to clinical between 1997–1998 (pre-PCV period) and 2001–2004 (post-PCV7 period), it was found that incidence of hospitalization went down by 39% (95% CI: 22–52%) in children <2 years of age ($p < 0.0001$) and by 17% (95% CI: 3–34%) in children <5 years of age. Similarly, incidence of hospitalization due to pneumococcal pneumonia went down by 65% (95% CI: 47–73%) in children <2 years of age ($p < 0.0001$) and by 73% (95% CI: 53–85%) in children <5 years of age ($p < 0.0001$). In age group of 18–39 years, also, there was a similar statistically significant reduction in hospitalization due to all-cause clinical pneumonia by 26% (95% CI: 4–43%) ($p = 0.021$) and due to pneumococcal pneumonia by 30% (95% CI: 9–47%) ($p = 0.008$).

The 10-valent pneumococcal conjugate vaccine has not shown her defects on pneumonia. Use of PCV13 in Nicaragua has shown 19% reduction in pneumonia hospitalization rates in 5–14 years of age (who were vaccine noneligible) suggesting her defects of PCV13 against pneumonia.

14. How about the safety of pneumococcal conjugate vaccine (PCV)?

Mild local reactions have been noted in 30–35% of patients vaccinated with PCV7 and include redness, warmth, pain, induration, and tenderness. Severe local reactions >2.5 cm in diameter are seen in 5–6% of patients. The reactions are less than those seen with inactivated diphtheria, tetanus, and whole-cell pertussis (DTwP) vaccine and comparable with those seen with combined vaccine against diphtheria, tetanus, and acellular pertussis (DTaP), *Haemophilus influenzae* type b (Hib)/measles, mumps, and rubella (MMR) vaccines. No increase in side effects with increasing serotypes or number of doses has been noted. Fever >38°C is seen in 25–35% of recipients whereas fever >39°C is seen in <5% of patients. Adverse reactions like febrile convulsion, breath-holding spasms are rare. Severe adverse reactions are unknown to occur with this vaccine.

15. What are the current recommendations on interchangeability of pneumococcal conjugate vaccine (PCV) in pediatric use?

Interchangeability is defined as an ability to use more than one PCV product without compromising or adversely affecting its safety of its effectiveness neither in the individual nor in the population as a whole. Currently due to coavailability of the two currently WHO-PQ PCV products (PCV10 and PCV13) in the NIP as well as with additional PCV products in development, doubts regarding the interchangeability have been risen. PCV products differ both biologically, including serotype composition, carrier protein, and conjugation methods, and programmatically, including presence of preservative and number of doses per container. These factors tend to affect immunogenicity, impact on disease occurrence, NP colonization, and other components described in total system effectiveness, including vaccine handling, storage, and delivery; safety; cost per dose delivered; and equity. Although there is substantial experience with interchangeability of the currently licensed PCVs globally, few studies have evaluated the effect of having more than one product available in a country or administration of a mixed schedule of PCV products in an individual child on outcomes listed above. Although limited, phase II safety and immunogenicity data on interchangeability between PCV13 and the investigational PCV10 (Pneumosil™, SIIPL-PCV) are available in toddlers primed with PCV13 in infancy. Therefore, the available data and similarities between products, including those under development and PCV10/13, allow inferences to be made concerning their interchangeability.

16. What is the World Health Organization (WHO) recommendation for pneumococcal conjugate vaccine (PCV)?

The position paper, published in February 2019 by the WHO, replacing the corresponding WHO position paper on pneumococcal vaccines published in the Weekly Epidemiological Record in 2012 focuses on use of PCV in infants and children <5 years of age. The WHO recommends the inclusion of PCVs in childhood immunization programs worldwide. Use of pneumococcal vaccine should be complementary to other disease prevention and control measures, such as appropriate case management, promotion of exclusive breastfeeding for the first 6 months of life, and reducing known risk factors such as indoor air pollution and tobacco smoke. For administration of PCV to infants, the WHO recommends a three-dose schedule administered either as 2p + 1 or as 3p + 0, starting as early as 6 weeks of age. Countries should consider programmatic factors, including timeliness of vaccination and expected coverage in choosing between the 2p + 1 and 3p + 0 schedules. The 2p + 1 schedule induces higher antibody levels in the second year of life, maintaining herd immunity as compared with 3p + 0, but no high-quality evidence is available. Previously unvaccinated or incompletely vaccinated children who recover from IPD should be vaccinated according to the recommended age-appropriate regimens. Interrupted schedules should be resumed without repeating the previous dose. Both PCV10 and PCV13 have substantial impacts against pneumonia, VT IPD, and NP carriage. PCV13 may have an additional benefit in settings where disease attributable to serotype 19A or serotype 6C is significant. The choice of product to be used in a country should be based on programmatic characteristics, vaccine supply, vaccine price, the local and regional prevalence of vaccine serotypes, and antimicrobial resistance patterns. Product switching is not recommended unless there are substantial changes in the epidemiological or programmatic factors that determined the original choice of product, e.g., an increasing burden of serotype 19A.

17. What is the recommendation for pneumococcal conjugate vaccine (PCV) in India?

Considering the greatest burden of pneumococcal disease among the underprivileged children in India, PCVs are of public health importance and ideally should be given to all children. But the major drawback of PCV is its high cost and limited coverage of the currently available vaccine. The GAVI has offered to supply PCV at a cost of 0.15–0.3 USD/dose to India, so as to include it in national immunization schedule and commits to extending this support until the year 2015. The Advisory Committee on Vaccines and Immunization Practices (ACVIP) of the IAP recommends to use PCV10/PCV13 in healthy children <2 years with catch-up for children up to 5 years of age. The benefit of the vaccine is likely to be lower in healthy children above 2 years of age because of lower risk of IPD in this age group. Vaccination with single dose of PCV vaccine may be considered in children aged 2–5 years. It is not recommended in children aged 5 years and above. The recommended dosage for PCV13 is 0.5 mL and the vaccination route is IM.

Both PCV10 and PCV13 are licensed for active immunization in healthy children from 6 weeks to 5 years. PCV13 also licensed for adults >50 years in India. The United States Food and Drug Administration (USFDA) has licensed PCV13 for use in the age group of 6–17 years also, but not as yet approved for this age group in India.

- According to the IAP immunization schedule, PCV should be given at 6, 14 weeks as primary doses and at 9 months as booster dose schedule (2 + 1).
- Previously unvaccinated infants aged 7–11 months should receive two doses, the second dose at least 4 weeks after the first, followed by a third dose in the second year of life.
- For PCV10, unvaccinated children 12 months to 5 years of age should receive two doses, with an interval between the first and second dose of at least 2 months.
- For PCV13, unvaccinated children aged 12–24 months should receive two doses at least 2 months interval. Children aged 2–5 years should receive a single dose; adults >50 years of age should receive a single dose.

The PCV13 has already been introduced in many states with 6, 14 weeks and 9-month schedule (2 + 1). These states are included: Bihar, Himachal Pradesh, Madhya Pradesh, Uttar Pradesh, and Rajasthan.

18. What precautions should one take while administering 13-valent pneumococcal conjugate vaccine (PCV13) with Menactra and influenza vaccines?

When PCV13 and influenza vaccine are coadministered, it is generally well-tolerated with no vaccine-related serious side effects. In a study conducted at Ohio, USA, a randomized, double-blind, and phase III trial found that all serotypes met the predefined IgG geometric mean concentration (GMC) ratio but was lower as compared when not administered together. PCV13 injection site reactions were similar and mostly mild whether given together or separately. Systemic events were more frequent when the vaccines are coadministered than when given separately ($p < 0.001$) but no vaccine-related serious adverse events occurred. Coadministration of PCV13 and trivalent inactivated vaccine (TIV) was well-tolerated, but associated with lower PCV13 antibody responses and is of unknown clinical significance. Given the positive immunologic attributes of PCV13, concomitant administration with TIV should be dictated by clinical circumstances.

Similar results were noted when PCV13 is coadministered with Menactra in a study done at Spain where they found ≥90% of the subjects in whom PCV13 and Menactra were coadministered achieved an antibody concentration ≥0.35 µg/mL after dose three in the infant series. Safety and tolerability were also similar. Immunogenicity results of MnCCV-CRM197 for PCV13 had lower geometric mean titers (GMTs), but the clinical significance of this is unknown as the proportion of infants achieving protective MenC antibody titers was comparable up to titers of 1:128. PCV13 has an acceptable safety profile in infants and toddlers, while providing expanded coverage against pneumococcal disease.

19. What are the serological correlates of protection for pneumococcal conjugate vaccines (PCVs)?

Any new PCV has to meet the following two criteria laid down by the WHO for its licensure:
1. Immunoglobulin G (for all common serotypes collectively and not individually) of ≥0.35 µg/mL measured by the WHO qualified enzyme-linked immunosorbent assay (ELISA) technique.

    The geometric mean IgG concentration, as measured by ELISA without 22F adsorption, in sera collected 4 weeks after a three-dose primary series is considered the principal licensing criterion. If an alternative ELISA is used, it should be bridged and calibrated to the recommended reference assay. For serotypes in the licensed vaccine, the percentage of responders to each serotype in the new vaccine should be compared with the percentage of responders to the same serotypes in the licensed vaccine. Noninferiority for all serotypes is desirable, but not an absolute requirement. For new serotypes, not included in the licensed

vaccine, noninferiority to the aggregate response to the serotypes in the licensed vaccine should be demonstrated. Failure of one or more serotypes should be considered on case-by-case basis. In addition to demonstrating noninferiority with respect to the primary endpoint, the functional activity of the antibody should be demonstrated by the use of the opsonophagocytic assay (OPA) with a subset of sera and evidence for the induction of immunological memory should be obtained.
2. Opsonophagocytic activity with OPA titers of 1:8 or higher.

20. Can we use 2 + 1 schedule or 3 + 0 schedule instead of 3 + 1 schedule in our practice?

Countries should consider programmatic factors, including timeliness of vaccination and expected coverage in choosing between 2p + 1 and 3p + 0 schedules. The 2p + 1 schedule by producing higher antibody levels in the second year of life and thus maintaining herd immunity has potential benefits over the 3p + 0 schedule, but no high-quality evidence is available. If the 3p + 0 schedule is used, a minimum interval of 4 weeks should be maintained between doses. If the 2p + 1 schedule is selected, an interval of ≥8 weeks is recommended between the two primary doses, but the interval may be shortened if there is a compelling reason to do so, such as timeliness of receipt of the second dose and/or achieving higher coverage when a 4-week interval is used. The booster dose should be given at 9–18 months of age.

21. Can we use 23-valent pneumococcal polysaccharide vaccine (PPSV23) in >2-year-old children for routine immunization instead of pneumococcal conjugate vaccine (PCV)?

The 23-valent pneumococcal polysaccharide vaccine being unconjugated vaccine does not induce quality immune response as it induces only IgM response, which is low in quantity and quality with poor avidity and short-lived without memory response. Hence, it is to be used only in high-risk patients and not for healthy children. Giving PPSV23 before PCV may induce hyporesponsiveness and can be hazardous.

22. What are the characteristics of 23-valent pneumococcal polysaccharide vaccine (PPSV23)?

There are two types of pneumococcal vaccines that are currently licensed against *Pneumococcus* (*S. pneumoniae*): (1) PPSV and (2) PCVs. While PPSV offers "broad-based", "add-on" protection, despite its limitations, to children who are at high risk to contract pneumococcal disease, PCVs have much greater public health importance as they *effectively* prevent "pneumococcal pneumonia", one of the leading killers of under-five children.

The unconjugated PPS visa 23-valent vaccine (PPSV23) that contains 25 μg per dose of the purified polysaccharide of the following serotypes, accounting for over 80% of serotypes associated with serious diseases in adults—1, 2, 3, 4, 5, 6B, 7F, 8, 9N, 9V, 10A, 11A, 12F, 14, 15B, 17F, 18C, 19F, 19A, 20, 22F, 23F, and 33F. It is a T-cell independent vaccine that is poorly immunogenic below the age of 2 years, has low immune memory, does not reduce NP carriage, and does not provide herd immunity. It has at best 70% efficacy against prevention of IPD in the high-risk population, but offers no protection against nonbacteremic pneumonia/otitis media. It is stored at 2–8°C and the dose is 0.5 mL subcutaneous/IM in deltoid. It is a safe vaccine with occasional local side effects. Not more than two life time doses are recommended as repeated doses may cause immunologic hyporesponsiveness. PPSV should be given at least 2 weeks before the start of any treatment that can weaken your immune system. PPSV is also given at least 2 weeks before you undergo a splenectomy (surgical removal of the spleen). It may be harmful to an unborn baby and generally should not be given to a pregnant woman.

23. What are the recommendations of vaccination for high-risk children?

It is recommended to offer both PCV and PPSV23 to all high-risk children. PPSV23 will cover additional 10–15% of serotypes causing IPD that are not covered by PCV10/13. Hence, for the common serotypes, PCV will induce robust protection; subsequent PPSV23 will provide protection against IPD caused by 11 additional serotypes as well as it will boost up immune response to the common serotypes. If PCV cannot be given due to cost constraint, at least PPSV23 should be given to high-risk children above 2 years of age (**Table 3**).

24. What is the vaccination schedule for high-risk children?

Both PCV13 and PPSV23 are recommended for at-risk children >2 years of age (**Table 4**). The order of vaccination should be PCV13 followed by PPSV23 and not the other way as it can lead to hyporesponsiveness to subsequent PCV13.

25. What is the status of pneumococcal conjugate vaccine (PCV) introductions in the national immunization schedules in the world?

So far, 149 countries have introduced PCV vaccine in their NIP so far, globally. Only 44 countries have not introduced this vaccine in their NIPs at all (**Fig. 4**).

26. What are the recommendations for revaccination with 23-valent pneumococcal polysaccharide vaccine (PPSV23) among children at highest risk?

A second dose of PPSV23 is recommended 5 years after the first dose of PPSV23 for children who have anatomic or functional asplenia, including sickle cell disease (SCD), HIV infection, or other immunocompromising condition. No more than two PPSV23 doses are recommended.

TABLE 3: Children at high risk for pneumococcal disease.

Risk groups	Condition
Immunocompetent children	Chronic heart disease (particularly cyanotic congenital heart disease and cardiac failure)
	Chronic lung disease (including asthma if treated with prolonged high-dose oral corticosteroids)
	Diabetes mellitus
	Cerebrospinal fluid leak
	Cochlear implant
Children with functional or anatomic asplenia	Sickle cell disease and other hemoglobinopathies
	Congenital or acquired asplenia or splenic dysfunction
Children with immunocompromising conditions	HIV infection
	Chronic renal failure and nephrotic syndrome
	Diseases associated with treatment with immunosuppressive drugs or radiation therapy (e.g., malignant neoplasms, leukemias, lymphomas, and Hodgkin disease, or solid organ transplantation)
	Congenital immunodeficiency includes B (humoral) or T-lymphocyte deficiency; complement deficiencies, particularly C1, C2, C3, and C4 deficiency; and phagocytic disorders (excluding chronic granulomatous disease)
Premature and VLBW babies*	—

*The IAP now stresses the need of treating prematurity (PT) and very low birth weight (VLBW) infants as another high-risk category for pneumococcal vaccination. These infants have up to ninefold higher incidence of IPD in VLBW babies as compared to full-size babies. PCV must be offered to these babies on a priority basis.

(HIV: human immunodeficiency virus; IAP: Indian Academy of Pediatrics; IPD: invasive pneumococcal disease; PCV: pneumococcal conjugate vaccine)

27. What dosing intervals should be observed when giving 13-valent pneumococcal conjugate vaccine (PCV13) and 23-valent pneumococcal polysaccharide vaccine (PPSV23) to patients (children and adults) who are recommended to receive both vaccines?

It is advised to give PCV13 before PPSV23 if possible and also to not give PCV13 and PPSV23 at the same visit (**Table 5**).

28. What are the recommendations for the use of 13-valent pneumococcal conjugate vaccine (PCV13) in adult population?

In India, PCV13 has been approved in adults who are ≥50 years of age for the prevention of pneumonia and IPD. It is recommended by various scientific

TABLE 4: Vaccination schedule for high-risk children.

Age groups	Associated medical conditions	Schedule
2–4 years old	No associated condition	One dose of PCV13
2–5 years old	<ul><li>Chronic heart disease</li><li>Diabetes mellitus</li><li>Chronic lung disease including asthma if treated with high-dose corticosteroid oral therapy</li><li>CSF leaks</li><li>Cochlear implants</li></ul>	<ul><li>Give two doses of PCV13 if they are unvaccinated or received an incomplete PCV13 series with <three doses. Give the second at least 8 weeks after the first dose</li><li>Give one dose of PCV13 if they have received three doses of PCV13 but none were given after 12 months of age</li><li>Give one dose of PPSV23 at least 8 weeks after the PCV13 series are complete.</li></ul>
	<ul><li>Sickle cell anemia or other hemoglobinopathies</li><li>Anatomic or functional asplenia</li><li>Congenital or acquired immunodeficiency</li><li>HIV infection</li><li>Chronic renal failure or nephrotic syndrome</li><li>Iatrogenic immunosuppression, including radiation therapy</li><li>Leukemia or lymphoma</li><li>Hodgkin lymphoma</li><li>Multiple myeloma</li><li>Generalized and malignant malignancies</li><li>Solid organ transplant</li></ul>	<ul><li>Give two doses of PCV13 if they are unvaccinated or received an incomplete PCV13 series with <three doses. Give the second at least 8 weeks after the first dose</li><li>Give one dose of PCV13 if they have received three doses of PCV13 but none were given after 12 months of age</li><li>Give two doses of PPSV23 after PCV13 series is complete. Give the first dose at least 8 weeks after any prior PCV13 dose, then give the second dose of PPSV23 at least 5 years after the first dose of PPSV23</li></ul>

Contd...

Age groups	Associated medical conditions	Schedule
6–18 years old	• CSF leaks • Cochlear implants	• Give one dose of PCV13 if they have not received any dose of PCV13. Give PCV13 before giving any recommended dose of PPSV23 • Give one dose of PPSV23 (if have not received any dose in childhood) at least 8 weeks after PCV13
	• Chronic heart disease • Diabetes mellitus • Chronic lung disease including asthma if treated with high-dose corticosteroid oral therapy • Alcoholism • Chronic liver disease.	• Give one dose of PPSV23 if not given earlier in childhood

Contd...

(CSF: cerebrospinal fluid; HIV: human immunodeficiency virus; PCV13: 13-valent pneumococcal conjugate vaccine; PPSV23: 23-valent pneumococcal polysaccharide vaccine)

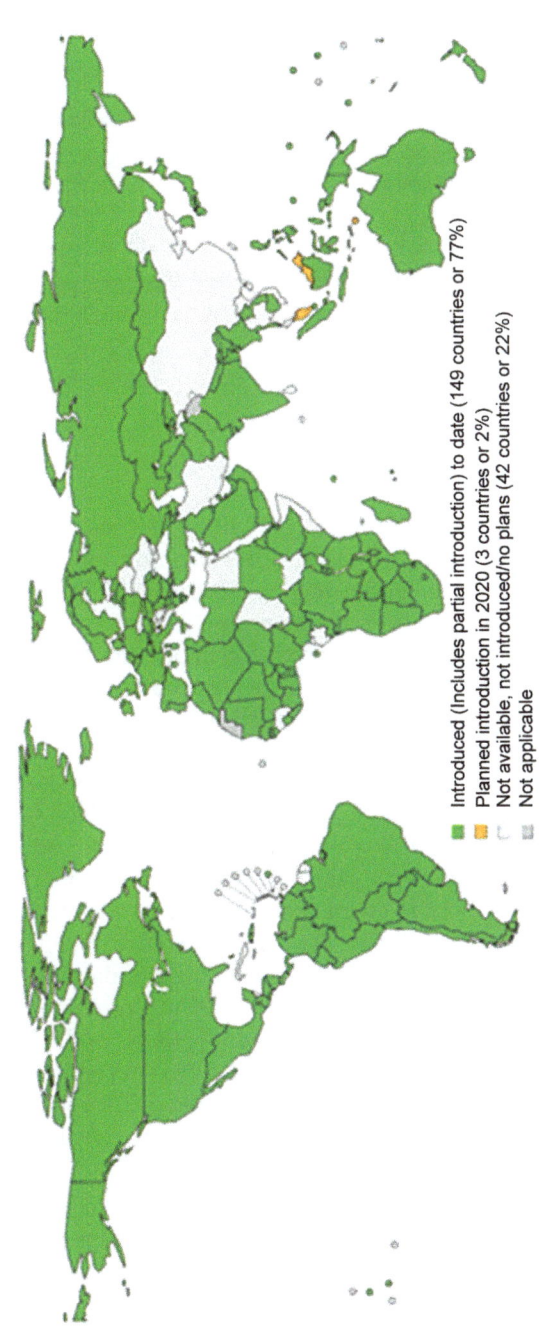

Fig. 4: Countries with pneumococcal conjugate vaccine (PCV) in the "National Immunization Program" and planned introductions in 2020.

TABLE 5: Recommendations for use of PCV 13 and PPSV 23 in children and adult.	
Population	Advice
Children who has already received PPSV23	Wait 8 weeks before giving PCV13
Adults at high risk of pneumococcal disease (immunocompromised, asplenia, CSF leak, and cochlear implants)	PCV13 followed by PPSV23 at least 8 weeks later
Adults 19–64 years with other high-risk conditions (e.g., chronic heart, lung or liver disease, diabetes, smoking, or alcoholism)	Give PPSV23 followed by an additional PPSV23 dose at age 65 years (at least 5 years after the first PPSV23 dose)
Age 65 years and above with no prior pneumococcal vaccination but no risk factors	Give PCV13 followed by PPSV23 1 year later
Adults who have already received PPSV23 and for whom PCV13 recommended	Wait 12 months before PCV13

(CSF: cerebrospinal fluid; PCV13: 13-valent pneumococcal conjugate vaccine; PPSV23: 23-valent pneumococcal polysaccharide vaccine)

bodies, including the Geriatric Society of India, for use in adults above 50 years of age keeping the increased predisposition and poor outcomes of pneumonia, observed in geriatric population. PPSV23 has been used in adults for 3 decades. However, the scientific evidence for the efficacy of PPSV23 in adults especially against prevention of pneumonia has been a very controversial issue, with more than 15 meta-analyses with conflicting results, having been published till date. Recently, in 2015, the Advisory Committee on Immunization Practices (ACIP) recommends spacing between PCV13 and PPSV23 in adults >65 years. According to the old ACIP recommendation, PPSV23 can be given after 6–12 months of PCV13. However, the new recommendation states that the recommended interval for adults receiving PCV13 and PPV23 to be at least 1 year, regardless of the sequence of the two vaccines that means PCV13 is given first followed by PPSV23 with spacing at least 1 year. If the adult above 65 years received PPSV23, then he will receive PCV13 after 1 year as per the older recommendation. However, the recommended intervals between PCV13 and PPSV23 remain unchanged for persons aged 2 years or older with medical indications and PPSV23 is to be given 8 weeks or more after PCV13 for those aged 19 years or older with certain underlying medical conditions. The new updated ACIP recommendations strongly support the usage of PCV13 as a routine vaccine in the adult population for prevention of pneumococcal disease.

29. What is the risk of febrile seizures associated with influenza and 13-valent pneumococcal conjugate vaccine (PCV13) vaccines?

There has been mixed evidence on risk of febrile seizures associated with influenza and PCV13 vaccines. Under the FDA-sponsored Sentinel Initiative, children aged 6–23 months were examined for the risk of febrile seizures after inactivated influenza vaccine (IIV) and PCV vaccine during the 2013–2014 and 2014–2015 influenza seasons. Adjusted for age, calendar time, and concomitant administration of the other vaccine, the incidence rate ratio (IRR) for risk of febrile seizures following IIV was found to be 1.12 (95% CI: 0.80, 1.56) and following PCV13 was found to be 1.80 (95% CI: 1.29, 2.52). The attributable risk for febrile seizures following PCV13 ranged from 0.33 to 5.16 per 100,000 doses by week of age. The age and calendar time-adjusted IRR comparing exposed to unexposed time were numerically larger for concomitant IIV and PCV13 (IRR 2.80, 95% CI: 1.63, 4.83) as compared to PCV13 without concomitant IIV (IRR 1.54, 95% CI: 1.04, 2.28) and the IRR for IIV without concomitant PCV13 suggested no independent effects of IIV (IRR 0.94, 95% CI: 0.63, 1.42), suggesting a possible interaction between IIV and PCV13. Thus, there could be an elevated risk of febrile seizures after PCV13 vaccine but not after IIV. The risk of febrile seizures after PCV13 is low compared to the overall risk in this population of children and the risk should be interpreted in the context of the importance of preventing pneumococcal infections.

30. What is the potential of pneumococcal conjugate vaccine (PCV) in the National Immunization Program (NIP) in India?

India accounts for 28 million infants born annually and yet to a large extent, these children do not benefit from the protection provided by a PCV immunization program. The Government of India, with support from GAVI, the Vaccine Alliance (in short, GAVI), has committed to a pilot implementation of PCV. With state-level PCV13 programs comprising 25% uptake across the country, approximately 1.9 million cases of pneumococcal disease and approximately 77,000 deaths could be prevented annually. An NIP with PCV13 could prevent approximately 7.6 million cases of pneumococcal disease and approximately 0.3 million pneumococcal deaths annually, compared with no vaccination, considering 100% vaccine uptake. These results are likely to have underestimated the additional potential benefits of herd effects in unvaccinated children and adults. GAVI funding of state-level programs is an important step toward achieving the full benefits of an NIP in India. Pneumococcus causes an enormous pneumonia disease and mortality burden is a number one cause of severe pneumonia-related cases and deaths and the effectiveness of PCV on pneumonia burden and child mortality, the WHO in 2007 recommended to include PCV in the NIP of any country with under-five mortality rate (UFMR) >50/1,000 live births or absolute child deaths >50,000 per year. With UFMR of 52 per 1,000 live birth and nearly 1.6 million under-five deaths per year, India merits to include PCV in NIP with high priority. There are 55 GAVI eligible countries, which can apply for GAVI support for inclusion of live saving vaccines in the NIP at a nominal cost sharing of few US cents per dose by these countries (and also 17 countries that have graduated who can also apply albeit they have to pay the entire GAVI cost of the vaccines). As on 2014, 10 million children have been vaccinated with PCV through GAVI support and 77 million immunized with

PCV by 2015 that is expected to avert 1.5 million deaths due to pneumococcal disease by 2020.

31. What are the future pneumococcal vaccines candidates? What role they can play?

Although with the availability of newer vaccines, PCV10- and PCV13-valent broadening the coverage of PCVs, the problem of serotype replacement still remains unresolved. Current conjugate vaccines are only capable of protecting against infection with bacteria that express polysaccharide capsule types that are included in the vaccine; it has the potential for replacement disease with nonvaccine serotypes, and lastly, the complexity of conjugate vaccines production. All these factors coupled with rapid increase in antibiotic resistance have led the researchers to search for novel pneumococcal vaccines that would not only be providing broader coverage but will also be much more affordable and easier to produce for many developing countries. The strategies being used for the development of newer pneumococcal vaccines include the following: individual or a combination of protein antigens produced by recombinant technology; pneumococcal protein carriers combined with traditional carriers produced by recombinant technology; traditional conjugate vaccines with added pneumococcal proteins; pneumococcal fusion proteins produced by recombinant technology; DNA vaccines; and attenuated whole-cell vaccines with low level expression of capsular polysaccharides. Intranasal immunization with various adjuvants induces strong antibody responses both in serum and on mucous membranes in mice and can protect them against lethal infections. Many different approaches have been tried so far, as yet the search for an ideal universal pneumococcal vaccine candidate is still far from over. Protein-based pneumococcal vaccines are the front runner as far as next generation pneumococcal vaccines is concerned. Low cost PCVs represent an exciting arena for future consideration. Protein-based vaccines are attractive for several reasons as they are expected to be immunogenic in early infancy and in the elderly due to their T-cell-dependent nature and their coverage should be at least, in theory, broader than that of conjugate vaccines. It is also suggested that they would offer stronger protection against colonization and by containing more than one species-specific antigen, they may be able to avoid the replacement phenomenon. In addition, they would be relatively simple to produce because they would have fewer components than multivalent conjugate vaccines; thus, protein-based vaccines are expected to be less expensive, allowing wide use in all areas of the world.

A new vaccine PCV20 has been under trials which was introduced by Pfizer Inc., who announced the USFDA granted Breakthrough Therapy Designation for 20vPnC for the prevention of invasive disease and pneumonia in adults age 18 years and older on September 20, 2018. 20vPnC candidate PF-06482077 includes the 13 serotypes contained in Prevnar 13 (1, 3, 4, 5, 6A, 6B, 7F, 9V, 14, 18C, 19A, 19F, and 23F) plus seven additional serotypes (8, 10A, 11A, 12F, 15BC, 22F, and 33F) to prevent IPD and pneumonia caused by *S. pneumoniae*. Three phase III trials (NCT03828617, NCT03835975, and NCT03760146) have been initiated for the purpose of evaluating 20vPnC in adults, including population with vaccine naïve adults and adults with prior pneumococcal vaccination. It is designed to compare immune responses after 20vPnC administration to responses in control subjects ≥60-year-old receiving PCV13 and PPSV23, evaluate the immunogenicity of 20vPnC in adults 18–59 years of age, and describe the 20vPnC safety profile in adults ≥18-year-old. Another phase III trial initiated on February 12, 2019 is designed to describe the safety and immunogenicity of 20vPnC in adults 65 years of age or older with prior pneumococcal vaccination. A third phase III trial initiated on February 14, 2019 is designed to provide additional safety data and evaluate three different lots of 20vPnC in adults 18 through 49 years of age.

Merck's PCV15 also called V114 have two additional STs 22F and 33F that are not contained in Prevnar 13 and are an emerging cause of pneumococcal infection and have been showing positive results in phase III clinical trials. The vaccine comprises pneumococcal polysaccharides from 15 serotypes conjugated to a CRM197 carrier protein. It includes 22F and 33F serotypes that are commonly related to IPD and not included in the PCV currently licensed for adults. Data from the PNEU-WAY (V114-018) trial revealed that V114 induce an immune response to all 15 serotypes included in the vaccine in adults aged 18 years or above with HIV.

Several pneumococcal proteins such as pneumococcal surface protein A (PspA), pneumococcal surface protein C (PspC), pneumococcal surface adhesin A (PsaA), pneumolysin (Ply), neuraminidase enzymes (Nan A and Nan B), pneumococcal histidine-triad proteins, etc., are found to possess immunogenic properties and they have been considered essential for bacterial virulence. Many trials are underway to explore their potential as pneumococcal vaccines—either as such or as carrier proteins for pneumococcal conjugates. However, the best future option would be to develop a protein vaccine that have a combination of more than one such protein antigens or even better would be to have a combination of a conjugate and a protein vaccine in order to get the best protection and the widest coverage. This type of futuristic pneumococcal vaccine will be most suited for developing countries obviating the need of "redesigning" vaccine every alternate year to reduce the risk of replacement with strains not included in the vaccine.

SUGGESTED READING

1. Centers for Disease Control and Prevention (CDC). (2019). Pneumococcal Vaccination: Summary of Who and When to Vaccinate. [online] Available from: cdc.gov/vaccines/vpd/pneumo/hcp/who-when-to-vaccinate.html. [Last accessed August, 2020].
2. Clarke E, Bashorun AO, Okoye M, Umesi A, Hydara MB, Adigweme I, et al. Safety and immunogenicity of a novel 10-valent pneumococcal conjugate vaccine candidate in adults, toddlers, and infants in The Gambia-Results of a phase 1/2 randomized, double-blinded, controlled trial. Vaccine. 2020;38(2):399-410.
3. Diez-Domingo J, Gurtman A, Bernaola E, Gimenez-Sanchez F, Martinon-Torres F, Pineda-Solas V, et al. Evaluation of 13-valent pneumococcal conjugate vaccine

and concomitant meningococcal group C conjugate vaccine in healthy infants and toddlers in Spain. Vaccine. 2013;31(46):5486-94.
4. Farooqui H, Jit M, Heymann DL, Zodpey S. Burden of severe pneumonia, pneumococcal pneumonia and pneumonia deaths in Indian states: modelling based estimates. PLoS One. 2015;10(6):e0129191.
5. Frenck RW, Gurtman A, Rubino J, Smith W, van Cleeff M, Jayawardene D, et al. Randomized, controlled trial of a 13-valent pneumococcal conjugate vaccine administered concomitantly with an influenza vaccine in healthy adults. Clin Vaccine Immunol. 2012;19(8):1296-303.
6. Indian Academy of Pediatrics Committee on Immunization (IAPCOI). Consensus recommendations on immunization, 2008. Indian Pediatr. 2008;45(8):635-48.
7. Lee H, Choi EH, Lee HJ. Efficacy and effectiveness of extended-valency pneumococcal conjugate vaccines. Korean J Pediatr. 2014;57(2):55-66.
8. Malik A, Taneja DK. Conjugate pneumococcal vaccines: need and choice in India. Indian J Community Med. 2013;38(4):189-91.
9. Rudan I, Boschi-Pinto C, Biloglav Z, Mulholland K, Campbell H. Epidemiology and etiology of childhood pneumonia. Bull World Health Organ. 2008;86(5):408-16.
10. Vashishtha VM. Pneumococcal vaccines—the future. Indian J Pediatr. 2015;82(11):S55-60.
11. World Health Organization (WHO). (2019). Summary of key points: WHO position paper on pneumococcal conjugate vaccines in infants and children under 5 years of age—February 2019. [online] Available from: https://www.who.int/immunization/policy/position_papers/who_pp_pcv_2019_presentation.pdf?ua=1. [Last accessed August, 2020].
12. Yewale V, Choudhary P, Thacker N. IAP Guidebook on Immunization 2009-2011. Mumbai: Indian Academy of Pediatrics; 2011. pp. 94-108.

CHAPTER 26

Rabies Vaccines

Omesh Kumar Bharti, Jaydeep Choudhury, Vipin M Vashishtha

1. Which animals transmit rabies?

All warm-blooded animals transmit rabies. Dog is the most common offender in urban setting. Apart from dog, the other culprits are cat, mongooses, fox, jackals, squirrels, wild rats, monkeys, horses, sheep, cows, buffaloes, donkeys, and pigs. The domestic animals like cow, buffalo, goat, pig, and sheep can transmit rabies after they are bitten and get infected by rabid animals. Monkey transmits rabies, if they are infected. Rarely, elephants, camels, and bears may lead to rabies, but rabies deaths due to home rodents have not been reported. Man-to-man transmission is not reported, except in cases of cornea/organ transplant from donors with undiagnosed rabies.

Bats infect each other in their roosts and there are few well-established incidences of bats infecting men or other animals. Apart from bites, direct infection by the virus in aerial route has been reported, but this mode of transmission has not been reported from India.

Two cycles of rabies exist: (1) sylvatic and (2) urban. Foxes, raccoons, skunks, jackals, mongooses, bats, etc., maintain the sylvatic cycle whereas dogs, cats, cattle, horses, sheep, pigs, etc., maintain the urban cycle.

2. What are the various modes of transmission of rabies?

The followings are the modes of transmission of rabies infection: (i) through broken skin—bites and scratches, (ii) licks on damaged skin and intact mucous membrane by rabid animals, (iii) aerosol spread, and (iv) organ transplant—cornea transplant.

- *Through broken skin*: The most common mode of transmission of virus to human population is the bite from infected dogs. Rabies virus cannot penetrate intact skin. Contamination of broken skin with saliva of rabid animal by simple licking can also become dangerous anytime. Scratches by rabid animals, even if not bleeding, are also considered another mode of transmission, which allow virus entry. So, biting, scratching, and licking of rabid animals on broken skin all are to be given importance.
- *Direct mucous membrane contact*: Rabies virus can penetrate intact mucous membrane, however drinking of raw milk of infected cow, buffalo, or goat is not considered as exposure and no postexposure prophylaxis (PEP)

is required. Contact of saliva of rabid animals in anal region or mouth cavity, i.e., moist mucous surfaces, is also considered to be dangerous.
- *Aerosol infection in bat-infested caves*: This has importance in North American countries not in India.
- *Organ transplants*: Mainly corneal transplant from undiagnosed infected humans (encephalitis) can also transmit rabies accidentally.

3. What is the incubation period of rabies in human?

It is highly variable. Incubation period may be as short as 4 days or as long as 3 years. Average incubation period varies between 3 weeks and 3 months. Prolonged incubation period is reported in relatively fewer cases. The size of virus inoculum and the bites on head and neck region due to proximity to brain and bites on hands due to excess innervations may have some significance in the early causation of the disease. Direct bites on face, large facial or sciatic nerves may cause early disease.

4. What are the clinical types of rabies?

Two distinct types of clinical rabies have been described. The common type is furious type, seen in 80% of cases and the other one is paralytic or dumb rabies which is seen in 20% of cases. Both types are common for human and canine rabies. The furious type of rabies presents with acute neurological phase characterized by hydrophobia, aerophobia, photophobia, dysphagia, etc. The presenting features are as follows:
- *Furious rabies*:
  - Tingling and numbness at bite site, paresthesia
  - Nonspecific symptoms like fever, malaise, and headache
  - Characteristic symptoms are hydrophobia, aerophobia, and photophobia related to spasms of gullet
  - Aggressiveness
  - Death due to cardiac and respiratory failure occurs in 3–5 days.
- *Paralytic rabies*:
  - Tingling and numbness at bite site
  - Nonspecific symptoms like fever, malaise, and headache
  - Progressive ascending paralysis. The order of involvement is lower limbs, abdominal muscles, upper limb, and thoracic muscles, followed by coma, respiratory failure
  - Death due to cardiac and respiratory failure occurs in 7–21 days
  - Mostly paralytic rabies is seen in patients having received incomplete rabies prophylaxis.

5. What are the various categories of exposure to rabies virus and management?

The World Health Organization (WHO) recommended management of animal exposure is described in **Table 1**.

TABLE 1: Management of animal exposure.

Category	Type of contact with suspected or confirmed domestic or wild animals* or animal unavailable for observation	Recommended treatment
I	Touching or feeding of animals, licks on intact skin	None, if reliable case history is available
II	Nibbling of uncovered skin, minor scratches or abrasions without bleeding, and licks on broken skin	• Administer vaccine immediately • Stop treatment, if animal remains healthy throughout an observation period of 10 days§ • Or, if the animal is euthanized and found to be negative for rabies by appropriate laboratory technique
III	Single or multiple transdermal bites or scratches, contamination of mucous membrane with saliva (i.e., licks)	• Administer rabies immunoglobulins and vaccine immediately • Stop treatment, if animal remains healthy throughout an observation period of 10 days§ • Or, if the animal is euthanized and found to be negative for rabies by appropriate laboratory techniques

*Exposure to rabbits, rodents, and hares seldom, if ever, require specific anti-rabies treatment.
§This observation applies only to dogs and cats.

6. Why are children at a higher risk for rabies?

Children are more at risk of rabies because of the following reasons:
- Short height of the children makes the vulnerable parts of the body like head, face, neck, and hands more accessible to the animals. Again due to short height, the traversing time of rabies virus from periphery to central nervous system is short.
- Tremendous curiosity regarding pets and other animals. Children love to play with dogs and cats and pets love to play with children.
- Children do not have any knowledge about the outcome and danger of encounter with animals.
- Children often do not report animal bites and scratches to their parents.

7. How to manage a child who has been exposed to an animal?

Exposure to an animal consists of bite, scratch, or lick on broken wounds in skin or directly on mucous membrane, i.e., on oral cavity or on anus by an animal. All warm-blooded animals are potentially rabid. Treatment follow in an exposure will consist of the following:
- *Step I: Proper wound management*: The most important steps in wound management are:
  - Thorough washing of wounds under running tap water for at least 15 minutes with the aim of physical elimination of the viral load and

application of soap or detergent for chemical treatment to kill the virus in the wounds.
- Application of disinfectants like povidone-iodine, spirit, household antiseptics, etc., to remove the remaining virus particles and prevention of secondary infection.
- Application of irritants to the wounds like chili, plant juices, etc., cauterization and suturing for wound closure should be avoided. If suturing is needed for the purpose of hemostasis, it can be done only after local wound infiltration of rabies immunoglobulin (RIG).
- *Step II: Rabies Immunoglobulin*: Infiltration/inundation of the entire wound surface till depth with RIG in all category III exposures. It neutralizes the virus and forms a coat around the virus thus obliterating virus entry into the nerve endings.
- *Step III: Anti-rabies vaccination* (ARV): PEP with ARV should be initiated as soon as possible and full course should be completed.
- *Step IV: Anti-tetanus prophylaxis and supportive treatment*: Administration of tetanus toxoid (TT or Td) as required depending on the child's immunization status. Supportive treatment is given for fever and pain with antipyretics and analgesics, local and/or systemic antibiotic as required.

8. How rabies immunoglobulin (RIG) is given? What are the different types of RIG available in the market?

Rabies immunoglobulin provides passive immunity in the form of readymade antibody to tide over the initial phase of the infection. RIG has the property of binding to rabies virus, thereby resulting in neutralization of the virus. Three types of RIGs are available:
1. *Equine rabies immunoglobulin (ERIG)*: ERIG is of heterologous source raised by hyperimmunization of horses. Currently, manufactured ERIGs are highly purified and enzyme refined. The dose of ERIG is 40 IU/kg body weight of patient up to a maximum of 3,000 IU. As per latest recommendations from the WHO, skin testing prior to ERIG administration is not recommended as skin tests do not accurately predict anaphylaxis risk and ERIG should be given whatever the result of the test.
2. *Human rabies immunoglobulin (HRIG)*: HRIG is prepared from the serum of people hyperimmunized with rabies vaccines. The dose of HRIG is 20 IU/kg body weight (maximum 1,500 IU). HRIG does not require any prior sensitivity testing.
3. *Rabies monoclonal antibodies (RmAbs)*: A single mAb product against rabies was licensed in India in 2017, Rabishield. It has been demonstrated to be safe and effective in clinical trials. This RmAb neutralizes a broad panel of globally prevalent rabies virus isolates. The comparative advantages of RmAb products include large-scale production with standardized quality elimination of the use of animals in the production process and reduction in the risk of adverse events. The dose is 3.33 IU/kg given like RIG.

Another RmAbs available recently is TwinRab. The two monoclonal antibodies (MAb), docaravimab and miromavimab are the active ingredients present in equipotent amounts in TwinRab. TwinRab neutralizes a broad range of rabies viruses and dose is 40 IU/Kg body weight of the patient.

The cost of RmAbs may be prohibitory to poor patients and equine rabies immunoglobulins (eRIGs) is equally effective and time tested option for PEP and only wound infiltration causes negligible side effects to the patients.

The WHO has recently recommended abolishing the skin sensitivity test as it is considered not predictive of adverse events/reactions to occur. But in India, it is obligatory on the part of physician to do it as mentioned in the product insert due to prevailing drug laws and until it is withdrawn.

Rabies immunoglobulin is to be infiltrated as much as possible into and around all the wounds. The remaining RIG, if any, needs not to be given intramuscular (IM) away from wound site, but to be given to next patient depending on the size of the wound. After calculation of the dose of RIG, if it is seen that RIG is insufficient by volume to infiltrate all the wounds, it should be diluted with normal saline to make it two or three times to required volume. If RIG could not be given when ARV was initiated, it should be administered as early as possible but no later than the 7th day after the first dose of anti-rabies vaccine. From the 8th day onward, RIG is not indicated since an antibody response to the vaccine is presumed to have occurred. RIG is also not indicated in individuals who have received pre-exposure or PEP in the past. Therefore, RIG is administered only once in lifetime.

9. Can equine rabies immunoglobulin (RIG) be used safely?

Most of the new ERIG preparations are potent, safe, highly purified, and less expensive as compared to HRIG/RmAb, but do carry a negligible risk of anaphylaxis.

10. Should rabies immunoglobulin (RIG) be given to all dog bite cases?

All category III exposures to rabies in endemic countries, i.e., in transdermal bites (single or multiple) or scratches, contact of patient's mucous membrane with animal saliva should immediately be treated with RIG along with ARV. If the administration of the RIG is delayed initially, it can be administered up to 7th day after the first dose of vaccine, i.e., along with third dose of vaccine. RIG needs not to be given after the 8th day because it results in suppression of the endogenous systemic antibody response to vaccination. If the volume of RIG is inadequate for infiltration of all wounds, it should be diluted with normal saline up to two- to three-fold to make up sufficient volume required.

11. What are the various anti-rabies vaccines?

Active immunization is done by administration of ARV. In India, nerve tissue vaccine (NTV) (Semple vaccine) was used for postexposure treatment.

The vaccine was highly reactogenic with potential neuroparalyticogenic effect and is no longer used. The currently available vaccines are the modern tissue culture vaccines (TCVs). All TCVs have almost equal efficacy and any one of these can be used. These vaccines induce protective antibodies in >99% of vaccinees following PrEP or PEP. The dosage schedule of cell culture rabies vaccine is same irrespective of the body weight or age of the children. The vaccines are available in lyophilized form and are stable for 3 years at 2–8°C. Rabies vaccines should be used within 6 hours of reconstitution. The main adverse effects are local pain, swelling and redness, and less commonly fever, headache, dizziness, and gastrointestinal side effects.

Types of anti-rabies vaccines:
- *Cell culture rabies vaccines (CCRV)*:
    - Purified chick embryo cell vaccine (PCECV)
    - Purified Vero cell rabies vaccine (PVRV).
- All CCRVs used for PEP should have potency, i.e., antigen content >2.5 IU per dose.

Reconstitution and storage: The lyophilized vaccine should be reconstituted with the diluent provided with the vaccine immediately prior to use. In case of unforeseen delay, it should be used within 6–8 hours of reconstitution.

12. Which one is the best "anti-rabies vaccine" available in the market?

All "TCVs" available in the market are equally effective, highly immunogenic, and safe. For all practical purposes, there is absolutely nothing to choose between all the available TCV as far as efficacy and safety are concerned. The WHO has now recommended abandoning old, crude "NTV" and replaces it by TCV.

13. What is the schedule of pre-exposure prophylaxis (PrEP) of rabies vaccination?

Pre-exposure prophylaxis (PrEP) is indicated for those people who are having high professional risk of acquiring rabies infection. It may be advisable to vaccinate children after they attain the age of 3 years and start playing in the streets and may come in contact with street or pet dogs.

Pre-exposure prophylaxis is recommended for certain high-risk groups enumerated below:
- *Continuous exposure*: Laboratory personnel involved with rabies research and production of rabies biologics.
- *Frequent exposure*: Veterinarians, laboratory personnel involved with rabies diagnosis, medical and paramedical staff treating rabies patients, dog catchers, zookeepers, and forest staff.
- *Infrequent exposure*: Postmen, municipality workers, garbage collectors, policemen, courier boys, and travelers to rabies endemic countries, particularly those who intend to trek.

- *Pets*: Children having pets at home.
- *Higher threat*: Children perceived with higher threat of being bitten by dogs.

Schedule of pre-exposure vaccination: The WHO recommends the following PrEP schedule:
- Two-site 0.1 mL intradermal (ID) vaccine administered on days 0 and 7.
- If IM administration is used, the WHO recommends a one-site IM vaccine administration on days 0 and 7.

Routine assessment of anti-rabies antibody titer after completion of vaccination is not recommended, unless the person is immunocompromised. It is desirable to monitor antibody titer every 6 months in those with continuous exposure and every year in those with frequent exposure. A booster is recommended, if antibody levels fall below 0.5 IU/mL.

It has been shown in several studies that pre-exposure vaccination elicits a good immune response and the memory cells generated lasts for many years. If such people are exposed to rabies by animal bites, two booster doses given on day 0 and on day 3 will elicit a rapid and stronger secondary immune response which will neutralize the virus. Alternatively, one time four-site 0.1 mL ID vaccination can also be done as booster vaccination. There is no need for administration of RIG in patients who had taken a complete course of PrEP.

14. Is there some change in new Indian Academy of Pediatrics-Advisory Committee on Vaccines and Immunization Practices (IAP-ACVIP) 2014 recommendations pertaining to rabies?

Yes, now the committee has recommended that practically all children need vaccination against rabies and following two situations to be included in "high-risk category of children" for rabies vaccination:
1. Children having pets at home
2. Children perceived with higher threat of being bitten by dogs such as hostellers, risk of stray dog menace while going outdoor.

These groups of children should be offered "PrEP" against rabies. This must be preceded by a one-to-one discussion with the parents. However, the "PrEP" is not included in the Indian Academy of Pediatrics (IAP) immunization schedule for all children. There is no change in the IAP recommendations for "PEP" of rabies.

15. A 4-year-old boy is bitten by a stray dog. He had received a full course (five doses) of postexposure prophylaxis only 3 months back. Does he need any shot of anti-rabies vaccine?

If an individual had a repeat exposure in <3 months after a previous exposure and has already received complete PEP within last 3 months, only wound treatment is required; neither vaccine nor RIG is needed. For repeat exposure occurring > 3 months till years after the last PEP, the PEP schedule for previously immunized individuals should be followed; RIG is not indicated.

16. What are the benefits of "pre-exposure prophylaxis (PrEP)" against rabies?

The advantages of the PrEP include elimination of the need for painful wound infiltration of RIG, reduction in the number of vaccine doses on exposure, and provision of immunity to individuals whose PEP is delayed. Further, the likelihood of lack of documentation of a dog bite among young children who may not report scratches and small playful bites from dogs and cats are other reasons why PrEP would be useful.

17. If there are so many benefits of "PrEP immunization" against rabies, why the Indian Academy of Pediatrics-Advisory Committee on Vaccines and Immunization Practices (IAP-ACVIP) has not included it in its routine immunization schedule?

The committee is of the opinion that inclusion of PrEP against rabies in only IAP schedule for office practice would not serve the desired purpose, since majority of deaths occur among children belonging to low socioeconomic strata and those living in remote areas. The committee has strongly recommended to the Government of India (GoI) to include PrEP against rabies in their Universal Immunization Program (UIP).

18. What are the World Health Organization (WHO) recommendations in this regard?

As per the WHO, "PrEP for entire populations is not cost-effective in most settings and is, therefore, not recommended; however, wide-scale PrEP should be considered in remote settings with limited access to PEP if the annual dog bite incidence is >5% or if exposure to vampire bats is prevalent".

19. What is postexposure prophylaxis (PEP) (Table 2)?

Postexposure prophylaxis is a medical emergency. PEP should be initiated as soon as possible and should not be delayed till results of laboratory tests or animal observation is available. Infancy, pregnancy, and lactation are never contraindications for PEP. Persons presenting several days, months, or even years after the bite should be managed in a similar manner as a person who has been bitten recently (with RIG, if indicated) as rabies has a long incubation period and the window of opportunity for prevention remains even in cases who present late for prophylaxis.

All category II and III animal bites merit rabies vaccine. Any of the TCV may be used IM in anterolateral thigh or the deltoid depending on the age. Rabies vaccine should never be injected in the gluteal region. The dose is same at all ages and is 1 mL IM for PCECV, and 0.5 mL for PVRV. The standard schedule, which is known as Essen protocol of four doses on days 0, 3, 7, and between days 14 and 28; with day "0" being the day of first vaccine injection.

Following rabies vaccine administration on days 0, 3, and 7 if the animal remains healthy over a 10-day observation period, further vaccination may be discontinued. Recent recommendation of the WHO is to give IM rabies vaccine four shots only on days 0, 3, and 7 and fourth between any day between 14 and 28.

TABLE 2: Postexposure prophylaxis (PEP) by category of exposure as per latest WHO guidelines 2018.

	Category I exposure	Category II exposure	Category III exposure
Immunologically naive individuals of all age groups	Washing of exposed skin surfaces No PEP is required	Wound washing and immediate vaccination Two-site ID on days 0, 3, and 7 Or One-site IM on days 0, 3, and 7 and between days 14 and 28 Or Two-site IM on day 0 and one-site IM on days 7, 21 RIG is not indicated	Wound washing and immediate vaccination Two-site ID on days 0, 3, and 7 Or One-site IM on days 0, 3, and 7 and between days 14 and 28 Or Two-site IM on day 0 and one-site IM on days 7, 21 RIG administration is recommended
Previously immunized individuals of all age groups	Washing of exposed skin surfaces No PEP is required	Wound washing and immediate vaccination At four-site ID on day 0 Or One-site ID on days 0 and 3 At one-site IM on days 0 and 3 RIG is not indicated	Wound washing and immediate vaccination One-site ID on days 0 and 3 Or At four-site ID on day 0 Or At 1-site IM on days 0 and 3 RIG is not indicated

(ID: intradermal; IM: intramuscular; PEP: postexposure prophylaxis; RIG: rabies immunoglobulin)

20. How many doses of tissue culture vaccine (TCV) should be administered for pre-exposure prophylaxis (PrEP)?

The WHO recommends the following PrEP schedule: two-site 0.1 mL ID vaccine administered on days 0 and 7. If IM administration is used, the WHO recommends a one-site IM vaccine administration on days 0 and 7.

21. Is there any alternate route of anti-rabies vaccine administration?

The ID schedules have been used successfully in many countries. ID regimen consists of administration of a fraction of IM dose of TCVs on multiple sites in the layers of dermis of skin. The use of ID route leads to considerable savings in terms of total amount of vaccine needed for full pre- or postexposure vaccination, thereby reducing the cost of active immunization.

22. Should initial dose of tissue culture vaccine (TCV) be doubled if rabies immunoglobulin (RIG) is not available?

If RIG is not available, then more emphasis should be given to proper wound management by washing with soap and water and later application of antiseptic and vaccination before referring the patient to the nearest facility/pooling center providing RIG so as to receive it within 7 days of starting rabies vaccine. There is no substitute to RIG as any amount of vaccine leaves a window period of 7–10 days for infection before active immune response is generated by the body's immune system.

23. Is observing the dog for 10 days without initiating treatment risky or justifiable?

Whether to observe the dog for 10 days following exposure or to start vaccination immediately after exposure is still a matter of controversy. However, in a hyperendemic country like India, it would be a sane approach to start treatment and discontinue it after the dog remains healthy or has been found laboratory negative.

24. What should be the treatment protocol for a patient who had exposure, but only goes for treatment after considerable delay (weeks to months)?

Since prolonged incubation period has been noted, persons who present themselves for evaluation and treatment even months after having been bitten should be dealt in the same manner as if the contact occurred recently.

25. What will be rabies postexposure treatment of previously vaccinated persons?

Patient who has been previously received PrEP or PEP with rabies vaccine should receive the treatment protocol as follows:
- Local treatment of wound.
- *Vaccination schedule*: One dose immediately and second on day 3, no RIG should be applied. Alternatively, one time four-site 0.1 mL vaccine can be given intradermally on day zero as booster.
- However, full treatment should be given to persons who have received pre- or postexposure treatment with vaccines of unproven potency with old NTV or people who have not demonstrated acceptable rabies neutralizing antibody titer.

26. What should be the management if a child is bitten by a vaccinated pet dog?

Up to 8% pet dogs do not seroconvert even after being regularly vaccinated. Therefore, pet vaccination is not reliable basis to not to start PEP. Immediate PEP should be started and pet observed for 10 days as explained above.

27. Can a vaccinated dog transmit rabies?

An adult dog effectively vaccinated against rabies cannot suffer and transmit the disease however rabies due to pup bites has been reported in India and pup need to be vaccinated before they are brought home then at 3 months and then yearly. However, it is very difficult to say with certainty that a particular dog immunized with a specific vaccine is immune against rabies. If a TCV is regularly given to a healthy dog, it should develop sufficient protection. But, in a recent survey, 8% of dogs having a reliable history of rabies vaccination need re-vaccination to prevent the re-establishment of rabies.

28. Can rabies be transmitted from man to man?

There has never been a well-documented case of human-to-human transmission, other than the few cases resulting from organ transplant. However, persons who have been exposed closely to the secretions of a rabid patient may be offered PEP as a precautionary measure. Hence, confirmation of cause of death particularly in neurological cases (encephalitis) is very important before corneal transplantation. Besides, it is also important to avoid contact with saliva and secretions of a patient diagnosed as having rabies.

29. Do modern rabies tissue culture vaccines interfere with other commonly used childhood vaccines?

No. They can safely be given with other childhood vaccines.

30. Is it possible to include rabies vaccines in Expanded Program on Immunization (EPI) schedule?

Yes. In fact, rabies vaccines had been administered along with diphtheria, tetanus, and pertussis-inactivated polio vaccine (DTP-IPV) in Vietnamese infants at 6, 10, and 14 weeks of age and have been found to be safe and efficacious. This could lead to future integration of pre-exposure rabies vaccination into the EPI of countries where rabies is enzootic and endemic for humans.

31. How are rabies neutralizing antibody titers estimated? Where in India are such facilities available?

Rabies neutralizing antibody titers are estimated utilizing the rapid fluorescent focus inhibition test (RFFIT). Routine estimations are not required if the WHO recommendations are followed and the four to five injections are taken on schedule. However, in certain circumstances (e.g., considerable delay in first dose, incomplete treatment, miscalculation of scheduled days of administration, etc.), it may be necessary to ensure that adequate antibody titers have been achieved.

Following centers in India are estimating these titers:
- National Institute of Mental Health and Neurosciences (NIMHANS), Bengaluru
- National Institute for Communicable Diseases, New Delhi.

32. If the patient has consumed milk of a cow or buffalo bitten by a rabid dog, is it necessary to give anti-rabies vaccine?

There is no need for PEP in case of consumption of raw milk from a rabid cow as rabies virus has not been demonstrated in the raw milk of a rabid cow/buffalo. However, boiling of the milk inactivates the virus.

33. Is there a carrier state of rabies in dogs?

There have been stray reports of carrier state of rabies in dogs. However, no report has convincingly demonstrated a carrier state in dogs and for all practical purposes this can be taken as nonexistent. However, in African countries, brain and saliva of healthy dogs slaughtered for meat have been found to carry rabies virus.

34. In the event of a rat bite, do we need to give anti-rabies vaccine?

Most rodents in India have been found to be free of rabies. Mongooses and squirrels have been shown to be suffering from rabies and it is possible for these animals to transmit the infection to other rodents and man. Cases of bites by rodents that are usually aggressive must be viewed with suspicion. Theoretically, all warm-blooded mammals are capable of suffering from rabies and transmitting it to man. In principal, house mice bite do not require any PEP, but wild rats and other animals may require PEP.

35. If an individual has been vaccinated with a cell culture vaccine (CCV) by intradermal (ID) route and later exposed again to rabies, what should be the booster schedule?

Four-site one time 0.1 mL rabies vaccination intradermally or two shots of IM rabies vaccination on days 0 and 3 as boosters.

36. What are the contraindications to rabies vaccination? How should allergic reactions to rabies vaccines be handled?

Because rabies is a lethal disease, any contraindication to postexposure treatment should be considered carefully before disqualifying an individual for PEP.

Individuals with histories of severe allergies are more prone to develop allergic reactions to rabies vaccine. When those individuals are vaccinated, prophylactic antihistamines should be given and epinephrine should be available. If an allergic reaction occurs, one may give an alternative vaccine of different tissue origin, e.g., PVRV in the case of a reaction to or PCECV.

37. Is pregnancy a contraindication to rabies vaccination?

No, pregnancy is not a contraindication to rabies vaccination. Follow-up of 202 Thai women vaccinated during pregnancy revealed no excess of medical complications or abnormal births.

38. What is "spirit test"?

Broken skin can be assessed by *spirit test*; if there is doubt, then a spirit swab is applied on the affected area and if there is tingling/burning sensation, it means that skin is broken and would require local RIG infiltration and vaccination after thorough wound wash and antiseptics.

39. Discuss "switch over from one brand or type of vaccine to the other".

Shifting from one brand or type of cell culture and embryonated egg-based rabies vaccines (CCEEVs) to other brand/type should not be encouraged in routine practice. However, under unavoidable circumstances, available brand/type of rabies vaccine may be used to complete the PEP.

40. Discuss suturing of wound.

It should be avoided as far as possible. If suturing after wound cleansing cannot be avoided, the wound(s) should first be thoroughly infiltrated with human or equine RIG and suturing delayed for several hours to allow diffusion of the immunoglobulin through the tissues before minimal loose sutures are done. Minimum loose sutures (one or two) to approximate the edges can be applied after proper infiltration of RIGs into wounds. Cauterization of wound is no longer recommended. Tetanus toxoid injection should be given to those children who have not received a booster dose in the last 5 years. To prevent sepsis in the wound, a suitable course of an antibiotic must be prescribed. A film has been made on only wound infiltration of RIG and is available on web link; https://www.youtube.com/watch?v=mtYGnRPGWv0&feature=youtu.be

41. Which route of rabies vaccination is more potent?

A very important question that is frequently asked is whether IM rabies vaccination is superior in eliciting an immune response than ID rabies vaccination or vice versa. For the first time, the WHO Weekly Epidemiological Record (WER 9316) has reported that intradermal (ID) rabies vaccination has efficacy equivalent to or higher than that of the same vaccine administered by the IM route. ID vaccination even in small doses is effective as we directly present the antigen to the lymph nodes that elicits a strong response through antigen presenting cells that are strong in skin than in muscles.

42. Is there a single dose rabies vaccine for PEP?

No, there is no single dose PEP and multiple vaccine doses with local wound infiltration are essential for complete PEP.

43. What is clinical management of rabid patient?

It is beyond the preview of this chapter to deliberate on the detailed management of rabid patients here. Since rabies is invariably fatal, we have to do just palliative management of patients with rabies. Most patients with rabies remain conscious and are aware of the nature and outcome of their illness. The patients are kept in a quiet room with dim light and are protected from all stimuli of sound, water, light and air currents. Mostly sedatives are given to control aggression and IV fluids are maintained. Milwaukee protocol have been found to be unreliable and may add to the pain of the patient.

44. Can RIG be injected into wounds if health facility has no rabies vaccine?

In case we have no rabies vaccine we should do vigorous wound washing with copious amount of water followed by antiseptic application. We need to clean the antiseptic soon thereafter so that it does not neutralize the RIG. After cleaning the antiseptic with spirit, let the wound dry before RIG is injected into the wound/s. Please refer the patient to nearby facility for vaccine administration as early as possible as vaccine gives long-term protection and is essential. In case of RIG shortage, same strategy should be adopted and patient may be referred to nearby facility for RIG administration after wound management and vaccination.

45. Some rabies vaccines are 0.5 mL and some 1 mL, which vaccine we should prefer?

Dose of vaccine administration is same irrespective of if it being 0.5 mL or 1 mL, e.g., dose for ID administration is 0.1 mL per site whether the vial being 0.5 mL or 1 mL while full volume of the vaccine vial is injected as one dose for IM administration whether the vial volume is 0.5 or 1 mL. For ID administration, 1 mL vials are preferred for use by more number of patients and for IM administration, 0.5 mL vials are preferred for having less volume of the vaccine.

46. What to do Rabies vaccine dose on schedule is missed?

If rabies vaccine schedule is missed the vaccination is to be resumed for remaining doses not reschedules afresh.

47. PEP for immunocompromised patients?

Mostly such individuals will probably respond to vaccine in the same way as people who are not severely immunocompromised or are healthy, as observed in studies conducted for routine vaccines. Clinical experience suggests that, whenever possible, the best PEP options available (the most immunogenic regimen, high-quality vaccines and RIG) should be used, regardless of the route of vaccine administration. Meticulous, very thorough wound-cleaning as first aid to bite victims is of utmost importance in immune-compromised patients.

48. What are the signs of animal rabies?

Animal rabies is typically described as furious rabies and paralytic rabies. furious rabies is described as animal having aggressive or combative behavior, irritability, viciousness and hyper-reaction to external stimuli and hyper-salivation A paralytic phase is characterized by weakness of one or more limbs, dribbling of saliva and dropping of jaw. Difficulty in making routine vocalizations leads to altered phonation/altered barking sound. Dog mostly do not run amok and remain to a limited geographical area biting people suddenly and unprovoked.

49. Safe handling of dead body of patients who died of Rabies.

Since the blood does not contain any virus (no viremia) only body secretions may be infectious like saliva, tears, urine, etc. and precautions should be taken to not to get spillage by these secretions. Tissues and organs may be infected and should not be transplanted. Early cremation or burial should be done.

50. What is risk of infection following bite by a rabid dog?

The risk of infection following bite by a rabid dog is about 15% and varies (0.1–60%) depending on site of bite and size of viral inoculum, number of bites and bite depth and area of rich/low nerve innervations.

51. Do we have some areas free of rabies?

Yes, we have Islands of Andaman and Nicobar and Lakshadweep free of rabies. There are no dogs in Lakshadweep but cats are there.

52. A child is bitten by a dog on 5th September. He is being advised 'ICMR-GoI' schedule of five-dose of rabies vaccines along with rabies immunoglobulins for post-exposure prophylaxis. His schedule is as follows: 5th, 8th, 12th, 19th September, and 2nd October. He comes for the 3rd dose on 15th instead of 12th September. When will you administer the 4th dose, 19th September (as scheduled) or 22nd September (7 days after dose 3)?

The correct answer is 22nd September. The first two doses are the most important and the later doses can be shifted according to specified intervals.

SUGGESTED READING

1. Beatriz Quiambao, et. al. Health economic assessment of a rabies pre-exposure prophylaxis program compared with post-exposure prophylaxis alone in high-risk age groups in the Philippines; International Journal of Infectious Diseases 97 (2020) 38-46; https://www.ijidonline.com/article/S1201-9712(20)30369-6/pdf
2. Bharti OK, Chand R, Chauhan A, Rao R, Sharma H, Phull A. "Scratches/Abrasions without bleeding" cause rabies: a 7 years rabies death review from Medical College Shimla, Himachal Pradesh, India. Indian J Community Med. 2017;42:248-9.
3. Bharti OK, Ramachandran V, Kumar S, Phull A. "Pup Vaccination Practices in India Leave People to the Risk of Rabies—Lessons from Investigation of Rabies Deaths Due to Scratch/Bite by Pups in Remote Hilly Villages of Himachal Pradesh, India," World Journal of Vaccines, 2014, doi: 10.4236/wjv.2014.41002. https://www.scirp.org/journal/paperinformation.aspx?paperid=42538
4. Bharti OK, Thakur B, Rao R. Wound-only injection of rabies immunoglobulin (RIG) saves lives and costs less than a dollar per patient by "pooling strategy". Vaccine. 2019;37:A128-31.
5. Chomchay P, Khawplod P, Wilde H. Neutralizing antibodies to rabies following injection of rabies immune globulin into gluteal fat or deltoid muscle. Available

from: J Travel Med, 7 (2000), pp. 187-188; https://pubmed.ncbi.nlm.nih.gov/11003730/
6. Denis M, Knezevic I, Wilde H, Hemachudha T, Briggs D, Knopf L. An overview of the immunogenicity and effectiveness of current human rabies vaccines administered by intradermal route. Vaccine. 2019;37 Suppl 1:A99-A106. doi:10.1016/j.vaccine.2018.11.072; https://pubmed.ncbi.nlm.nih.gov/30551985/
7. Jeon S, Cleaton J, Meltzer MI, Kahn EB, Pieracci EG, Blanton JD, et al. Determining the post-elimination level of vaccination needed to prevent re-establishment of dog rabies. PLoS Negl Trop Dis. 2019;13(12): e0007869.
8. Kessels JA, Recuenco S, Navarro-Vela AM, Deray R, Vigilato M, Ertl H, et al. Pre-exposure rabies prophylaxis: a systematic review. Bull World Health Organ. 2017;95:210-9C.
9. Serum Institute of India Pvt. Ltd. (2020). Rabishield™—rabies human monoclonal antibody. [online] Available from: https://www.seruminstitute.com/product_ind_rabishield.php. [Last accessed June, 2020].
10. WHO/Department of Control of Neglected Tropical Diseases. Rabies vaccines: WHO position paper—April 2018. Wkly Epidemiol Rec. 2018;93:201-20.
11. Wilde H, Sirikawin S, Sabcharoen A, Kingnate D, Tantawichien T, Harischandra PAL, et al. Failure of postexposure treatment of rabies in children. Clin Infect Dis 1996;22(2):228-32. http://cid.oxfordjournals.org/content/22/2/228.full.pdf
12. World Health Organization (WHO). (2018). Rabies vaccines: WHO position paper—April 2018. [online] Available from: https://apps.who.int/iris/bitstream/handle/10665/272371/WER9316.pdf?ua=1. [Last accessed June, 2020].
13. World Health Organization (WHO). (2018). WHO Expert Consultation on Rabies, Third Report (WHO Technical Report Series, No. 1012). [online] Available from: https://apps.who.int/iris/bitstream/handle/10665/272364/9789241210218-eng.pdf?sequence=1&isAllowed=y. [Last accessed June, 2020].

CHAPTER 27

Japanese Encephalitis Vaccines

Vipin M Vashishtha, Chandra Mohan Kumar

1. What is Japanese encephalitis?

Japanese encephalitis (JE) is a serious neurological infection caused by JE virus, a zoonotic mosquito-borne flavivirus. It occurs in certain rural parts of Asia mainly South East Asia and Western Pacific regions. JE spreads through the bite of infected mosquitoes. It cannot spread directly from one person to another.

2. What are the key features of the JE disease?

Japanese encephalitis virus (JEV) can cause:
- Mild infections with fever and headache
- Severe infections with encephalitis.

Symptomatic JE, most commonly manifest as encephalitis, is rare and thought to occur in approximately 1 in 250 infections. About 1% of the infected develop encephalitis, another 10% develop minor illness. JEV is the main cause of viral encephalitis in many countries of South East Asia with an estimated 68,000 clinical cases every year. The case-fatality rate among those with encephalitis can be as high as 30%. Permanent neurologic or psychiatric sequelae can occur in 30–50% of those with encephalitis. Symptoms of more severe infection are headache, high fever, neck stiffness, stupor, disorientation, abnormal movements, occasional convulsions (especially in infants), coma, and paralysis. There is no antiviral treatment for patients with JE, and supportive care is the mainstay of the management of a case of JE encephalitis.

3. How is JE transmitted?

Conventionally, it is believed that the JEV is transmitted by *Culex* mosquitos (primarily *Culex tritaeniorhynchus*) and circulates in an enzootic cycle between mosquitoes, pigs, and/or aquatic birds that serve as amplifying hosts. Therefore, it is not possible to eliminate JE completely owing to these animal reservoirs; however, it can be controlled by large-scale vaccination along with other measures. *Culex* mosquitoes that breed in paddy fields, ditches, and ground pools are the main vector of the disease. Humans are dead-end reservoirs, but noninfectious since viremia is only very brief. Furthermore, since human infection does not contribute to transmission and vaccination of

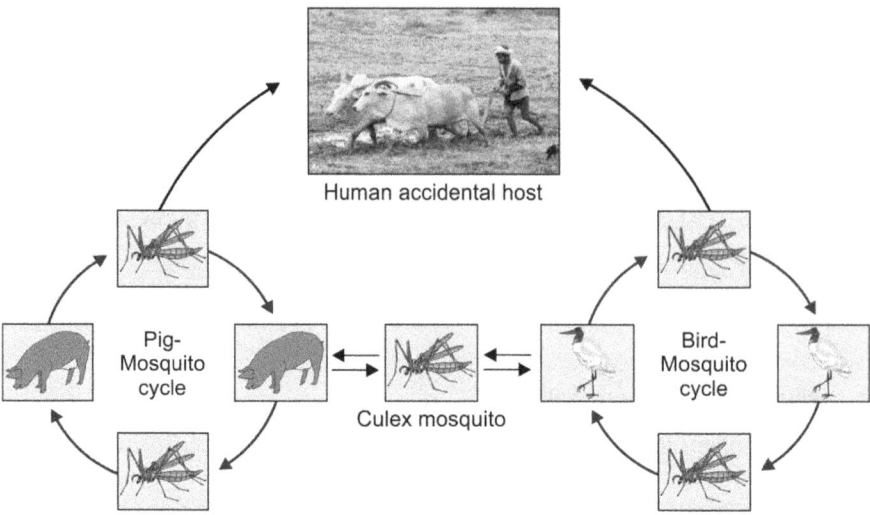

Fig. 1: Japanese encephalitis (JE) virus transmission cycle.

humans does not reduce transmission of JEV in the reservoir community, no herd immunity is generated, and vaccination must be sustained indefinitely **(Fig. 1)**. Human-to-human transmission is not documented till quite recently. This transmission cycle was proposed by many investigators who conducted ecological studies in Japan that primarily involved *Culex* mosquitoes, pigs, and, to a lesser extent, ardeid birds.

4. What is the "conventional" basic transmission cycle?

Mosquitoes become infected by feeding on domestic pigs and wild birds infected with the JEV. Infected mosquitoes then transmit the JEV to humans and animals during the feeding process. The JEV is amplified in the blood systems of domestic pigs and wild birds.

5. Could you get the JE from another person?

No, JEV is not transmitted from person-to-person. For example, one cannot get the virus from touching or kissing a person who has the disease, or from a health care worker who has treated someone with the disease. However, though the chances of JEV transmission from person-to-person is extremely low, recently rare case/s JEV transmission from person-to-person through the transfusion of blood product has been confirmed in Hong Kong.

6. Could you get JE from animals other than domestic pigs?

Yes. Recently, there has been new thinking regarding transmission of JEV has emerged. On studying epidemiology and the high burden of JE in many Asian countries like India and Bangladesh that do not practice intensive pig farming

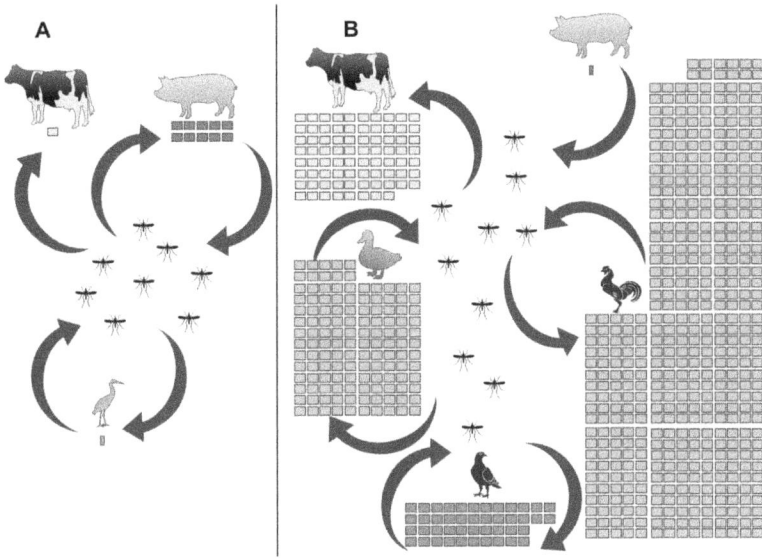

Figs. 2A and B: Rethinking Japanese encephalitis (JE) virus transmission: Implications for control.

and have comparatively lesser number of pig population in comparison to Japan, a new hypothesis is proposed in a recent study from Bangladesh. According to this hypothesis, the domesticated birds like ducks, pigeon, and chickens may play a major role than ardeid birds in JEV transmission, and cattle were found to be far more important in maintaining JEV transmission than pigs. Ducklings and chicks have shown to have high viremia for prolonged duration. In countries like Bangladesh and India, the density of cattle far outnumbers that of pigs. Not only domesticated birds like ducks, pigeon, and chickens, recent serological surveys have demonstrated that animals like dogs, goats, sheep, buffaloes, boars, bats, etc. can be subclinically infected and their potential role still in disease transmission needs further studies **(Figs. 2A and B)**. Additionally, vector-free, direct transmission of JEV between animals has been demonstrated in animals like pigs and mice.

7. **Conventionally, it is believed that *Culex* mosquitoes are the main vectors for transmission of JE. Can one also get infected by the bites of other mosquitoes?**

Till quite recently, only the *Culex* mosquitoes were considered as the only vector. There are reports of JE virus being detected in the field from the experimentally inoculated non-*Culex* species like *Anopheles*, *Aedes*, and *Mansonia* mosquitos also. This supports the occurrence of JE in nonpaddy areas or urban areas. JEV can also be transmitted from infected *Culex* or non-*Culex* mosquitoes to her eggs indicating transovarian transmission by which virus is maintained in the environment for long periods. The above-mentioned recent additions to our knowledge regarding transmission of JE may help to explain JEV outbreaks in the regions not having usual vectors. The results may have major implications on the future preventive measures against the JEV.

8. What is the incubation period for JE?

Usually 5–15 days.

9. What is the epidemiology of JE? What is the global burden of JE?

According to WHO, nearly 50,000 cases of JE occur worldwide per year and 15,000 of them die. In endemic areas, the annual incidence of disease ranges from 10–100/100,000 population. There are total 24 countries at risk of JE risk; however, only 22 countries are having well-established JE surveillance program. Of the 24 countries of Asia-Pacific region considered endemic to JE, 10 have no JE vaccination program **(Fig. 3)**. As per the most recent estimates,

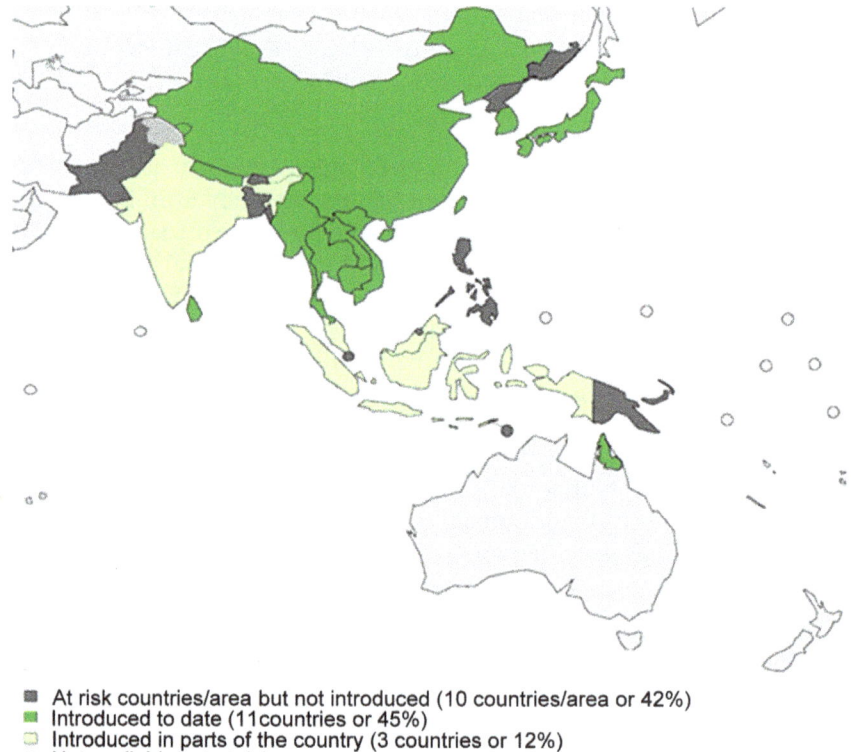

■ At risk countries/area but not introduced (10 countries/area or 42%)
■ Introduced to date (11countries or 45%)
▢ Introduced in parts of the country (3 countries or 12%)
▢ Not available/not at risk
▨ Not applicable

Fig. 3: Countries and territories at risk of JE disease and using JE vaccine in their national programs.

Source: World Health Organization. Vaccines in National Immunization Programme update, October 2019. [online] Available from www.who.int/immunization/monitoring_surveillance/VaccineIntroStatus.pptx [Last accessed September, 2020).

TABLE 1: Global burden of disease in few high-burden countries: cases reported to WHO, 2012–2019.

Countries	2012	2013	2014	2015	2016	2017	2018	2019
India	745	1,078	1,657	1,620	1,627	2,043	1,707	2,496
China	1,763	2,178	858	624	1,130	1,147	1,800	369
Nepal	75	118	1,304	937	98	63	98	71
Bangladesh	52	23	183	76	1,294	19	96	86
Vietnam	183	224	421	368	357	200	313	196
Myanmar	14	3	50	113	393	442	126	115
Philippines	0	24	69	115	312	361	204	143
Malaysia	22	12	47	39	59	20	28	48
Cambodia	55	41	60	48	10	5	11	01
Sri Lanka	60	70	21	17	18	23	29	—
Indonesia	0	0	72	40	43	281	0	—
Republic of Korea	20	14	26	40	0	9	—	34
Laos	23	9	4	13	19	9	11	96
Japan	2	9	2	2	11	3	0	09
Australia	1	4	1	3	0	1	0	03

Source: World Health Organization. (2020). Japanese encephalitis reported cases. [online] Available from: http://apps.who.int/immunization_monitoring/globalsummary/timeseries/tsincidencejap-enc.html [Last accessed September, 2020].

nearly 3 billion people are living in at-risk areas and as per the WHO estimates, 67,900 cases are reported annually with approximately 13,600–20,400 deaths, with an overall incidence rate of 1.8/100,000 in the 24 countries with JE risk. There is gross underreporting of JE cases, and WHO thinks that only 10% of cases are being reported. Considering the above evidence, the actual number of JE cases in India could be around 15,000–20,000 per year. As per the WHO data, India, Nepal, China, and Vietnam have contributed 87% of all JE cases recently with India topping the list **(Table 1)**.

10. What is the epidemiology of JE in India?

Japanese encephalitis viral activity has been widespread in India. The first evidence of presence of JE virus dates to 1952. First case was reported in 1955; Outbreaks have been reported from different parts of the country. Presently out of total 268 JE endemic districts across 22 states, campaign activity has been completed in 231 districts and JE vaccination has been started as a part of routine immunization.

Japanese encephalitis has been reported from all states and union territories in India except Arunachal, Dadra, Daman, Diu, Gujarat, Himachal, Jammu, Kashmir, Lakshadweep, Meghalaya, Nagar Haveli, Odisha, Punjab, Rajasthan, and Sikkim. Highly endemic states include Assam, Bihar, Tamil

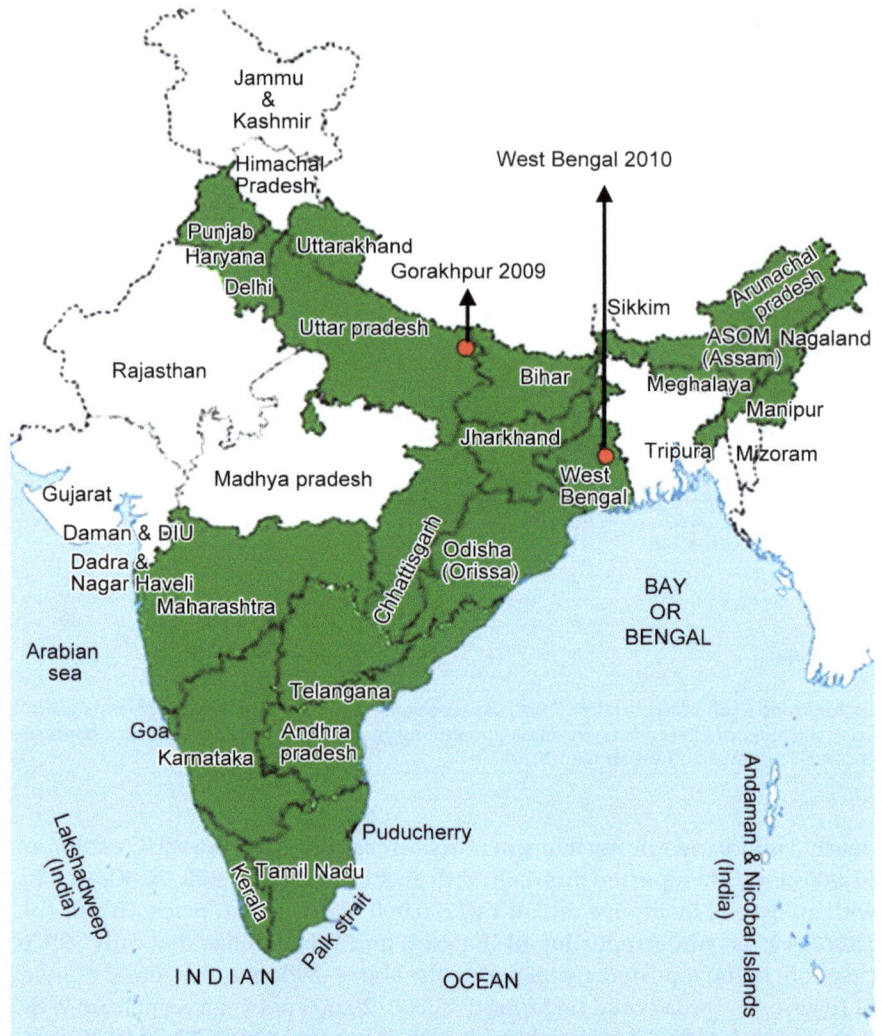

Fig. 4: Japanese encephalitis endemic states in India, 2017.

Nadu, Uttar Pradesh, Odisha, West Bengal, and Karnataka. These states are reporting more than 80% of all JE cases in India **(Fig. 4)**. According to the National Vector Borne Disease Control Programme (NVBDCP) India, a total of 10,082 cases of acute encephalitis syndrome (AES) were reported in 2019 till 30th September, and JE constituted 1,656 (16.4%) cases. Considering the gross underreporting, the actual number of JE cases in India could be around 15,000–20,000 per year.

As per the data available at NVBDCP, India JE constitutes around 9–18% of all cases of AES from 2008–2019 **(Fig. 5)**. There is an upward trend in the total number of JE cases reported to NVBDCP **(Fig. 5)**. The main reasons are: increasing surveillance efforts, spread of JE to newer states like Jharkhand,

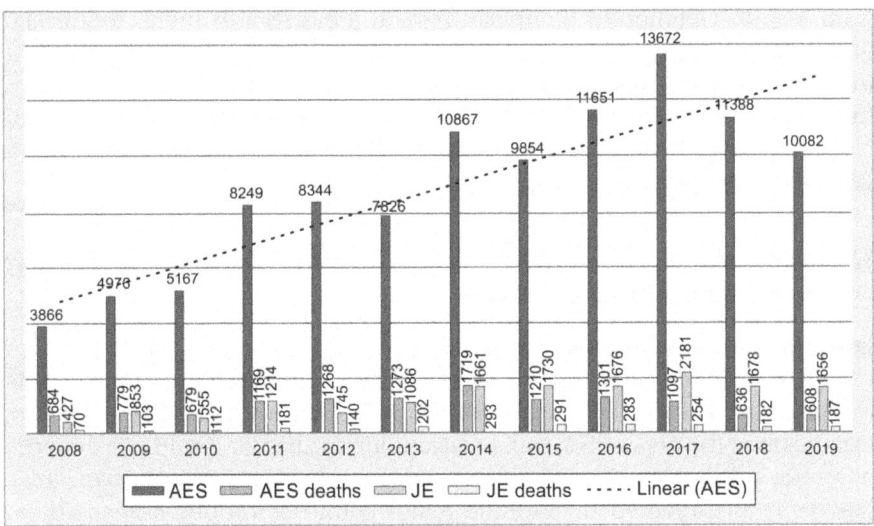

Fig. 5: Acute encephalitis syndrome (AES) and Japanese encephalitis (JE) cases and deaths in India, 2008–2019.

Source: National Vector Borne Disease Control Programme, Ministry of Health and Family Welfare, Government of India.

Odisha, Manipur, Meghalaya, spread of JE to newer districts within the same state such as in states like Bihar, Uttar Pradesh, West Bengal, Maharashtra, and Tamil Nadu, and increasing number of cases from older children and adults in states like Uttar Pradesh, West Bengal, and Assam. In Maharashtra, during 2017 out of 27 JE cases reported, 21 cases were from nonendemic regions. AES surveillance during 2018 has found 108 JE cases in Maharashtra (actual reported cases were only 8). In 2018, NVBDCP has recommended identified seven new endemic districts for JE in Maharashtra including Pune. There is an observation that the JE is now spreading beyond the endemic zones, and cases have been reported from states like Madhya Pradesh, Rajasthan, Gujarat, and Himachal Pradesh which were considered free of JE.

Japanese encephalitis is still an important cause of AES in India. Various studies in the past identified JE as a major identifiable etiology of AES. According to a recent laboratory-based surveillance study conducted in three states (Uttar Pradesh, Assam, and West Bengal) between 2014 and 2017 among 10,107 patients with AES, etiology could be identified in 49.2% of cases. Among the identified etiologies, JE (16%), scrub typhus (16%), and dengue (5.2%) accounted for 75% of cases.

11. Is the disease seasonal in its occurrence? What seasonal pattern is seen in India?

Patterns of JE transmission vary within individual countries and from year to year. In endemic areas, sporadic cases occur throughout the year. In North temperate area (Japan, Taiwan, Nepal, Northern India), large epidemics occur from May to October. In Southern tropical areas (South India, Indonesia, Sri Lanka), the disease is endemic, but peak starts after rains that is from July to December. Within India, it is seen from July to December in North India. It occurs during May to October in Goa, October to January in Tamil Nadu, August to December in Karnataka, September to December in Andhra Pradesh, and July to December in Northern States.

12. Traditionally, the JE is considered to be a disease of rural people. Is there any recent change in its epidemiology?

Japanese encephalitis is predominantly, although not exclusively, a rural disease. However, the JE cases have been detected in cities, such as Kathmandu and New Delhi, in the absence of rural travel, possibly suggesting expansion of the area of JEV transmission due to changing land use patterns or vector adaptation. The increased risk of suburban or periurban areas has been documented in multiple Asian countries (South Korea, China, Singapore, Taiwan, etc.). As per the recent epidemiological studies, 25% of JE cases are reported from urban regions from the cities like Kolkata, Patna, Ranchi, Lucknow, Goa, Trivandrum, Chennai, Bangaluru, Ranga Reddy district (Hyderabad), etc. The Ministry of Health and Family Welfare, Government of India is vaccinating children both from rural and urban areas through Universal Immunization Programme (UIP).

13. Most of the cases of JE infections and disease are usually found in pediatric population ranging from 5–15 years. Is there any indication of age shift? What is the latest trend as far as different age group involvement is concerned?

Conventionally, the JE is considered as a disease of children and adolescents in the age group of 1–15 years. However, in last few years, cases of adult JE have been reported from identified JE endemic districts. Accordingly, 31 endemic districts were identified across 3 states where adult JE vaccination campaigns were recommended. The adult JE campaigns, covering adults aged 15–65 years, have been completed in these 31 districts wherein 33 million adults were vaccinated against JE. The epidemiological shift of JE to older children and adults is mainly due to introduction routine JE vaccination in younger children only (9 months–2 years). Epidemiological shift indicates the need for a vaccine and schedule which provides sustained protection for long term. As per the study by the National Institute of Epidemiology, the Indian Council of Medical Research (ICMR) Chennai, India and the data from the virus research and diagnostic laboratories (VRDLs), the median age of JE cases in India is 13 years. Out of total 1,231 cases, 37.5% cases were in the age group of 5-14 years **(Fig. 6)**. The study was conducted from centers all over the India between January 2014 to April 2017.

Not only in India, but the available data suggest that in many areas of the world JE is a disease of all ages. As the numbers of cases in children decrease due to successful vaccination programs, there is frequently a shift to a greater

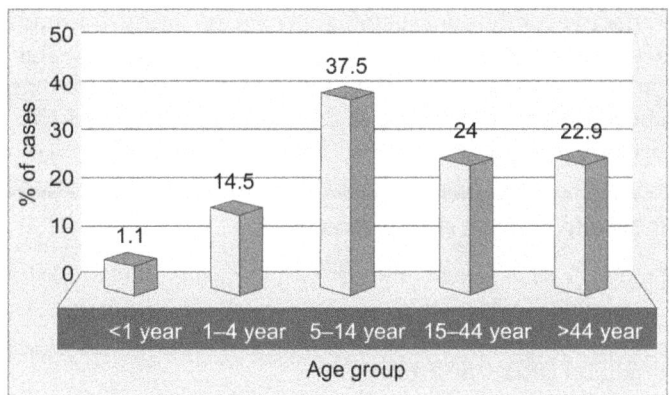

Fig. 6: Age distribution of JE cases in India (January 2014 to April 2017).

proportion of cases in older, unvaccinated age groups. But even in some areas without vaccination programs, such as Bangladesh, over 50% of cases are in the adult age groups. In Thailand, approximately 10% of the population above 40 years of age did not have protective levels of antibody titers against JEV. In Philippines also, the seroprevalence rate was just 44% among a sample of 12–18-year-olds. This means an important proportion of adults is still susceptible to JE. How severity differs by age group is not yet well recognized because of lack of follow-up of many cases.

14. What are the personal preventive measures against JE?

As with any disease transmitted by mosquitoes, one can prevent exposure to JE virus by:
- Remaining in well-screened areas.
- Wearing clothes that cover most of the body, and
- Using an effective insect repellent, such as those containing up to 30% N,N-diethyl-meta-toluamide (DEET) on skin and clothing. Use of permethrin on clothing will also help prevent mosquito bites.
- Japanese encephalitis vaccine can prevent JE; however, even though JE vaccine is not 100% effective still vaccination of humans is the most effective means of preventing JE in addition to mosquito protection.

15. How can JE be controlled at community level?

The control of JE is based essentially on three interventions:
- Mosquito control
- Avoiding human exposure to mosquitoes
- Immunization.

Mosquito control, although regarded as most important step as a part of NVBDCP, has been difficult to achieve in rural settings and avoidance of exposure is difficult as *Culex* mosquitoes bite during daytime. Immunization is the only effective method for sustainable control. Routine immunization of school-age children is currently in use in Korea, Japan, China, Thailand, and Taiwan. The introduction of the JE vaccine into the Expanded Programme on Immunization (EPI) has helped curb the disease in countries like Thailand, Vietnam, Sri Lanka, and China.

16. What is the current status of JE vaccines?

Approximately, 15 JE vaccines are currently in use globally. All vaccines are based on genotype 3 virus strains. Given the large number of vaccines in use, focus was placed on vaccines that are internationally distributed and/or WHO prequalified **(Box 1 and Table 2)**.

> **BOX 1:** An overview of globally available Japanese encephalitis vaccines.
>
> **Live, Attenuated JE Vaccines (LA-JEV):**
> - Live attenuated vaccine based on the SA 14-14-2 strain **(CD-JEV)**
> - Live recombinant (chimeric) vaccines **(JE-CV)**
>
> **Inactivated Vero cell-based JE vaccines (JE-VC):**
> - SA 14-14-2 strain:
>   – IXIARO®/JESPECT® (Valneva, Austria) and JEEV® (BE, India)
> - Kolar 821564XY strain:
>   – JENVAC® (BBIL, India)
> - Beijing-1 viral strain:
>   – ENCEVAC® (Kaketsuken, Japan) and JEBIKV® (Biken, Japan)
> - Beijing P-3 strain:
>   – CVI-JE, JEVAC® (Liaoning Chengda Biotechnology Co., China)

17. What is the status of mouse brain inactivated JE (JE-MB) vaccines?

The older generation of JE vaccine, the inactivated mouse brain vaccine (JE-MB) was available since 1930s, mainly produced in Russia and Japan. There were two strains available worldwide, i.e., Nakayama strain and Beijing-1 strain. In India, the vaccine was earlier manufactured at Kasauli from Nakayama strain. However, considering the various limitations and drawbacks, the JE-MB is gradually removed from the immunization schedule of almost all the countries. Still, a handful of countries are employing this vaccine for the mass vaccination.

18. What were the drawbacks of mouse brain inactivated JE vaccines?

The drawbacks and limitations of the JE-MB vaccines include the following:
- High cost of production
- Complicated dosing schedule
- Limited duration of protection
- Requirement of boosters
- Concerns about some rare serious side effects
- Reliance on neurological tissue.

CHAPTER 27 Japanese Encephalitis Vaccines

TABLE 2: Key differentiating features of available JE vaccines, globally.

	Names	Manufacturers	Strain	Age (first dose)	Dose Schedule	Licensure
Inactivated (Vero Cell)	IXIARO IC51/(JE-VC)/JESPECT	Austria: Valneva, distributed by Novartis and Bio CSL	SA-14-14-2	2 months	Primary 2 doses (0/28D) Booster 1Y	US, EU, Canada, Australia, HK, Switzerland, Israel, Singapore, New Zealand, PNG, Pacific Islands
	JEEV*	India: Biological E	SA-14-14-2	1 year onward (India 1–49 years)	Primary 2 doses (0/28D) Booster?	India, Bhutan, Pakistan, Nepal
	JENVAC	India: Bharat Biotech	Kolar Strain (JEV821564XY)	≥ 1 year (1–50 years)	Primary 2 doses (0/28D) Booster?	India
Live Attenuated (PHK)	LA SA-14-14-2 (CD JEVAX)*	China: Chengdu Institute of Biological Products	SA-14-14-2	≥ 8 months	Primary 1 dose Booster 9M-12 M, or age 2 Y In some countries	India, South Korea, Thailand, Nepal, Sri Lanka, DPRK, Laos, Cambodia, Burma, Malaysia, Vietnam
Live Chimeric (Vero)	IMOJEV* (JE-CV)	France: Sanofi pasteur	SA-14-14-2/ Yellow fever 17D	> 1 year	Primary 2 doses (Paediatric age) Adults: 1 dose	Australia, Malaysia, Thailand, Brunei

*WHO prequalified vaccines.

Furthermore, the availability of far more safe and efficacious new generation JE vaccines, the JE-MB, and primary Hamster kidney cells-P3 are no longer being produced.

19. The live attenuated cell culture-derived SA 14-14-2 vaccine (CD-JEV/CD.JEVAX®) has been in use in India's National Immunization Program (NIP) for more than a decade now. What are the key characteristics of this vaccine?

This vaccine is based on the genetically stable, neuroattenuated SA 14-14-2 strain of the JE virus, which elicits broad immunity against heterologous JE viruses. Reversion to neurovirulence is considered highly unlikely. WHO technical specifications have been established for the vaccine production. Chengdu Institute of Biological Products (CDIBP) is the only manufacturer authorized to export this vaccine from China. Two other live attenuated vaccines based on the SA 14-14-2 strain are manufactured in China but not exported. The SA 14-14-2 strain used in CD-JEV is produced in primary Hamster kidney cells **(Box 2)**.

The CD-JEV vaccine was licensed in China in 1989. Since then more than 700 million doses have been distributed globally. Currently, more than 50 million doses of this vaccine are produced annually. Extensive use of this and other vaccines has significantly contributed to reducing the burden of JE in China from 2.5/100,000 in 1990 to <0.5/100,000 in 2004. This vaccine is also licensed for use in Nepal (since 1999); South Korea (since 2001); India (since 2006); Thailand (since 2007), and Sri Lanka. The price per dose of the vaccine is comparable to the EPI measles vaccine. The CD-JEV attained WHO prequalification in October 2013.

> **BOX 2:** Key characteristics of CD-JEV vaccine.
>
> **SA 14-14-2 live attenuated, JE vaccine (CD-JEV):**
> - Minimum age: 8 months
> - Dose is 0.5 mL **subcutaneously** for all ages
> - Two doses are needed
> - Can be coadministered with MMR/MR vaccine
> - Not be used as an "outbreak response vaccine"
> - Contains gelatin, saccharose, human serum albumin, and sodium glutamate as excipients
> - **Shelf life:** 24 months

20. What is the biology of CD-JEV vaccine?

It contains gelatin, saccharose, human serum albumin, and sodium glutamate as excipients. A standard dose is not less than 5.7 log plaque-forming units (PFUs) per mL. The shelf life is 24 months.

21. What are the doses and administration schedule?

The dose of CD-JEV is 0.5 mL subcutaneously for all ages, and it can be coadministered with measles-containing vaccine/s, measles-rubella (MR)/

measles-mumps-rubella (MMR). In China, the vaccine is licensed for 0.5-mL dose to be administered subcutaneously to children at 8 months of age and a second opportunity again at 2 years. In some areas, a booster dose is given at 7 years. It should not be used as an "outbreak response vaccine". It can also be offered to all susceptible children up to 15 years as catch-up vaccination.

22. How stable is the CD-JEV vaccine?

The infectious titer of the vaccine is not appreciably changed after storage at 37°C for 7–10 days, at room temperature for 4 months, or at 2–8°C for at least 1.5 years.

23. Is there a known correlate of protection for this vaccine? What is the immunogenicity?

A neutralization antibody titer of more than 1:10 is generally accepted as evidence of protection and postvaccination seroconversion. After a single dose, antibody responses are produced in 85–100% of nonimmune 1–12 yeas-old children.

24. How efficacious is this vaccine? Do we have efficacy/effectiveness data?

A case-control study performed in 1993 in Sichuan Province China in children < 15 years measured effectiveness of routinely delivered SA 14-14-2 vaccine at 80% for a single dose and 97.5% for two doses given at 1-year interval. Five major efficacy trials of SA 14-14-2 vaccine, completed in China from 1988–1999 in 1–10 years-olds, consistently yielded high protection rates, above 98%. Case control studies and numerous large-scale field trials in China have consistently shown an efficacy of at least 95% following two doses administered at an interval of 1 year.

However, due to the passage of time since the studies were completed, the nonrandomized design, limited detail in the methods sections, possible minor variations in the vaccine, and use of a two-dose schedule in some studies, focus was given to studies of the CDIBP live attenuated vaccine that have been published more recently, especially those employing good manufacturing practice (GMP)-compliant vaccine lots.

25. What are the results of recent studies with CD-JEV, conducted in new GMP-compliant facilities?

Immunogenicity of a single dose: In infants, when the CD-JEV was given as a single dose at 8–12 months of age, seroprotection rates after 1 month of vaccination ranged from 90.6–92.1% among children in different age groups. The seroprotection rate was 97.3% for the CD-JEV vaccine when used as a comparator vaccine in a randomized controlled trial (RCT) of IMOJEVTM, a live recombinant JE vaccine in children aged 9–18 months and 99.1% in children aged 12–24 months. In a similar study in children in

Korea, the seroprotection rate was 99.1%. These results are consistent with immunogenicity results from observational studies in children in Korea and Thailand. All trials were from the endemic regions involving children.

26. What were the results of PATH-sponsored RCTs of CD-JEV in the Philippines and Bangladesh?

In the two PATH-sponsored RCTs of CD-JEV in the Philippines and in Bangladesh among children with a single dose of vaccine at ages 8–12 months, the seroprotection rates were 92.1% and 90.6%, respectively. In the Philippines trial, measles vaccine was administered 1 month prior the CD-JEV.

In the Bangladesh trial, a lot-to-lot consistency was observed in the vaccine produced from a new GMP-compliant facility except for two lots that have a difference of −4.33 (−11.94–3.31) in the seroprotection rates. However, the WHO disregarded this minor variation in granting the WHO prequalification status to CD-JEV. Overall, the seroprotection rates ranged between 80.2 and 86.3%.

27. What was the efficacy/effectiveness of CD-JEV in Nepal?

In a field trial in Nepal in 1999, involving more than 160,000 subjects 1–15 years of age, reported efficacy of a single dose of 99.3% in the same year and 98.5% 1-year later. At 5 years, the protective efficacy was 96.2%. Vaccine in this study contained 105.8 PFU/0.5 mL. The study provides evidence that SA 14-14-2 will be useful to combat epidemics.

28. What was the effectiveness in China?

A case-control study performed in 1993 in Sichuan Province China in children < 15 years found 80% effectiveness with single dose and 97.5% with two doses administered at 1-year interval. Five major efficacy trials of SA 14-14-2 vaccine, completed in China from 1988–1999 in 1–10 year-olds, consistently yielded high protection rates, above 98%. Data is also emerging from Sri Lanka and South Korea where this vaccine is used in public health.

29. What is the Indian experience with the CD-JEV vaccine?

In India, SA 14-14-2 CD-JEV vaccine was imported from China, and was used in many states including Eastern Uttar Pradesh, Bihar, and Assam since 2006 and children between the age group of 1–15 years were vaccinated as a single dose of vaccine. Mass campaigns were continued in the endemic districts during 2008 and 2010 also. Following the campaigns targeting all children in the age group of 1–15 years in the high-risk districts, the vaccine is integrated into the UIP of endemic districts in 2011. Children at 16–24 months of age [with diphtheria, pertussis, and tetanus (DPT)/oral polio vaccine (OPV) booster] are targeted for one dose of this vaccine in select endemic districts after the campaign. In 2013, a two-dose JE vaccination strategy was introduced, with first dose given between 9 and 12 months along with measles vaccine.

30. Do we have any effectiveness data on CD-JEV from India?

A small case-control study from Lucknow, India found an efficacy of 94.5% after a single dose of this vaccine within 6 months after its administration. However, data from post marketing surveillance (PMS) in India (ICMR unpublished study) showed that protective efficacy of the vaccine in India is not as high as that seen in Nepal. The PMS study showed that virus neutralizing antibodies were seen in 45.7% of children before vaccination. Seroconversion against Indian strains 28 days after vaccination was 73.9% and 67.2% in all individuals and in those who were nonimmune prevaccination, respectively. The protective efficacy of the vaccine at 1 year was 43.1% overall and 35% for those who were nonimmune prevaccination, respectively.

Another recently published retrospective case-control study conducted during single dose JEV campaign during 2006–2007 from India, found an unadjusted protective effectiveness of 72.2% in those with any report of vaccination, either vaccination history or card/record. According to this report, the JE vaccine effectiveness (VE) was lower in Uttar Pradesh (65.7%) as compared with Assam (86.7%) based on any evidence of vaccination **(Table 3)**. The VE was higher in older age groups and against severe disease. The effectiveness was lower in the first year following vaccination but remained stable in the second year. The retention of vaccination cards was more common in Assam than in Uttar Pradesh. Following this report, the ICMR recommended a study on the impact of two doses versus single dose of CD-JEV in Assam.

A case-control study in India estimated VE at 84% at 0–38 months postvaccination in the four districts of Gorakhpur division in Uttar Pradesh in 2013. However, the coverage of CD-JEV was only 51% in the entire division.

TABLE 3: Vaccine efficacy estimates after single dose campaign among children aged 1–15 years in India during 2006–2007.		
Estimates	Vaccine effectiveness (VE)	VE (95% CI)
Overall (n = 149 case-control sets)		
Written (card or record)	43.8%	1.9–67.8
Any (written or verbal)	72.4%	56.2–82.4
Assam (n = 34)		
Written (card or record)	78.8%	39.9–92.5
Any	86.7%	62.5–95.3
Uttar Pradesh (n = 115)		
Written (card or record)	6.6%	−18.4–52
Any	65.7%	42.9–79.4

31. Conventionally, boosters are unlikely to be required as with most live, attenuated vaccines, one dose will provide lifelong protection. In Nepal and China, even a single dose of CD-JEV was found efficacious and to provide long-term protection. However, in India, two doses of this vaccine are administered. What is the current recommendation on the need of booster doses?

Studies have already documented ongoing protection from a single dose for a minimum of 5 years in a JE-endemic area. However, after analyzing recent Indian efficacy/effectiveness data, it is concluded that there is need of a second dose of the vaccine to provide more complete and more sustained protection.

According to a comprehensive review of the CD-JEV, a single dose of the vaccine protects against clinical JE disease for at least 5 years, providing a longer duration of protection in comparison to MB-JE vaccines.

32. There are always a doubt about the safety and efficacy of Chinese vaccines. How safe is this vaccine?

An estimated 300 million children have been immunized with this vaccine without apparent complication. WHO's Global Advisory Committee on Vaccine Safety (GACVS) acknowledged the vaccine's "excellent" safety profile. Transient fever may occur in 5–10%, local reactions, rash, or irritability in 1–3%. Neither acute encephalitis nor hypersensitivity reactions have been associated with the use of this vaccine. A recent review on the safety of CD-JEV reports that the serious adverse events have been reported, the independent experts and health agencies have not found enough evidence for causality based on the available data.

33. What are the different inactivated JE vaccines available?

Table 4 provides details about the available inactivated JE vaccines along with the strains used to develop them.

TABLE 4: Inactivated Vero cell-based JE vaccines (JE-VC).		
Strain	Vaccine	Developer
SA 14-14-2 strain	IXIARO® JESPECT®	Valneva, Austria
SA 14-14-2 strain	JEEV®	Biological Evans Ltd., India
Kolar 821564XY strain	JENVAC®	BBIL, India
Beijing-1 viral strain	ENCEVAC®	Kaketsuken, Japan
Beijing-1 viral strain	JEBIKV®	Biken, Japan
Beijing P-3 strain	CVI-JE, JEVAC®	Liaoning Chengda Biotechnology Co., China

34. The only inactivated JE vaccine available for the travelers in US and many other western countries is IXIARO™ (JE-VC). Tell us more about this vaccine.

This is an inactivated vaccine (JE-VC) derived from the attenuated SA 14-14-2 JEV strain propagated in Vero cells. The vast majority of publicly available data on inactivated Vero cell-based vaccines have been generated for a single product, IXIARO®, developed by Valneva (earlier called Intercell AG from Austria). This vaccine has been evaluated in several clinical trials conducted in India and abroad in both adults and children. The one JE vaccine available in private sector in India, JEEV™ is also derived from this product.

35. What are the recommendations on its use?

IXIARO® has now been approved by the US Food and Drug Administration (FDA) and EU for use in children from the age of 2 months onward. There is no efficacy data for IXIARO®, and the vaccine has been licensed in pediatric age group especially for travelers to Asian countries on the basis of a phase III RCT conducted in the Philippines, and favorable interim data from a second phase III trial in EU, US, and Australia. The safety profile of the test vaccine was good, and its local tolerability profile was more favorable than that of the mouse brain vaccines.

36. What are the dose and recommended schedule?

Each 0.5-mL dose contains approximately 6 µg of purified, inactivated JEV proteins and 0.1% aluminum hydroxide as an adjuvant. The finished product does not include gelatin stabilizers, antibiotics, or thimerosal.* The vaccine should be stored at 2–8°C; it should not be frozen. The vaccine should be protected from light. The vaccine is administered by intramuscular (IM) route. **Box 3** provides the details schedule of the vaccine based on recent CDC's Advisory Committee on Immunization Practices (ACIP) recommendations.

BOX 3: CDC's ACIP recommendations on IXIARO® dose and schedule, by age group.

Dose and schedule, by age group:
- 2–35 months: 2 doses (0.25 mL) administered on days 0 and 28[†]
- 3–17 years: 2 doses (0.5 mL) administered on days 0 and 28
- 18–65 years: 2 doses (0.5 mL) administered on days 0 and 7–28[§]
- >65 years: 2 doses (0.5 mL each) administered on days 0 and 28
- For all age groups, the two-dose series should be completed at least 1 week before potential exposure to JE virus

Booster dose, by age group (if ongoing exposure or re-exposure is expected):
- <3 years: 1 dose (0.25 mL) at ≥1 year after the second dose[†] [¶]
- ≥3 years: 1 dose (0.5 mL) at ≥1 year after the second dose[¶]
- Clinical trial data show high rates of seroprotection for at least 6 years after a booster dose

[†] To administer a 0.25-mL dose, expel and discard half of the volume from the 0.5-mL prefilled syringe.
[§] Studies showing the second dose can be administered as early as 7 days after the first dose only included adults aged 18–65 years.
[¶] No data are available on the response to a booster dose administered > 2 years after the second dose.

---

*The final preparation contains residues of protamine sulfate.

> **BOX 4:** Key characteristics of JEEV® vaccine by Biological E Ltd.
>
> **JEEV® inactivated Vero cell culture-derived SA 14-14-2, IC51 JE vaccine:**
> - Similar to IC51 (IXIARO) in terms of raw materials and development process
> - M/s Valneva (Intercell) established a partnership with Biological E Ltd. for production and distribution in India
> - Licensed in India: September 2011; launched in 2012
> - Age range: Initially, the age range approved: 1–3 years-old children and 18–49 years; now from 1–49 years
> - Two doses are mandatory for primary immunization
> - Route of Administration: IM
> - Shelf life: 24 months
> - First WHO prequalified JE vaccine (July 2013)
> - Also marketed in Bhutan, Nepal, and Bangladesh

37. An Indian variant of IXIARO® is available in Indian market. Tell us more about this vaccine.

M/s Biological E Ltd. has launched a vaccine for the Indian market under the trade name JEEV® based on Intercell's technology. Valneva (Intercell) established a partnership with Biological E Ltd. for production and distribution in India. JEEV® (6 µg/0.5 mL) is the first WHO prequalified JE vaccine (July 2013). JEEV® and IC51 (IXIARO®) are similar in terms of raw materials (cell banks and virus seed banks), and have same process of development and release specifications. It was launched in Indian market in 2012 by Biological E Ltd. JEEV® pediatric 3 µg/0.5 mL is also now WHO prequalified for children between ≥ 1 and < 3 years. Initially, the age range approved was 1–3 year-old children and 18–49 years; however, following a new trial, the JEEV® is now approved for subjects from 1–49 years. It is now also marketed in Bhutan, Nepal, and Bangladesh **(Box 4)**.

38. Did Biological E Ltd. conduct any trial of JEEV® in India?

Yes, in 2011, the Biological E Ltd. India conducted a multicentric open-label randomized controlled phase II/III study to evaluate safety and immunogenicity of JEEV® vaccine in ~450 children (≥1 to <3-year-old) and compared to control Korean Green Cross Mouse Brain Inactivated (KGCC) vaccine. This study demonstrated seroconversion [seroconversion rate (SCR)] of 56.28% on day 28 and 92.42% on day 56 in JEEV® vaccinated group. Geometric mean titers (GMTs) in JEEV® group were significantly higher than GMTs achieved in KGCC-JE vaccine group (218 vs. 126). Bases on the results of this trial, the Drugs Controller General of India (DCGI) licensed JEEV® in India.

Another multicentric study conducted in the age group of 3–18 years among 107 subjects. Out of 107 subjects, none of the subjects have seroprotection titers ≥ 1:10 PRNT50 at day 0 (prevaccination) and the proportion of subjects seroprotected postvaccination at day 56 (postvaccination) were 95.33%. The GMT in overall study population was 209.24 and the GMT in subset-1

(≥ 3 to < 8 years) was 280.66, subset-2 (≥ 8 to < 12 years) was 140.87, and in subset-3 (≥ 12 to < 18 years) was 233.59. Based on the above study results, DCGI has approved JEEV 6 µg/0.5 mL in children ≥ 3 to < 18 years.

39. Can one use a single dose of JEEV® for primary immunization?

No. As mentioned above, the seroconversion rate after first dose was only 56.28%. Hence, two doses are must for primary immunization.

40. What are the key characteristics of JENVAC® by M/s Bharat Biotech, the only indigenously-developed Indian JE vaccine?

JENVAC® is a Vero cell culture derived, inactivated, adjuvanted [aluminum hydroxide (0.25 mg) and thiomersal (0.025 mg)] containing vaccine developed by M/s Bharat Biotech International Limited (BBIL). The original virus strain used in the vaccine was isolated from a patient in the endemic zone in Kolar, Karnataka, India by National Institute of Virology (NIV), Pune and later transferred to BBIL for vaccine development. Two doses of 0.5 mL (5 µg) are administered intramuscularly at 0 and 28 days. The vaccine was launched in India in October 2013 **(Box 5)**.

> **BOX 5:** Key characteristics of JENVAC® vaccine by M/s BBIL.
>
> **Inactivated Vero cell culture-derived Kolar strain, 821564XY, JE vaccine (JENVAC®):**
> - Obtained from: NIV, Pune, India
> - Strain: Thermostable Kolar strain (JEV 821564XY)
> - Adjuvant: Aluminum hydroxide (0.25 mg)
> - Preservative: Thiomersal (0.025 mg)
> - Administration: IM
> - 5 µg/0.5 mL two doses at 0 and 28 days
> - Even a single dose may suffice for primary immunization
> - Launched in India in October 2013

41. What are the key takeaways from the pivotal trials?

Preclinical animal studies were conducted at Mahidol University, Thailand where almost 100% serocoversion was seen after two doses.

A phase II/III, randomized, single-blinded, active controlled study to evaluate the immunogenicity and safety of the vaccine was conducted among 644 healthy subjects. Out of 644 subjects, 212 were between the age of ≤50 to >18 years, 201 subjects were between the age of ≤18 to >6 years, and 231 subjects were between the age of ≤6 to >1 years. Subjects received two doses of the test vaccine or a single dose of a reference vaccine (live attenuated, SA 14-14-2 Chinese vaccine) as the first dose and a placebo as the second dose.

The results revealed that even a single dose of the test vaccine was sufficient to elicit the immune response. On 28th day, the subjects who had received a single dose were 98.67% seroprotected and 93.14% seroconverted (4-fold) for ≤50 to ≥1 years, whereas the corresponding figures for the reference vaccine were 77.56% and 57.69%, respectively (p-value < 0.001). There was no statistically significant difference in all the three groups. The seroconversion (93.14 and 96.90%) and seroprotection (98.67 and 99.78%) percentages on the 28th and 56th day were not significantly different and similarly, no statistically significant difference in these rates was noted among different age groups. Higher GMTs were achieved in younger age groups. After the second dose of the test vaccine, the GMTs increased exponentially from day 28 (145) to day 56 (460.5) in ≤50 to ≥1 years.

42. Can JENVAC® be used as a single dose in primary schedule?

Following receipt of two doses of JENVAC®, 61.17% of subjects retained seroprotection titers at 24 months. However, there was waning of both seroconversion and GMTs in both the test vaccine and reference vaccine groups at 18 months **(Figs. 7A and B)**. Seroprotection reduced to <80% at 12 months and 61% at 24 months, and the GMTs declined rapidly within 12 months (8-fold reduction).

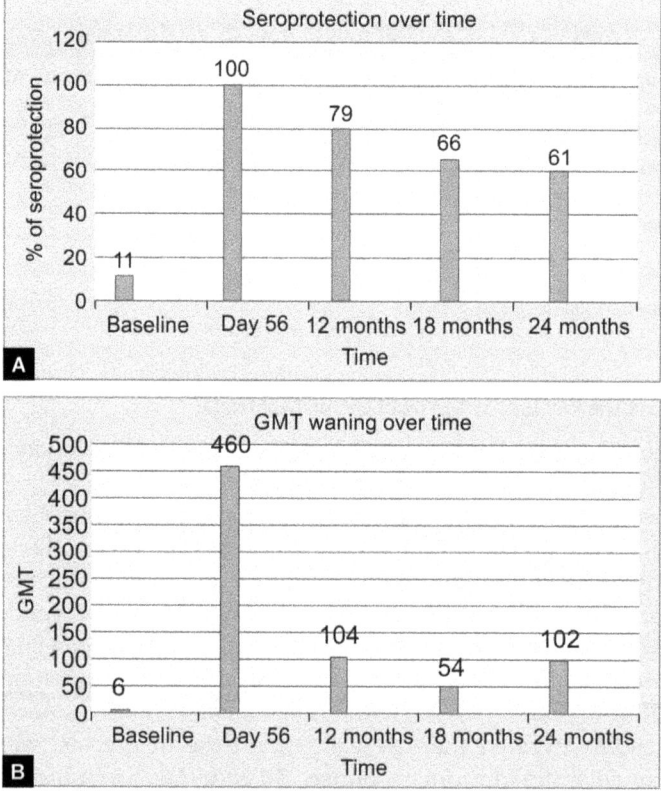

Figs. 7A and B: Long-term persistence of immune responses following two doses of JENVAC®.

TABLE 5: A comparative evaluation of open-label randomized, active controlled immunogenicity study of a single dose of JENVAC versus CD-JEV (live attenuated JE vaccine) vaccine with 1-year follow-up in healthy volunteers.

Parameter	JENVAC	Live SA 14-14-2	p-value
Subjects	180	180	
Seroprotection (PRNT50 equal or > 1:10)			
Day 28	92.4%	71.4%	$p = 0.0001$
Day 360	81.7%	47.9%	$p = 0.0001$
Seroconversion (4 fold or greater increase)			
Day 28	81.8%	50.3%	$p = 0.0001$
GMTs			
Day 28	83.2	24.6	
Day 360	33.7	12.2	

A phase IV, open-labeled, comparative, randomized, active controlled study was conducted to evaluate the immunogenicity and safety of a single dose of BBIL's JENVAC versus Chinese SA 14-14-2 (LA-JEV, CD-JEV) vaccine in healthy volunteers. After 1 month, the seroprotection rate was 92.4% in the test vaccine group and 71.4% in the control group. After 1 year, the corresponding figures were 81.7% and 47.9% in the test and control vaccine group. Similarly, the seroconversion (4-fold or greater increase) rates were 81.8 and 50.3% after 1 month, and 61.6 and 29.1% after 1 year, respectively in the test and control vaccine group. The GMTs were 83.2 and 33.7, and 24.6 and 12.2 after 1 month and 1 year, respectively in the two groups **(Table 5)**.

Additionally, in the original trial of JENVAC, immunogenicity data in subset of subjects who withdrew after the first dose showed that seroprotection rate (81.82%) and GMT (40.90) was higher in subjects receiving JENVAC (n = 22) compared to seroprotection rate of 44.44% and GMT of 29.44 in subjects receiving SA 14-14-2 (n = 9), after 1 year from vaccination.

In summary, 2-year follow-up is data available for JENVAC. Comparing with JEEV (which requires at least two doses for primary induction of immunity), it is evident that even a single dose of JENVAC may suffice to induce adequate seroprotection in most vaccines. There is definite waning of immunity following one or two doses; however, no difference is seen in seroprotection rates following one or two doses after 1 year (81.7% vs. 79%) of following primary series. A booster dose will be needed after 1 year of primary schedule.

43. Immunologically, it is believed that inactivated vaccines generally require multiple doses for primary immunization. The WHO has also recommended this in their TRS (WHO TRS. No. 963, 2011 (Section C.2.3 Dose and Schedule) to JE vaccine manufacturers. What is your take on this issue?

Yes, it is true that a single dose of inactivated vaccine fails to generate germinal centers thereby limiting the induction of memory responses and high affinity, long half-life plasma cells. Based on the past experience with inactivated JE vaccines, it is anticipated that more than one dose will be needed to achieve and maintain protection. There is definitely a need of more data, i.e., booster responses in 1- and 2-dose recipients of JENVAC vaccine after 1 year.

44. What is a chimeric vaccine? Tell us more about a new chimeric JE vaccine known as IMOJEV®.

Chimera is a gene or protein consisting of parts from two different genes or proteins that are normally distinct, sometimes derived from two different species. JE-CV is a novel recombinant chimeric virus vaccine, developed using the Yellow fever virus (YFV) vaccine vector YFV17D, by replacing the cDNA encoding the envelope proteins of YFV with that of an attenuated JEV strain SA 14-14-2. Resulting recombinant virus grows on Vero cells **(Fig. 8)**. The JE-CV (IMOJEV™) was found to be safe, highly immunogenic, and capable of inducing long-lasting immunity in both preclinical and clinical trials. Moreover, a single dose of IMOJEV was sufficient to induce protective immunity, which was similar to that induced in adults by three doses of JE-VAX®, a mouse brain-derived inactivated JE vaccine. It was previously known as ChimeriVax™-JE. This vaccine is administered by

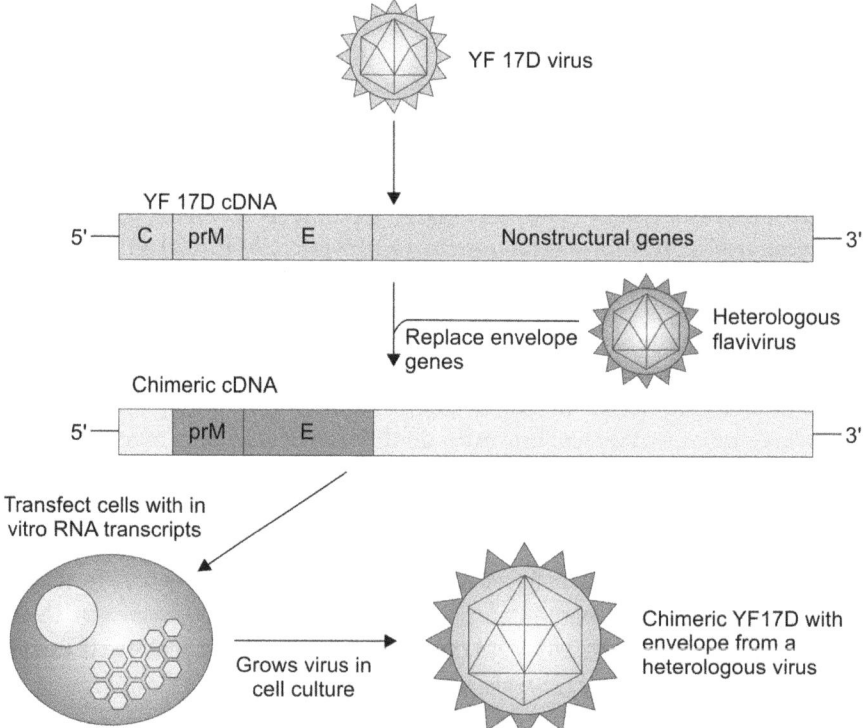

Fig. 8: A diagrammatic representation of the various steps involved in the development of a chimeric vaccine.

subcutaneous route. It is free from preservatives and other excipients and has a shelf life of 36 months. The JE-CV has been licensed for use in Australia, Malaysia, Philippines, and Thailand for the prevention of JE in children and adults and is currently licensed in 14 endemic countries. The JE-CV was WHO prequalified in September 2014.

45. How many doses of IMOJEV needed for primary immunization? Do booster doses are also needed?

A single dose of IMOJEV (JE-CV) administered to children in endemic settings has evidence of seroprotective neutralizing antibody titers for at least 5 years after immunization. Available immunogenicity data indicate children vaccinated at ≥12 months of age have adequate seroprotective titers at 2 years. One small study shows adequate seroprotective titers up to 5 years in nonendemic regions in adults. However, another study showed some evidence of waning in seroprotection rates after a single dose in endemic region in children.

In Australia and Malaysia, JE-CV is licensed as a two-dose vaccine for the pediatric population, and single-dose vaccine for the adult population. In studies from Thailand and Philippines, the researchers found JE antibody persistence for up to 5 years following a booster dose of JE-CV (IMOJEV) in children aged 36–42 months who received a single JE-CV dose 2 years earlier. Hence, a booster dose 12–24 months after primary vaccination is necessary in pediatric populations to confer long-term protection.

46. M/s Sanofi Pasteur had initiated a trial of IMOJEV® in India also. What is the status of that trial in India?

Yes, it is true that M/s Sanofi Pasteur had conducted an immunogenicity study in 9-month to 10-year-old children of their chimeric JE vaccine (JE-CV) known as IMOJEV® in India. However, lower seroprotection rates were found with some serological assays in the study in (e.g., as compared against Nakayama strain and Indian strains (Kolar 821564XY strain), both genotype 3). However, similar results were obtained with the comparator vaccine, a Nakayama mouse brain-derived vaccine. The virus stock used for testing was reportedly not good. Though good immunogenicity results were obtained with other two assays. Later, M/s Sanofi Pasteur withheld the further trials of the vaccine in India.

47. There are five different genotypes of JE virus. Most of the current JE vaccines are derived from G3 genotype. Are the available JE vaccines equally effective against all genotypes?

The JEV is categorized in 5 genotypes. The major JEV genotypes have varying overlap in geographical distribution, but all belong to the same serotype and are similar in terms of virulence and host preference. While genotype 3 used to be the predominantly circulating genotype, there has been a shift toward circulation of genotype type 1.

Most of the current JE vaccines derived from G3 genotype of JE virus and can induce protective immune response against G1-G4 genotypes. In some recent studies, low levels of neutralizing antibodies induced by the current JE vaccine against the G5 genotype was noticed. Hence, there is a need to establish cross-protection against the emerging G5 genotype of JE virus.

48. What are the key recommendations of Government of India and IAP on the use of JE vaccines?

Boxes 6 and 7 show recommendations of Ministry of Health and Family Welfare, Government of India and Advisory Committee on Vaccines and Immunization Practices (ACVIP) of Indian Academy of Pediatrics (IAP) on the use of JE vaccines.

BOX 6: Government of India recommendations on use of JE vaccines.

Live attenuated SA 14-14-2 (LA-JEV, CD-JEV/CD.JEVAX®)
Dosage and schedule:
Current recommendations:
- GoI-UIP now recommends a booster of CD-JEV
- 1st dose can be administered at 9 months along with measles vaccine
- 2nd dose at 16–18 months at the time of 1st booster of DTP vaccine

---

BOX 7: IAP's ACVIP recommendations on use of inactivated JE vaccines.

IAP's ACVIP recommendations
Routine and catch-up vaccination:
- Children (up to 14 years) living in JE endemic areas
- Travelers to endemic/epidemic areas
- For catch-up vaccination, the upper age has been increased to 14 years and the schedules are two doses 28 days apart for inactivated JE vaccines

Primary schedule
JEEV®:
- Two doses of 0.25 mL (3 µg) for children aged ≥ 1 to ≤ 3 years
- Two doses of 0.5 mL (6 µg) for children > 3 years, adolescents and adults administered intramuscularly on days 0 and 28

JENVAC®:
- Two doses of the vaccine (0.5 mL each) administered intramuscularly at 4 weeks interval for office practice starting from 1 year of age onward

Boosters:
- Long-term persistence of protective efficacy and need of boosters are still undetermined; need of booster dose

---

49. What are the new Government of India recommendations on JE vaccination?

For newer vaccines with limited follow-up time in endemic areas, it is unclear for how long protective level of antibodies will last, and whether natural boosting contributes to maintaining protective antibody level.

> **BOX 8:** Government of India (GoI) revised recommendations on use of JE vaccines.
>
> **Revised JE Vaccination Guidelines: July 2019**
> **Routine vaccination (under UIP):**
> - Any of the three vaccines (LA-JEV, JEEV, and JENVAC) will be used as two doses schedule
>   - 1st dose at 9–12 months, 2nd at 16–24 months
>   - For programmatic purpose interchangeability between live and inactivated JEVs is accepted
>   - ICMR is going to study the interchangeability between all three vaccines
>
> **Campaign vaccination:**
> - Any of the three vaccines (LA-JEV, JEEV 6 µg, and JENVAC): 1 dose
> - Campaign vaccination: children—1–15 years, adults—15–65 years

Source: Japanese encephalitis vaccination guidelines in India, Ministry of Health and Family Welfare (MoHFW), July 2019.

Some countries, including China, and recently India, administer CD-JEVAX as a two-dose series. Informal discussions with countries suggest much of the rationale for a two-dose schedule comes from programmatic reasons, primarily enhancing coverage and vaccinating missed children rather than a concern about protection with one dose.

Following the NTAGI February 2019 recommendations, all the three JE vaccines [live attenuated SA 14-14-2 (CD-JEV), JEEV, and JENVAC] will be used both in routine immunization (two-dose schedule 9–12 and 16–24 months) and campaign immunization (one dose of live or one dose of JEEV 6 µg or JENVAC) **(Box 8)**. These guidelines are issued in the July 2019 *(Japanese encephalitis vaccination guidelines in India, MoHFW, July 2019)*. Almost 17 million doses of inactivated JEV shall be used in 2019–2020 out of total 37 million used in India. ICMR is taking up the interchangeability studies between these three JE vaccines.

50. Can the available JE vaccines be coadministration other vaccines?

Yes, the data support coadministration of live attenuated JE (CD-JEV) vaccine with measles vaccine. Immunogenicity studies are needed for coadministration with MR and MMR. However, for programmatic reasons it may be considered acceptable to coadminister CD-JEV with MR or MMR vaccines, although data are not yet available. Following the same rationale, coadministration of MMR and JE-CV (IMOJEV) is acceptable although slightly lower anti-JEV GMT values, but nonetheless seroprotective, were obtained in the coadministration group at 12 months after vaccination. Immunogenicity studies, including long-term studies, are needed for coadministration of JE-CV with measles and MR vaccines.

51. What is the public health impact of JE vaccines? Which JE vaccine is the being employed by the most countries in their national immunization program?

Data on the population impact of vaccination programs show significant reductions in JE cases. When high coverage is achieved in populations at risk

> **BOX 9:** Country-specific use of different types of JE vaccines.
>
> **JE vaccines use in national programs:**
> - 8 countries are using live attenuated CD-JEV
> - 3 countries using live chimeric JE-CV vaccine
> - 1 country is using inactivated Vero cell culture-derived vaccine
> - 3 countries, Vietnam, South Korea, and Taiwan are still using JE-MB vaccine

of disease, JE in humans can be significantly controlled while the virus remains in circulation. Many countries with JE surveillance systems have been able to track JE trends over time, before and after vaccination. Vaccination of the susceptible population has been demonstrated to be cost-effective strategy in China, Nepal, Japan, and Thailand. Significant impact of mass JE vaccination on disease burden was seen with live attenuated (CD-JEV) and older mouse-brain (JE-MB) vaccines in China, Japan, Taiwan, Malaysia, Nepal, and Thailand. Most of the recent disease impact data are available with the use of JE-VC since live, chimeric vaccine (JE-CV) are not yet used in widespread areas. The live attenuated SA 14-14-2 JE vaccine (CD-JEV) is being used by the most countries in their immunization programs. **Box 9** displays the country-specific use of different types of JE vaccines.

52. Are the new generation JE vaccines cost-effective?

Japanese encephalitis vaccination, even with more expensive inactivated products requiring multiple doses, was nearly always cost-effective regardless of the vaccination strategy. One dose of live attenuated, CD-JEV vaccine was found to be very cost-effective by WHO criteria of cost-saving. The cost per DALY averted was highly sensitive to the prevaccination incidence and the cost of the vaccine. Cost-effective studies from many Asian countries including from Indonesia and Cambodia have found JE vaccination a cost-effective intervention.

53. What is the risk of JE to travelers traveling to endemic countries?

The travelers from US, Europe, and other Western countries are constantly at risk of JE infection and disease on traveling to endemic regions. Risk of JE in travelers is rare, however very dangerous. Risk of disease among travelers in Asia is 1 in 1000,000. Susceptibility does not decrease with mass immunization. The risk will be more if one travels during monsoon season, to rural places, and involve in outdoor activities.

Usually endemic disease is not noted, and epidemics are detected late hence vaccination should be recommended for selected travelers to Asia who are at high risk. Last dose should be given 7-10 days before travel. Travelers to South East Asia (SEA) and Western Pacific countries need JE vaccination depending on travel duration, transmission season, visiting rural places, outdoor activities, and staying under poor mosquito control conditions.

54. What are the new recommendations on use of JE vaccines for the travelers coming to endemic regions?

Till quite recently, the JE vaccine was only "recommended" for travelers who plan to "spend a month or longer in endemic areas during the transmission season. The criterion of 1 month was arbitrary.

However, the epidemiology of JE and risk to the traveler has changed in recent times and continues to evolve. However, a recent review of JE cases globally found that at least half the cases reported were in travelers of <30 days. A report on the US International travelers through 2014 included 87 cases of JE and only 50% of them had visits of over 30 days. There are recent incidents from Bali and Thailand where even a short 10-day stopover with very little rural exposure, outside transmission season resulted in JE infection.

Considering the changing epidemiology of JE and the publication of above reports, the CDC in its 2019 guidelines has strengthen the JE recommendation by recommending JE vaccine even for the travelers who visit the endemic areas for short term also provided they visit during transmission season, visit rural places, go for outdoor activities. For adults, vaccination schedule has been changed to 0 and 7–28 days (previously 0 and 28 days). A booster dose should be (previously may be) given for people who are the risk of re-exposure **(Box 10)**.

BOX 10: Japanese encephalitis vaccine: recommendations of the CDC's Advisory Committee on Immunization Practices.

CDC' ACIP 2019 recommendations:
- Should be given for travelers staying in endemic area for ≥1 month
- JE vaccine also should be considered for shorter-term (e.g., <1 month) travelers with an increased risk of JE based on planned travel duration, season, location, activities, and accommodations
- Vaccination also should be considered for travelers to endemic areas who are uncertain of specific duration of travel, destinations, or activities (previously it was "may be considered")
- In adults aged 18–65 years, the primary vaccination schedule is two doses administered on days 0 and 7–28 (previously it was 0 and 28 days)
- For adults and children, a booster dose (i.e., third dose) should be given at ≥1 year after completion of the primary IXIARO series if ongoing exposure or re-exposure to JE virus is expected (previously it was/may be given)

Source: Hills SL, Walter EB, Atmar RL, Fischer M. Japanese encephalitis vaccine: recommendations of the Advisory Committee on Immunization Practices. MMWR Recomm Rep. 2019;68(2):1-33.

55. What are the novel approaches to produce new generation of JE vaccines?

Recent advances in recombinant DNA technology have made it possible to explore a novel approach for developing live attenuated flavivirus vaccines against other flaviviruses. Full length complementary DNA (cDNA) clones allow construction of infectious virus bearing attenuating mutations or deletions incorporated in the viral genome.

It is also possible to create chimeric flavivirus in which the structural protein genes for the target antigens of a flavivirus are replaced by the corresponding genes of another flavivirus. By combining these molecular techniques, the DNA sequences of Dengue virus 4 (DEN4) strain 814669, Dengue virus 2 (DEN2) PDK-53 candidate vaccine, and YF17D vaccines have been used as the genetic backbone to construct chimeric flaviviruses with the required attenuation phenotype and expression of the target antigens. Encouraging results from preclinical and clinical studies have shown that several chimeric flavivirus vaccines have the safety profile and satisfactory immunogenicity and protective efficacy to warrant further evaluation in humans. The chimeric flavivirus strategy has led to the rapid development of novel live attenuated vaccines against dengue, tick-borne encephalitis (TBE), JE, and West Nile viruses. Many arthropod-borne flaviviruses are important human pathogens responsible for diverse illnesses, including dengue, JE, yellow fewer, and TBE. Other approaches to JE vaccines including naked DNA, oral vaccination, and recombinant subunit vaccines are also being currently reviewed. Vaxfectin, a recently developed adjuvant, was found to have an ability to enhance immunogenicity of DNA vaccines in experimental models.

56. Tell us about new generation of future JE vaccines?

Broadly, three types of new JE vaccines are undergoing clinical trials. They include:

1. *Recombinant JE vaccines*: The E protein of JEV has a great potential for use as an immunogenic substance capable of eliciting protective immunity, since JEV-neutralizing antibodies alone are sufficient to confer protection against infection. In *Escherichia coli*, antigenic portions of the E protein have been expressed that generate a wide range of neutralizing antibody titers in mice. In a baculovirus-insect cell system, the E protein has also been expressed alone or together with another viral protein, prM or NS1, that elicits neutralizing antibodies and protects mice against a challenge with JEV. Moreover, in mammalian cells, coexpression of the prM and E proteins has been shown to produce a secreted form of subviral particles capable of inducing JEV-neutralizing antibodies and generating JEV-specific cytotoxic T cells in animals.

2. *Poxvirus-based vaccines*: Recombinant poxviruses have been used as viral vectors to deliver JEV antigens (e.g., prM, E, and/or NS1) that can induce protective immunity in mice. Three major poxviruses that have been demonstrated the potential for JE vaccine development are NYVAC (an attenuated vaccinia), ALVAC (an attenuated canarypox), and MVA (the modified vaccinia Ankara). In a clinical trial, NYVAC- and ALVAC-based JE vaccines were found to be well tolerated, but their immunogenicity did not appear to be satisfactory; in particular, the NYVAC-based vaccine elicited JEV-neutralizing antibodies in vaccinia-nonimmune volunteers but not in vaccinia-immune volunteers, suggesting that preexisting poxvirus immunity may suppress the induction of immune responses to JEV antigens. In addition to these poxviruses, adenoviruses have also been explored as a viral vector to express JEV antigens in animals.

3. *Plasmid DNA-based vaccines*: In mice and pigs, immunization of a plasmid encoding the prM and E proteins can induce a range of protective immune responses that include JEV-specific B cells and cytotoxic T cells. In addition to the two structural proteins (prM and E), immunization with a plasmid encoding the viral nonstructural protein NS1 can also induce an antibody response with cytolytic activity in a JEV-specific, complement-dependent manner. The NS1 immunization thus has been shown to be sufficient to protect mice against a lethal infection with JEV, despite having no detectable neutralizing antibodies induced.

SUGGESTED READING

1. Buescher EL, Scherer WF, Rosenberg MZ, Gresser I, Hardy JL, Bullock HR. Ecologic studies of Japanese encephalitis virus in Japan. II. Mosquito infection. Am J Trop Med Hyg. 1959;8:651-4.
2. Centers for Disease Control and Prevention. (2019). Japanese encephalitis [online] Available from: https://www.cdc.gov/japaneseencephalitis/vaccine/index.html [Last accessed September, 2020].
3. Muniaraj M, Rajamannar V. Impact of SA 14-14-2 vaccination on the occurrence of Japanese encephalitis in India. Hum Vaccin Immunother. 2019;15(4):834-40.
4. National Vector Borne Disease Control Programme, Ministry of Health and Family Welfare, Government of India. State wise number of AES/JE cases and deaths from 2013-2019 (till Sept). [online] Available from: https://www.nvbdcp.gov.in/WriteReadData/l892s/67972593411571401755.pdf [Last accessed September, 2020].
5. Operational Guide: Japanese Encephalitis Vaccination in India, November 2017. Immunization Division, Department of Family Welfare, Ministry of Health and Family Welfare, Government of India. 2017.
6. Scherer WF, Buescher EL. Ecologic studies of Japanese encephalitis virus in Japan. I. Introduction. Am J Trop Med Hyg. 1959;8:644-50.
7. Vashishtha VM, Ramachandran VG. Vaccination policy for Japanese encephalitis in India: tread with caution! Indian Pediatr. 2015;52(10):837-9.
8. Vashishtha VM. Japanese Encephalitis Vaccines. In: Vashishtha VM (Ed). IAP Textbook of Vaccines, 2nd edition. 2020 New Delhi: Jaypee Brothers Medical Publishers (P) Ltd; 2020. pp. 478-501.
9. World Health Organization. Japanese encephalitis vaccines: WHO position paper—February 2015. 2015;90:69-88.
10. Yun SI, Lee YM. Japanese encephalitis: the virus and vaccines. Hum Vaccin Immunother. 2014;10(2):263-79.

CHAPTER 28

Rotavirus Vaccines

Rakesh Bhatia

1. Why rotavirus (RV) disease is so important?

Worldwide, rotavirus (RV) infection is the leading cause of severe, dehydrating diarrhea in young children. Almost all children will suffer from at least one episode of RV infection by the age of 5 years. Many of them will have more than one episode, of which the first one is the most severe, leading to dehydration and hospitalization, and may be potentially fatal.

Despite improvements in public hygiene and sanitation, a corresponding decline in RV disease burden has not been observed. This is because of universal presence of virus, its small infectious dose, and its environmental stability—all of which greatly facilitate transmission. Therefore, the incidence of this "democratic virus" is the same the world over. Unfortunately, what differs is the outcome of severe RV disease; the chances of death following RV diarrhea are estimated to be 1:50,000 in USA and 1:200 in developing countries.

2. What is the global burden of rotavirus disease?

According to latest available World Health Organization (WHO) estimates, 215,000 child deaths occurred due to RV infection in 2013 as compared to 528,000 in the year 2000. Almost 90% of all RV-associated fatalities occurred in low-income countries in Asia and Africa. Four countries (India, Pakistan, Nigeria, and Democratic Republic of Congo) accounted for approximately half (49%) of all RV deaths under the age of 5 years. A sentinel hospital-based RV surveillance report from 35 nations representing each of six WHO regions concluded that 40% hospitalizations for diarrhea in under-five children were attributable to RV infection.

More recent figures from the Institute for Health Metrics and Evaluation (IHME, 2018) reveal a significant reduction in RV-associated mortality among children below 5 years of age. Thus, in a seminal study by Troeger et al in 2016, RV infection was responsible for 128,500 deaths worldwide, with approximately 104,000 deaths occurring in sub-Saharan Africa. Almost 30% of deaths from diarrhea in this age group were attributable to RV infections. RV was the third leading pathogen associated with under-five mortality in 2016, behind malaria and *Pneumococcus*.

3. What is the rotavirus disease burden in India?

According to the WHO, India accounts for 22% of global deaths due to rotavirus gastroenteritis (RVGE). Combining the data from Million Death Study and Indian Rotavirus Strain Surveillance Network (IRSSN), it was estimated that in 2013, in India, RV was responsible for 11.37 million episodes of GE in under-five children, requiring 3.27 million outpatient visits and 827,000 hospitalizations. There were 78,000 deaths due to RVGE, with the majority (75%) in the first 2 years of life. In an exhaustive study of RVGE in under-five Indian children hospitalized for diarrhea between 2012 and 2016, 35.5% were positive for rotavirus by enzyme immunoassay (EIA). G1P[8] (36%), G9P[4] (11.4%), G2P[4] (11.2%), and G12P[6] (8.4%) were the most common genotypes in Northern India while G1P[8] (56.3%), G2P[4] (9.1%), and G9P[4] (7.6%) were most common in Southern India.

4. What is the efficacy of currently licensed rotavirus (RV) vaccines?

Currently licensed rotavirus vaccines effectively prevent severe rotavirus gastroenteritis (SRVGE), although they are less efficacious against mild RVGE or RV infection. In developed, high-income countries like USA, UK, and Australia, vaccine efficacy against SRVGE has been above 90%; in middle-income countries of Latin America like Mexico and Brazil, observed efficacy is around 80%. These countries have witnessed substantial decline in RV and/or diarrhea-related hospitalizations and deaths following Vaccine Implementation Programs. Unfortunately, similar efficacy has not been demonstrated in low-income countries of Asia and Africa. Trials in Africa have yielded efficacy rates between 50 and 80%. In Indian studies, overall efficacy against SRVGE in first year of life was 53.6%, which declined to 48.9% in second year of life.

5. Why vaccine efficacy is lower in resource-poor countries?

Live, oral viral vaccines like polio, cholera, and RV have significantly lower efficacy in developing countries as compared to developed countries. The possible reasons for this difference in immune response include widely prevalent malnutrition, deficiencies of zinc, vitamin A and vitamin D, coinfection with multiple enteral pathogens, interference by maternal antibodies (either transplacental or via breast milk), and coadministration of two live, oral vaccines. Disturbances in intestinal microbiota, possibly a result of high rates of tropical enteropathy, are also likely to play an important role. But as the disease burden is very high in poor countries, the morbidity and mortality averted by rotavirus vaccines (RVVs) are likely to be much higher despite lower vaccine efficacy.

6. Which are the rotavirus (RV) vaccines available in India?

At present, there are four different types of vaccines available in India. All of these are oral, live attenuated vaccines and are WHO prequalified.

Out of these, two vaccines (RotaTeq™ and Rotarix™) are available worldwide and are routinely used in several National Immunization Programs (NIPs). The other two vaccines Rotavac™/Rotasure™ and Rotasiil™ are available in India and have been used in Universal Immunization Program (UIP) for last many years (**Table 1**).

All the vaccines are administered to infants in a three-dose schedule, except Rotarix™ which is given in a two-dose schedule. RVV should ideally be given at an interval of 4–8 weeks, starting at 6–8 weeks of age. Currently, in India, three doses of vaccine are given at 6 weeks, 10 weeks, and 14 weeks of age.

RotaTeq™ (Merck) is a pentavalent human-bovine reassortant vaccine, which contains human G1, G2, G3, G4, and P8 strains reassorted with WC3 bovine strain. It is a liquid vaccine, available in a ready-to-use formulation in a single dose squeezable tube (latex free).

Rotavac™ (Bharat Biotech) is a monovalent neonatal human rotavirus vaccine (nHRV) strain 116E, classified as G9P[11]. It is currently available in a low-dose liquid formulation (0.5 mL)—Rotavac-D—as a single dose, prefilled

TABLE 1: Currently licensed RV vaccines in India.

Vaccine manufacturer	RotaTeq™ (Merck)	Rotarix™ (GSK)	Rotavac™ (Bharat Biotech)	Rotasiil™ (Serum Institute)
Composition	Pentavalent human-bovine reassortant	Monovalent human	Monovalent human	Pentavalent human-bovine reassortant
Serotypes/strain	G1P7[5], G2P7[5], G3P7[5], G4P7[5], and G6P1A[P]	G1P[8] and RIX4414 strain	G9P[11] and neonatal 116E strain	G6P[5] bovine RV backbone with human genes of serotypes G1, G2, G3, G4, and G9
Presentation	Liquid vaccine in squeezable tube	Lyophilized vaccine reconstituted with calcium carbonate buffer	Liquid vaccine single dose prefilled syringe (0.5 mL); multidose vial in UIP	Lyophilized vaccine reconstituted with citrate bicarbonate buffer
Storage	2–8°C (not frozen)	2–8°C (not frozen)	Frozen at –20°C. May be stored at 2–8°C for final 6 months before expiry	Heat stable at 37°C for 2 years. Can be stored below 25°C for 36 months
Dose schedule	Three-dose	Two-dose	Three-dose	Three-dose
Availability in UIP	No	No	Yes	Yes

- All are oral, live attenuated vaccines and are WHO prequalified
- Rotarix™ and RotaTeq™ are licensed in more than 100 countries in world
- Rotavac™ and Rotasiil™ are licensed only in India
- Neonatal 116E (Bharat Biotech) is also marketed by Abbott as *Rotasure*.

(GSK: GlaxoSmithKline; RV: rotavirus; UIP: Universal Immunization Program; WHO: World Health Organization) syringe ensuring ease of administration with no spit-ups. Previously available single-dose vials are being phased out while multidose glass vials are being used in UIP. This vaccine is also being marketed by Abbott with the brand name *Rotasure*™.

Rotasiil™ (Serum Institute) is a pentavalent vaccine constituted by five human-bovine reassortant strains of serotype G1, G2, G3, G4, and G9 reassorted with bovine (UK) RV. It is a thermostable vaccine and can be stored at a temperature below 25°C for 36 months. It is available as a vial of freeze-dried vaccine, which is reconstituted with the liquid diluent just prior to administration. Each dose is 2.5 mL in volume.

Rotarix™ [GlaxoSmithKline (GSK)] is a monovalent vaccine with G1 serotype/genotype and P[8] genotype, using human rotavirus RIX4414 strain. It is supplied as a lyophilized powder in a glass vial with rubber stopper that requires reconstitution with 1 mL liquid diluent just before oral administration. A fully liquid preparation is likely to be introduced in India in the near future.

7. Can rotavirus vaccines be used interchangeably?

Ideally, RV vaccine series should be completed with the same brand whenever possible. However, vaccination should not be deferred because the product used for a previous dose is either not available or is unknown. In such a situation, the series should be completed with the available product.

If any dose in the series was RotaTeq™ or the vaccine brand is unknown for any dose in the series, a total of three doses of available RVV should be administered.

There are no studies addressing the interchangeability of two RVVs. However, according to the Advisory Committee on Immunization Practices (ACIP), no theoretical reason exists to expect that the risk for adverse events would be increased if the series included more than one product. Further, although it is possible that effectiveness of a series that contains both products could be reduced compared with a complete series with one product, the effect of a series that contains both products is likely to be greater than an incomplete series with one product.

Currently, there is no published data on the interchangeability of Rotavac™ and Rotasiil™ used in UIP in India. The National Technical Advisory Group on Immunization has not raised any safety concern for mixed Rotavac™ and Rotasiil™ course. It has recommended that in case of interstate migration, the RVV course will be completed with whichever vaccine is available.

8. At present, there are four different types of vaccines available in India. Which is the best among these?

There is no head-to-head trial of all these RVVs in India. In some industrialized countries, RotaTeq™ had some edge over Rotarix™. However, Rotarix™ did slightly better in low-to-middle-income countries (LMIC) of Africa. In LMICs, maximum experience for rotavirus disease

TABLE 2: Different rotavirus (RV) vaccines in India: Comparative vaccine efficacy against severe rotavirus gastroenteritis (SRVGE) (Vesikari score ≥ 11).

Vaccine	Vaccine type	Included STs	Africa	Asia	India	WHO PQ
Rotarix™	Natural human strain	G1P[8]	49.4%	48%	NA	January, 2007
RotaTeq™	Bovine-human reassortant	G1-4 and P[8]	39.3%	48.3%	NA	October, 2008
Rotavac™	Bovine-human naturally occurring reassortant	G9P[11]	NA	–	53.6%	January, 2018
Rotasiil™	Bovine-human reassortant (G6P[5] bovine RV backbone)	G1-4 and G9	66.7%	–	39.5%	September, 2018

TABLE 3: Comparative efficacy of available rotavirus vaccines (RVVs) against very severe rotavirus gastroenteritis (VSRVGE) (Vesikari score ≥ 16).

	Rotavac™	Rotasiil™	Rotarix™	RotaTeq™
Efficacy	India = 54.4%	• Niger = 78.8% • India = 54.7%.	• Finland = 85% • Asia = 48.3%.	• USA and Finland = 98% • Africa = 39.3%.

prevention has been with Rotarix™; it now accounts for 80% of all RVVs supplied to the Global Alliance for Vaccines and Immunization (GAVI) for LMICs. However, in India, no efficacy data for RotaTeq™ and Rotarix™ exist. In India, only two vaccines, Rotavac™ and Rotasiil™, have undergone large scale efficacy trials. Rotavac™ has 48.9% efficacy after 2 years in India whereas Rotasiil™ has got 39.5% efficacy against SRVGE **(Table 2)**. However, when Rotasiil™ was studied in Niger, the efficacy against severe and very severe RV diarrhea was 66.7% and 78.8%, respectively. Against very severe rotavirus gastroenteritis (VSRVGE), both Rotavac™ and Rotasiil™ have got almost similar efficacy (54.4% vs. 54.7%) **(Table 3)**. According to the manufacturer of the Rotasiil™, the reason behind the low efficacy of its vaccine was indiscriminate use of the Vesikari score whose application may have differed widely across studies and even across sites within a given study. The Government of India (GOI) is not discriminating between the two available Indian products and is using both these brands in the Universal Immunization Program (UIP).

9. What are the upper age limits for the first and the last doses of rotavirus vaccines?

The first dose of RVV should not be given after the age of 14 weeks 6 days because there is a greater risk of intussusception (IS) in children given the first dose after 15 weeks of age.

According to the ACIP and the Advisory Committee on Vaccines and Immunization Practices (ACVIP) of the Indian Academy of Pediatrics (IAP), 8 months (32 weeks) is the upper limit for the last dose of RVV. Thus, the "window period" for administration of this crucial vaccine is very small; many children in developing countries who come late for vaccination may, therefore, miss this vaccine. These limits prescribed by regulatory bodies are different from those recommended in UIP (vide infra).

10. If the first dose of rotavirus (RV) vaccine is accidentally given to a baby above the age of 15 weeks, should we continue the series?

After inadvertent administration of first dose to an infant older than 15 weeks, the remaining doses of the series should be given as per routinely recommended intervals. This will not affect the safety and efficacy of the remaining doses. RVV should not be given after the age of 8 months, even if the series is incomplete.

11. When should preterm babies receive the rotavirus (RV) vaccine?

A preterm baby should receive RVV according to the same schedule and with the same precautions as a full-term baby, provided the baby is clinically stable and his chronological age meets the age requirements for the RVV. For instance, an 18-week old preterm baby, who has not received any dose of RVV, should not be given the vaccine because this baby has crossed the maximum permissible chronological age for the first dose (14 weeks 6 days).

12. What if the baby spits out or vomits the dose?

General recommendation is that there is no need to repeat the vaccine dose. However, in the unlikely event that an infant spits out or regurgitates most of the vaccine dose, a single replacement dose may be given at the same vaccination visit. Guidelines for the administration of oral vaccines should be followed.

13. Can the baby be breastfed immediately before/after rotavirus vaccine?

Breastfeeding can be given immediately before or after the administration of RV vaccination. Clinical trials in India, Pakistan, and South Africa, in which breastfeeding was withheld for 30 minutes to 1 hour before and after vaccination, revealed similar seroconversion rates in these babies compared to control groups with unrestricted breastfeeding. Similar findings were reported in a European study using Rotarix™; breastfeeding did not interfere with the efficacy of vaccine.

14. Does oral polio vaccine (OPV) interfere with the uptake of rotavirus vaccine?

Ideally two live, oral vaccines should not be given together as they can interfere with each other's uptake and efficacy. While RVVs do not influence the response to oral polio vaccine (OPV), immune responses to RV vaccination are lower when coadministered with OPV, especially after the first dose. In a Bangladesh study, concomitant OPV administration resulted in lower immunogenicity compared to a schedule in which OPV and Rotarix™ doses were staggered. Despite the lower immunogenicity, a large study of 6,500 infants conducted across six Latin American countries revealed no decrease in protective efficacy of RVV in infants receiving concomitant OPV.

15. If a baby has received the first dose of rotavirus (RV) vaccine and later develops laboratory-confirmed rotavirus gastroenteritis (RVGE), should the course be discontinued?

No. Even if the baby develops RVGE before the completion of full course of RVV, the course should be completed according to age-appropriate schedule and interval recommendations. The reason behind this recommendation is that the initial RV infection might provide only partial protection against subsequent RV infections.

16. What are the common adverse effects of rotavirus vaccines?

Apart from the dreaded complication of IS, several other common adverse events have been reported after RV vaccination. In a clinical trial of RotaTeq™, a small but statistically significant rate of diarrhea and vomiting were reported during the first week after any dose. During the 6 weeks postvaccination following any dose, significantly higher rates of diarrhea, vomiting, otitis media, nasopharyngitis, and bronchospasm were observed compared with placebo recipients.

Similarly in a Rotarix™ clinical trial, statistically significant occurrence of moderately severe cold and rhinitis was reported; irritability and flatulence were other notable adverse events.

17. What is the risk of intussusception with current rotavirus vaccines?

RotaShield®, a quadrivalent Rhesus-human reassortant vaccine, introduced in USA in 1998, had to be withdrawn in the next year due to a slightly increased risk of IS (1:10,000). This was a major setback for the immunization programs worldwide. Because of grave concerns about safety, two new vaccines were introduced, almost after 2 decades, following extensive efficacy and safety studies. Both were tested in >60,000 children in Latin America and Europe and demonstrated excellent efficacy against severe RVGE, without any significant risk of IS.

Postlicensure studies conducted in several countries confirmed that risk of IS with both RotaTeq™ and Rotarix™ was in the range of 1:20,000 to 1:100,000 only. A seven country study from Africa using Rotarix™ did not find any increased risk indicating that population background may also play a role in determining risk of vaccine-associated IS. Similar, reassuring findings have been reported for Rotavac™ and Rotasiil™ in the Indian studies.

The Global Advisory Committee on Vaccine Safety (GACVS) of the WHO (2017) concluded that there is a definite, but small risk of acute IS following use of current generation of RVVs. However, the benefits of RV vaccination against severe diarrhea and death from RV infection far exceed the miniscule risk of IS.

18. What are the contraindications and precautions with the use of rotavirus vaccines?

- Rotavirus vaccines should not be given to infants with a history of severe allergic reaction like anaphylaxis to a previous dose of RVV or to a vaccine component. Those with latex allergy should not be given Rotarix™.
- Severe combined immunodeficiency (SCID) and a history of IS are absolute contraindications for the use of RVVs.
- Risk-benefit ratio should be considered before administration of RVV to following categories of patients:
  - Infants with primary and acquired immunodeficiency, cellular immune deficiency, and hypo- and dysgammaglobulinemia.
  - Infants with blood dyscrasias, leukemias, and lymphomas.
  - Infants on immunosuppressive therapy including high-dose systemic steroids.
  - Human immunodeficiency virus (HIV)-exposed or infected infants.

  These infants may experience severe and prolonged RVGE.

19. Can a monovalent vaccine protect from other rotavirus (RV) serotypes?

An important study conducted in Mexico tracked the natural history of RV infection (symptomatic as well as asymptomatic). It was observed that every child developed at least one RV infection by 2 years of age, 65% had two infections, 40% developed three infections, and 30% developed four to five infections by 2 years of age.

A crucial observation was that the first infection was usually moderate-to-severe, second infection was mild, and all subsequent infections were asymptomatic; the repeat infections were usually caused by different RV serotypes. These observations led to the conclusion that first RV infection protects against severe, subsequent RV infections even when caused by different serotypes. Monovalent RV vaccines mimic this process exactly and provide protection against severe RV infection. However, in case of RV vaccination, even the first infection caused by vaccine virus is asymptomatic.

Similarly, concerns were raised about homotypic and heterotypic protection provided by RVVs. Data from clinical trials revealed that both Rotarix™ and RotaTeq™ exerted similar effectiveness against homotypic and heterotypic RV strains. Rotarix™ provided broad clinical efficacy and field effectiveness against homotypic G1P[8] and also against fully heterotypic G2P[4] strains.

RotaTeq™ also provided broad efficacy and effectiveness against both RotaTeq™ as well as non-RotaTeq™ strains. Strain diversity did not seem to play an important role in varying efficacy of RVVs.

20. What are the World Health Organization (WHO) recommendations for rotavirus vaccination?

Rotavirus vaccines have shown significant efficacy even in the developing countries. According to current recommendations of the WHO, RVVs should be included in NIPs of all countries and should be considered a priority, especially in developing countries with high RVGE-associated mortality. The RV vaccination of target population should be part of a comprehensive strategy to control diarrheal diseases including promotion of breastfeeding, improved water supply and sanitation, oral rehydration solution (ORS), and zinc administration. Introduction of RV vaccination should be accompanied by measures to ensure high vaccination coverage and timely administration of each dose.

The WHO recommends that the first dose of RVV should be administered as soon as possible after 6 weeks of age, preferably along with the first dose of diphtheria, pertussis, and tetanus vaccine (DPT1) to ensure induction of protection prior to natural RV infection. The remaining doses of the vaccine should also be given with subsequent doses of DPT. Because of the typical age distribution of RVGE, administration of RVV to children above the age of 24 months is not recommended.

21. What are the recommendations of the Indian Academy of Pediatrics for rotavirus vaccination?

For the protection of individual children, the recommendations of the ACVIP of the IAP are in accordance with the guidelines of the WHO. It is a well-established fact that the first dose of RVV administered at 6 weeks of age is poorly immunogenic. Studies conducted to evaluate the response to an early (6–10 weeks) vis-à-vis delayed schedule (10–14 weeks) of administering RVVs have yielded variable/conflicting results. In the South African study, the anti-RV immunoglobulin A (IgA) antibody seroconversion rates were higher for 10–14 weeks schedule (55–61%) compared to 6–10 weeks schedule (36–43%), although the difference was not statistically significant. But in a study from Pakistan giving Rotarix™ in a three-dose schedule (6–10–14 weeks) did not lead to a significantly higher rotavirus IgA seroconversion compared to a two-dose schedule of 6–10 weeks. Similarly, Indian studies found no evidence that delaying the first dose from 6 to 10 weeks helped in achieving any significant improvement in immune response.

Reviewing the available data, the ACVIP observed that although it seems that the 6–10 weeks schedule is not as immunogenic as 10–14 weeks schedule, these differences might be due to random variability.

As the recommended upper age limit for the first and the last doses is very rigid, a delayed schedule will lead to incomplete course of RV vaccination because of a small window period for administration of vaccine. This will make many of these children vulnerable to RV infections. Therefore, the ACVIP recommendations (2018–2019) have clearly stated that RVVs should be given in a 6–10–14 weeks schedule along with DPT vaccines, except Rotarix™ which should be administered in a 6–10 weeks schedule. This will ensure that babies with highest risk of exposure are protected at the earliest possible opportunity. Recommended upper age limits for the first dose and the last doses are 15 weeks and 32 weeks, respectively. RVVs should not be given beyond 8 months of age.

22. What are the guidelines for rotavirus vaccination in Universal Immunization Program?

Rotavirus vaccine used in UIP (neonatal 116E strain) is a liquid vaccine and is supplied in a five-dose vial and does not require reconstitution. Each dose is 0.5 mL (five drops). The RVV in UIP is administered in a three-dose schedule at 6, 10, and 14 weeks of age along with other UIP vaccines. No booster dose is recommended. The upper age limit for administering the first dose of RVV in UIP is 12 months. During the initial phase of RVV introduction, only the infants coming for the first dose of OPV and pentavalent vaccine will be administered RVV. These children will receive the second and the third doses in subsequent visits as per schedule. If the child has received the first dose by 12 months of age, two more doses of the vaccine should be given at an interval of 4 weeks to complete the series. Similar guidelines are applicable for Rotasiil™ vaccine.

In 2016, India became the first country in Asia to launch RVV in UIP. Initially introduced in four states, by September, 2019, the program has been extended to all states and union territories of the country.

23. What is the rationale behind unrestricted schedule for administration of rotavirus vaccines?

In view of the serious consequences of RV infection in underprivileged children and minimal impact of public hygiene and sanitation measures, it is widely agreed that vaccination is the most promising preventive strategy against this disease. Ideally, vaccination schedule should be designed to provide benefits to those at the highest risk of severe disease and death. Thus, to maximize its impact, RVV should be given before RVGE occurs and before a significant proportion of target population acquires natural infection.

It was realized that adherence to a very rigid schedule for RVV because of the fear of IS deprived many vulnerable children who would have benefitted from RV vaccination. A model was used to predict the number of deaths prevented by RV vaccination and the number of IS deaths caused by RV vaccination in a restricted (start before 15 weeks, complete by 32 weeks) versus unrestricted schedule (up to 3 years). The model revealed that the restricted schedule will prevent 155,800 deaths while causing 253 IS deaths. Vaccination without age restrictions would prevent 283,000 deaths while causing 547 IS deaths.

Thus, removing the age restrictions would avert an additional 47,200 deaths and cause an additional 294 IS deaths; this would mean an incremental benefit-risk ratio of 154 deaths averted for every death caused by vaccine. Thus, in developing countries, extra lives saved by removing age restrictions for RV vaccination would far outnumber the excess vaccine-associated IS deaths.

24. What is the impact of RV vaccination in developing countries?

Despite lower VE in developing countries, introduction of RVVs in NIPs was predicted to have a major impact in view of high disease burden and mortality. Several countries which have implemented RV vaccination programs have documented fewer cases of SRVGE and RV-associated hospitalizations and reduction of 22–50% in diarrhea-associated mortality.

RotaTeq™ was reported to reduce the number of SRVGE cases in Asia (Bangladesh and Vietnam) by 48% and 39% in Africa (Ghana, Kenya, and Mali), during a 2-year follow-up. A recent modeling study in India that compared a strategy of nationwide 116E vaccination to one of no vaccination estimated that an established 116E vaccination program will reduce RV hospitalization by 28% and mortality by 34%, saving over 34,000 lives every year.

25. What are the new approaches to rotavirus vaccination?

Although live, attenuated RVVs are generally safe and effective for preventing RVGE, there are continuing concerns about serious adverse effects like IS and lower efficacy in developing countries. This has stimulated interest in alternative strategies including inactivated RV particles and nonreplicating RV proteins. The potential advantages of nonreplicating, parenterally delivered vaccines are:

- An improved safety profile with respect to IS, which is believed to be triggered by replication of oral vaccines.
- Improvement in efficacy due to circumventing the proposed interference by environmental enteropathy and maternal antibodies.
- And, probably lower manufacturing costs of the subunit RVV candidates.

The most advanced of the nonreplicating candidates is a recombinant subunit parenteral RVV P2-VP8 candidate from the National Institutes of Health (NIH) and the Population Assessment of Tobacco and Health (PATH). An inactivated whole virus approach is being developed by the Centers for Disease Control and Prevention (CDC), USA. Other novel approaches include virus-like particles (VLPs), cold-adapted strains, and deoxyribonucleic acid (DNA) vaccines.

SUGGESTED READING

1. Bhandari N, Rongsen-Chandola T, Bavdekar A, John J, Antony K, Taneja S, et al. Efficacy of a monovalent human-bovine (116E) rotavirus vaccine in Indian children in the second year of life. Vaccine. 2014;32:A110-6.
2. Burke RM, Tate JE, Kirkwood CD, Steele AD, Parashar UD. Current and new rotavirus vaccines. Curr Opin Infect Dis. 2019;32:435-44.
3. Carvalho MF, Gill D. Rotavirus vaccine efficacy: current status and areas for improvement. Hum Vaccine Immunother. 2019;15:1237-50.
4. Giri S, Nair NP, Mathew A, Manohar B, Simon A, Singh T, et al. Rotavirus gastroenteritis in Indian children <5 years hospitalized for diarrhea, 2012 to 2016. BMC Public Health. 2019;19:69.
5. Kasi S, Shah AK. Rotavirus vaccines. In: Balasubramanian S (Ed). IAP Guidebook on Immunization 2018-2019. New Delhi: Jaypee Brothers Medical Publishers (P) Ltd; 2020:207-26.
6. Kirkwood CD, Ma LF, Carey ME, Steele AD. The rotavirus vaccine development pipeline. Vaccine. 2019;37:7328-35.

7. Madhi SA, Cunliffe NA, Steele D, Witte D, Kirsten M, Louw C, et al. Effect of human rotavirus vaccine on severe diarrhea in African infants. N Engl J Med. 2010;362:289-98.
8. Ministry of Health and Family Welfare, Government of India (2019). Operational Guidelines: Introduction of Rotavirus Vaccine in the Universal Immunization Programme. [online] Available from: https://nhm.gov.in/New_Updates_2018/NHM_Components/Immunization/Guildelines_for_immunization/Operational_Guidelines_for_Introduction_of_Rotavac_in_UIP.pdf. [Last accessed July, 2020].
9. Troeger C, Khalil IA, Rao PC, Cao S, Blacker BF, Ahmed T, et al. Rotavirus vaccination and the global burden of rotavirus diarrhea among children younger than 5 years. JAMA Pediatr. 2018;172:958-65.
10. Vesikari T, Matson DO, Dennehy P, van Damme P, Santosham M, Rodriguez Z, et al. Safety and efficacy of a pentavalent human-bovine (WC3) reassortant rotavirus vaccine. N Engl J Med. 2006;354:23-33.
11. World Health Organization (WHO). Rotavirus vaccines: WHO position paper—January 2013. Wkly Epidemiol Rec. 2013; 88:49-64.
12. Zachariah KR, Kang G. Rotavirus vaccines. In: Vashishtha VM, Kalra A (Eds). IAP Textbook of Vaccines, 2nd edition. New Delhi: Jaypee Brothers Medical Publishers (P) Ltd; 2008:323-47.

CHAPTER 29

Human Papillomavirus Vaccines

Jaydeep Choudhury, Srinivas G Kasi

1. What is the cause of cervical cancer?

Human papillomavirus (HPV) has a predilection for mammalian epithelial cells. There are multiple HPV genotypes with a tropism for cutaneous or mucosal squamous surfaces. A subset of it infects the anogenital tract and are true human carcinogens and cause carcinoma of cervix. HPV infection has been linked to the development of almost all cases of cervical cancer.

These viruses are classified on the basis of their deoxyribonucleic acid (DNA) sequence into various genotypes. One group is responsible for most genital warts and is known as "low risk" as they do not cause cancer. This group is typified by the closely related species HPV 6 and HPV 11. There is another group of 30 oncogenic or high-risk (HR) HPV which are responsible for cervical cancer. Of this, HPV 16 and HPV 18 account for 70% cases and along with HPV 31, 33, and 45 for over >80% cases.

2. How does human papillomavirus (HPV) cause cervical cancer?

Human papillomavirus infects the transformation zone which lies between the columnar epithelium of the endocervix and the squamous epithelium of the ectocervix. The virus infects basal keratinocytes probably via microabrasions of the epithelial surface that leaves the basal lamina intact. The subsequent event in the viral cycle is linked with the differentiation of the keratinocytes as it moves up through the epithelium. This intraepithelial life cycle causes no inflammation, thus no danger signals are sent to alert the innate immunity. HPV does not kill the infected cells—the life cycle is carried out in the keratinocytes which are destined for death from natural cause. Also, there is no viremia hence the adaptive immunity is also not stimulated.

In the cervix, persistent infection can cause dysplastic changes that are termed as low-grade squamous intraepithelial lesion (LSIL) or high-grade squamous intraepithelial lesion (HSIL) on cytology and cervical intraepithelial neoplasia I (CIN I) and CIN II/III on histopathology, respectively. These precancerous lesions may take 2–5 years to progress. Cervical cancer is a late consequence of persistent HPV infection and may take over 10–20 years to develop. The most common form is the squamous cell carcinoma followed by the adenocarcinoma (10%) and adenosquamous carcinoma (2%).

Human papillomavirus is known to infect women in the prime of their reproductive age, though the disease spectrum may unfold in the later years. It is believed that women are likely to be infected with the virus in certain period of their reproductive life, but they may remain asymptomatic and be cleared of the infection over a period of 2 years or they may develop neoplastic changes over more than a decade later.

Also, 80–90% of genital HPV infections resolve with time. About 10–20% of the individuals do not become HPV-DNA negative and develop persistent infection. During persistent HR-HPV infection, there is expression of the oncogenes E6 and E7 that lead to uncontrolled growth of host cells leading to carcinogenesis.

The following cofactors help in causing persistent infection:
- Young age of sexual initiation, particularly below 25 years
- Multiple sex partners
- Multiple pregnancies
- Smoking
- Oral contraceptive use
- Lack of circumcision of male partner.

The HPV is known to be associated with neoplastic changes in the anus, cervix, vulva, and vagina. In addition, they can predispose to esophageal cancer, penile cancer, and recurrent respiratory papillomatosis.

3. How does human papillomavirus (HPV) get transmitted?

Oncogenic HPV can spread via skin-to-skin genital contact and does not necessarily require penetrative sexual intercourse. Thus, unlike other sexually transmitted diseases (STDs), condom cannot prevent HPV infection. Unlike other sexually transmitted infections, female-to-male transmission appears greater that male-to-female transmission.

The various modes of transmission are as follows:
- *Sexual contact*:
  - Through sexual intercourse
  - Genital-genital, manual-genital, and oral-genital
  - Genital HPV infection in virgins is rare, but may result from nonpenetrative sexual contact
  - Proper condom use may help reduce the risk, but is not fully protective against infection.
- *Nonsexual routes*:
  - Mother to newborn (vertical transmission)
  - Fomites (e.g., undergarments, surgical gloves, and biopsy forceps).

These are hypothesized but not well-documented.

4. What is the burden of cervical cancer in India?

Cervical cancer is the second most frequent cancer in women in India after breast cancer and it accounts for 23.5% of all cancers in women in India. The crude incidence rate of cervical cancer in India is 14.9 per 100,000 women/

year compared to 26.2 per 100,000 women/year for breast cancer. India has a population of 0.469 billion women aged 15 years and older who are at a risk of developing cervical cancer. Current estimates indicate that every year 96,922 women are diagnosed with cervical cancer and 60,078 die from the disease. The prevalence (%) of HPV 16 and/or HPV 18 among women with normal cytology is 5%.

About 7.9% of women in the general population are estimated to harbor cervical HPV infection at a given time and 82.5% of invasive cervical cancers are attributed to HPVs 16 or 18. In India, the estimated HPV 16/18 positive fraction was 83.2% (81.5-84.8) in women with invasive cervical carcinoma (ICC), 62.8% (56.7-68) with high squamous intraepithelial lesion, 28.2% (22.1-35.3) with low squamous intraepithelial lesion, and 5% (4.6-5.5) in women with normal cytology/histology. Overall HPV prevalence in India was similar to the HR areas in Latin America, but lower than that observed in some parts of sub-Saharan Africa. One out of four women who die due to cervical cancer in the world is an Indian.

5. Will everybody who gets human papillomavirus (HPV) infection develop cervical cancer?

Over 80% of HPV infections are transient, asymptomatic, and resolve spontaneously.

The vast majority of HPV infections are transitory and become undetectable in 12-24 months. The presence of persistent infection with an oncogenic HPV type is the main risk factor for progression from CIN1 to CIN3 and cancer. Certain HR-HPV types 33 and 16 were associated with the highest risk, followed by HPV 18, HPV 31, and HPV 45.

Over 70-80% of CIN1 lesions spontaneously regress without treatment or become undetectable. Apart from the presence of the HR serotypes mentioned above, long-term oral contraceptive use, smoking, and multiparity are associated with progression.

Cervical intraepithelial neoplasia 2 (CIN2) is less commonly progresses to cancer, with an annual regression rate ranging from 15 to 23%, with up to 55% regressing by 4-6 years. Approximately, 2% of CIN2 lesions develop to CIN3 within the same period.

Cervical intraepithelial neoplasia 3 is considered a true precancer which progresses to cervical cancer at a rate of 0.2-4% within 12 months.

Untreated CIN3 has a 30% probability of becoming invasive cancer over a 30-year period, although only about 1% of properly treated CIN3 will become invasive.

6. What are the common human papillomavirus (HPV) serotypes that affect human?

Human papillomavirus 16 and 18 account for 70% of squamous cell carcinoma and high-grade invasive cancer worldwide. Of the two, HPV 16 prevalence is 57% in Asia and 58% in Europe. HPV 18 is the second most common cause of cervical cancer. Other HPV causes <5% of cervical cancers. Six most common

HR types are 31, 33, 35, 45, 52, and 58. Together these, eight serotypes account for 90% of cervical cancers. HPV16/18 is slightly higher in Australia, Europe, and North America (74–79%) than in Africa, South and Central America, and Asia (65–70%). HPV 52 and 58 are more prevalent in Asia than elsewhere. In a study on the prevalence of HR-HPV infection among apparently healthy populations in various regions of India, the most common HPV types reported were (in descending order) HPV 16, 18, 31, 33, 35, 39, 45, 51, 52, 56, 58, 59, and 68.

7. Does natural infection with human papillomavirus (HPV) give immunity?

Natural HPV infection induces a weak immune response. Genital HPV is followed eventually by seroconversion and type-specific antibody to L1 but not to the L2 protein. It generally occurs 6–18 months after the initiation of infection. The antibody concentrations after natural infections are very low. The lack of a viremia and the fact that viral particles are shed from the surface of squamous epithelia with poor access to vascular and lymphatic channels may explain the poor antibody response. Only 20–25% of women remain antibody positive over 10 years. These low levels of antibodies may not be protective against future infections. In a natural infection, the route of entry of HPV and the initial intraepithelial localization markedly reduce the exposure of HPV to the host immune system. This may be the reason for the generally poor immune response to natural infection.

8. What are the mechanisms of vaccine-induced immunity?

An immune correlate of protection has not yet been established in the efficacy trials due to the very low failure rates of vaccines. It is postulated that neutralizing antibodies are the primary, if not the exclusive, immune effectors for the virus-like particle (VLP) vaccines. The role of cell-mediated immunity (CMI) and memory B-cells is uncertain. VLP-L1 vaccines induce very high levels of specific antibodies. Antibody concentrations in cervical secretion are usually very low, 10–1,000 times less than those in the serum and likely to be undetectable in many subjects 18–24 months postvaccination. Microabrasion of the genital epithelium that results in epithelial denudation but retention to the epithelium basement membrane favors HPV binding to this exposed basement membrane by a primary receptor in L1 before binding to and entering keratinocytes. This occurs presumably when the keratinocytes migrate along basement membrane to re-epithelialize the small wound. Rapid serous exudation occurs in the wound. In the vaccinated, this exudate contains high levels of specific antibodies. This results in rapid virus neutralization and also provides an opportunity to encounter with circulating memory B-cells to initiate memory response. High levels of VLP-L1 antibodies prevent infection by blocking association with basement membrane heparan sulfate proteoglycans (HSPGs) whereas low levels of VLP-L1 antibodies prevent infection by blocking transfer from basement membrane HSPGs to the keratinocyte surface receptors.

9. What are the currently available vaccines against human papillomavirus (HPV)? How do they differ?

Presently, three HPV vaccines are available. All are manufactured by recombinant DNA technology that produces noninfectious VLPs comprising of the HPVL1 protein, the major capsid protein of HPV. The quadrivalent vaccine is a mixture of L1 proteins of HPV serotypes 16, 18, 6, and 11 with aluminum-containing adjuvant. The second is a bivalent vaccine. It is a mixture of L1 proteins of HPV serotypes 16 and 18 with AS04 as an adjuvant. The third vaccine is a nonavalent vaccine containing the L1 protein of 6, 11, 16, 18, 31, 33, 35, 52, and 58 with aluminum-containing adjuvant.

Types 6 and 11 account for >90% of genital warts.

Human papillomavirus vaccines licensed for clinical usage are described in **Table 1**.

TABLE 1: Human papillomavirus (HPV) vaccines licensed for clinical usage.

	B-HPV: Cervarix™	Q-HPV: Gardasil™	Gardasil 9™
Serotypes included	16:20 µg 18:20 µg	6:20 µg 11:40 µg 16:40 µg 18:20 µg	6:30 µg 11:40 µg 16:60 µg 18:40 µg 20 µg each of 31, 33, 45, 52, and 58
Adjuvant	AS04 50 µg of the 3-O-desacyl-4'-monophosphoryl lipid A (MPL) and 0.5 mg of aluminum hydroxide	Amorphous aluminum hydroxyphosphate sulfate (AAHS)	AAHS
Preservative	Nil	Nil	Nil

None of the vaccines contains live biological products or viral DNA and are, therefore, noninfectious; they do not contain antibiotics or preservative agents.

10. Are there any differences in the immunological responses elicited by these vaccines?

Both vaccines are highly immunogenic with the highest immune responses being observed in young girls aged 9-15 years. Titers for HPV 16 and 18 antibodies produced are several folds higher than after natural infection. Geometric mean titers (GMTs) were highest 1 month after the third dose. This was followed by a step fall in GMTs over the next 2 years followed by a plateau. Titers observed during the plateau phase are generally well above those seen after natural infection.

For the B-HPV vaccine titers of antibodies against 16 and 18 remain at least 11-fold higher than that observed after a natural infection for at least 5 years.

For the Q-HPV vaccines, while the antibody titers against type 16 remain elevated, 18 months after first vaccination, the antibody titers for HPV 18 return to the level of natural infection, with a further reduction in seropositivity over time.

In a head-to-head immunogenicity trial comparing Cervarix™ and Gardasil™, using an in vitro pseudovirion neutralization assay, Cervarix™ was found to induce 24-month GMT titers that were, depending on age group, 2.4- to 5.8-fold higher against HPV 16 and 7.7- to 9.4-fold higher against HPV 18. The higher titers were observed till 60 months of follow-up. Whether the higher titers would translate into longer-term protection against vaccine-targeted or -related types is debatable, as there was no indication that protection to HPV 18 was preferentially waning in Gardasil™-vaccinated women.

11. What is the efficacy of these vaccines?

Clinical trials with both vaccines have used efficacy against CIN2/3 and adenocarcinoma in situ (AIS) caused by HPV strains contained in the concerned vaccine as primary endpoints. In addition, Q-HPV has demonstrated efficacy against genital warts, vulvar intraepithelial neoplasia (VIN) 1 and 2 and vaginal intraepithelial neoplasia (VaIN) 1 and 2 **(Table 2)**.

In the FUTURE trial, 99.0% (95.8–99.7) efficacy was seen against vaccine type-related genital warts.

12. Is there any cross-protection against nonvaccine oncogenic serotypes?

Immunity to HPV is type-specific. However, HPV 16 is phylogenetically related to HPV types 31, 33, 52, and 58 (A9 species) and HPV 18 is related to HPV 45 (A7 species).

At study end of the PATRICIA study (average 34.9 months), for B-HPV, significant cross-protection against 6 months persistent infection was seen against HPV 31: 78.7% (70.2–85.2), HPV 33: 45.7% (25.1–60.9), and HPV 45: 75.7% (60.4–85.7).

At 6.4 years, the efficacy of the bivalent vaccine against incident infection with HPV 31 was 59.8% (20.5–80.7) and 77.7% (39.3–93.4) against HPV 45.

In the combined phase III analysis of FUTURE I and II studies, the vaccine efficacy (VE) against persistent infection was 40.3% (13.9–59.0) against HPV types 31 or 45 and VE against five most common HR serotypes was 25.0% (5.0–40.9).

However, cross-protection does not last for long as in the long-term follow-up of B-HPV, up to 6.4 years, the VE against HPV 45 remained at 94.2% (63.3–99.9) and HPV 31 remained at 54.5% (11.5–77.7). No protection was seen against HPV types 33, 52, and 58 at 8 years of follow-up, indicating the shorter duration of protection with cross-reactive antibodies.

13. What is the role of gender-neutral vaccination or vaccination of boys/men?

The only study conducted in men showed a VE of 90.4% [95% confidence interval (CI): 69.2–98.1] for per protocol (PP) and 65.5% (95% CI: 45.8–78.6)

TABLE 2: Vaccine efficacy (VE) of Cervarix and Gardasil.		
	VE (%) Cervarix™	VE (%) Gardasil™
CIN 2+		
ATP[1]/PP[2]	92.9 (79.9–98.3) 98.1 (88.4–100) ATP-E[5]	98.2 (93.3–99.8)
TVC/ITT[3]	52.8 (37.5–64.7)	51.5 (40.6–60.6)
TVC naïve[4]	98.4 (90.4–100)	100 (91.9–100)
CIN 3		
ATP/PP	80.0 (0.3–98.1)	96.8 (88.1–99.6)
TVC/ITT	33.6 (1.1–56.9)	45.1 (29.8–57.3)
TVC naïve	100 (64.7–100)	100 (90.5–100)
HPV naïve		
Genital warts	–	96.4 (91.4–98.8)
VIN 1/VaIN 1	–	95.2 (70.0–99.9)
VIN 2/VaIN 2	–	95.4 (71.5–99.9)
Intention to treat		
Genital warts	–	79.5 (73.0–84.6)
VIN 1/VaIN 1	–	76.0 (54.2–88.3)
VIN 2/VaIN 2	–	78.5 (55.2–90.8)

(CIN: cervical intraepithelial neoplasia; HPV: human papillomavirus; VaIN: vaginal intraepithelial neoplasia; VE: vaccine efficacy; VIN: vulvar intraepithelial neoplasia)

[1] According to protocol (ATP): Received three vaccinations, seronegative/deoxyribonucleic acid (DNA) negative to respective HPV types at day 1; DNA negative to respective HPV types at month 6; normal or low-grade Pap test at day 1; case counting began 1 day after vaccine dose 3.

[2] Per protocol (PP): Received three vaccinations, seronegative/DNA negative to vaccine HPV types; remained DNA negative through 1 month postdose 3; case counting started 1 month after dose 3.

[3] Total vaccinated cohort (TVC) and intention to treat (ITT): Received at least one vaccination, regardless of baseline HPV-related infection or disease; case counting began after day 1.

[4] Total vaccinated cohort-naïve and HPV-naïve: Received at least one dose; polymerase chain reaction (PCR) negative at entry for HPVs 16, 18, 31, 33, 35, 39, 45, 51, 52, 56, 58, and 59 (and 66 and 68 for TVC-naïve); seronegative for vaccine types and Pap cytology normal at day 1; case counting after day 1.

[5] ATP-E: Analysis in which probable causality to HPV type was assigned in lesions infected with multiple oncogenic types (ATP-E cohort).

for intention to treat (ITT). A VE of 60.2% (95% CI: 40.8–73.8) was observed in the ITT cohort against external genital lesions, irrespective of HPV type. In a subset of men who have sex with men (MSM) in the above study, VE against HPV 6/11/16/18-related anal intraepithelial neoplasia (AIN) of any grade and AIN2+ was 77.5% (95% CI: 39.6–93.3) and 74.9% (95% CI: 8.8–95.4), respectively, in the PP group. PP efficacy against persistent anal infection by the vaccine types was 94.9% (95% CI: 80.4–99.4).

Human papillomavirus infections are responsible for a range of noncervical diseases in both sexes that have serious morbidity and contribute to a substantial healthcare burden. HPV vaccination of boys alongside girls would facilitate the eradication of HPV and protect boys from infection, reduce transmission, increase herd immunity, and effectively prevent HPV-associated diseases. Limiting HPV vaccination to girls will not lead to eradication. However, it is believed that vaccinating males provides only small additional benefit and is not cost-effective, especially if female programs obtain high (>75%) coverage.

14. Should screening be continued in women who have received human papillomavirus (HPV) vaccine?

Vaccination is primary prevention while screening is secondary prevention. Hence, need for both should be stressed. The available HPV vaccines protect against HPV types 16 and 18 which are responsible for about 70% of cervical cancer. Periodic screening for cervical cancer has to be continued even in vaccinated women because women may get infected with other oncogenic HPV types. The integration of the vaccination of women against HPV types 16 and 18, with cervical screening at 3-yearly intervals, could reduce the incidence of cervical cancer by 94% compared with no intervention. Hence, cervical cancer screening should be continued in women who have received HPV vaccines.

15. What is the safety profile of the human papillomavirus (HPV) vaccines?

Most of the adverse effects described with the HPV vaccines are all minor adverse effects and no serious vaccine-related adverse events have been reported either in trials or postmarketing surveillance studies. Syncope, which is common in adolescents, can be avoided by administering the vaccine in sitting or lying down position and 15 minutes after vaccination.

Serious adverse effects (SAEs), such as adverse pregnancy outcomes, autoimmune conditions, multiple sclerosis (MS), venous thromboembolism (VTE), Guillain-Barré syndrome (GBS), anaphylaxis, and stroke, were extensively studied and showed no increase in the incidence of these AEs compared with background rates.

There is no evidence to suggest a causal association between HPV vaccine and complex regional pain syndrome (CRPS), postural orthostatic tachycardia syndrome (POTS), or the diverse symptoms that include pain and motor dysfunction.

The Centers for Disease Control and Prevention (CDC) and the Food and Drug Administration (FDA) have found no evidence that Gardasil™ may be causing premature ovarian failure and continue to monitor for vaccine safety.

16. Are human papillomavirus (HPV) vaccines effective in the immunocompromised?

The immunogenicity of HPV vaccines in persons with human immunodeficiency virus (HIV) is, in general, inferior to that in HIV-negative subjects. Reduced efficacy has been demonstrated in some studies.

In a four-arm vaccine randomized controlled trial (RCT), with both HIV-positive and HIV-negative women, who were randomized 1:1 to receive Cervarix™ or Gardasil™ and serology measured using a pseudovirion-based neutralizing antibody assay, Cervarix™ was superior to Gardasil™ in the HIV-positive females, for HPV 16 by 2.74-fold (CIs: 1.83–4.11) and for HPV 18 by 7.44-fold (4.79–11.54) in GMTs. Memory B-cell responses were inferior in the HIV positive, more so with Gardasil™. These results may be explained by the superior adjuvant in Cervarix™.

17. Are boosters needed?

A 14-year of follow-up of Q-HPV has shown undiminished protection against cases of cervical/genital disease related to HPV types 6, 11, 16, and 18. Similar undiminished protection has been demonstrated for the B-HPV vaccine till 9.4 years of follow-up.

At present, there is no data to support use of boosters.

18. Are there other human papillomavirus (HPV) diseases that the two vaccines may prevent?

Studies have shown that the quadrivalent vaccine prevents cancers of the vagina and vulva, which like cervical cancer, can be caused by HPV types 16 and 18.

Published studies have not looked at other health problems that might be prevented by HPV vaccines. It is possible that HPV vaccines will also prevent cancers of the head and neck, penis, and anus due to HPV 16 or 18. The quadrivalent vaccine might prevent recurrent respiratory papillomatosis (RRP), a rare condition caused by HPV 6 or 11 in which warts grow in the throat.

In the Costa Rica Vaccine Trial of the B-HPV, in a restricted cohort of women, with both cervical HPV 16/18 DNA negative and HPV 16/18 seronegative prior at enrollment, VE against prevalent HPV 16/18 anal infection measured 4-year postvaccination was 83.6% (95% CI: 66.7–92.8%) (N = 1,989) and in the full cohort (all women with an anal specimen), the VE was 62.0% (95% CI: 47.1–73.1%).

19. Can pregnant women be vaccinated?

Pregnant women are not included in the recommendations for HPV vaccines. Studies show neither vaccine caused problems for babies born to women who got the HPV vaccine while they were pregnant. Getting the HPV vaccine when pregnant is not a reason to consider ending a pregnancy. But, to be on the safer side until even more is known, a pregnant woman should not get any doses of either HPV vaccine until completion of pregnancy.

20. What should a woman do if she realizes she received human papillomavirus (HPV) vaccination while pregnant?

If a woman realizes that she got any shots of an HPV vaccine while pregnant, she should wait until her pregnancy has completed and complete the schedule.

21. Can one use both these vaccines interchangeably?

Whenever feasible, the same HPV vaccine should be used for the entire vaccination series. No studies address interchangeability of HPV vaccines. However, if the vaccine provider does not know or does not have the HPV vaccine product administered previously, either HPV vaccine can be used to complete the series to provide protection against HPV 16 and 18. For protection against HPV 6 or 11-related genital warts, a vaccination series with <three doses of HPV 4 might provide less protection against genital warts than a complete three-dose HPV 4 series.

22. What is the Indian Academy of Pediatrics-Advisory Committee on Vaccines and Immunization Practices (IAP-ACVIP) recommendation regarding use of human papillomavirus (HPV) vaccination?

The Indian Academy of Pediatrics-Advisory Committee on Vaccines and Immunization Practices (IAP-ACVIP) has included HPV vaccination in routine immunization. Minimum age for vaccination is 9 years. As of current licensing regulations in India, catch-up vaccination is up to the age of 45 years.

According to new 2014 recommendations, two doses of HPV vaccine are advised for adolescent/preadolescent girls aged 9–14 years while for girls 15 years and older, current three-dose schedule will continue. For two-dose schedule, the minimum interval between doses should be 6 months. The interval between the first and second dose may be extended up to 12 months, should this facilitate administration—say in school settings. Those >15 years and the immunocompromised, irrespective of age, should receive three doses.

This recommendation is valid for both the vaccine brands available in the market.

23. Why is the thrust on adolescent vaccination for a condition which is essentially an adult disease?

Since the present HPV vaccines are prophylactic vaccines, they should be given prior to beginning of sexual activity.

Moreover, vaccination in young adolescents elicits a significantly superior immune response compared to the vaccine administration in older adolescents and young adults.

Vaccination in early adolescence needs only two doses, making it more cost-effective especially in national programs.

24. How many doses of human papillomavirus (HPV) vaccine a 15-year and 4-month-old girl should take now? She has received her first HPV shot when she was 14 years and 10-month-old.

Only one dose. According to both the ACVIP and the World Health Organization (WHO), for girls, primed before the age of 15 years, even if older at the time of boosting (second dose), a two-dose schedule will be applicable.

25. An adolescent girl is inadvertently administered the second dose 4 months after dose 1. What is the schedule to be followed?

The minimum acceptable interval between dose 1 and dose 2, of a two-dose schedule, is 5 months. The early second dose is an invalid dose and should be repeated at least 5 months after dose 1 and 12 weeks after the invalid dose.

26. Why has the Indian Academy of Pediatrics-Advisory Committee on Vaccines and Immunization Practices (IAP-ACVIP) changed its recommendations on human papillomavirus (HPV) vaccination?

The move to revise HPV vaccine immunization schedule for adolescent girls from existing three to two doses is in tune with the recommendations of the WHO and the Advisory Committee on Immunization Practices (ACIP). The reduced dose regimen would not only be cost saving, but would also simplify logistics like increased flexibility of the intervals and annual doses for school-based delivery. Hence, the revised recommendations may help in improving acceptance, facilitating delivery, and enhancing coverage of the vaccine.

27. Is there enough evidence for this change in recommendations?

Yes, there is now enough evidence emanating from various countries and different trials favoring this shortened schedule. The main source of evidence for the revised recommendations is provided by a systematic review commissioned by the WHO-Strategic Advisory Group of Experts (SAGE) Working Group. The systematic review has identified various studies that include both randomized and nonrandomized trials of both the vaccines, bivalent and quadrivalent, from various high-income group countries like Canada, Australia, Sweden, Denmark, and Germany and low middle-income (LMI) countries like Uganda, Mexico, and India. The other sources include nonsystematic review of the data from observational studies on two- versus three-dose schedule and proceedings of an Ad Hoc Expert Consultation on HPV vaccine schedules organized in Geneva, 2013. All these studies have shown an immunological noninferiority of two-dose versus three-dose schedules in those between 9 and 15 years of age.

28. The recommendations of shortened schedule are based entirely on comparisons of immunogenicity and geometric mean concentration (GMC) levels achieved after vaccination. There is no data about clinical efficacy. Is this sufficient justification to have a reduced dose schedule?

Human papillomavirus vaccines were licensed based upon the demonstration of their clinical efficacy in young adult women.

The age extension for adolescent girls, in whom efficacy trials would not be feasible, was granted because studies demonstrated that antibody responses in adolescent girls were not inferior to those elicited in women ("immunological bridging"). Alternative adolescent vaccine schedules should, thus, demonstrate that their immunogenicity is similarly noninferior. To seek licensing, a phase III immunogenicity study of the quadrivalent HPV vaccine was conducted in adolescents with the objective of bridging the efficacy findings in young women to preadolescents and adolescents. The neutralizing anti-HPV GMTs at month 7 were noninferior in adolescents and indeed 1.7–2.7-fold higher than in the group of 16–23-year-old females in whom efficacy was demonstrated. Similar observations were made for the bivalent vaccine and for the nonavalent vaccines currently in clinical development.

The magnitude of the vaccine response is determined by the age at the first dose. The review of different trials has shown that 100% adolescents can be primed with a single dose of the vaccine and the second dose after 6 months results in higher (almost twice) peak titers in adolescents than in adults. These antibodies then plateau for about 12 months after the peak and decline very slowly providing a long-lasting protection.

In fact, strong 4 year protection was reported in Costa Rican women who received just one dose of bivalent vaccine.

Hence, there are enough evidence to justify correlation of antibodies level with ultimate clinical protection against HPVdisease.

29. Can we have shorter, e.g., 2 months interval for two-dose schedule?

No, the available data strongly favor long interval between two doses. In a recent RCT, different intervals (0, 2 months vs. 0, 6 months vs. 0, 12 months) between doses of HPV vaccine were compared. The results revealed that the 6-month interval resulted in superior GMCs compared with the 2-month interval 1 month after the last vaccine dose in all the age groups enrolled (9–14, 15–19, and 20–25 years). There are no data as yet publicly available from the other trial comparing 0, 6 months with 0, 12 months interval.

30. What has been the impact of human papillomavirus (HPV) vaccines?

Data on vaccine impact on HPV-associated cancers will not be available for many more years.

A 10-year impact data is available for Q-HPV vaccine from nine high-income countries. Maximal reductions of approximately 90% for HPV 6/11/16/18 infection, approximately 90% for genital warts, approximately 45% for low-grade cytological cervical abnormalities, and approximately 85% for high-grade histologically proven cervical abnormalities have been reported. The highest decreases were seen in the younger birth cohorts. Declines were detected within 4 years after vaccine availability, even in settings with comparatively low vaccine coverage.

There was a significant decline of 40.1% in the prevalence of four-valent vaccine-type HPV among women who were unvaccinated indicating a significant herd immunity. Similar findings have been reported from Australia, Scotland, and England.

31. Why was the four-valent vaccine upgraded to a nine-valent vaccine?

In USA, 4-HPV protected against 70% of CC. Addition of five serotypes has increased the coverage to 90%. Gardasil™ 9 has 6, 11, 16, 18, 31, 33, 45, 52, and 58. The additional cost of the nonavalent vaccine was considered to be a cost-effective intervention.

The nonavalent vaccine was studied in the pivotal study (protocol 001). It showed noninferiority to 6, 11, 16, and 18 as compared to 4-HPV. The VE was 97.4% (85–99.9) against cervical/vulvar/vaginal disease, 97.1% (83.5–99.9) against CIN2/3, and AIS and 100% (39.4–100) against CIN3, caused by the five additional serotypes.

4-HPV is no longer used in USA.

32. Which are the newer human papillomavirus (HPV) vaccines under development?

The major disadvantages of the present HPV vaccines are a virus-type restricted protection, the high cost of the manufacture, and an absence of therapeutic activity on the established lesions. The second-generation prophylactic HPV vaccines, using capsomere or minor capsid HPV L2 protein or made by more cost-effective strategies of production, are undergoing evaluation.

Four vaccines have reached the stage of human studies: (1) *Escherichia coli (E. coli)*-based HPV 16 and 18 L1-VLPs (Celcolin™) in phase III, (2) *E. coli*-based HPV 6, 11 L1-VLPs (Gelcolin™) in phase I, (3) *Pichia pastoris*-based HPV 16, 18 VLPs in phase I, and (4) *Hansenula polymorpha*-based HPV 6, 11, 16, and 18 VLPs in phase I.

L2, the minor HPV capsid protein, is highly conserved among the different HPV types. L2 increases the formation of cross-neutralizing antibodies, extending the protection also against LR-HPV types. Moreover, this protein can be obtained by bacteria.

L2-based vaccines result in transient and lower antibody titers than L1-based VLPs. This is being overcome by the use of newer adjuvants.

Chimeric L1-L2 VLPs are being investigated. This combines the immunogenicity of L1-based vaccines and the broad cross-protection of L2.

Combined prophylactic or therapeutic vaccines are being studied by fusion of the L2 protein with the early HPV proteins such as E6 or E7.

33. What is the duration of protection after human papillomavirus (HPV) vaccination? Does it last for lifelong?

Subsequently, after vaccination, the antibody titer gradually wanes off in case of HPV 18 but vaccine efficacy remains near 100% probably due to immune memory. The immune response mounted after third dose of vaccine schedule is maximal and gradually decline by 2 years and then remains unaltered for next 5 years. Computer modeling of the response to HPV 16 L1 vaccine suggested that immune response persists for 12 years to near lifelong after third dose of vaccine administration. The same should be hold true for a two-dose schedule.

For three-dose schedule quadrivalent vaccine, no breakthrough cases of cervical/genital disease related to pertinent four types were observed among vaccinated preadolescents and adolescents during 10 years follow-up. For the bivalent vaccine, immunogenicity and efficacy of a three-dose schedule against HPV 16 and 18 have been demonstrated up to 8.4 and 9.4 years, respectively. It is still unknown whether booster doses will be required in long run.

34. What is the current status of human papillomavirus (HPV) vaccine use in a single-dose schedule?

Many studies are underway to explore the feasibility of using a single dose of HPV vaccine in immunization schedules that should facilitate better coverage along with lower cost. An Indian study concluded that a single dose of quadrivalent HPV vaccine was immunogenic and provided lasting protection against HPV 16 and 18 infections like the three- and two-dose vaccine schedule. A national cohort analysis from Australia found one dose had comparable effectiveness as two or three doses in preventing high-grade disease in a high coverage setting. Earlier, the Costa Rica Vaccine Trial provided the initial data that one dose of the HPV vaccine could provide durable protection against HPV infection. According to a recent systematic review of data from national immunization programs, almost half found some effectiveness with one dose. All these studies hint that one-dose vaccination may be a viable strategy when working toward the global elimination of cervical cancer.

35. There is lot of talk on therapeutic vaccines. What is the progress made in this field pertaining to human papillomavirus (HPV)-induced cervical cancer arena?

E6 and E7 are two early proteins that get expressed in all HPV-infected cells and are upregulated in cancer cells. So, these proteins have been an area of interest to develop therapeutic vaccines by using viral/bacterial vectors, peptides, DNA, and dendritic cells. A phase I trial has concluded using recombinant HPV16 E7 and HPV18 E7 and after seeing encouraging safety profile has progressed to phase II trial.

SUGGESTED READING

1. Barra F, Maggiore ULR, Bogani G, Ditto A, Signorelli M, Martinelli F, et al. New prophylactics human papilloma virus (HPV) vaccines against cervical cancer. J Obstet Gynaecol. 2019;39:1-10.
2. Bosch FX, Lorincz A, Muñoz N, Meijer CJ, Shah KV. The casual relation between human papillomavirus and cervical cancer. J Clin Pathol. 2002;55:244-65.
3. Brotherton JM, Budd A, Rompotis C, Bartlett N, Malloy MJ, Andersen RL, et al. Is one dose of human papillomavirus vaccine as effective as three? A national cohort analysis. Papillomavirus Res. 2019;8:100177.
4. Doorbar J. The papilloma virus life cycle. J Clin Virol. 2005;32:S7-15.
5. FUTURE II Study Group. Quadrivalent vaccine against human papillomavirus to prevent high-grade cervical lesions. N Engl J Med. 2007;356:1915-27.
6. Garland SM, Kjaer SK, Muñoz N, Block SL, Brown DR, DiNubile MJ, et al. Impact and effectiveness of the quadrivalent human papillomavirus vaccine: a systematic review of 10 years of real-world experience. Clin Infect Dis. 2016;63:519-27.
7. Gilca V, Sauvageau C, Panicker G, De Serres G, Ouakki M, Unger ER. Immunogenicity and safety of a mixed vaccination schedule with one dose of nonavalent and one dose of bivalent HPV vaccine versus two doses of nonavalent vaccine—a randomized clinical trial. Vaccine. 2018;36:7017-24.
8. Giuliano AR, Harris R, Sedjo RL, Baldwin S, Roe D, Papenfuss MR, et al. Incidence, prevalence, and clearance of type-specific human papillomavirus infections: The Young Women's Health Study. J Infect Dis. 2002;186:462-9.
9. GLOBOCAN 2002. In: Preedy VR, Watson RR (Eds). Handbook of Disease Burdens and Quality of Life Measures. Springer, New York, NY. https://doi.org/10.1007/978-0-387-78665-0_5729.
10. Kreimer AR, Herrero R, Sampson JN, Porras C, Lowy DR, Schiller JT, et al. Evidence for single-dose protection by the bivalent HPV vaccine—Review of the Costa Rica HPV vaccine trial and future research studies. Vaccine. 2018;36:4774-82.
11. Markowitz LE, Drolet M, Perez N, Jit M, Brisson M. Human papillomavirus vaccine effectiveness by number of doses: systematic review of data from national immunization programs. Vaccine. 2018;36:4806-15.
12. McIntosh N. (2000). Jhpiego strategy paper 8. [online] Available from: http://www.jhpiego.jhu.edu/scripts/pubs/category_detail.asp?category_id=4. [Last accessed July, 2020].
13. Moscicki AB, Schiffman M, Kjaer S, Villa LL. Updating the natural history of HPV and anogenital cancer. Vaccine. 2006;24:S42-51.
14. Munoz N, Castellsague X, de Gonzaleza B, Gissman L. HPV in the etiology of human cancer. Vaccine. 2006;24:S3-10.
15. Muñoz N, Manalastas R, Pitisuttithum P, Tresukosol D, Monsonego J, Ault K, et al. Safety, immunogenicity, and efficacy of quadrivalent human papillomavirus (types 6, 11, 16, 18) recombinant vaccine in women aged 24-45 years: a randomised, double-blind trial. Lancet. 2009;373:1949-57.
16. Paavonen J, Naud P, Salmerón J, Wheeler CM, Chow SN, Apter D, et al. Efficacy of human papillomavirus (HPV)-16/18 AS04-adjuvanted vaccine against cervical infection and precancer caused by oncogenic HPV types (PATRICIA): final analysis of a double-blind, randomized study in young women. Lancet. 2009;374:301-14.

17. Parkin DM, Bray F. The burden of HPV-related cancers. Vaccine. 2006;24:S13-25.
18. Petrosky E, Bocchini JA, Hariri S, Chesson H, Curtis CR, Saraiya M, et al. Use of 9-valent human papillomavirus (HPV) vaccine: updated HPV vaccination recommendations of the Advisory Committee on Immunization Practices. MMWR Morb Mortal Wkly Rep. 2015;64:300-4.
19. Sankaranarayanan R, Joshi S, Muwonge R, Esmy PO, Basu P, Prabhu P, et al. Can a single dose of human papillomavirus (HPV) vaccine prevent cervical cancer? Early findings from an Indian study. Vaccine. 2018;36:4783-91.
20. Schiller JT, Frazer IH, Lowy DR. Human papillomavirus vaccines. In: Plotkin S, Orenstein W, Offit P (Eds). Vaccines, 5th edition. Philadelphia: Elsevier; 2008. pp. 243-58.
21. Stanley M, Lowy DR, Frazer I. Chapter 12: Prophylactic HPV vaccines: underlying mechanisms. Vaccine. 2006;24:S106-13.
22. Vashishtha VM, Choudhury P, Kalra A, Bose A, Thacker N, Yewale VN, et al. Indian Academy of Pediatrics recommended immunization schedule for children aged 0 through 18 years—India, 2014 and updates on Immunization. Indian Pediatr. 2014;51:785-800.

CHAPTER 30

Influenza Vaccines

Sanjay Srirampur, Pritesh Nagar, Vipin M Vashishtha

1. What is influenza?

Influenza, also commonly known as "the flu", is a viral respiratory tract infection. It is caused by a ribonucleic acid (RNA)-based virus; the influenza virus belongs to the Orthomyxoviridae virus family. It is an airborne infection and patient is infectious for 5–10 days from a day before the onset of symptoms.

2. What are the causes of flu?

There are four main types of influenza viruses—A, B, C, and D. Influenza A and B are the main causes of seasonal epidemics in humans. When a new strain of influenza A appears, it can lead to global pandemics. Type C infection usually causes either a very mild respiratory illness or no symptoms at all; it does not cause epidemics.

3. What are the key characteristics of influenza virus?

Influenza viruses are RNA viruses of the Orthomyxoviridae family and are classified into types A, B, or C. The great majority of human infections are associated with types A and B. Influenza A viruses are further subtyped based upon characterization of two surface proteins: (1) hemagglutinin (HA) and (2) neuraminidase (NA). Among influenza A viruses that circulate among humans, three major subtypes of HAs (H1, H2, and H3) and two subtypes of NAs (N1 and N2) have been described **(Fig. 1)**.

Influenza A viruses have a remarkable ability to undergo changes in the antigenic characteristics of their envelope glycoproteins, especially the HAs. Influenza B viruses circulate widely only among humans, but have a lesser propensity for antigenic changes; two antigenic lineages (Victoria and Yamagata) of influenza B have been shown to cocirculate in recent years. Burden of influenza B in India varied from 5 to 15% in last 5–10 years.

4. What do the terms "antigenic shift" and "antigenic drift" mean?

Influenza viruses have cell envelope glycoproteins HA (HA—18 types) and NA (NA—11 types). Influenza viruses are constantly changing and evolving. Smaller changes in the genetic material over a period of time are known as

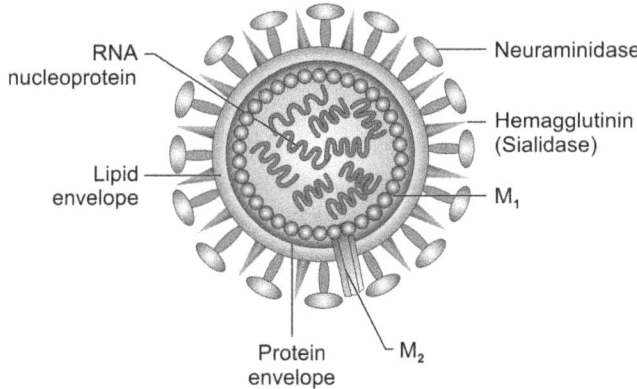

Fig. 1: Schematic diagram of influenza virus.
(RNA: ribonucleic acid)

antigenic drifts and sudden changes are known as antigenic shifts. When an antigenic drift occurs, the newer virus is slightly different form the older parent virus but is located closely on the phylogenetic tree. Due to the changes in the surface glycoproteins, the person may not have immunity for the newer virus. This is the reason for epidemics and also need to change the vaccine composition each year. A sudden major change in the virus (antigenic drift) leads to pandemics. One of the ways a drift happens is when an influenza virus from an animal gains ability to infect humans or there is genetic reassortment between human and animal influenza viruses, as it occurred in the 2009 pandemic. There are at least four documented pandemics in the last 100 years.

5. What are the symptoms of influenza?

Infection from poultry and pigs occurs usually by direct contact. Human-to-human transmission is by inhaling aerosols from an infected person. A person is infective for 5–10 days from a day before onset of symptoms. A majority of patients tend to be asymptomatic or have only mild symptoms. Incubation period ranges from 1 to 3 days. The common symptoms of influenza are fever, running nose, cough, sore throat, myalgia, body pain, headache, and fatigue. Most of the patients recover in a few days to about 2 weeks. Sinusitis and middle ear infections are the most common complications of influenza. In severe cases, it can lead to pneumonia and sometimes acute respiratory distress syndrome (ARDS), which can be fatal.

6. What can be the serious complications of influenza?

Rarely, influenza can lead to other life-threatening complications such as myocarditis, encephalitis, rhabdomyolysis, or even sepsis. In children, high fever can even trigger a febrile seizure. Children <5 years of age, adults >65 years of age, and those with chronic conditions such as asthma, diabetes, and renal or cardiac conditions are at higher risk for morbidity and mortality. Progressive pneumonia leading to ARDS or secondary bacterial infections are the usual causes of death. Avian influenza (H5N1) and porcine influenza remain zoonosis and sustained human-to-human transmission is questionable. The illness appears to be more severe with a majority of them progressing to ARDS and respiratory failure in the avian influenza.

7. What are emergency or danger signs of flu in children?

Any sick child who has fast or troubled breathing, bluish or gray skin color, not drinking enough fluids, severe or persistent vomiting, not waking up or not interacting, being so irritable that the child does not want to be held. In addition, children with fever of 104°F or more, an infant <3 months of age, or underlying chronic medical conditions also need to seek urgent medical care.

8. What is the epidemiological trend of influenza and how is it monitored across the world?

Influenza affects millions of people worldwide every year. According to the World Health Organization (WHO), the estimated global mortality is around 650,000 every year. This number is significantly higher as compared to estimates made around a decade ago. Influenza in both the hemispheres peaks in the respective winter seasons. It is slightly different in India due to its latitude of location, tropical climate, and distinct environmental factors. Northern most places like Srinagar experience peak of influenza during winter (January) whereas most of the other places experience peak with the onset of monsoon (July to September). Certain Southeastern states, which have a late onset of monsoon, experience peak around October.

Currently, India is having the following circulating strains:
- Influenza A H1N1 (pandemic 2009-like virus)
- Influenza A H3N2
- Influenza B.

The WHOs Global Influenza Surveillance and Response System (GISRS) through its network of laboratories across the world monitors the evolution of influenza viruses and provides recommendations in areas including diagnostics, vaccines, antiviral susceptibility, and risk assessment on weekly and twice-weekly basis.

9. What is the status of burden of influenza in India? Is there a significant burden of the disease in India?

Influenza imposes a substantial burden among under-fives in India. However, adequate data on the prevalence and burden of influenza in India is lacking. According to published data in India, it contributes to around 5–10% of all acute respiratory infections (ARIs). As per a recent meta-analysis, influenza-associated acute respiratory illness (ARI) incidence was estimated as 132 per 1,000 child-years. The patients positive for influenza among ARI in outpatients and inpatients were estimated to be 11.2% and 7.1%,

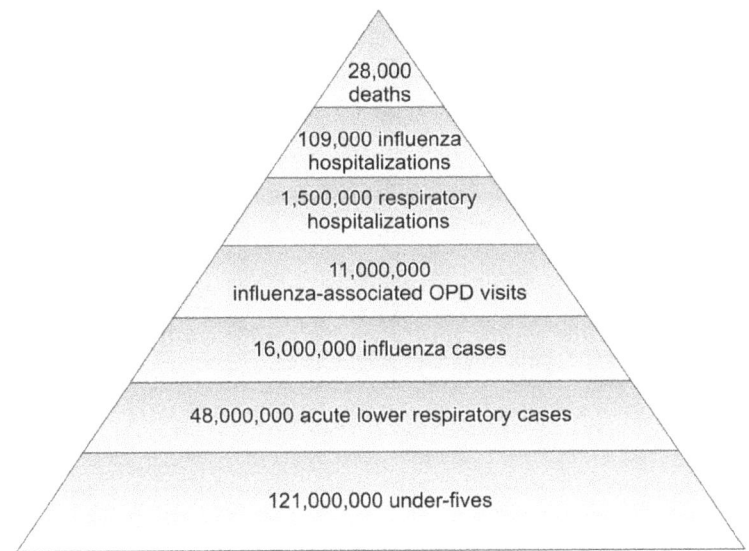

Fig. 2: Estimated burden of influenza in under-fives in India in the year 2016.
(OPD: outpatient department)

respectively. As per the researchers of the meta-analysis, the estimated total influenza cases were 16,009,207 in India during 2016. Influenza accounted for 10,913,476 outpatient visits and 109,431 hospitalizations. A total of 27,825 influenza-associated under-five deaths were estimated in India in 2016 **(Fig. 2)**.

Community burden: According to a household-based healthcare utilization survey of 69,369 residents in rural north India during 2011 to estimate rates of community-level influenza-like illness (ILI) and influenza-associated ILI. The study identified 150 ILI episodes with a rate of 38 ILI episodes/1,000 per year. Among 1,372 ILI cases enrolled from clinics, 126 cases (9%) had laboratory-confirmed influenza [A (H3N2) = 72; B = 54]. After adjusting for age, month, and clinic type, overall influenza-associated ILI rate was 4.8/1,000 per year; rates were highest among children <5 years and persons ≥60 years.

National Centre for Disease Control (NCDC)/Integrated Disease Surveillance Program (IDSP) data: According to data from 10 sentinel surveillance sites, 14% of all ILI during a season are due to one of the flu viruses. As per last updated data from the NCDC at the time of writing, 85,793 cases of H1N1 have been reported in the last 5 years. Year 2017 saw the highest peak with 38,811 cases. There are 4,897 reported deaths, amounting to a case fatality rate of 5.7%. **Figure 3** depicts the number of influenza cases and deaths in India from 2011 to 30th September 2020.

10. How can influenza be diagnosed in patients suffering from flu-like illness?

Diagnosis of influenza depends on epidemiological, clinical, and laboratory considerations. During an epidemic, any child with fever without focus and

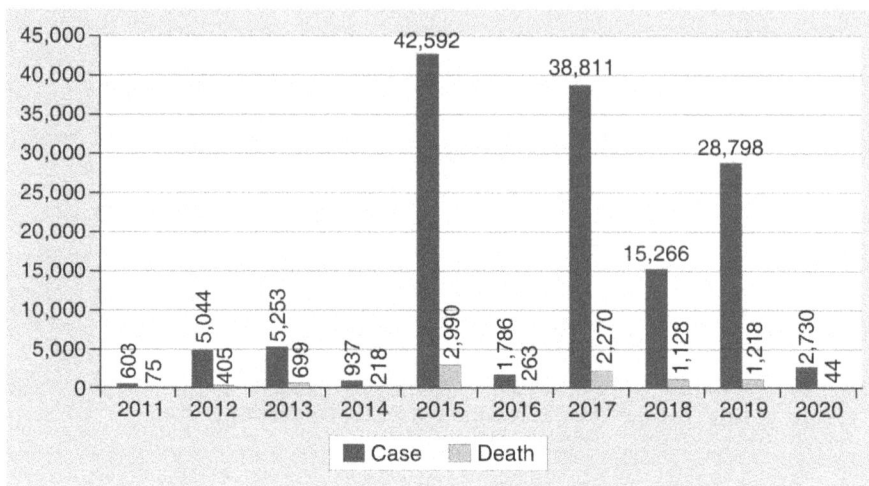

Fig. 3: Integrated Disease Surveillance Program (IDSP) data on seasonal influenza cases and deaths from 2011 to 2020 (till 30th September 2020)

Source: National Centre for Disease Control (NCDC). Seasonal Influenza A (H1N1): State/UT wise number of cases and deaths. Available from: https://ncdc.gov.in/showfile.php?lid=280 [Last accessed October 22,2020].

having respiratory symptoms with systemic features, diagnosis can be made to a certain degree clinically and treatment started. In seasonal flu, laboratory diagnosis of suspected cases is based on virus isolation from nasopharynx in early stages. Reverse transcription-polymerase chain reaction (RT-PCR) is other method for confirmation of diagnosis. Rapid influenza diagnostic tests, direct immunoassay, and paired sera for antibodies are other possible ways of diagnosis, but they are not readily available in India. In addition, serological diagnosis is of little value for a clinician in terms of treatment.

11. What types of influenza vaccines are available?

Currently available seasonal influenza vaccines include trivalent inactivated vaccine (TIV), quadrivalent influenza vaccine (QIV), and live attenuated influenza vaccines (LAIVs). These vaccines contain:
- Influenza A H1N1 (pandemic 2009-like virus)
- Influenza A H3N2
- Influenza B Victoria lineage
- Influenza B Yamagata lineage (only QIV contains this strain).

The vaccines contain 15 µg of HA vaccine of each strain of the virus in 0.5 mL of vaccine. The vaccines are approved for used in children above 6 months of age. The LAIVs are approved for children above 2 years of age. Pregnant women, high-risk individuals, and children below 2 years should not be given LAIV. The vaccines are generally safe. Transient local reactions are common and mild systemic adverse events occur in a few of the vaccine recipients. There have been reports of increase incidence of Guillain–Barré syndrome (GBS) following influenza vaccination, but there is no substantial evidence of cause and effect. People with allergy to egg can also receive the influenza vaccine with monitoring in an outpatient or in patient setup.

12. What is the basis of the World Health Organization (WHO) recommendations on the composition of the influenza vaccines?

The antigenic composition of the influenza vaccines is revised twice annually and adjusted to the antigenic characteristics of circulating influenza viruses obtained within the WHOs GISRS to ensure optimal vaccine efficacy against prevailing strains in both the Northern and Southern Hemispheres. The WHO meets twice in a year to issue recommendations on the antigenic composition of influenza vaccines: February (for Northern Hemisphere) and September (for Southern Hemisphere). The most recent WHO recommendations are for Southern and Northern Hemispheres are given in **Box 1**.

13. What are the different approaches to produce influenza vaccines?

Conventionally, only egg-based flu vaccines were developed. However, in recent times, many new approaches have adopted by the vaccine manufacturers. They include the following:

BOX 1: Flu vaccine recommendations for Northern Hemisphere (NH) 2020–2021 season and Southern Hemisphere (SH) 2020–2021.

2020–2021 NH (issued on 28 February, 2020)
It is recommended that *quadrivalent vaccines* for use in the 2020–2021 NH influenza season contain the following:
- *Egg-based vaccines*:
  - An A/Guangdong-Maonan/SWL1536/2019 (H1N1) pdm09-like virus
  - An A/Hong Kong/2671/2019 (H3N2)-like virus
  - A B/Washington/02/2019 (B/Victoria lineage)-like virus
  - A B/Phuket/3073/2013 (B/Yamagata lineage)-like virus.
- *Cell- or recombinant-based vaccines*:
  - An A/Hawaii/70/2019 (H1N1) pdm09-like virus
  - An A/Hong Kong/45/2019 (H3N2)-like virus
  - A B/Washington/02/2019 (B/Victoria lineage)-like virus
  - A B/Phuket/3073/2013 (B/Yamagata lineage)-like virus.

2021 World Health Organization (WHO) SH (issued on 25 September, 2020)
It is recommended that *quadrivalent vaccines* for use in the 2021 SH influenza season contain the following:
- *Egg-based vaccines*:
  - An A/Victoria/2570/2019 (H1N1) pdm09-like virus
  - An A/Hong Kong/2671/2019 (H3N2)-like virus
  - A B/Washington/02/2019 (B/Victoria lineage)-like virus
  - A B/Phuket/3073/2013 (B/Yamagata lineage)-like virus.
- *Cell- or recombinant-based vaccines*:
  - An A/Wisconsin/588/2019 (H1N1) pdm09-like virus
  - An A/Hong Kong/45/2019 (H3N2)-like virus
  - A B/Washington/02/2019 (B/Victoria lineage)-like virus
  - A B/Phuket/3073/2013 (B/Yamagata lineage)-like virus.

Flowchart 1: Conventional and novel platforms for influenza vaccine production.

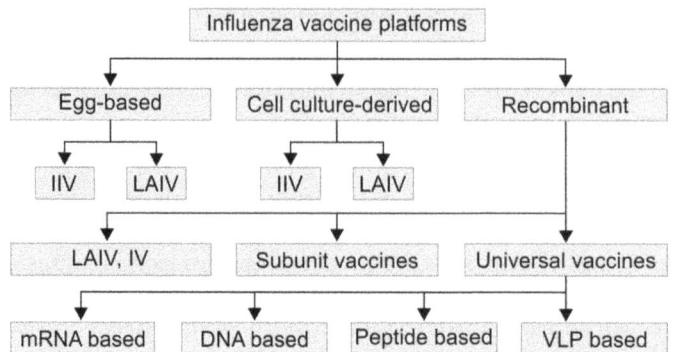

(DNA: deoxyribonucleic acid; IIV: inactivated influenza vaccine; LAIV: live attenuated influenza vaccine; mRNA: messenger ribonucleic acid; VLP: virus-like particle)

- Egg-derived vaccines
- Cell culture-derived vaccines
- Recombinant or synthetic flu vaccines **(Flowchart 1)**.

14. What are the characteristics of egg-based flu vaccines?

The most common way to produce flu vaccines is by egg-based technology. This technique has been used for >70 years. Egg-based vaccine manufacturing is used to make both inactivated (killed) vaccine and live attenuated vaccine (usually called the "nasal spray flu vaccine"). The inactivated seasonal flu vaccines (IIV) are of four types: (1) split virus, (2) subunit, (3) whole-virus inactivated, and (4) recombinant HA-based protein vaccine.

The egg-based production process begins with laboratory partner in the WHO GISRS providing private sector manufacturers with candidate vaccine viruses (CVVs) grown in eggs per current the Food and Drug Administration (FDA) regulatory requirements. These CVVs are then injected into fertilized hen's eggs and incubated for several days to allow the viruses to replicate. The fluid-containing virus is harvested from the eggs. For IIVs, the vaccine viruses are then inactivated and the virus antigen is purified. The manufacturing process continues with quality testing, filling, and distribution. For the nasal flu vaccine (i.e., the LAIV), the starting CVVs are live, but weakened viruses that go through a different production process.

15. What are the advantages of cell culture-derived influenza vaccines?

Cell-based flu vaccine production does not require chicken eggs because the vaccine viruses used to make vaccine are grown in animal cells. Cell-based technology also has the potential for a faster startup of the flu vaccine manufacturing process. Compared to egg-based technology, cell culture-derived influenza vaccines reduce the vaccine production time and risk of contamination during production, are safe for those with an allergy to eggs, and an animal component-free production is feasible.

Prior to the 2019–2020 season, some of the viruses provided to the manufacturer had been originally derived in eggs. For the 2019–2020 influenza season, all four influenza viruses (H1N1, M3N2, and two B groups) used in the cell-based vaccine are cell derived, making the vaccine egg free. In some respect, the novel cell-based vaccines are considered superior to conventional egg-based technique since in the latter some alterations in the antigenicity may occur owing to egg-adapted mutations. The reverse genetic approach employed in cell-based technique avoids this drawback associated with egg-based vaccines. Flucelvax™ was the first flu vaccine based on the cell-based technology which was licensed by the USFDA.

16. What are the latest group of flu vaccines, the recombinant or synthetic influenza vaccines? Tell us in detail the different processes being adopted to develop them.

Recombinant technology is the latest to develop influenza vaccines that was approved for use in the US in 2013. It involves plasmid-based reverse genetics techniques to engineer recombinant flu viruses entirely from full-length complementary deoxyribonucleic acid (DNA) copies of the viral genome. Recombinant flu vaccines do not require having a CVV sample to produce. Instead, recombinant vaccines are created synthetically. To make a recombinant vaccine, developers first obtain DNA, i.e., genetic instructions for making a surface protein called HA. This DNA for making flu virus HA antigen is then combined with a baculovirus, a virus that infects invertebrates. This results in a "recombinant" virus. Baculovirus helps in transporting the DNA instructions for making HA antigen of influenza virus into a host cell. After entering the host cell line, the recombinant virus instructs the cells to rapidly produce the HA antigen. This antigen is grown in bulk, collected, purified, and then packaged as recombinant flu vaccine.

This production of flu vaccines with this technique does not require an egg-grown vaccine virus and does not use eggs at all in the production process. This production process is the fastest because it is not limited by the selection of vaccine viruses that are adapted for growth in eggs or the development of cell-based vaccine viruses.

17. What do you mean by "universal influenza vaccine (UIV)"?

A universal flu vaccine is the one that provides strong, durable protection against multiple subtypes of influenza virus, rather than a select few. Such a vaccine would eliminate the need to update and administer the seasonal flu vaccine each year and could provide protection against newly emerging flu strains, potentially including those that could cause a flu pandemic **(Box 2)**.

18. Are there any universal flu vaccine available anywhere?

No. But several different approaches to develop universal flu vaccine are underway globally. There are now several "universal" flu vaccine candidates, using a variety of technologies, in phase II and phase III clinical trials. With the advent of coronavirus disease 2019 (COVID-19) pandemic, there are more

> **BOX 2:** Key characteristics of a universal influenza vaccine.
>
> *Key characteristics of universal influenza vaccines*:
> - Should be at least 75% efficacious
> - Should provide protection against groups I and II influenza A viruses
> - Have long-lasting protection
> - Should have protection from antigenic drift/shift
> - Should be suitable for all age groups
> - Boosters should not be needed frequently.

demand to develop such vaccines at a rapid pace since there is a remarkably high potential for the cocirculation of these two respiratory viruses.

19. What are the key immunological strategies to develop universal flu vaccines?

The current influenza vaccines employ complete HA antigen of the virus as only immunogen eliciting a lasting immunity. These vaccines target the globular domain (head) of the HA (subunit HA1) that constitutes the immunodominant antigen because it hosts on its surface most variable epitopes (glycosylation patterns). However, because it is the most accessible and external area of the virus, which determines the binding to the cellular receptor, it is the one that presents a higher rate of antigenic diversity due to the intense selection pressure of the human immune system. The variability of the globular head of HA and the immune system's preference for these epitopes have led to the search for more conserved epitopes across multiple influenza strains. If vaccines can focus the immune response against viral regions that undergo less mutation, there is a greater probability of protection on a near-universal level. Two of these strategies center on conserved regions found within HA: (1) recombinant stalk-specific HA and (2) chimeric recombinant HA.

20. What are the different vaccine platforms to design a "universal influenza vaccine (UIV)"?

Various approaches are adopted to target conserved epitopes of key influenza virus antigens such as HA, NA, M2, etc., to elicit immune response that consists of cross-reactive cellular and humoral immunity. There are several vaccine platforms that include few novel strategies such as nucleic acid vaccines (mRNA and DNA), vaccine-like particles (VLPs), nanoparticles-based peptides, chimeric vaccines, viral vector vaccines, etc. (*see* **Flowchart 1**).

21. What is the chimeric universal influenza vaccine (UIV)?

Multiple vaccine platforms as described above are being pursued. Vaccines targeting conserved epitopes of HA stem are more promising. Chimeric HA (cHA) with a stem common to a certain subtype and heads belonging to unusual subtypes have been constructed with this stem. The progressive immunization with them increases and reinforces the immunity against the stem showing cross-reaction with all those belonging to the same genetic groups (H1 or H2), obtaining a protection almost similar to the classic vaccine based on complete HA.

22. What is the coverage of influenza vaccines in India?

There is no recommendation to use influenza vaccines in the Universal Immunization Program (UIP) in India. However, recently, the Indian Academy of Pediatrics (IAP) has recommended routine administration of influenza vaccines in the age group of 6 months to 5 years of age. However, there is no data on the coverage of influenza vaccines even in the private sector.

Influenza vaccine uptake within Asia is generally low and a systematic review focused on Asian countries reported a median uptake of 14.9% among the general population and 37.3% among high-risk groups—far below the WHO target of 75%.

23. How long does immunity from influenza vaccine last?

Protection from influenza vaccine is thought to persist for at least 6 months. Following vaccination, anti-HA antibody titers peak 2–4 weeks postvaccination in primed individuals but may peak 4 weeks or later in unprimed individuals or older adults. Serum antibody titers may fall by 50% or more by 6 months after vaccination, with the degree of reduction being proportional to the peak titers achieved.

Protection declines over time because of waning antibody levels and because of changes in circulating influenza viruses from year to year. For persons who require only one dose of influenza vaccine for the season, yearly vaccination is likely to be associated with suboptimal immunity before the end of the influenza season, particularly among older adults.

However, there are reports of even shorter duration of protection of influenza vaccines. According to a recent study from Australia, the vaccine effectiveness (VE) estimates were highest for patients immunized within 2 months prior to symptom onset [VE: 60%; 95% confidence interval (CI): 26–78%] and lowest for patients immunized >4 months prior to symptom onset (VE: 19%; 95% CI: 73–62%).

24. Why do the influenza vaccines have such a low duration of protective immunity?

The goal of vaccination is to generate long-lasting protection against infection. Most vaccines in clinical use achieve this protection, at least in part, through the generation of pathogen-specific antibody responses. Antibody levels peak in the months following vaccination, followed by a decline to a plateau level which may be maintained for decades with minimal decline. Animal models have shown that these plateau antibody levels are maintained by nondividing, bone marrow-resident long-lived plasma cells. Studies of antibody synthesis rates have suggested that bone marrow plasma cells (BMPCs) are likely to produce the majority of total serum immunoglobulin G

(IgG) in humans as well. Consistent with this, total and antigen-specific serum antibody levels correlate closely with BMPC numbers in humans. Antibody titers and protective immunity decline rapidly following seasonal influenza vaccination, suggesting that the vaccine may fail to elicit BMPC or that these BMPC fail to become long-lived.

25. I am a middle-aged healthcare professional. Can I get myself vaccinated against influenza twice in the same calendar year?

Interesting query. Though there are no official recommendations from any academic body to prescribe flu vaccine twice in the same year, however, considering the current state of evidence or lack of it, an off-label use of flu vaccine twice in a year would not be a bad idea. One can go for flu vaccination with new vaccines having strains recommended for Northern and Southern Hemisphere (which are usually launched at 6-month interval) as soon as they become available. However, this would be an entirely a personal, case-based practice and cannot be recommended to general population.

26. What is the ideal time for influenza vaccination in India?

Although, India lies within the Northern Hemisphere, parts of the country have distinct tropical environment being located closer to the equator and behave much like Southern Hemisphere. Northern most places like Srinagar experience peak of influenza during winter (January) whereas most of the other places experience peak with the onset of monsoon (July to September). Certain Southeastern states, which have a late onset of monsoon, experience peak around October. Based on these epidemiological data, the ideal time for vaccination is May to June for most of the country. In certain parts such as Srinagar and Chennai, a winter vaccination strategy can be used.

However, in last few years, the epidemiology of influenza has changed. Now, there is a large peak of influenza activity during the first quarter of the year (i.e., from January to April) from almost all the places barring few. Hence, it would be reasonable to vaccinate at around September to November to cover this peak.

27. There are two different types of inactivated influenza vaccines launched every year, i.e., one carrying strains from Northern Hemisphere and other with Southern Hemisphere strains. I am confused which vaccine should I get to get optimal protection?

Influenza vaccines elicit a relatively strain-specific humoral response, have reduced efficacy against antigenically drifted viruses, and are ineffective against unrelated strains. It is of utmost importance, therefore, that vaccine should incorporate the current strain prevalent during that time. Influenza vaccination is recommended annually to ensure optimal match between the vaccine and prevailing influenza strains and because, unlike the long-lasting, strain-specific immunity following natural infection, influenza vaccines induce protection of relatively short duration, particularly in the elderly.

To ensure optimal vaccine efficacy against prevailing strains in both the Northern and Southern Hemispheres, the antigenic composition of the vaccines is revised twice annually and adjusted to the antigenic characteristics of circulating influenza viruses obtained within the global influenza surveillance network. The WHO classifies India under the "South Asia" transmission zone of influenza circulation and reviews strain circulation in the country during both the meetings. Though India lies within the Northern Hemisphere, parts of the country have a distinct tropical environment being located close to the equator and behave much like Southern Hemisphere seasonality with almost year round circulation and monsoon months peak, still Northern India experiences another peak during winter just like Northern Hemisphere pattern. But these patterns and strain circulation dynamics are not fixed and exclusive to one particular hemisphere and strains usually "spill" from one to another. Hence, it will not be prudent to stick to strain formulations recommended for one hemisphere, but one should use the vaccine that has the "most recent strains" irrespective of the hemisphere-specific formulations.

28. What are the guideline and protocol for administering influenza vaccines?

The following is the recommended schedule for vaccination in India as per the IAP:
- *Minimum age*: 6 months for IIV and 2 years for LAIV
- *Recommended for*: Children 6 months to 5 years and high-risk population. The high-risk population includes healthcare workers, people with chronic diseases, congenital and acquired immunodeficiency, and children on long-term salicylate therapy
- *Number of doses at first visit*: Two doses for below 9 years and one dose for above 9 years
- *Annual*: Single dose each year
- *Dose*: 0.25 mL for below 3 years and 0.5 mL for 3 years and above. It is to be noted that as of February 2020, the QIV vaccine manufactured by Abbott India is approved for a dose of 0.5 mL across all age groups.

The vaccine is administered by the intramuscular (IM) route (usually deltoid) to most children and adults. For infants and young children, the anterolateral aspect of the thigh is a preferred site. QIV and TIV vaccines should be stored at 2–8°C and should not be frozen.

Live attenuated influenza vaccine is designed for intranasal administration only and cannot be given by any other route. Half the content of a pre-filled syringe is sprayed into each nostril with the child positioned upright. The sprayer (device) has a dose-divider clip which ensures that more than half the dose cannot be inadvertently sprayed into any nostril. The vaccine is stored at 2–8°C. However, currently the LAIV is not available in India.

29. How efficacious are the available influenza vaccines?

Most of the reported data on efficacy/effectiveness of flu vaccines are from industrialized countries having temperate climate. There is no data on efficacy/effectiveness of influenza vaccines from India.

The reported efficacy/effectiveness of influenza vaccines varies substantially with factors such as the case definition (*e.g.*, laboratory-confirmed influenza disease or the less specific ILI), the "match" between the vaccine strains and prevailing influenza strains, vaccine preparation, dose, prior antigenic experience, and age or underlying disease conditions of an individual. Flu vaccines, however, often do not exactly match the rapidly evolving influenza virus, so their effectiveness changes each year. In the United States between 2009 and 2019, it ranged from a low of 19% to a high of 60% **(Fig. 4)**.

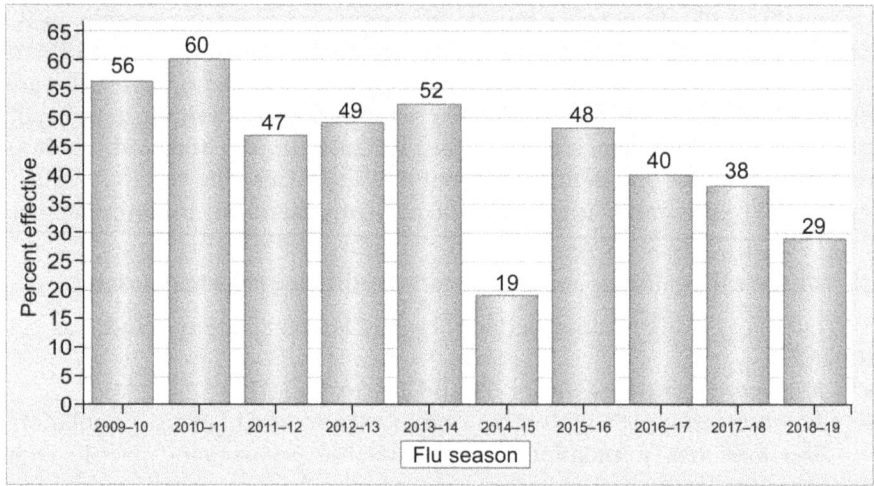

Fig. 4: Effectiveness of seasonal flu vaccines from the 2009 to 2018 flu seasons in the United States.
Source: Centers for Disease Control and Prevention (CDC). (2020). CDC Seasonal Flu Vaccine Effectiveness Studies. [online] Available from https://www.cdc.gov/flu/vaccines-work/effectiveness-studies.htm. [Last accessed October, 2020].

While VE can vary, recent studies show that flu vaccination reduces the risk of flu illness by between 40 and 60% among the overall population during seasons when most circulating flu viruses are well-matched to the flu vaccine. In general, current flu vaccines tend to work better against influenza B and influenza A (H1N1) viruses and offer lower protection against influenza A (H3N2) viruses.

According to a systematic review and meta-analysis, conducted on the data from 2004 to 2015, it was concluded that influenza vaccines had provided substantial protection against H1N1pdm09, H1N1 (pre-2009) and type B, and reduced protection against H3N2. The estimated VE was 33% (95% CI: 26-39%) for A H3N2, 61% (95% CI: 57-65%) for A H1N1pdm09, and 54% (95% CI: 46-61%) for type B. The VE against A H3N2 for antigenically matched viruses was 33% (95% CI: 22-43%) and for variant viruses were 23% (95% CI: 2-40%).

30. Why is flu vaccine typically less effective against influenza A (H3N2) viruses?

There are a number of reasons why flu VE against influenza A (H3N2) viruses may be lower.

- While all influenza viruses undergo frequent genetic changes, the changes that have occurred in influenza A (H3N2) viruses have more frequently resulted in differences between the virus components of the flu vaccine and circulating influenza viruses (i.e., antigenic change) compared with influenza A (H1N1) and influenza B viruses. That means that between the time when the composition of the flu vaccine is recommended and the flu vaccine is delivered, H3N2 viruses are more likely than H1N1 or influenza B viruses to have changed in ways that could impact how well the flu vaccine works.
- Growth in eggs is part of the production process for most seasonal flu vaccines. While all influenza viruses undergo changes when they are grown in eggs, changes in influenza A (H3N2) viruses tend to be more likely to result in antigenic changes compared with changes in other influenza viruses. These so-called "egg-adapted changes" are present in vaccine viruses recommended for use in vaccine production and may reduce their potential effectiveness against circulating influenza viruses. Other vaccine production technologies, e.g., cell-based vaccine production or recombinant flu vaccines, circumvent this shortcoming associated with the use of egg-based candidate vaccine viruses in egg-based production technology.

31. What are the adverse effects following immunization with inactivated influenza vaccines (IIVs)?

Transient local reactions at the injection site occur frequently (>1/100) and fever, malaise, myalgia, and other systemic adverse events may affect persons without previous exposure to the influenza vaccine antigens, trivalent influenza vaccines are generally considered safe. No vaccines against seasonal influenza contain the AS03 adjuvant which has been associated with rare cases of narcolepsy/cataplexy following large-scale use of an AS03-adjuvanted pandemic H1N1 vaccine, primarily in the Nordic countries and in England.

During some influenza seasons, seasonal trivalent as well as monovalent influenza A (H1N1)pdm 2009 vaccines have been associated with a slight increase in the risk of GBS. However, there is no definite cause and effect relation with GBS. A brand of seasonal IIV from M/s CSL 2010 batch was associated with febrile seizures in children <5 years of age in Australia. In US also, a higher risk for febrile seizures was found from Fluzone™, another brand of M/s CSL during December 2010 to January 2011. Analysis of these observations concluded that risk was only present among 6–23-month-old when trivalent vaccine was given along with 13-valent pneumococcal conjugate vaccine (PCV13).

Children allergic to egg proteins can have severe adverse events such as anaphylaxis, angioedema, allergic bronchial asthma, and urticaria. As per current recommendations, such children should receive vaccine under close supervision with availability of facilities to manage an anticipated allergic reaction.

Apart from these few product-specific issues, there are no generic safety issues for influenza vaccines in young children.

32. For whom is inactivated influenza vaccine (IIV) contraindicated?

Persons who have experienced a severe allergic reaction to a prior dose of influenza vaccine or who are known to have a severe allergy to a vaccine component (except egg) should not be vaccinated.

Precautions to vaccination include moderate or severe acute illness and history of GBS within 6 weeks of a dose of influenza vaccine.

33. What is the latest Centers for Disease Control and Prevention-Advisory Committee on Immunization Practices (CDC-ACIP) guidance on influenza vaccination and egg allergy?

The Advisory Committee on Immunization Practices (ACIP) recommends that people with a history of egg allergy who have experienced only hives after exposure to egg should receive influenza vaccine without specific precautions (except a 15-minute observation period for syncope). Any age-appropriate vaccine (IIV, Recombinant Influenza Vaccine (RIV) or LAIV) may be used.

People who report having had an anaphylactic reaction to egg (more severe than hives) may also receive any age-appropriate influenza vaccine (IIV, RIV, or LAIV). The vaccine for these individuals should be administered in a medical setting (such as a physician office or health department clinic). Vaccine administration should be supervised by a healthcare provider who is able to recognize and manage severe allergic conditions.

Although not specifically recommended by the ACIP, providers may prefer an egg-free inactivated vaccine (Flucelvax™ Quadrivalent, Seqirus, licensed for people age 4 years and older) or recombinant vaccine (Flublok™, Sanofi Pasteur, licensed for people age 18 years and older) with severe egg allergy.

A previous severe allergic reaction to influenza vaccine, regardless of the component suspected to be responsible for the reaction, is a contraindication to future receipt of the vaccine.

34. What is "target group prioritization"?

Prioritization is based on contribution of risk group to the overall influenza disease burden in population, disease severity within individual risk group, and VE in different age groups and categories.

Prioritization of target groups (1-highest priority, 4-lowest priority):
1. Elderly individuals (>65 years) and nursing home residents (the elderly or disabled)
2. Individuals with chronic medical conditions including individuals with HIV/acquired immunodeficiency syndrome (AIDS) and pregnant women (especially to protect infants 0–6 months)

3. *Other groups*: Healthcare workers including professionals, individuals with asthma, and children from ages 6 months to 2 years
4. Children aged 2–5 years and 6–18 years and healthy young adults.

Among pediatric population, apart from the children with chronic medical conditions (see prioritization of target groups), the children below 2 years of age should be considered a target group for influenza immunization because of a high burden of severe disease in this group **(Table 1)**.

Age group/category	Burden of disease	Fatalities/severe disease	Effectiveness/efficacy of vaccine	Level of evidence	Prioritization
0–6 months	High (+++)	Very high (++++)	Not eligible	NA	2*
6–23 months	High (+++)	High (+++)	Not effective/very low	Moderate	3
2–5 years	Substantial (++)	Moderate (++)	Moderate	Limited	4
6–64 years	Low (+)	Low (+)	Moderate to high	Moderate	4
>65 years	High (+++)	Very high (++++)	Low	Low	1
Pregnant women	Substantial (++)	High (+++)	Moderate **	Limited to high **	2
Individual with asthma	Not known	Moderate (++)	Not effective	Limited	3
Individuals with HIV/AIDS	Not known	High (+++)	Moderate	Low	2
Individuals with other underlying medical conditions	Not known	High (+++)	Low	Limited	2
Healthcare workers	Substantial (++)	Moderate (++)	High	High	3

TABLE 1: Summary of disease burden, efficacy/effectiveness of IIVs, and prioritization of influenza vaccination in different age groups and categories of target population.

*Not eligible to receive currently licensed influenza vaccines and should be protected through vaccination of their mothers during pregnancy
** Effectiveness varies for maternal and neonatal protection; Prioritization 1. Highest; 2. High; 3. Moderate; 4 Low
(AIDS: acquired immunodeficiency syndrome; HIV: human immunodeficiency virus; IIVs: inactivated influenza vaccines)
Source: Adapted from Vashishtha VM, Kalra A, Choudhury P. Influenza vaccination in India: position paper of Indian Academy of Pediatrics, 2013. Indian Pediatr. 2013;50(9):867-74.

35. What are the recent Indian Academy of Pediatrics-Advisory Committee on Vaccines and Immunization Practices (IAP-ACVIP) recommendations on influenza vaccines?

Recently, in December 2018, the Advisory Committee on Vaccines and Immunization Practices (ACVIP) of the IAP has recommended IIV (either trivalent or quadrivalent) routinely to all children below 5 years of age starting from 6 months of age annually (2–4 weeks before influenza season).

36. Which flu vaccines are more suitable for older people?

Aging decreases the body's ability to develop a good immune response after getting influenza vaccine, which places older people at greater risk of severe illness from influenza. A higher dose of antigen or an adjuvanted vaccine should give older people a better immune response and therefore provide better protection against influenza. There are two products which should be more efficacious for elderly people (>65 years): (1) Fluad™ (Seqirus), a trivalent, MF59-adjuvanted IIV and (2) Fluzone™ high-dose (Sanofi Pasteur) flu vaccine **(Fig. 5)**.

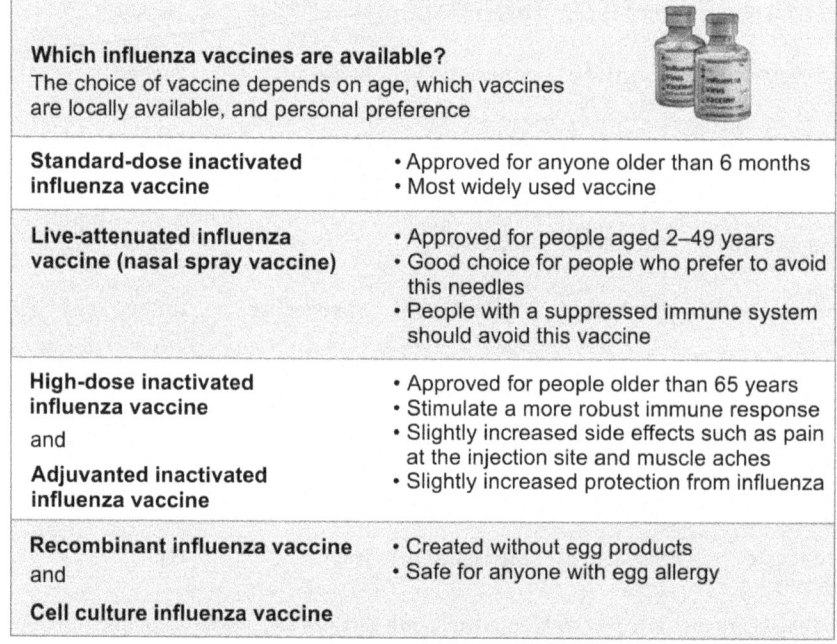

Fig. 5: Globally available different influenza vaccines for different categories of people.

Fluad™ is the first adjuvanted influenza vaccine marketed in the US. Fluad™ has been used in Europe since 1997 and is approved in 38 other countries. In contrast to Fluzone™ high dose, Fluad™ is a standard-dose vaccine, containing 15 µg of HA per virus per dose (total of 45 µg). In a small observational study among adults age 65 years and older, Fluad™ was about 63% more effective than unadjuvanted trivalent IIV. However, despite published evidence of better protection from Fluzone™ high dose when compared to standard-dose Fluzone™, the ACIP has not stated a preference for this vaccine for people age 65 years and older.

37. If a patient was vaccinated earlier in the influenza season and later becomes pregnant during the same season, should she be revaccinated due to her pregnancy?

No. The ACIP does not recommend more than one dose of influenza vaccine per season, except for certain children being vaccinated for the first time.

38. What are the problems in formulating universal recommendation for influenza vaccination in India?

There are various factors which prevent formulation of universal recommendation in India such as:
- Exact burden of disease regarding morbidity and mortality is not known
- Attack rates are highest in young children but fatality is more in elderly population, so target population cannot be defined well
- Limited data on effectiveness of vaccine in our country; moreover, optimum timing and optimum strain of vaccination are often not clear.

SUGGESTED READING

1. Advisory Committee on Vaccines and Immunization Practices. IAP Guidebook on Immunization 2018–2019. In: Vashishtha VM, Kalra A (Eds). Influenza Vaccines, 3rd edition. New Delhi: Jaypee Brothers Medical Publishers (P) Ltd; 2020. pp. 315-32.
2. Belongia EA, Simpson MD, King JP, Sundaram ME, Kelley NS, Osterholm MT, et al. Variable influenza vaccine effectiveness by subtype: a systematic review and meta-analysis of test-negative design studies. Lancet Infect Dis. 2016;16(8): 942-51.
3. Centers for Disease Control and Prevention (CDC). (2020). Influenza (Flu). [online] Available from: https://www.cdc.gov/flu/index.htm. [Last accessed October 2020].
4. Chadha MS, Potdar VA, Saha S, Koul PA, Broor S, Dar L, et al. Dynamics of influenza seasonality at sub-regional levels in India and implications for vaccination timing. PLoS One. 2015;10(5):e0124122.
5. Davis CW, Jackson KJL, McCausland MM, Darce J, Chang C, Linderman SL, et al. Influenza vaccine-induced human bone marrow plasma cells decline within a year after vaccination. Science. 2020;370(6513):237-41.
6. Dharmapalan D. Influenza. Indian J Pediatr. 2020;11:1-5.
7. Grohskopf LA, Alyanak E, Broder KR, Walter EB, Fry AM, Jernigan DB. Prevention and Control of Seasonal Influenza with Vaccines: Recommendations of the Advisory Committee on Immunization Practices—United States, 2019–20 Influenza Season. MMWR Recomm Rep. 2019;68(3):1-21.
8. Iuliano AD, Roguski KM, Chang HH, Muscatello DJ, Palekar R, Tempia S, et al. Estimates of global seasonal influenza-associated respiratory mortality: a modelling study. Lancet. 2018;391(10127):1285-300.
9. Kiseleva I. New points of departure for more global influenza vaccine use. Vaccines (Basel). 2020;8(3):E410.
10. Ministry of Health and Family Welfare (MoHFW). (2016). Seasonal Influenza: Guidelines on categorization of Seasonal Influenza cases during screening for home isolation, testing, treatment and hospitalization (Revised on

18.10.2016). [online] Available from: https://main.mohfw.gov.in/sites/default/files/394697031477913837.pdf. [Last accessed October, 2020].
11. National Centre for Disease Control (NCDC). (2020). Seasonal Influenza A (H1N1): State/UT-wise number of cases and deaths from 2016 to 2020* (As on 30.09.2020). [online] Available from: https://ncdc.gov.in/showfile.php?lid=280. [Last accessed October, 2020].
12. Ram Purakayastha D, Vishnubhatla S, Rai SK, Broor S, Krishnan A. Estimation of burden of influenza among under-five children in India: a meta-analysis. J Trop Pediatr. 2018;64(5):441-53.
13. Vaccines against influenza WHO position paper—November 2012. Wkly Epidemiol Rec. 2012;87(47):461-76.
14. Vashishtha VM, Kalra A, Choudhary P. Influenza vaccination in India: position paper of Indian Academy of Pediatrics. Indian Pediatr. 2013;50(9):867-74.
15. World Health Organization (WHO). (2018). Influenza (Avian and other zoonotic). [online] Available from: https://www.who.int/news-room/fact-sheets/detail/influenza-(avian-and-other-zoonotic). [Last accessed October, 2020].
16. World Health Organization (WHO). (2020). Recommended composition of influenza virus vaccines for use in the 2020-2021 northern hemisphere influenza season. [online] Available from: https://www.who.int/influenza/vaccines/virus/recommendations/2020-21_north/en/. [Last accessed October, 2020].
17. World Health Organization (WHO). (2020). Up to 650,000 people die of respiratory diseases linked to seasonal flu each year. [online] Available from: https://www.who.int/news/item/14-12-2017-up-to-650-000-people-die-of-respiratory-diseases-linked-to-seasonal-flu-each-year. [Last accessed October, 2020].

![Chapter 31]

Meningococcal Vaccines

Parang N Mehta

1. What are meningococci?

Meningococci, or *Neisseria meningitidis* (*N. meningitides*), are Gram-negative cocci. They are associated with some very serious illnesses. Chief among them are meningitis, purpura fulminans, shock, and sepsis. About 30% or more of purulent meningitis in children is caused by meningococci. Meningococci also cause focal disease like arthritis and pneumonia.

An important feature of meningococci is the presence of a polysaccharide capsule. This capsule protects them against destruction by the host's complement system as well as from phagocytosis.

Meningococcal disease is endemic in most parts of India, but occurs in deadly epidemics also. The disease is most common in infants 3–12 months of age. Case fatality rates are 9–12% with invasive meningococcal disease, but can be as high as 30% with purpura fulminans. Meningitis also has a high mortality and survivors have a significant incidence of sequelae.

2. Are there different types of meningococci?

Yes, there are 13 known serotypes of meningococci. Of them, only five commonly cause human disease (types A, B, C, W-135, and Y). In India, meningococcal disease is endemic and most of it is caused by type B. Meningococcal disease also occurs in epidemics sometimes and these are usually type A.

Type B is the problem type all over the world. It causes about 50% of meningococcal cases and effective vaccines against it have only recently become available. Not only are the strains variable antigenically, but there is molecular similarity between some of them and human nervous system components.

3. What are the vaccines available?

Three types of vaccines are available:
1. The unconjugated polysaccharide vaccine
2. The meningococcal conjugate vaccines (MCVs)
3. The meningococcal recombinant protein vaccines.

4. What is the unconjugated polysaccharide vaccine?

The unconjugated polysaccharide vaccine has been available for many years. Like pneumococci, meningococci also have a capsular polysaccharide, which makes this vaccine effective only in children above the age of 2 years. This vaccine, the unconjugated meningococcal polysaccharide vaccine 4 (MPSV4), covers four types of meningococci (A, C, W-135, and Y). These vaccines are available in lyophilized form, to be kept at 2–8°C, and reconstituted with water just before use. Administration is subcutaneous.

These vaccines induce antibodies to the included serotypes in 7–10 days. Serotype A can sometimes induce antibodies in infants as young as 3 months, but type C is poorly immunogenic below 2 years. All four serotype vaccines are safe and immunogenic. Protection rates of 85–90% have been shown with types A and C. In young children, antibody levels decrease after 3 years.

These vaccines are T-cell independent, which means they are ineffective in children younger than 2 years. Antibodies induced are only immunoglobulin M (IgM) type and levels fall after some years. Another problem with these vaccines is that they do not induce immunological memory. There is no booster effect of another dose. Now that the conjugated vaccine is widely available, MPSV4 is not recommended for general use.

5. Is there a better vaccine?

Conjugated meningococcal vaccines are the more recent vaccines. Meningococcal antigens are conjugated with proteins like the CRM197 or tetanus toxoid, which induce a T-cell response.

Such vaccines are effective in younger children also and are approved for use from 9 months onward. Considering the high incidence of meningococcal disease in infants, this vaccine can do much good. Conjugate vaccines are more immunogenic than unconjugated polysaccharide vaccines and are the recommended choice. Conjugate vaccines are also expected to provide herd effect and reduce nasopharyngeal carriage of meningococci. The conjugated vaccines also provide protection against four types of meningococci: types A, C, W-135, and Y. Like the MPSV4 vaccine, these vaccines are also quadrivalent and do not protect against type B.

The protective efficacy of these vaccines is 69–97% 1 month after the vaccine is given. The protection wanes after 5 years in many adolescents.

6. What are different meningococcal conjugate vaccines available in India?

Currently, following different MCVs are available in Indian market:
- MenACWY-D (Menactra™) by Sanofi Pasteur
- MenACWY-CRM (Menveo™) by GlaxoSmithKline (GSK)
- Monovalent, serogroup A vaccine (MenAfriVac™) by Serum Institute of India.

The main difference between the two MCVs, Menactra™ and Menveo™, is the type of carrier protein used to conjugate polysaccharide moiety with protein. While the former employs diphtheria toxoid, the latter employs CRM197.

MenACWY-D (Menactra™): This vaccine contains 4 mg each of A, C, Y, and W-135 capsular polysaccharide (CPS) conjugated to 48 mg of diphtheria toxoid. The minimum age of administration is 9 months.

MenACWY-CRM (Menveo™): This vaccine consists of two portions: 10 µg of lyophilized meningococcal serogroup A (MenA) capsular polysaccharide conjugated to CRM197 and 5 µg each of capsular polysaccharide of serogroup C, W, and Y (MenCWY) conjugated to CRM197 in 0.5 mL of phosphate buffered saline. Although it is licensed in India to use in children 2 years and above, in US and other countries, the minimum age of administration is 2 months.

Monovalent, serogroup A vaccine (MenAfriVac™): This monovalent, serogroup A MCV is produced by Indian company, Serum Institute of India for African countries. This vaccine contains 10 µg of serogroup A polysaccharide conjugated to 10–33 µg tetanus toxoid with alum as adjuvant and thimerosal as preservative. The vaccine should be given as single intramuscular dose of 0.5 mL to individuals 1–29 years of age. The possible need for a booster dose has not yet been established. However, this vaccine is not available for private use in India **(Table 1)**.

7. What are the recombinant protein vaccines?

These vaccines fill the long-standing gap in meningococcal disease prevention by providing protection against meningococci type B. One of the available vaccines contains recombinant *Neisserial adhesin* A (NadA), Neisserial Heparin Binding Antigen (NHBA) and factor H binding protein (fHbp), and outer membrane vesicles (OMVs), along with excipients. The other vaccine contains recombinant versions of two lipidated fHbp variants along with excipients.

These proteins are strong antigens that are recognized by the immune system, which then produces antibodies against them. This is protective against meningococcal disease. The protective efficacy has been found to be 63–94% 1 month after completion of the schedule. The duration of protection is yet not well-known.

The recombinant protein vaccines require two doses (0, 6 months) or three doses (0, 1 month, and 6 months) for protection.

8. What are the different serogroup B meningococcal vaccines available globally?

Vaccines against serotype B meningococcal disease have proved difficult to produce and require a different approach from vaccines against other serotypes. Whereas effective polysaccharide vaccines have been produced against types A, C, W-135, and Y, the CPS on the type B bacterium is too similar to human neural adhesion molecules to be a useful target. Recently, two

TABLE 1: Licensed meningococcal vaccines in India.

Type	Valency/strains covered	Brand/manufacturer	Nature and diluent	Dose and scheduel	Cost
Polysaccharide (MPSV: Meningococcal polysaccharide vaccine)	**Quadrivalent** (serogroups A, C, W-135, and Y; contain individual capsular polysaccharides 50 μg each)	Mencevac, GSK; Quadri Meningo, BioMedd MPV A +C, GSK	Lyophilized, sterile distilled water	0.5 mL by SC or IM, recommended in children > 2 years#, revaccination after 3–5 years in high-risk children and adolescents	Rs 1,050/-
	Bivalent (serogroups A and C contains individual capsular polysaccharides 50 μg each)	Bi Meningo, BioMed			Rs 650/-
MCV: Meningococcal conjugate vaccines	**Quadrivalent** (serogroups A, C, W-135 and Y: contain 4 μg each of A, C, Y, and W-135 polysaccharide conjugated to 48 μg of diphtheria toxoid)	Menactra, Sanofi Pasteur	Lyophilized, sterile distilled water	0.5 mL by deep IM as single dose in children >2 years and two doses 4–6 weeks apart in children 9–23 months, revaccination after 3–5 years in high-risk children and adolescents	Rs 3,600/-
	Quadrivalent Consist of two portions: 10 μg of lyophilized meningococcal serogroup A (MenA) capsular polysaccharide conjugated to CRM 197, and 5 μg each of capsular polysaccharide of serogroup C, W, and Y (MenCWY) conjugated to CRM 197 in 0.5 mL of phosphated buffered saline	Menveo® by GlaxoSmithKline	Supplied in 2 vials; reconstitute the MenA lyophilized component with the MenCYW-135 liquid component	0.5 mL by IM injection, approved for single dose use in >2 years in India (for people age 2 months through 55 years by US FDA)	Rs 3,600/-
	Monovalent (serogroup A: 10 μg of group A polysaccharide conjugated to 10–33 μg tetanus toxoid, with alum as adjuvant and thimerosal as preservative)	Serum Institute of INdia, Ltd	Lyophilized vaccine, distilled water as diluents	0.5 mL Intramuscular single administration for individuals 1–29 years of age	Not disclosed

#In infants aged 3 months to 2 years, MPSV may be given if risk for meningococcal disease is high, e.g., outbreaks/close household contacts: two doses 3 months apart.
(IM: intramuscular; SC: subcutaneous; USFDA: United States Food and Drug Administration)

serogroup B vaccines are available globally, Bexsero® and Trumenba®. Bexsero® was approved for use in Europe in January 2013 and by the Food and Drug Administration (FDA) in February 2015. In October 2014, Trumenba® was approved by the FDA. These products are not available in India.

- *Bexsero® by GSK*: Each 0.5-mL dose of Bexsero® contains: 50 µg each of recombinant proteins NadA, NHBA, and fHbp; 25 µg of OMVs and 5 mg aluminum hydroxide (0.519 mg of Al^{+++} and 125 mg sodium chloride, 776 mg histidine, and 10 mg sucrose at pH 6.4–6.7). Each dose contains <0.01 µg kanamycin (by calculation).
- *Trumenba® by Pfizer*: Each 0.5-mL dose of Trumenba® contains: 60 µg each of two lipidated fHbp variants (total of 120 µg of protein), 018 mg of polysorbate 80, 25 mg of Al^{+++}, and 10 mM histidine buffered saline at pH 6.0.

Recommendations for use by the Centers for Disease Control and Prevention-Advisory Committee on Immunization Practices (CDC-ACIP): MenB vaccine may be administered based on individual clinical decision to adolescents not at increased risk age 16–23 years (preferred age 16–18 years):

Bexsero®: Two-dose series at least 1 month apart.

Trumenba®: Two-dose series at least 6 months apart; if dose two is administered earlier than 6 months, administer a third dose at least 4 months after dose two.

Available data on MenB vaccines suggest that protective antibodies decrease quickly (within 1–2 years) after vaccination.

9. How should the meningococcal conjugate vaccines be stored and administered?

These vaccines and their diluents should be stored at 2–8°C. The supplied diluent only should be used for reconstitution.

The vaccines are meant for intramuscular administration and should be given into the vastus lateralis muscle in the anterolateral aspect of the thigh. Older children and adolescents may be given the injection in the deltoid area. The MCVs are given as a single dose, with a booster 4–5 years later.

10. What are the side effects with these vaccines?

Most adverse reactions are mild and short-lived. Local reactions consist of pain, redness and swelling, and are rarely severe. Fever, headache, and malaise occur in a small proportion of recipients in the first few days. Only symptomatic treatment is required.

11. Are there any serious side effects?

Some cases of Guillain-Barré syndrome (GBS) have been reported after the use of MCV. The incidence is low and it is difficult to say whether it is higher than the background incidence of this rare disease.

12. Are there any contraindications to vaccination?

Children who have had a severe allergic (anaphylactic) reaction to the vaccine or a component of it, in the past, must not receive it again. In children with moderate or severe acute illness, the vaccine should be deferred. Breastfeeding and immunosuppression are not contraindications.

13. What specific precaution should be taken when MenACWY-D (Menactra™) is administered along with PCV13 (Prevnar)?

These two vaccines should not be given together, as the response to pneumococcal vaccine will be reduced. The PCV vaccine series should be completed first, and the meningococcal vaccine should be given after an interval of at least 4 weeks.

In children with anatomic or functional asplenia, Menactra should not be given at all before age 2 years, as it reduces the response to Prevenar. Menveo does not interfere with the immunological response to Prevenar, and is recommended in this situation.

14. Adults who are asplenic, need PCV13 and MenACWY. Does the recommendation to separate PCV13 and MenACWY-D (Menactra™) apply to adults as well as children?

We know that Menactra reduced the response to PCV7 (Prevenar-7), from studies done in children. As a matter of caution, then, Prevenar-13 should not be coadministered with Menactra, though studies have not been performed. If they have to be both used, Menactra should be given 4 weeks after PCV13. If both have been administered together, or at an interval of less than 4 weeks, the PCV should be repeated when 4 weeks have elapsed after Menactra.

Menveo does not interfere with the immune response to PCV13, and can be used before PCV13 or simultaneously with it.

15. Is meningococcal vaccine recommended in India?

Unfortunately, we have very little data on the incidence and prevalence of disease. We do know that most endemic cases are caused by type B meningococci, against which a vaccine is not yet available in India. However, most of the recurring, large outbreaks are caused by type A meningococci, which could be prevented by this vaccine.

Though the conjugated meningococcal vaccine is now available, the Indian Academy of Pediatrics (IAP) recommends this vaccine only for:
- High-risk group of children
- During disease outbreaks
- International travelers, including people going for Haj and students going abroad for studies. Travelers to certain African countries where meningococcal meningitis is endemic must also be vaccinated.

At present, the meningococcal vaccine is not recommended for general use in children in India.

16. Who are considered children at risk?
- Children with asplenia, functional or anatomic
- Children with congenital or acquired immunodeficiencies, particularly children with terminal complement component deficiencies
- Children with cerebrospinal fluid (CSF) leaks, cochlear implants, or malignancies
- Children on long-term steroid, salicylate, immunosuppressive, or radiation therapy.

It is also recommended for:
- Together with chemoprophylaxis in close contacts of patients with meningococcal disease (household contacts, school and daycare contacts, and healthcare workers)
- Laboratory personnel and healthcare workers who are exposed routinely to *N. meningitidis*.

17. What are the recommendations for meningococcal vaccination for children with anatomical or functional asplenia?

The CDC-ACIP has offered following recommendations for MCVs in this specific category:
- *Menactra™*:
  - *Age 9–23 months*: Not recommended
  - *24 months or older*: Two doses at least 8 weeks apart
  - Menactra™ must be administered at least 4 weeks after completion of PCV13 series.
- *Menveo™*:
  - *Dose one at age 2 months*: Four-dose series at 2, 4, 6, and 12 months
  - *Dose one at age 7–23 months*: Two-dose series (dose two at least 12 weeks after dose one and after the first birthday)
  - *Dose one at age 24 months or older*: Two-dose series at least 8 weeks apart.

18. A child with functional asplenia has received a dose of MenACWY-D (Menactra™) when she was 3-year-old. Does she need any booster doses?

Yes, these patients are at risk for overwhelming sepsis with encapsulated organisms. Meningococcal vaccine booster doses must be given.

The primary series is two doses in people with asplenia. The second dose should be given now, if 8 weeks have elapsed since the first dose. After this, booster doses are required.

If the child is less than 7 years old, a booster must be given 3 years after the last dose of the primary series. Once the age is over 7 years, booster doses must be given every 5 years.

19. **Menveo™ (MenACWY-CRM) is approved by the Food and Drug Administration (FDA) for use in children as young as 2 months of age. What is the Advisory Committee on Immunization Practices (ACIP) recommendations for use of this vaccine?**

MenACWY-CRM is approved for people age 2 months through 55 years. For children beginning the vaccination series at age 2 months, the schedule is four doses at age 2, 4, 6, and 12–15 months. Fewer doses are recommended for children beginning the vaccination series at age 7 months or older.

The ACIP recommends the use of MenACWY-CRM in high-risk children 2 through 23 months of age [children with persistent complement deficiency including children taking eculizumab (Soliris) or ravulizumab-cwvz (Ultomiris), functional or anatomic asplenia, human immunodeficiency virus (HIV) infection, who travel to or reside in regions where meningitis is epidemic or hyperendemic, or who are at risk during a community outbreak attributable to a vaccine serogroup].

Menactra™ (MenACWY-D) can be given to children 9 months and older at increased risk of meningococcal disease.

20. **If a healthy child received meningococcal polysaccharide vaccine 4 (MPSV4) or conjugate vaccine (MenACWY) prior to international travel at age 9 years, will two additional doses of meningococcal conjugate vaccine (MCV) be needed?**

Yes. The protection provided by these vaccines is not lifelong. A dose of MenACWY at 11 or 12 years and a booster dose at age 16 years is required.

21. **Why should chemoprophylaxis and vaccine both be given to contacts of cases?**

The vaccine is not immediately protective. Development of an antibody response takes 7–10 days and the person is at risk of developing a dangerous disease during this period. Contacts should, therefore, be given both chemoprophylaxis and the vaccine. Chemoprophylaxis alone is an acceptable solution, but vaccination alone is not.

22. **Are meningococcal vaccines effective in preventing or controlling epidemics?**

Many factors need to be considered in answering this question. The type of the organism, the age group mainly involved, and the population density all have a bearing. In India, type B organisms are frequent and vaccines are not yet available in our country.

The usual strategy is to give both the vaccine and chemoprophylaxis to populations where there have been a cluster of cases.

23. **If vaccine has been given once, is revaccination needed?**

Yes. The immunity induced by both polysaccharide and conjugated meningococcal vaccines wanes over time. An additional dose is recommended

3–5 years after the primary dose. Beyond the age of 21 years, revaccination is not recommended for healthy people.

24. Are the two MenACWY vaccines, Menactra™ and Menveo™ interchangeable?

MenACWY-D (Menactra™) is only approved for children older than 9 months, so only MenACWYCRM (Menveo™) should be used for children age 2 through 8 months. For children aged 9 months and older, and adults, the vaccines are interchangeable.

25. What are the recommendations for use of meningococcal serogroup B vaccines in high-risk conditions?

Certain people are at high risk for meningococcal infections:
   Complement component deficiencies, or taking complement inhibitor drugs. Anatomic or functional asplenia, including sickle cell disease.
   These persons should be given protection against meningococci serogroup B, in addition to the quadrivalent vaccine, as follows:
- Bexsero®: Two-dose series at least 1 month apart
- Trumenba®: Three-dose series at 0, 1–2, and 6 months.

Bexsero® and Trumenba® are not interchangeable; the same product should be used for all doses in a series.

26. What are the recommendations for human immunodeficiency virus (HIV)-positive individuals?

It is now known that these people have an increased risk for meningococcal disease, and should be vaccinated. A single dose is not considered adequate in this population; two doses 8–12 weeks apart should be given. Boosters are recommended after 3 years for children under 7 years age, and every 5 years for older individuals. This recommendation is for the quadrivalent conjugate vaccine.

27. Should all adolescents receive a routine booster dose of MenACWY?

That is the high-risk age for meningococcal disease. The first dose of meningococcal conjugate vaccine should be given at 11–12 years, and a booster at 16–18 years, since immunity is known to wane.
   If the first dose is given at age 16 years or later, a booster is not recommended. Both the quadrivalent and serogroup B vaccines can be given at the same visit.

28. Should people with continued high risk of meningococcal disease receive additional doses of meningococcal vaccine beyond the 3- or 5-year booster?

The immunity derived from meningococcal vaccines lasts only a few years, and booster doses should be given every 5 years, if the high-risk situation continues.

SUGGESTED READING

1. Centers for Disease Control and Prevention (CDC). (2019). Meningococcal disease. Chapter 4: Travel-Related Infectious Diseases. [online] Available from: https://wwwnc.cdc.gov/travel/yellowbook/2020/travel-related-infectious-diseases/meningococcal-disease. [Last accessed July, 2020].
2. John TJ, Gupta S, Chitkara AJ, Dutta AK. An overview of meningococcal disease in India: knowledge gaps and potential solutions. Vaccine. 2013;31:2731-7.
3. Leach JP, Davenport RJ. Neurology-bacterial meningitis. In: Ralston SH, Penman ID, Strachan MWJ, Hobson RP (Eds). Davidson's Principles and Practice of Medicine, 23th edition. London: Elsevier; 2018. pp. 1118-23.
4. Meningococcal vaccines: WHO position paper, November 2011. Wkly Epidemiol Rec. 2011;86:521-39.
5. Pollard AJ, Sadarangani M. *Neisseria meningitidis* (meningococcus). In: Kleigmann RM, Stanto BF, St Geme JW, Schor NF (Eds). Nelson Textbook of Pediatrics, 1st edition. India: Reed Elsevier; 2016. pp. 1356-65.
6. Sinclair D, Preziosi MP, John TJ, Greenwood B. The epidemiology of meningococcal disease in India. Trop Med Int Health. 2010;15:1421-35.
7. Trestioreanu AZ, Fraser A, Gafter-Gvili A, Paul M, Leibovici L. Antibiotics for preventing meningococcal infections. Cochrane Database Syst Rev. 2011;8:CD004785.
8. Vashishtha VM, Choudhury P, Kalra A, Bose A, Thacker N, Yewale YN, et al. Indian Academy of Pediatrics (IAP) recommended immunization schedule for children aged 0 through 18 years—India, 2014 and updates on immunization. Indian Pediatr. 2014;51:785-800.
9. World Health Organization (WHO). (2018). Meningococcal meningitis. [online] Available from: https://www.who.int/en/news-room/fact-sheets/detail/meningococcal-meningitis. [Last accessed July, 2020].

CHAPTER 32

Cholera Vaccines

Nupur Ganguly

1. What is cholera?

Cholera is profuse watery diarrhea caused by cholera toxin (CT) producing strains of the gram negative bacteria *Vibrio cholerae*.

It remains an important cause of death in developing countries, especially Asia, Africa and South and Central America. The disease is also a risk to travelers to these areas of the world. It spreads by feco-oral route. Transmission occurs through consumption of contaminated food and water. When the contaminated food is kept at room temperature *V. cholerae* multiplies and can gives rise to an outbreak. The environmental water becomes contaminated with human feces during epidemic and contamination further spreads the epidemic. If sanitation is adequate, secondary cases do not occur.

Severe cholera is characterized by acute diarrhea, passing rice watery stools and vomiting, giving rise to moderate to profound dehydration within 4–18 hours. However, not all patients with cholera will have severe diarrhea and may remain asymptomatic or have only mild diarrhea. The case-to-infection ratio (number of symptomatic cases per asymptomatic people infected) ranges from 1:3 to 1:100 depending upon the geographical region, biotype, phase of epidemic and size of inoculum. In epidemic situation, the case to infection ratio increases. Establishment of adequate personal hygiene, food safety and sanitation along with vaccination can bring down the incidence of asymptomatic cases and control this life-threatening disease. Vaccination against cholera was first tested in the 19th century and played a role in controlling epidemics. Injected (parenteral) whole-cell vaccines were used in the 1960s and 1970s, but they went out of favor as their efficacy was thought to be low and short-lived, high titers of serum vibriocidal antibodies were thought not to provide sufficient intestinal immunity to prevent infection, and there was high rate of adverse effects.

Cholera epidemics have shown that there is a requirement for an effective vaccine against this major disease. Understanding the importance of stimulating local intestinal immunity in the prevention of the disease both killed and live oral vaccines are licensed now.

2. What is the disease burden of cholera in India?

There is a lack of proper data of disease burden in India due to under reporting. Cholera occurs over a wider geographic area in India. National Institute of

Cholera and Enteric Diseases (NICED), Kolkata, West Bengal, India, is a World Health Organization (WHO) collaborating Center for Diarrheal Diseases Research and Training. It receives about more than 1,500 strains of *V. cholerae* every year from about 30–40 institutions from India and a few from outside the country for biotyping, serotyping and phage typing. In this center, one of the largest studies (18 year study) was conducted from 1990 to 2007. During this period, 24 of the 35 states and union territories in India had sent strains at least once. Andhra Pradesh, Delhi, Goa, Gujarat, Karnataka, Madhya Pradesh, Maharashtra, Punjab, Rajasthan, Tamil Nadu and West Bengal had sent strains for three consecutive years. Highest numbers of strains were received from Maharashtra, followed by West Bengal. No strains were submitted from Puducherry during this period. From 2004 onward, strains were also received from Kerala and Sikkim. Of the total strains received, 96.5% strains were serotyped as Ogawa and the remaining 3.5% were Inaba. From 1997 to 2006, there were 68 outbreaks in 18 states, and 222,038 cases were detected overall in 7 out of the 10 years. This figure is about six times higher than the number reported to WHO (37,783) over the same period. The states of Odisha, West Bengal, Andaman and Nicobar Islands, Assam and Chhattisgarh accounted for 91% of all outbreak-related cases as per the analysis report of NICED. It shows there is considerable disease burden throughout the country, and the annual number of cholera cases reported to WHO by the government was several times lower than the numbers obtained through strains received at the phage typing unit. This may be due to lack of surveillance as well as proper laboratory.

3. What are the various serotypes types of *V. cholerae* as per the O antigen of its lipopolysaccharide causing cholera?

There are over 200 distinct serological groups of *V. cholerae*, classified on the basis of the "O" antigen present on the cell surface. Out of these, only two are known to cause epidemics that are serogroups O1 and O139. *V. cholerae* O1 can be further classified into two biotypes— (1) classical and (2) El Tor, each of which can be divided into three serotypes: Ogawa, Inaba and Hikojima. The epidemic strains currently in circulation worldwide are the El Tor biotype of *V. cholerae* O1, which was first recognized in Indonesia in 1961 and has now spread to many other countries in Asia, Europe, Africa and Latin America; and the Bengal strain of *V. cholerae* O139, which began in 1992 in India and Bangladesh, remains restricted to Asia. The classical biotype of *V. cholerae* O1 is also known to cause epidemics, though these are now uncommon, and non-O1/non-O139 strains occasionally cause sporadic cases of gastroenteritis **(Flowchart 1)**.

4. What is the difference between epidemic and endemic cholera?

In areas of high endemicity, the infection is usually seasonal and peaks before and after rainy seasons. It is highest in children below 5 years due to lack of protective immunity.

Flowchart 1: Serotypes, biotype sand serogroups of *V. cholerae*.

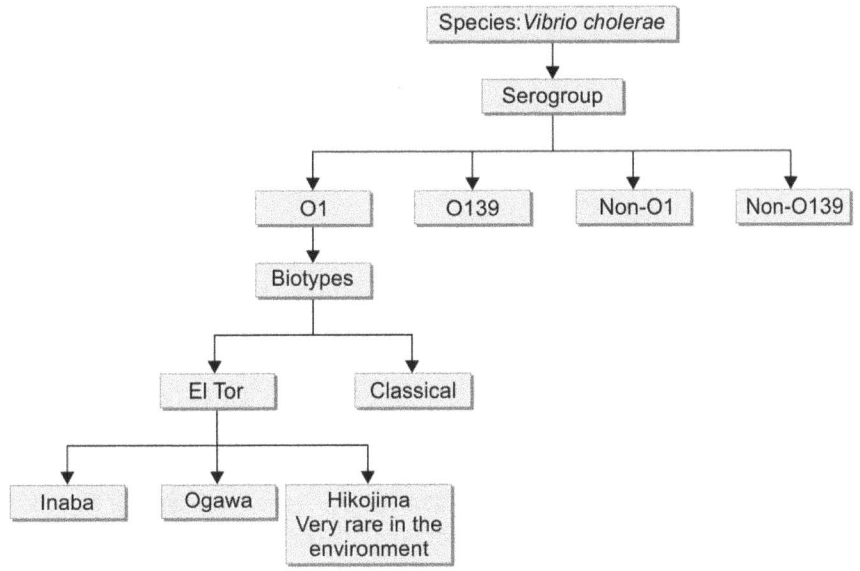

However in endemic regions, epidemic outbreaks may occur during breakdowns in safe water supply, poor hygiene, mass gatherings or *melas* with lack of proper health facilities. Epidemic occurs in areas with more limited immunity in the population. It may occur with similar attack rates in children and adults.

5. In which countries cholera infection is prevalent?

Due to considerable underreporting, the true global figures are not available. It is endemic in approximately 50 countries (defined by reporting of cholera cases in at least three of the last 5 years) mostly in Africa and Asia. However, epidemics have been reported throughout Africa, Asia, Middle East, South and Central America and the Caribbean. Outbreak in Haiti was associated with outbreak in Dominican Republic, Cuba and Mexico. Sporadic cases occur along the US, Gulf coast and are due to undercooked shellfish especially crabs.

6. How is the protective immunity in cholera mediated? What type of vaccine will be helpful—oral or parenteral?

The main virulence factor for cholera is mediated through cholera toxins (CTs). It is responsible for massive watery diarrhea characteristic of cholera. Mainly antibodies produced locally in the intestinal mucosal surface mediate protective immunity. These antibodies are directed against bacterial components including CT, protect by inhibiting bacterial colonization and multiplication and by blocking toxin action. Immunoglobulin A (IgA), IgG and IgM antibodies to cholera antigens have been demonstrated in the intestinal lumen; although in terms of protective immunity, intestinal IgA antibodies are the most important one. Oral vaccine is always preferable as it has been seen that the efficacy of injectable vaccine is around 50% only, and moreover it does not prevent introduction of cholera into a country or interrupt transmission (no herd immunity). For all these reasons, parenteral vaccine is not recommended by WHO for controlling epidemics.

7. Why old killed parenteral whole-cell cholera vaccine is withdrawn?

During 1960s, different controlled studies from India, Bangladesh, Philippines and Indonesia showed that the vaccine had only 50% efficacy, duration of protection lasted for only 6 months and it had to be given every 6–12 months to maintain clinically significant protection. It had higher rates of side effects and it did not prevent transmission. In 1970s, it was withdrawn.

8. What is whole-cell recombinant B-subunit (WC/rBS) vaccine (Dukoral)? What is its schedule and its effectivity and safety? Can this oral cholera vaccine (OCV) help to prevent cholera in our country?

It is a newer generation killed oral O1 vaccine marketed since 1990. It contains both Ogawa and Inaba serotypes of classical and El Tor biotypes with a recombinant B-subunit of oral CT. Field trial in Bangladesh and Peru showed that it provides 80–90% protection during first 6 months in all age groups after administration of two doses 1–2 weeks apart. Because heat labile toxin of enterotoxigenic *Escherichia coli* (ETEC) cross reacts with CT, the vaccine provides short-term protection against ETEC, which is an added benefit for the travelers. It is currently licensed in 60 industrialized countries and mostly used by Western tourists. The limitation of the vaccine is that the vaccine is supplied with a buffer [as cholera toxin B subunit (CTB) is sensitive to stomach acid], which is to be dissolved in a glass of water. This needs safe drinking water and it also needs to be stored at 2–8°C. In developing country with poor sanitation, safe drinking water may not be easily available. Further, this vaccine does not have O139 strain which has been found as a causative pathogen in West Bengal and Bangladesh, causing epidemic in West Bengal in 1994, this vaccine is not recommended in India.

9. Which cholera vaccine is available in India?

Shanchol™ is the killed oral vaccine currently available in India. It is a variant of WC-r BS whole-cell vaccine without beta subunit. It is a bivalent vaccine against *V. cholerae* O1 and O139, found to be safe and conferred significant protection against El Tor cholera in both children and adults. This vaccine was further been reformulated by the International Vaccine Institute (IVI) to meet WHO requirements. Large phase III study of the vaccine was carried out in Kolkata, India, in over 120,000 participants aged from 1 year and above.

Results of the study showed vaccine gives over 60% protection against cholera. The vibriocidal antibody response rate was 80% in children and 53% in adults. The reformulated vaccine was found to be safe and immunogenic in Indian children as well as adults. In India, the vaccine was produced in the name of Shanchol and it has been licensed in India in April 2009. It is approved by Drug Controller General of India (DCGI), Central Drug Laboratory, Kasauli, India, to be used in children above 1 year. It received WHO prequalification in November 2011. The vaccine is now being marketed in India and is available at an affordable price for the developing countries. Shanchol and Euvichol (Eu Biologics) are essentially the same vaccine.

10. What is the recommendation of use of Shanchol?

Shanchol is recommended for children above 1 year in two doses. Two doses are given 15 days apart. A booster dose is recommended after 2 years. Duration of immunity and protection has been demonstrated to provide sustained protection >60% to last for 3 years after 2 doses. A single dose provides a good short-term protection for at least 6 months. As per WHO position paper, it should be used in areas of endemic cholera, in humanitarian crisis with high risk of cholera, as a prevention of an outbreak where resources are limited In India, children aged 1–5 years are at highest risk of cholera in endemic setting. Immunization should be targeted in children above 1 year. The vaccine should always be used in conjunction with other cholera control and prevention strategies.

11. Is herd immunity conferred by killed oral cholera vaccines?

Analyzing data from a field trial in Bangladesh and Peru to ascertain the evidence of indirect protection from killed whole-cell oral cholera vaccines and B-subunit killed whole-cell vaccine in children and adult women showed in addition to providing direct protection to vaccine recipients; killed oral cholera vaccines confer significant herd protection to neighboring nonvaccinated individuals. This effect was attributed to vaccine-induced reduction of fecal excretion of vibrios in vaccinated individuals giving rise to less environmental contamination and thus reducing feco-oral transmission. Use of these vaccines could have a major effect on the burden of cholera in endemic settings.

12. What is CVD 103-Hg R vaccine? How efficacious and safe it is?

The CVD103-HgR (Vaxchora®) is a single dose live attenuated oral vaccine consisting of genetically manipulated classical *V. cholerae* O1 strain available since 1994. It is safe and safety profile is due to its poor colonization in the human intestine. As the vaccine strain is live, maintenance of cold chain is needed to preserve the bacteria. The bacteria must also be protected from stomach acid, which is achieved by formulating and packaging of the vaccine with a buffer. In a randomized, placebo-controlled field trial in Indonesia; a single dose conferred 60% protection in first 6 months, only 24% during the first year. However, it does not confer significant long-term protection during 4 years of observation. Being a live vaccine, it is not recommended for immunocompromised individual. Moreover, it does not confer any protection against O139 strain.

The FDA approved a single-dose Vaxchora® for adults 18–64 years old who are traveling to an area of active cholera transmission, a province, state, or other administrative subdivision within a country where cholera infections may be reported regularly (endemic) or where a cholera outbreak is occurring (epidemic), and includes areas with cholera activity within the past year.

No country or territory currently requires vaccination against cholera as a condition for entry.

Vaxchora® has been reported to reduce the chance of severe diarrhea in people by 90% at 10 days after vaccination and by 80% at 3 months after vaccination. The safety and effectiveness of Vaxchora® in pregnant or breastfeeding women is not yet known, and it is also not known how long protection lasts beyond 3–6 months after getting the vaccine. Side effects from Vaxchora® are uncommon and may include tiredness, headache, abdominal pain, nausea and vomiting, lack of appetite, and diarrhea.

There is ongoing phase 4 study of Vaxchora® to evaluate the safety and immunogenicity of children aged 2–18 years in developed countries.

13. What is the role of available cholera vaccine Shanchol in epidemic situation?

Experience shows that, once a cholera outbreak has begun, a reactive vaccination campaign with a two-dose vaccine is almost impossible; a single-dose vaccine requiring no buffer and no cold chain, easy to administer and providing long-term protection would provide the ideal solution. Limitation of the currently available and two-dose vaccine is that it needs administration in two doses 10–14 days apart, which needs to reach the same population twice. However, efforts should be made to find ways of overcoming the limitations of the currently available vaccine. A mass vaccination campaign cannot be improvised at the last moment; it needs careful advance preparation and needs to be given before-hand for proper protection. If an outbreak is about to start or has already started, use of oral cholera vaccine may not be appropriate. The current available Shanchol is recommended for preparedness to prevent epidemic situation.

14. What are the future vaccines in pipeline?

A number of other killed and live oral vaccines are under development. Results are promising. Live oral vaccine against O139 is also undergoing safety and efficacy trials. A research on polysaccharide conjugate vaccine for cholera is currently being conducted in France and USA for parenteral use and evaluations are planned in countries with endemic cholera.

SUGGESTED READING

1. CDC for Disease Control and Prevention. Cholera. [online] Available from: https://www.cdc.gov/cholera/general/index.html. [Last Accessed August, 2020].
2. World Health Organization. Background Paper on the Integration of Oral Cholera Vaccines into Global Cholera Control Programmes (2009). [online] Available from: http://www.who.int/immunization/sage/1_Background_Paper_Cholera_Vaccines_FINALdraft_13_oct_ v2.pdf. [Last Accessed August, 2020].
3. World Health Organization. WHO position paper on Cholera August 2017 Recommendation Vaccine. Geneva: WHO; 2018. pp. 3418-20.

CHAPTER 33

Dengue Vaccines

Dipti Agarwal

1. What is the burden of dengue disease globally?

Dengue, the fastest spreading viral infection in the world, is also the number one concern not only for India, but to entire Southeast Asia (SEA) region. The number of dengue cases reported to the World Health Organization (WHO) increased over eightfold over the last 2 decades from 505,430 cases in 2000 to over 2.4 million in 2010 and 4.2 million in 2019. Reported deaths between the year 2000 and 2015 increased from 960 to 4,032.

Dengue affects nearly 390 million people globally with a large majority occurring in tropical areas of SEA, South America, Africa, and Pacific region. Nearly 500,000 people are admitted each year and 20,000 deaths occur due to severe dengue each year. The case fatality rate ranges from 5% to 20%.

2. How serious is the burden in India?

Dengue poses a substantial economic and disease burden which is higher than that of 17 other conditions including Japanese encephalitis (JE), upper respiratory infection (URI), and hepatitis B.

It has been estimated that in India about 188,401 and 89,974 dengue cases and 325–144 dengue deaths occurred in the year 2017 and 2018, respectively (**Fig. 1**).

Few states such as Karnataka, Kerala, West Bengal, Maharashtra, Uttar Pradesh, Tamil Nadu, etc., have high disease burden (**Fig. 2**).

3. Do you have any data to demonstrate community-wise burden, i.e., seroprevalence of the dengue fever in India? What are the age-stratified rates?

According to a report published in Lancet Global Health 2019, the overall seroprevalence of dengue virus (DENV) infection in India was 48.7% [95% confidence interval (CI): 43.5-54], increasing from 28.3% (21.5-36.2) among children aged 5-8 years to 41% (32.4-50.1) among children aged 9-17 years and 56.2% (49-63.1) among individuals aged between 18 and 45 years. The seroprevalence was high in the Southern [76.9% (69.1-83.2)], Western [62.3% (55.3-68.8)], and Northern [60.3% (49.3-70.5)] regions. According to a recent systematic review and meta-analysis, the age distribution of laboratory-confirmed

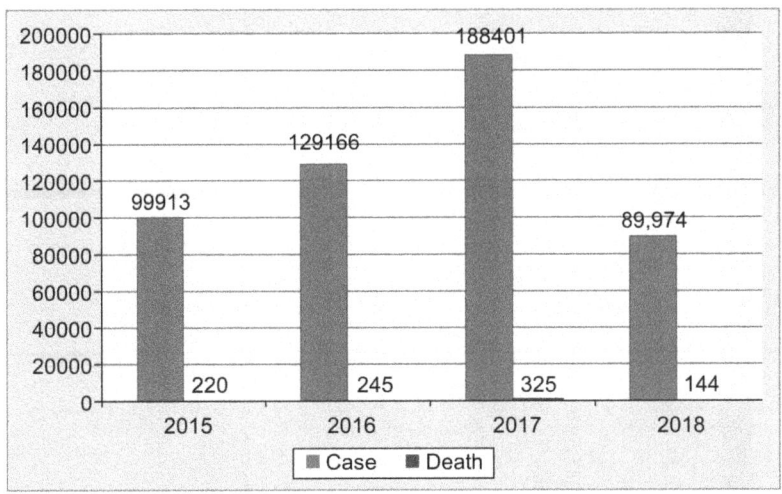

Fig. 1: Dengue cases and deaths in India since 2015–2018.v

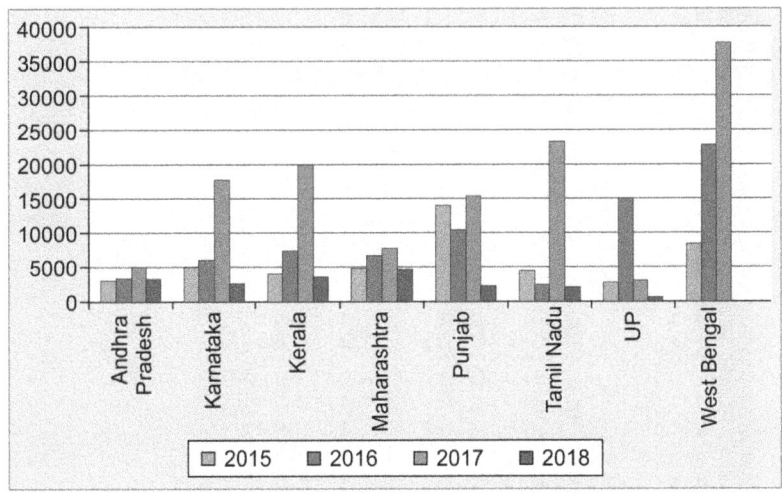

Fig. 2: State-wise distribution of dengue cases in India, 2015–2018 (*data till September 30, 2018*).

dengue patients was available from 52 out of 180 studies. The pooled median age of laboratory-confirmed dengue cases in these studies was 22 years (**Table 1**).

4. What are the preventive measures for dengue?

Dengue vaccines and vector control are the key methods of preventing the disease. According to the WHO prevention of vector-borne diseases, it requires effective surveillance, vector control measures, and vaccines, so as to decrease the burden of the disease.

TABLE 1: Seroprevalence of IgG antibodies against dengue in different geographic regions of India.

	Northern region (n = 2402)	Northeastern region (n = 2360)	Eastern region (n = 2486)	Western region (n = 2336)	Southern region (n = 2716)	All regions (n = 12300)
Age group, years						
5–8	794 (47.0% [33.7–60.7])	722 (1.6% [0.5–5.1])	815 (5.4% [3.0–9.8])	768 (27.0% [17.5–39.1])	960 (46.4% [36.3–56.9])	4059 (28.3% [21.5–36.2])
9–17	826 (57.8% [41.0–73.0])	805 (1.2% [0.3–4.8])	874 (7.4% [4.2–12.6])	824 (48.5% [39.4–57.8])	936 (69.6% [56.7–80.0])	4265 (41.0% [32.4–50.1])
18–45	782 (64.4% [47.7–78.2])	833 (7.3% [5.0–10.5])	797 (25.4% [20.3–31.3])	744 (76.4% [67.6–83.4])	820 (84.0% [71.9–91.5])	3976 (56.2% [49.0–63.1])
Sex						
Male	1145 (59.5% [52.2–66.3])	1028 (8.7% [4.3–16.8])	1192 (24.4% [19.8–29.9])	1159 (63.7% [56.4–70.4])	1289 (75.9% [66.3–83.5])	5813 (50.9% [46.8–55.1])
Female	1257 (61.3% [46.7–74.1])	1332 (3.3% [1.4–7.9])	1294 (14.7% [11.1–19.2])	1177 (61.5% [53.6–68.9])	1427 (77.7% [69.9–83.9])	6487 (47.5% [40.8–54.3])
Area of residence						
Rural	1117 (53.1% [381.1–67.5])	1196 (4.6% [2.8–7.5])	1280 (17.1% [13.3–21.7])	1229 (58.3% [49.7–66.5])	1415 (72.4% [62.3–80.6])	6237 (42.3% [36.0–48.9])
Urban	1285 (75.9% [64.7–84.4])	1164 (9.8% [5.6–16.6])	1206 (27.8% [20.6–36.2])	1107 (79.1% [72.3–84.6])	1301 (87.3% [79.6–92.4])	6063 (70.9% [64.3–76.6])
All age groups, years						
5–45	2402 (60.3% [49.3–70.5])	2360 (5.0% [3.3–7.6])	2486 (18.3% [14.8–22.4])	2336 (62.3% [55.3–68.8])	2716 (76.9% [69.1–83.2])	12300 (48.7% [43.5–54.0])

Data are n (%[95% CI]), where n is the number of sera tested and % is the Seroprevalence. An optimized cut off was used and sera samples with ≥ 15 Panbio units were considered as positive

(CI: confidence interval; IgG: immunoglobulin G)

5. Why is vaccine for dengue required?

As there is no specific treatment for dengue available at present, preventive measures and vaccination are the mainstay for controlling disease. Vaccine effective against all four strains of virus with long duration of protection is required for reducing burden of the disease. Vaccine would serve as important tool for achieving goal set by the WHO of reducing dengue morbidity by at least 25% and mortality by at least 50% by 2020.

6. How does immunity against dengue virus develop? What are the challenges in the development of vaccine?

Dengue is caused by four DENVs (DENV-1 to DENV-4). The mechanism of protective immunity against dengue is not fully understood. Neutralization antibody against DENV plays an important role in protection. Role of cytotoxic T cells in immune response is not very clear. The virions have a lipid envelope which is modified by the insertion of envelope (E) proteins and premembrane/membrane (prM/M) proteins. The amino acid sequence resembles each other in the four serotypes by only 60–70%. Antibodies directed against the DENV virion are mostly targeted at the E and prM proteins. Research to determine the most suitable target epitopes for vaccines is ongoing.

Infection by one of the four DENV serotypes has been shown to confer lasting protection against same serotype. Secondary dengue infection has increased risk of severity due to increased antigen uptake, cross-neutralization antibody, and cytokine storm which is known as antibody enhancement. Due to this complex immune response, there is difficulty in development of vaccine. Vaccine needs to be aimed at providing long-term protection against all virus serotypes. Additional challenges in the vaccine development include lack of animal model for the disease. Poor growth of the virion in cell culture adds to the difficulty in development of vaccine.

7. What are the characteristics of an ideal dengue vaccine?

An ideal dengue vaccine should have the following characteristics:
- Should be safe in children and adults
- Should not induce antibody-dependent enhancement
- Should be able to incorporate in the national immunization schedule
- Should have high immunogenicity with low reactogenicity
- Should be genetically stable
- Should be able to induce neutralizing antibodies and cell-mediated immunity
- Should be able to induce long-lasting immunity
- Should be able to form neutralizing immunity to all four serotypes
- Should be widely available at affordable cost.

8. What are technologies used for development of dengue vaccine?

Vaccine technologies used in the development of dengue vaccine include live attenuated vaccine, inactivated vaccines, recombinant subunits, virus-like particles (VLPs), and plasmid or viral vectors.

- Live attenuated virus vaccines have demonstrated long-lasting immunity. Both humoral and cellular immune responses have been shown to develop. The challenge primarily faced in this technology is to produce adequate level of attenuation to provide immunogenicity with low reactogenicity. These live attenuated vaccine should have the ability to grow in cell culture to aid in its production. Attenuation for the vaccine can be done by serial cell passage using dog kidney cells. Selected mutations created by recombinant deoxyribonucleic acid (DNA) technology can also be used. Majority of the live attenuated vaccines are in the clinical stage of vaccine development.
- Inactivated vaccines have shown decreased reactogenicity, but the immune responses are weaker and shorter lasting as compared to live attenuated vaccine. It can, however, be used safely in immunocompromised people. Inactivated dengue vaccines contain DENV structural proteins and viral ribonucleic acid (RNA). Immune response can be shown against the virion structural proteins. Although the killed dengue vaccines have not got much success, they have demonstrated formation of neutralizing antibody in primates.
- Recombinant DNA vaccines are developed by inserting viral genes into nonreplicative adenovirus vector. The recombinant virus expresses the protein membrane (prM) and structural protein sequence of the virus from both DENV-1 and DENV-2 and DENV-3 and DENV-4 each. The two recombinants have been tested and demonstrated neutralizing antibodies to the four DENV serotypes. It has been tested in primates and exhibited formation of protective antibody against all four DENV serotypes.
- Recombinant subunit dengue vaccines have been produced in a variety of protein expression systems such as bacterial, yeast, insect, and mammalian cells. These vaccines exhibit low reactogenicity and immunogenicity and need use of adjuvants. These vaccines are in preclinical development and some of them have reached the phase I of clinical trial.
- Virus-like peptides vaccines are VLPs that can present antigens similar to the structure of the virus. It, however, does not have the ability to replicate, which is thought to increase immunogenicity of the virus. Presently, VLP vaccines are in preclinical stages.

9. What are the initiatives taken in the development of pediatric dengue vaccines?

The Pediatric Dengue Vaccine Initiative has accelerated the development of vaccine against DENV. The Bill and Melinda Gates Foundation and the WHO have collaborated with the Pediatric Dengue Vaccine Initiative for development of DENV.

The key objectives of the program are as follows:
- To assess global burden of dengue
- To estimate the costs of dengue vaccine introduction
- To select sites for phase III vaccine trials in various countries where dengue is endemic
- To build local capacity for dengue research
- To fund research on safety of DENV.

10. Is there a licensed dengue vaccine available?

Yes, Dengvaxia™ (CYD-TDV) is the world's first licensed DENV. It was licensed for use in 2015. This vaccine is developed and marketed by M/s Sanofi Pasteur.

11. What are the key attributes of this vaccine?

CYD-TDV is obtained by replacing the genes encoding the prM and E proteins of the attenuated yellow fever (**Fig. 3**). It has been evaluated in phase III clinical trials. CYD14 has been conducted in five countries in Asia and CYD15 has been conducted in five countries in Latin America and CYD23 has been conducted in Thailand. In these trials, there were about 35,000 participants aged 2–16 years. First vaccination was given at the age of 2–14 years in the CYD14 trial and 9–16 years in CYD15 trial. The ratio of participants who

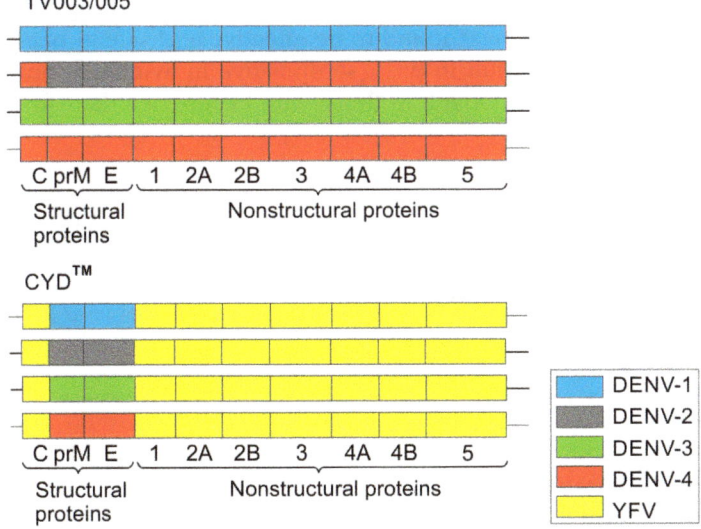

Fig. 3: Graphical representation of live-attenuated tetravalent dengue vaccines TV003/TV005 and Dengvaxia™ (CYD). The four serotypes are represented by different colors [DENV-1 = Blue, DENV-2 = Gray, DENV-3 = Green, DENV-4 = Red, and Yellow fever virus (YFV) = Yellow].

Source: Whitehead SS. Development of TV003/TV005, a single dose, highly immunogenic live attenuated dengue vaccine; what makes this vaccine different from the Sanofi-Pasteur CYD™ vaccine? Expert Rev Vaccines. 2016;15(4):509-17.

received vaccination to placebo was 2:1. Vaccine efficacy against confirmed dengue pooled across both these trials was 59.2% in the year following the primary series. During this initial period, cumulative efficacy against severe dengue was 79.1%. There was difference in efficacy in different types of serotype. Higher efficacy has been reported against serotypes 3 and 4 (71.5% and 76.9%, respectively) than for serotypes 1 and 2 (54.7% and 43%, respectively).

12. What are the schedule, limitations, and contraindications of Dengvaxia vaccine?

Dengvaxia™ (CYD-TDV) is a live-attenuated tetravalent dengue vaccine. It is recommended to be used between 9 and 45 years of age in endemic areas. It is to be given as a three-dose schedule (0–6–12 months). If vaccine dose is delayed, the next dose is given immediately. There is no recommendation for booster dose (**Box 1**).

It is contraindicated in individuals with history of allergic reaction to any component of the vaccine. It is also contraindicated in individuals with immune deficiency and human immunodeficiency virus (HIV) infection that impair cell-mediated immunity. The vaccine is not to be given in pregnant or breastfeeding women. The vaccine is also not recommended for the travelers.

13. What are the World Health Organization (WHO) recommendations on Dengvaxia™?

The WHO recommends that countries should consider introduction of the DENV CYD-TDV (Dengvaxia™) only in regions with high burden of the disease. The vaccine was found to be effective and safe in persons who have had a DENV infection in past (seropositive individuals), but showed increased risk of severe dengue in those who experience their first natural

---

BOX 1: Summary findings of some key characteristics and limitations of Dengvaxia™ vaccine.

Dengvaxia™: First licensed dengue vaccine:
- Recombinant, live, attenuated, and tetravalent chimeric yellow fever 17D vaccine dengue vaccine (CYD-TDV)
- Safe yet moderately effective
- *Recommended age*: 9–45 years
- *Schedule*: Three doses at 0, 6, and 12 months.

Vaccine efficacy:
- 65.6% for 9–16 years and 44.6% for 2–8 years (original trials)
- Currently licensed in 20 countries.

Limitations:
- Poor immune response against type 2 strain of DENV
- Moderate efficacy
- Multidose schedule
- Effective only in the age group of 9–45 years
- A real risk of developing severe disease in seronegative individuals.

dengue infection after vaccination (seronegative individuals). Countries which introduce vaccine should conduct prevaccination screening. The present recommendations are:
- Screening for past dengue infection has to be done before vaccination. Evidence of a past dengue infection is determined by presence of immunoglobulin G (IgG).
- If screening is not possible, vaccination could be considered in selected areas with seroprevalence rates of at least 80% by the age of 9 years.

14. Which is the other dengue vaccine whose phase III trial has been published?

TAK-003 is a new tetravalent dengue vaccine developed by Japanese company, Takeda Pharmaceutical Company Limited. It is based on a live-attenuated DENV-2 virus that provides genetic structure for all four serotypes (*see* Fig. 3). Takeda's TDV dengue vaccine is probably most advanced vaccine currently in pipeline. It is intended to be given in two doses, 90 days apart. Takeda began its phase III trial in September 2016. In its first phase III trial, a large 5-year study in Asia and Latin America was conducted to test how the vaccine prevents dengue fever and the long-term side effects of the vaccine in children. It began a second phase III trial in December 2017. This 12-month study was conducted on 400 healthy adolescents in nonendemic areas in Mexico. TDV was found to be safe and immunogenic in children aged 2–17 years, irrespective of previous exposure to dengue. The primary efficacy data from part 1 of ongoing phase III randomized trial was conducted on 20,071 participants of age 4–16 years. Overall, vaccine efficacy was found to be 80.9% (95% CI: 75.2–85.3). The incidence of serious adverse events was similar in the vaccine and placebo group (3.1% and 3.8%, respectively). Overall vaccine efficacy across all ages was found to be between 72.3% and 82.3% among seronegative cases. The trials showed highest neutralization antibody against DENV-2 serotype. These results support benefit in subjects regardless of previous exposures. Tetravalent Dengue Vaccine in Healthy Children (TIDES) is the ongoing phase III trial to assess efficacy and safety of vaccine.

15. What are the potential vaccine candidates in pipeline?

Dengue vaccine development has made enormous progress in recent years. The main vaccine candidates have entered phase III clinical trial and many other vaccines have reached stage of clinical evaluation while Dengvaxia™ is the first vaccine to be licensed against dengue. The details of the potential vaccine candidates are given below:
- CYD live recombinant vaccine is based on a yellow fever vaccine 17D backbone. It uses DENV-1 and -4 prM/E3 doses as the antigen. It is given in three-dose schedule (0/6/12 months). It is being developed by M/s Sanofi Pasteur company. It has completed phase III clinical trial.
- TV003/TV005 is a tetravalent live, attenuated/recombinant vaccine. It uses DENV-1, -3, and -4 as the whole genome and DENV-2 prM/E as the antigen. It is funded by US Government National Institutes of Health (NIH).

It is given as single dose and completed phase III clinical trial. TV005 has 10 times more dengue serotype 2 component than the latter.
- DENVAX is a tetravalent live, attenuated, and recombinant vaccine. It uses DENV2 as the whole genome and DENV-1/-3/-4 prM/E as the antigen. It is given in two doses (0/90 days). It has been developed by Takenda. It has completed phase II clinical trial.
- Dengue purified inactivated vaccine (DPIV) is a tetravalent purified inactivated vaccine. It uses DENV-1 and -4 as the whole genome as well as antigen. It is given in two doses (0/28 days). It has been developed by the Walter Reed Army Institute of Research/Fiocruz/GlaxoSmithKline (GSK). It has completed preclinical and clinical phase I clinical trial.
- DEN-80E tetravalent E-protein in subunit vaccine uses soluble DEN-1/-2/-3/-4 prM/E proteins as antigen. It is given in three doses (0/1/2 months). It has been developed by Merck and has reached phase I of clinical trial.
- TVDV tetravalent "shuffled" has used prM/E expressed from plasmid vector DNA vaccine. It uses plasmid DNA expressing DENV-1/-2/-3/-4 prM/E. It is given in three doses (0/1/3 months). It has been developed by US Naval Medical Research. The vaccine has completed phase I clinical trial.

16. What are the vaccines being developed in India?

There are two vaccine candidates being developed in India:
1. TetraVax-DV—the vaccine is based on live-attenuated TV0003/005 developed by the NIH. The four DENV serotypes are based on prM and E genes as seen in **Figure 4**. The C structured protein is not important for the formation of vaccine. The vaccine is engineered by deletion at

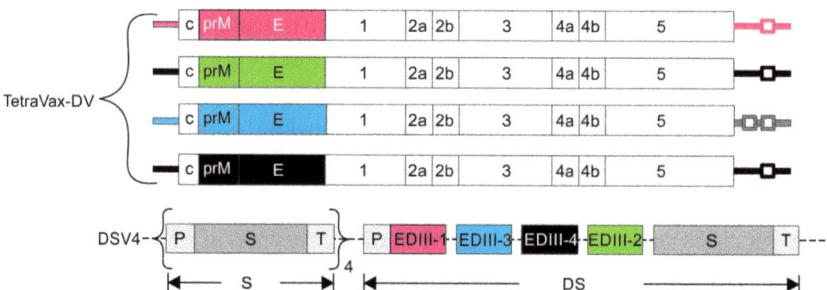

Fig. 4: Graphical representation of TetraVax-DV and DSV-4 (the DENV serotypes are: DENV-1 = Magenta, DENV-2 = Green, DENV-3 = Blue, and DENV-4 = Black). The empty box is C gene encoding for structural protein and NS proteins (1, 2a, 2b, 3, 4a, 4b, and 5). The short horizontal lines show 50 and 30 NTRs. DSV-4 shows S gene with promoter (P) and terminator (T). DS gene encodes for EDIIIs of the four DENV serotypes.

(DENV: dengue virus; NS: nonstructural)

Source: Swaminathan S, Khanna N. Dengue vaccine development: Global and Indian scenarios. Int J Infect Dis. 2019;84S:S80-6.

3'NTR end of the virus. An additional deletion is required for acceptable attenuation of the virus. The DENV-2 vaccine is a DENV-2/DENV-4 intertypic chimera. This vaccine virus expresses viral antigen in the host.
2. DSV4 vaccine—it is indigenously developed protein-based tetravalent dengue subunit vaccine. The DNA is integrated with the yeast *Pichia pastoris*. It encodes four copies of the S and one copy of fusion gene DS. The S and DS protein coassemble as mosaic VLPs.

17. What are the newer generations of vaccines?

Next-generation dengue vaccines may use prime-boost approach combining live and nonreplicating vaccine to balance the relative shortcomings of the vaccines. These vaccines could have more shorter schedule that can make them more suitable for certain target groups such as immunocompromised individuals, travelers, etc. These vaccines could generate cost-effective vaccines, which would facilitate their use particularly in endemic countries. India has joined the global efforts of developing a superior and safe, next-generation dengue vaccines in recent years and is poised to initiate the clinical development of such vaccine.

18. Do you think the dengue vaccine should be included as an important adolescent vaccine in endemic regions?

With the availability of more "refined" dengue vaccines, its integration in the list of essential adolescent vaccines would make sense.

The WHO recommends human papillomavirus (HPV) vaccine in 0 and 6 months schedule targeting adolescent females and in some cases adolescent males <15 years of age. With some newer vaccines having two-dose schedule, a combination of HPV and dengue vaccine can be implemented in different settings like in schools, health facilities, outreach sessions, etc. In countries using HPV vaccine, dengue vaccine can be combined with the 0 and 6 months HPV doses in targeted populations.

SUGGESTED READING

1. Biswal S, Borja-Tabora C, Vargas LM, Velásquez H, Alera T, Sierra V, et al. Efficacy of a tetravalent dengue vaccine in health children aged 4-16 years: a randomised, placebo-controlled, phase 3 trial. Lancet. 2020;395(10234):1423-33.
2. Biswal S, Reynales H, Saez-Llorens X, Lopez P, Borja-Tabora C, Kosalaraksa P, et al. Efficacy of a Tetravalent Dengue Vaccine in Healthy Children and Adolescents. N Engl J Med. 2019;381(21):2009-19.
3. Ganeshkumar P, Murhekar MV, Poornima V, Saravanakumar V, Sukumaran K, Anandaselvasankar A, et al. Dengue infection in India: a systematic review and meta-analysis. PLoS Negl Trop Dis. 2018;12(7):e0006618.
4. Murhekar MV, Kamaraj P, Kumar MS, Khan SA, Allam RR, Barde P, et al. Burden of dengue infection in India, 2017: a cross-sectional population based serosurvey. Lancet Glob Health. 2019;7(8):e1065-73.

5. Swaminathan S, Khanna N. Dengue vaccine development: global and Indian scenarios. Int J Infect Dis. 2019;84S:S80-6.
6. Tricou, V, Sáez-Llorens X, Yu D, Rivera L, Jimeno J, Cecilia A, et al. Safety and immunogenicity of a tetravalent dengue vaccine in children aged 2-17 years: a randomised, placebo-controlled, phase 2 trial. Lancet. 2020;395(10234):1434-43.
7. Verma S, Kalra A. Vaccines against dengue. In: Vashistha VM (Ed). IAP Textbook of Vaccines, 2nd edition. New Delhi: Jaypee Brothers Medical Publishers (P) Ltd; 2020. pp. 521-8.
8. World Health Organization. (2018). Dengue vaccine: WHO position paper–September 2018. [online] Available from: https://apps.who.int/iris/bitstream/handle/10665/274315/WER9336.pdf?ua=1. [Last accessed September, 2020].
9. World Health Organization. Dengue vaccine: WHO position paper, July 2016-Recommendations. Vaccine. 2017;35(9):1200-1.
10. Whitehead SS. Development of TV003/TV005, a single dose, highly immunogenic live attenuated dengue vaccine; what makes this vaccine different from the Sanofi-Pasteur CYD™ vaccine? Expert Rev Vaccines. 2016;15(4):509-17.

CHAPTER 34

Malaria Vaccines

Abhay K Shah

1. How malaria is transmitted?

Malaria is a vector-borne disease transmitted through the bite of *Anopheles* mosquitoes. Several species of the *Plasmodium* protozoan parasite can infect humans [*P. falciparum* (Pf), *P. vivax, P. ovale, P. malariae*, and *P. knowlesi*].

2. How serious is malaria?

Malaria represents one of the most important public health problems all over the world. It is the most common mosquito-borne disease and is a leading contributor to child morbidity and mortality. It is especially common and more troublesome in resource-poor tropical and subtropical regions. Malaria is associated with significant morbidity and mortality, especially in tropical counties. An estimated 219 million malaria cases and 438,000 malaria-related deaths were reported in 2017. Out of this, nearly 90% of deaths were contributed by sub-Saharan Africa. Most of these deaths are mainly caused by Pf and mortality is high in children under the age of 5 years. PF causes mild febrile illness like any other similar illnesses, but at times, it leads to life-threatening disease with cerebral malaria, respiratory distress, severe anemia, hypoglycemia, or circulatory shock.

3. What is the Indian scenario?

A total of 0.84 million confirmed malaria cases and 194 related deaths were reported by the National Vector Borne Disease Control Programme (NVBDCP) in 2017, contributing nearly 4% of the global malaria burden and 87% of the total malaria cases in Southeast Asia. Odisha, Chhattisgarh, Madhya Pradesh, and Jharkhand states accounted for 74.1% of the total malaria cases reported in the country. The highest number of malaria cases (40%) was reported from the Odisha state (**Fig. 1**). India has set targets for malaria-free status by 2030.

4. Which are the components of malaria elimination program?

The Global Technical Strategy for Malaria Elimination framed by the World Health Organization (WHO) has recommended a three-pillar system for elimination on emphasizing universal access to malaria diagnosis and treatment, strengthen surveillance, and accelerate toward elimination.

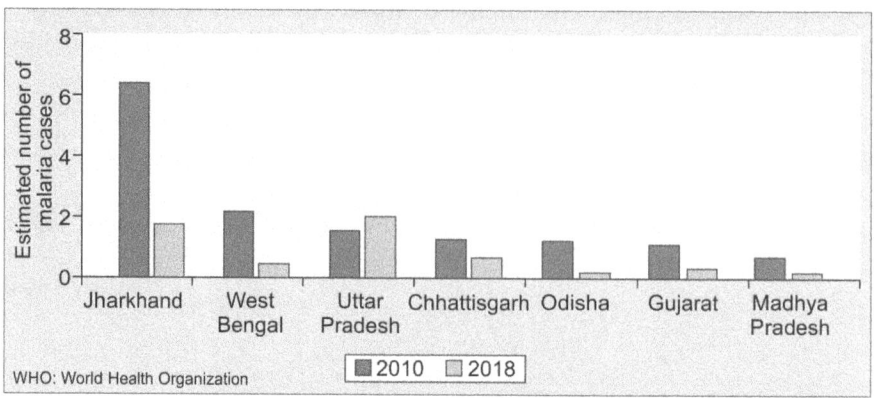

Fig. 1: Estimated malaria cases in India in seven key states: comparative analysis of cases in 2010 versus 2018.
Source: World Health Organization (WHO) estimates.

5. Which are the various modalities used for malaria control and prevention?

Various malaria control activities have proved successful in substantially reducing the incidence rates of malaria and malaria deaths.

Such interventions include widespread distribution and use of insecticidal nets having long duration of protective effect, the use of indoor residual spraying of insecticides in some settings, prompt diagnosis of malaria using rapid tests, and treatment with highly effective antimalarials like artemisinin derivatives used in combination with other drug. Vaccine against malaria is a much needed and awaited preventive modality to fill the gap left by all these interventions.

6. Why malaria vaccine is important in spite of such interventions?

In spite of various interventions of malaria transmission, morbidity and mortality remain high in many endemic settings. Prevention still needs to be strengthened further and new tools are needed. Vaccines have been proved to be an effective tool for disease attenuation, prevention, elimination, and eradication for number of vaccine-preventable diseases and malaria is not an exception to it as well. It is important to remember the limitations of various interventions used currently toward malaria elimination. Emerging resistance to antimalarial drugs and also mosquitoes developing resistance to insecticides are the major hurdles in malaria control and prevention. So, both antimalarial agents and insecticides are not foolproof. With this background reality, malaria vaccine, even if moderately efficacious, will be definitely a useful tool to protect substantial number of people from disease each year.

7. Do we have natural protection in endemic areas?

Yes. Persons residing in malaria-endemic areas do develop natural immunity to malaria, but this takes some years of exposure and is imperfect.

8. What is the timeline for malaria vaccine development?

Vaccine development efforts have focused on preventing illness from Pf and to a lesser extent on *P. vivax*. Significant roles for both humoral and cell-mediated effectors have been demonstrated in animal models and both humoral and cell-mediated immune responses are induced in humans after natural malaria infection and following inoculation of many candidate malaria vaccines.

The RTS,S was created in 1987 by scientists working at GlaxoSmithKline (GSK) laboratories. Early clinical development was conducted in collaboration with the Walter Reed Army Institute of Research. In January 2001, GSK and PATH Malaria Vaccine Initiative (MVI) grant funds from the Bill and Melinda Gates Foundation **Table 1** provides the details of timeline of malaria vaccine development.

TABLE 1: Timeline of malaria vaccine.

1940–1984	Malaria immunization studies are conducted with aim at developing vaccines
1984 onward	RTS,S, the first malaria vaccine candidate developed
1998 onward	First RTS,S vaccine trials in Africa are conducted in Gambia
2001	The GlaxoSmithKline (GSK)/PATH Malaria Vaccine Initiative (MVI) partnership was initiated, with grants from the Bill and Melinda Gates Foundation to PATH, for developing RTS,S vaccine for young children living in malaria-endemic regions in sub-Saharan Africa
2003	RTS,S/AS02A malaria vaccine candidate phase IIb clinical trial is conducted in children from 1 to 4 years of age in Mozambique. The vaccine shows to be safe, immunogenic, and efficacious, reducing *Plasmodium falciparum* clinical malaria cases by 30% and episodes of severe disease by up to 58%, and protection expected to lasts for an 18-month follow-up period
2007	Phase II results in African children and infants are published in The Lancet and The New England Journal of Medicine
2009–2014	RTS,S vaccine phase III study is launched in Kisumu, Kenya, involving 15,459 infants and young children at 11 sites in seven African countries, being the largest malaria vaccine trial in Africa to date
2014	Initial phase III result at 18 months of RTS,S trial introduction shows the vaccine efficacy of 46% in children and 27% among young infants against the clinical malaria
2016	The World Health Organization (WHO) implemented a pilot project using the four-dose schedule of the RTS,S/AS01 vaccine in three to five distinct epidemiological settings in sub-Saharan Africa. This project was covering moderate-to-high transmission settings, with three doses administered to children between 5 and 9 months of age, followed by a fourth dose 15–18 months later
2017	The WHO-Regional Office for Africa (AFRO) announces on April 24 that Ghana, Kenya, and Malawi will partner with WHO in the Malaria Vaccine Implementation Programme (MVIP) and the RTS,S vaccine can be available in selected areas of these countries

Source: Adapted and modified from Wikipedia. (2019). Timeline of malaria vaccine. [online] Available from: https://timelines.issarice.com/wiki/Timeline_of_malaria_vaccine. [Last accessed July, 2020].

SECTION 2 Licensed Vaccines

> **BOX 1:** Vaccine approaches explored for malaria vaccine.
> - Sporozoite subunit vaccine, using the CS protein, e.g., RTS,S in adjuvant
> - Irradiated sporozoite or genetically attenuated sporozoite immunization either by mosquito bite or using injected purified sporozoites
> - DNA and/or viral vectors to induce T cells against the liver-stage parasites or to target other stages in life cycle of malaria parasite
> - Using whole blood-stage malaria parasites as immunogens
> - Use of protein in adjuvant vaccines to reduce the growth rate of blood-stage parasites
> - Use of protein (or long peptide) in adjuvant vaccines to induce antibody-dependent cellular inhibition (ADCI) of blood-stage parasites
> - Use of peptide-based vaccines, mainly against blood-stage parasites, e.g., SPf66, PEV3a
> - Development of anti-disease vaccines based on parasite toxins, e.g., GPI based
> - Immunization with parasite adhesion ligands such as PfEMP1
> - Use of parasite antigens, such as the Var2 protein, preferentially expressed in the placenta to prevent malaria in pregnancy
> - Immunization with sexual stage parasite antigens as transmission-blocking vaccines
> - Use of mosquito antigens as transmission-blocking vaccines.

(CS: circumsporozoite; DNA: deoxyribonucleic acid; GPI: glycosylphosphatidylinositol)
Source: Hill AV. Vaccines against malaria. Philos Trans R Soc Lond B Biol Sci. 2011;366:2806-14.

9. Which are the vaccine approaches explored for malaria vaccine development?

They are described in **Box 1**.

More than 30 Pf malaria vaccine candidates are at advanced preclinical and clinical stages of evaluation. Approaches that use recombinant protein antigens and target different stages of the parasite life cycle are being developed. The RTS,S/AS01 vaccine has completed phase III evaluation and received a positive regulatory assessment.

10. Which are various types of malaria vaccines?

Malaria vaccines are developed on the basis of its life cycle in human beings.
- Pre-erythrocytic vaccines
- Vaccines acting on blood stage
- Vaccines capable of blocking malaria transmission, i.e., transmission-blocking vaccines (TBVs).

11. What is pre-erythrocytic vaccine? Which are they?

Pre-erythrocytic vaccines act by targeting the spores of Pf. The antibodies produced by them are capable to kill infected liver cells. They also interfere with the malaria parasite during liver cell proliferation and halt the subsequent release of infectious merozoites. Currently, the main research is focused on the development of subunit vaccines against parasite proteins such as the *Plasmodium falciparum* circumsporozoite protein (PfCSP), the thrombospondin-related adhesive protein (TRAP), and the liver-stage antigen (LSA). CSP is the predominant surface protein of malarial parasite and hence is the most researched candidate vaccine antigen till date.

It includes:
- *Plasmodium falciparum circumsporozoite protein vaccine*:
  - This is a deoxyribonucleic acid (DNA) vaccine against CSP. It has been studied for years and is a simple and stable vaccine, but being a DNA vaccine is still in the developmental stage.
  - *RTS,S/AS01 and RTS,S/AS02*:
    - RTS,S/AS01 is presently a leading recombinant candidate vaccine against malaria
    - AS01 and AS02 are the adjuvants and it is found that both RTS,S/AS01 and RTS,S/AS02 vaccines exhibited better CS-specific immune responses than nonadjuvanted RTS,S.
  - *Plasmodium falciparum circumsporozoite protein bacteria vaccines*:
    - Bacterial vectors are one of the most common delivery vectors for malaria vaccines. For example, *Salmonella enterica serovar typhi* live vector vaccines have been used widely since 2009.
- *Thrombospondin-related adhesive protein vaccine*: TRAP, also known as the *Plasmodium falciparum* sporozite (PfSPZ) surface protein-2 (SSP-2), is a major antigen that plays an important role in SPZ invasion of mosquito salivary glands and hepatocytes.
- *Liver-stage antigen vaccine*: LSA-1 immune response resembles closely to naturally transmitted parasites, hence, this antigen has become an attractive vaccine candidate.

Plasmodium SPZs undergo multiplication in the human liver after they are carried in the bloodstream following a bite from a female *Anopheles* mosquito. Accordingly, pre-erythrocytic vaccines against malaria need to be highly effective at killing liver SPZs. It is important to remember that even a single SPZ can initiate a malaria infection. Maintaining effective antibody levels and sustaining T cell-specific response are really a major challenge for the development of PfSPZ vaccine.

12. What is blood-stage vaccine? Which are they?

Clinical signs and various complications related to malaria are attributed to blood-stage parasites in the red blood cells of the human body. Once the merozoites are released from the liver, they will try to enter red blood cells. After entering the red blood cells, the surface protein of the Pf merozoite remains in the red blood cell membranes and stimulates T cell and B cell immune responses. Research on blood-stage malaria vaccines has been a "hot spot" area of vaccine development.
- *Merozoite surface protein-1 (MSP-1) vaccines*: MSP-1 is located on the merozoite surface where it plays a key role in erythrocyte invasion.
- *Apical membrane antigen-1 (AMA-1) vaccines*: AMA-1 is expressed in the SPZ, hepatic, and erythrocytic stages where it plays an essential role in parasite survival.

13. What are transmission-blocking vaccines (TBVs)?

Transmission-blocking vaccines (TBVs) are designed to control the transmission of malaria parasites from human hosts to the mosquito vectors. The TBV candidates include the Pfs25, Pfs48/45, and Pfs230 and they have shown transmission-blocking immunity in model systems in different stages of development.

14. What is RTS,S/AS01? What does the acronym RTS mean?

It is the most effective malaria vaccine tested so far. This vaccine has completed phase III evaluation and results are also promising from regulatory point of view.

The "R" stands for the central repeat region of CSP protein in Pf, the "T" indicates T-cell epitopes of the CSP, and the "S" stands for hepatitis B surface antigen (HBsAg). These are combined in a single fusion protein ("RTS") and coexpressed in genetically engineered *Saccharomyces cerevisiae* yeast cells with free HBsAg. Thus, RTS is a chimeric protein derived from the genetic fusion of the carboxy-terminal half of the CSP (designated RT) to the hepatitis B virus gene encoding the virus surface protein (designated S). The RTS and S proteins when simultaneously expressed in yeast cells assemble into virus-like particles (VLPs) that display at their surface CSP and S sequences. AS01 is a liposome-based adjuvant.

15. Where the phase III trials conducted for RTS,S/AS01 and in which age groups?

The phase III trial of RTS,S/AS01 (RTS,S) was conducted over 5 years (2009–2014) in seven sub-Saharan African countries: (1) Burkina Faso, (2) Gabon, (3) Ghana, (4) Kenya, (5) Malawi, (6) Mozambique, and (7) the United Republic of Tanzania. The trials were conducted in these countries involving different areas having high, medium, and low malaria transmission.

The phase III trial enrolled approximately 15,500 infants and young children comprising of two different groups:
1. Older children who received first dose of the malaria vaccine between 5 and 17 months of age.
2. Infants who received the malaria vaccine together with other routine childhood vaccines at 6, 10, and 14 weeks of age.

16. What were the vaccine efficacy trial results?

The efficacy of the RTS,S vaccine was established in a phase III clinical trial that concluded in 2014.
- *Children aged 5–17 months:* In children aged 5–17 months who received three doses of RTS,S administered at 1-month interval, followed by a fourth dose 18 months later, the vaccine reduced malaria by 39%, equivalent to preventing nearly 4 in 10 malaria cases. In addition, the four-dose vaccine schedule reduced severe malaria by 31.5% in this age group, which was associated with reduction in hospitalizations due to

malaria, all-cause hospitalizations, and the need for blood transfusions. In children aged 5–17 months who did not receive a fourth dose of the vaccine, the protection against severe malaria was lost (26% over an average 48 months of follow-up) and this signifies the usefulness of the fourth dose of this vaccine to maximize its benefits.
- *Infants:* Among the younger infants, the malaria vaccine did not work sufficiently well to justify its further use in this age group. This may be attributed to factors such as interference by concomitant administration of diphtheria, tetanus, and pertussis (DTP)-containing vaccines, the presence of maternally acquired antibodies to malaria in this age group, and immaturity of the immune system in the 6–12 weeks old compared to the 5–17 months age group.

17. What was the scientific opinion from the European Medicines Agency (EMA)?

The European Medicines Agency (EMA) found RTS,S to have an acceptable safety profile. As with other new vaccines and in line with national regulations, the safety profile of RTS,S will continue to be monitored as the vaccine is made available. The opinion indicated that, in EMA's assessment, the quality of the vaccine and its risk-benefit profile was favorable from a regulatory perspective. This opinion did not consider other aspects such as feasibility for implementation, cost-effectiveness, etc.

18. What were the safety results for the vaccine in phase III trial?

The RTS,S/AS01 vaccine showed an acceptable safety and tolerability profile during the entire phase III study period. In both age groups, common, adverse events after vaccination included local reactions (such as pain or swelling), which were observed more frequently after RTS,S/AS01 administration compared to the comparator vaccine. Among children in the older age group, there was an increased risk of febrile seizures (within 7 days after any of the vaccine doses) without any long-lasting consequences. Among the younger infants, this risk was only apparent after the fourth dose. Among children in the older age group, a modest increase in the number of cases of meningitis and cerebral malaria was found in the group receiving the malaria vaccine compared to the control group. It is unclear whether there is a causal link between these findings and the RTS,S vaccinations; this will be further monitored in the pilot implementation program. This observation was not seen in infants aged 6–12 weeks.

19. What are the World Health Organization (WHO) recommendations related to RTS,S?

In October 2015, the WHO jointly convened the Strategic Advisory Group of Experts (SAGE) on Immunization and the Malaria Policy Advisory Committee (MPAC) to review all evidence regarding RTS,S relevant for global policy. The SAGE/MPAC recommended that pilot implementation of RTS,S occurs in three to five settings in sub-Saharan Africa, administering three doses of the vaccine to children beginning as close to 5 months of age as possible and a fourth dose 15–18 months after the third dose. The SAGE and the MPAC were not supportive of vaccine use among infants aged 6–12 weeks due to the lower efficacy seen in this age group. The SAGE/MPAC recommended large-scale implementation pilots to evaluate the extent of protection observed in children aged 5–17 months in the phase III trial and whether this can be replicated in routine health system, particularly to evaluate the need for a four-dose schedule that requires new immunization contacts. Other objectives of this pilot implementation are as under:

- To assess the mortality impact of the RTS,S vaccination as the overall mortality in the trial setting was very low.
- To address the issues of excess number of cases of meningitis and cerebral malaria, identified during the phase III trial, and to find out the causal relationship, if any to RTS,S vaccination.

This pilot program will be of great importance to generate critical evidence in 3–5 years' time. This will provide a better insight about the possible use of this vaccine on a larger scale.

The WHO has officially adopted the SAGE/MPAC recommendations in January 2016 and has strongly emphasized the need to go ahead with this pilot as the next step for the RTS,S malaria vaccine.

20. Why was RTS,S developed for and tested in Africa?

This is because the children in sub-Saharan Africa, especially under 5 years of age, are found to be the greatest victims of Pf and majority of deaths belong to this age group, i.e., African children. It is scientific and logical to study this vaccine in such a high-risk region.

21. Why is RTS,S only for children and infants? Why not adults?

This vaccine has been aimed to reduce morbidity and mortality related to Pf in children living in malaria-endemic regions of sub-Saharan Africa as the incidence of Pf cases and its mortality are significant in African children under 5 years of age.

22. What is so special and remarkable with RTS,S as compared with other malaria vaccine candidates currently under development?

The RTS,S is the first, and to date, the only vaccine that has demonstrated its effectiveness in significantly reducing malaria, life-threatening severe malaria, in young African children. The vaccine was introduced in the beginning of year 2019 in selected areas of moderate-to-high malaria transmission areas in three sub-Saharan African countries—(1) Ghana, (2) Kenya, and (3) Malawi—as part of a large-scale pilot program coordinated by the WHO with a aim to vaccinate about 360,000 children per year in the selected areas across the three countries. Vaccinations are being provided through each country's routine immunization program.

23. What is Malaria Vaccine Implementation Programme (MVIP)?

The Malaria Vaccine Implementation Programme (MVIP) was designed in coordination with the WHO. Its aim is to address the following issues:
- Feasibility of administering the recommended four doses of the vaccine in children
- The vaccine's potential role in reducing childhood deaths
- Its safety in the context of routine use
- Ghana, Malawi, and Kenya are the three countries participating in the MVIP. Each of these countries selected the areas to be included in the pilot program.

24. Who developed and who manufactures the vaccine?

A 5-year phase III efficacy and safety trial was conducted between 2009 and 2014 through a partnership that involved GSK, MVI (with support from the Bill and Melinda Gates Foundation). GSK is the vaccine manufacturer.

25. Does RTS,S/AS01 protects against *P. vivax*?

No, it does not.

26. What is the trade name for this vaccine?

Mosquirix™ is the name trademarked by GSK for the RTS,S/AS01 malaria vaccine.

27. What is the way forward for RTS,S/AS01 vaccine?

The pilot implementation was designed as a 6-year program and the results are expected to be available by 2023. GSK is conducting phase IV studies in parts of the pilot areas in terms of its safety and effectiveness. Data collected through the phase IV studies will complement data from the pilot evaluations led by the WHO. The PATH is also working with the WHO in several areas, including on economic assessments and the qualitative assessment of behavior change that may occur during vaccine introduction. GSK is donating up to 10 million doses for use in the MVIP.

SUGGESTED READING

1. European Medicines Agency (EMA). (2015). First malaria vaccine receives positive scientific opinion from EMA. [online] Available from: https://www.ema.europa.eu/en/news/first-malaria-vaccine-receives-positive-scientific-opinion-ema#:~:text=First%20malaria%20vaccine%20receives%20positive%20scientific%20opinion%20from%20EMA,-Press%20release%2024&text=The%20European%20Medicines%20Agency's%20Committee,the%20European%20Union%20(EU). [Last accessed July, 2020].
2. Ghosh SK, Rahi M. Malaria elimination in India—The way forward. J Vector Borne Dis. 2019;56:32-40.

3. Hill AV. Vaccines against malaria. Philos Trans R Soc Lond B Biol Sci. 2011; 366:2806-14.
4. National Vector Borne Disease Control Programme (NVBDCP). (2012). Malaria situation. [online] Available from: http://nvbdcp.gov.in/Doc/malaria-situation-august12.pdf. [Last accessed July, 2020].
5. RTS,S Clinical Trials Partnership. Efficacy and safety of RTS,S/AS01 malaria vaccine with or without a booster dose in infants and children in Africa: final results of a phase 3, individually randomised, controlled trial. Lancet. 2015;386:31-45.
6. Wikipedia. (2019). Timeline of malaria vaccine. [online] Available from: https://timelines.issarice.com/wiki/Timeline_of_malaria_vaccine. [Last accessed July, 2020].
7. World Health Organization (WHO). (2016). Malaria vaccine: WHO position paper. [online] Available from: https://www.who.int/wer/2016/WER9104.pdf?ua=1. [Last accessed July, 2020].
8. World Health Organization (WHO). (2016). WHO Position Paper on Malaria Vaccine. [online] Available from: https://www.who.int/life-course/news/events/malaria-vaccine/en/. [Last accessed July, 2020].
9. World Health Organization (WHO). (2020). Q&A on the malaria vaccine implementation programme (MVIP). [online] Available from: https://www.who.int/malaria/media/malaria-vaccine-implementation-qa/en/. [Last accessed July, 2020].
10. Zheng J, Pan H, Gu Y, Zuo X, Ran N, Yuan Y, et al. Prospects for malaria vaccines: pre-erythrocytic stages, blood stages, and transmission-blocking stages. Biomed Res Int. 2019;2019:9751471.

CHAPTER 35

Combination Vaccines

Ashok K Dutta

1. What is combination vaccine and simultaneous vaccines?

A combination vaccine consists of two or more separate immunogens that have been physically combined in a single preparation by the manufacturer. On the other hand, simultaneous vaccines are those which are administered concurrently but are physically separate. Simultaneous vaccines are either injected at separate sites or are administered by separate routes. Simultaneous vaccination is as effective and as safe as administering various vaccines alone.

2. How does nomenclature of combination vaccines is represented while writing?

The hyphen (-) is intended to indicate that the antigens are mixed together by the manufacturer before the product is sold and the forward slash (/) indicates that the two products are to be reconstituted by the user. For example, pentavalent diphtheria, pertussis, and tetanus (DPT), *Haemophilus influenzae* type b (Hib), and hepatitis B (Hep B) combination vaccine are expressed as DPT-Hib-Hepatitis B. On the contrary, if two vaccines are physically combined as per the manufacturer's instruction in levels, e.g., DPT and Hib, it is expressed as DPT/Hib.

3. What are the types of combination vaccines?

Combination vaccines are either single pathogen or multiple pathogen vaccines. Single pathogen vaccines contain various antigens or serotypes of a pathogen while multiple pathogen vaccines contain various antigens or serotypes from multiple pathogens **(Table 1)**.

TABLE 1: Types of combination vaccines.

No.	Types of vaccine	Examples
1.	Single pathogen	Oral polio, IPV, influenza, pneumococcal, rotavirus, HPV, and meningococcal
2.	Multiple pathogen	DTwP, DTaP, DT, Td, Tdap, MMR, DTwP-Hib, DTwP-Hep B, DTwP-Hib-Hep B, DTaP-Hib, DTaP-Hib-IPV, DTaP-Hib-Hep B-IPV, Hep A-Hep B, MMRV and DTaP-IPV

(DTaP: diphtheria, tetanus, and acellular pertussis; DTwP: diphtheria, tetanus, and whole-cell pertussis; Hep A: hepatitis A; Hep B: hepatitis B; Hib: *Haemophilus influenzae* type b; HPV: human papillomavirus; IPV: inactivated poliovirus vaccine; MMRV: measles, mumps, rubella, and varicella; Td: tetanus and diphtheria; Tdap: tetanus, diphtheria, and acellular pertussis)

4. What about adverse events after combination vaccines as compared to monocomponent vaccines?

The available combination vaccines are safe and usually no serious adverse reactions are reported than the monocomponent vaccines. However, in some of the combination vaccines, certain side effects, e.g., fever has been reported to be more than monocomponent but was not very significant. However, the local injection site reactions may be slightly higher but the advantage is that reaction would be localized to one site only.

5. What are the advantages of combination vaccines?

There are various advantages of combination vaccines from the viewpoint of consumer as well as health planner of a country **(Table 2)**.

TABLE 2: Advantages of combination vaccines with regard to consumer and health planner.

Advantages to consumer	Advantages to health planner
• Reduced number of injections and less number of painful jabs	• Reduced burden on shipping, handling, cold chain, and storage of vaccines
• Reduced parental and patient anxiety	• Decreased possibility of errors
• Reduced vaccination visits	• Reduced paper work
• Decreased likelihood of missed vaccinations	• Increased compliance of vaccination program
• Increased satisfaction	• Economic benefit from one (above), reduced cost for labor and supplies, and reduced vaccination visits
• Timely completion of indicated vaccinations	• Successful immunization program for the country

6. What are the issues and challenges of combination vaccines?

There are several challenges from manufacturing, developmental, and researcher's point.

Manufacturing issues include:
- Antigenic compatibility with different antigens that needs to be combined
- Immunological tolerance with live virus vaccines
- Volume of the vaccine that can be given in an infant and children
- Use of right amount of adjuvant in the combination vaccine.

Developmental issues:
- Each component of the antigen in the combination vaccine has to be indicated at the same time in the immunization schedule
- The product should remain stable after combination of antigen for at least 18–24 months.

Researcher's issues:
- Potential to reduce antigenic response by antigenic compatibility and epitope suppression which needs to be adequately tackled

- Increased antigen: adjuvant ratio
- Competition for B cells.

Following are some examples of the above challenges but are adequately tackled:
- The antibody level which develops following separately administered antigens may be often different and combining whole-cell pertussis vaccine to diphtheria and tetanus toxoid improves the antibody level since whole-cell pertussis is an excellent property to improve the immunogenicity of the other two antigens.
- On the contrary combination of diphtheria, whole-cell pertussis, and tetanus (DwPT)-Hib may yield less antibody response than if given separately but it has been observed that although the geometric mean titer of Hib in combination vaccine is less still it produces critical level of antibody of >1 µg which gives long-term protection against invasive Hib disease.
- Competition among viruses can lead to altered immune responses in case of combination vaccines containing live attenuated viruses. This problem is tackled either by increasing the number of doses of vaccine [e.g., oral polio vaccine (OPV)] or increasing the concentration of the individual viral strain [e.g., increased varicella component in measles, mumps, rubella, and varicella (MMRV)].
- Live vaccines can interfere immunologically with each other by one vaccine stimulating interferon production which inhibits replication of another viral vaccine strain, e.g., in case of OPV, type 2 strain replicated faster than type 1 and 3 inducing interferon and hence interfered with growth of the latter viruses. To overcome this problem, the quantity of type 1 and 3 viruses was increased in mixture. This led to partial success but the administration of multiple doses became necessary to ensure optimal intake of all three serotypes.

7. **There is a fear in the minds of many physician and parents that using multiple antigens together as combination vaccine may cause immunological overload and may harm the infants and children. Is the concept true?**

There is no scientific evidence to support such an assertion and there is much evidence to refute it. It should be explained that newborn is naturally exposed to thousands of antigens in first few months of life and simultaneous exposure to multiple vaccine antigens will not overwhelm the infant immune system. In fact, infant immune system requires fairly intense challenge to develop normally and insufficient stimulation leads to increased risk of autoimmune disorders.

8. **Is there any association between use of combination vaccines and future development of asthma and type 1 diabetes mellitus in the recipient?**

There is no evidence to state that any of the disease occurs following administration of combination vaccine.

9. What are the practical issues concerning the administration of combination vaccines?

There are various issues regarding administration of combination vaccines.
- *Administration of superfluous antigen*: As numerous combination vaccines are available, one may have to give an extra dose of an antigen which patient may not need (as he has already received the recommended doses of that antigen). It has been demonstrated for many antigens that giving an extra dose involves no adverse consequence. Low reactogenicity of Hib, inactivated poliovirus vaccine (IPV), and Hep B makes it unlikely that giving an extra dose would cause a problem. When patients have received the recommended immunizations for some of the components in a combination vaccine, administering the extra antigen(s) in the combination vaccine is permissible if they are not contraindicated and doing so will reduce the number of injections required. One should be careful about some antigens which are known to be associated with increased adverse effects if administered too frequently, e.g., diphtheria and tetanus toxoid leading to extensive local reactions. For example, in spite of giving Hep B vaccine at birth when pentavalent or hexavalent combination vaccines are used in routine immunization is recommended even if an extra dose of Hep B is given.
- *Brand interchangeability*: The question of whether vaccines from different manufacturers can be used interchangeably also applies to monocomponent vaccines. It is reassuring to know that interchanging one brand of vaccine for another has never been shown to result in performance that is outside the range expected for the vaccine in question. The Advisory Committee on Immunization Practices (ACIP) has recognized diphtheria, tetanus, and whole-cell pertussis (DTwP) (and it is individual components), IPV, OPV, Hib (as long as one uses complete three doses), and Hep B as interchangeable. For the vaccines for which robust data on the interchangeability is not available [e.g., diphtheria, tetanus, and acellular pertussis (DTaP), newer combination vaccines], this committee has recommended that same product may preferably be used throughout the primary series. Still it is recommended that the opportunity to administer a vaccine, for which the child is eligible, should not be missed even if earlier brand is not available or if its identity is not known.

10. Can a healthcare worker mix two separate antigens in the same syringe and make a combination vaccine?

The providers should not make their own combination by mixing various vaccines in one vial or syringe unless it is recommended by the manufacturer in their package inserts. Such mixing may influence safety, stability, and immunogenicity of the vaccines used.

11. What is meant by second shot combination vaccines?

Combination vaccines that incorporate conjugate pneumococcal and conjugate meningococcal antigens are known as second shot combination vaccines.

12. What are various combination vaccines available today?

Combination vaccines currently licensed in India are:
- *DTwP-Hib-IPV-Hep B, DTaP-Hib-IPV-Hep B, DTwP-Hib-IPV, DTaP-Hib-IPV, DTwP-Hib, DTaP-IPV-MMRV, and Hep A-Hep B*: These are either available as ready to use or lyophilized form. Though antibody response to Hib is reduced, there is no reduced efficacy as most subjects achieve the seroprotective level of 1 µg/mL. They have good immunogenicity and safety profile for both primary and booster immunization.
- *DTaP-Hib, DTaP-Hib-IPV*: The primary concern in these combinations is reduced Hib immunogenicity noted specially for primary immunization and when vaccines were administered earlier in life and in premature babies. This lower immunogenicity to Hib was conclusively attributed mainly to no administration of booster dose at 18 months. The United States Food and Drug Administration (USFDA) and the ACIP have approved this pentavalent vaccine for primary immunization.
- *Hep A-Hep B*: Available in both pediatric and adult (for those aged 18 and above) formulations. Dosing schedule is 0, 1, and 6 months (three doses).

Combination vaccines available internationally are:
- In addition to all the above vaccines, DTaP-IPV, Hib-Meningococcal AC, and several other permutations of combinations are available.

13. Can combination vaccines be used in children who have fallen behind with their vaccinations as per schedule? If so, what schedule should we follow?

Combination vaccines can be used for children who have missed their schedule vaccination. All combination vaccines are recommended to be used when any of the components are indicated and none are contraindicated. The minimum interval between doses is the greatest interval between any of the individual antigens. For example, the minimum interval between the first and second doses of MMR is 4 weeks and the minimum interval between the first and second doses of varicella vaccine is 12 weeks. When the two vaccines are combined in MMRV, the minimum interval between MMRV dose 1 and dose 2 is 12 weeks, which is the greatest of the minimum intervals of the two vaccines if given separately.

14. A 4-month-old infant recently came to India from USA where the baby was given separate diphtheria, acellular pertussis, and tetanus (DaPT), Haemophilus influenzae type b (Hib), inactivated poliovirus vaccine (IPV), and hepatitis B (Hep B) and reports your clinic for the second dose of all these vaccines. Can you administer combination vaccine containing above antigens safely?

Switching between separate antigens with combination vaccines are permissible provided they are indicated and licensed for use and minimum interval is met with. In this case, any of the licensed hexavalent vaccine can be safely administered.

15. What are the Indian Academy of Pediatrics (IAP) recommendations for use of combination vaccines?

The Indian Academy of Pediatrics-Advisory Committee on Vaccines and Immunization Practices (IAP-ACVIP) concludes that all currently licensed combination vaccines in India have an immunogenicity, efficacy, and safety profile comparable to separately administered vaccines as of currently available data. However, it recommends strict observance of manufacturer's instructions regarding mixing of vaccines in same syringe.

SUGGESTED READING

1. Balasubramaniam S. IAP Guidebook on Immunization 2018-2019. New Delhi: Jaypee Brothers Medical Publishers (P) Ltd; 2018.
2. Decker MD, Edwards KM, Bogearets HH. Combination vaccines. In: Plotkin S, Orenstein W, Offit P (Eds). Vaccines, 7th edition. New York: Elsevier; 2018.
3. Dutta AK. Combination vaccines. In: Dutta AK (Ed). Childhood Vaccination, 2nd edition. New Delhi: Jaypee Brothers Medical Publishers (P) Ltd; 2018.
4. Dutta AK. Combination vaccines. In: Vashishtha VM, Kalra A (Eds). IAP Textbook of Vaccine. Mumbai: Indian Academy of Pediatrics; 2020.
5. Kimberlin W, Brady MT, Jackson MA, Long SS. Red Book 2018-2021: Report of the Committee on the Infectious Diseases, 31st edition. United States: American Academy of Pediatrics; 2018.

CHAPTER 36

Yellow Fever Vaccines

Chandra Mohan Kumar, Obeid Shafi, Shweta Singh

1. What is yellow fever?

Yellow fever is an infectious viral hemorrhagic fever caused by a virus that is spread by the bite of an infected *Aedes aegypti*, sometimes referred as Yellow Fever mosquito.[1]

2. Where does yellow fever virus occur and how does one get yellow fever?

Yellow fever virus is endemic in 47 countries in tropical and subtropical areas in South America and Africa. Around 90% of cases reported every year occur in Sub-Saharan Africa **(Fig. 1)**.[2]

The yellow fever virus is a member of the Flaviviridae family (group B arbovirus). The Flavivirus genus is composed of more than 70 viruses, mostly arthropod-borne, out of which 30 are known to cause human disease.

It is transmitted by infected mosquitoes, most commonly from the Aedes species—the same mosquito that spreads the Zika, chikungunya and dengue virus. Another species of mosquitoes, *Haemagogus* and *sabethes* mosquitoes also spread yellow fever and are mostly found in the jungle. Mosquitoes become infected with the virus when they bite an infected human or monkey.

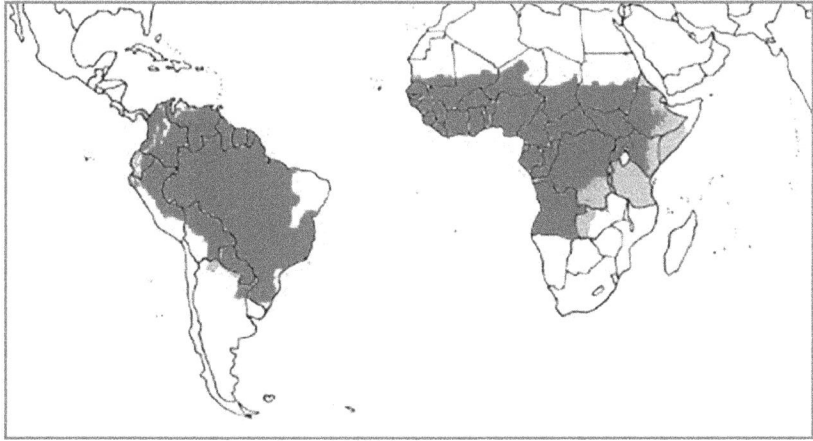

Fig. 1: Endemic countries for yellow fever.

3. What are the symptoms of yellow fever?

The incubation period after infection is usually 3-6 days. Yellow fever can manifest on a wide spectrum, ranging from asymptomatic illness to acute-onset viral hepatitis and hemorrhagic fever. Initial symptoms of yellow fever include sudden onset of fever, chills, severe headache, back pain, general bodyaches, nausea and vomiting, fatigue and weakness. Most people improve after these initial symptoms. However, roughly 15-20% of people have a brief period of hours to a day without symptoms and then develop a more severe form of yellow fever disease. In severe cases, a person may develop high fever, jaundice, bleeding (especially from the gastrointestinal tract), and eventually shock and multiorgan system failure. Roughly 20-50% of people who develop severe illness may die.

4. How is yellow fever diagnosed?

Diagnosis is usually based on blood tests. In acute stages, direct viral diagnosis is made by:
- Detection of yellow fever antigen using monoclonal enzyme immunoassay in serum specimens
- Detection of viral genome sequences in tissue or in blood or other body fluid using reverse-transcription polymerase chain reaction (RT-PCR) assay: Useful in early illness only (first 3-4 days). By the time overt symptoms are present, viral RNA is undetectable. Current recommendations are to test blood samples collected within the first 10 days of symptom onset.[3]

5. Is there any vaccine for yellow fever?

Yes, there is a vaccine available against yellow fever. In 1930s, a live attenuated 17D vaccine was developed by International Health Division of Rockefeller Institute, USA under Dr Max Theiler, who won Noble Prize for that in 1950.[4]

6. What type of vaccine is available?

The vaccine currently being used 17D vaccine is a live attenuated vaccine. Previously there was another vaccine, developed by Pasteur Institute, Tunis, called French Vaccine, but that was discontinued after 1982.

7. How does this vaccine work?

Immunization with this live attenuated viral vaccine produces long-term "active" immunity. The immune system develops a defense against the antigen. This defense is known as the immune response and usually involves the production of protein molecules by B lymphocytes, called antibodies (or immunoglobulins), and to facilitate the elimination of such antigens on subsequent exposure.[5]

8. What are contents in the vaccine?

It contains a freeze-dried powder of a live, attenuated yellow fever virus 17D-204 strain. The powder is mixed with sterile water before use.

When reconstituted (mixed with the sterile water supplied with the vaccine), each 0.5 mL dose of the vaccine contains the equivalent of not less than ≥4.74 log10 plaque-forming units/0.5 mL. The vaccine also contains polymyxin B sulfate, neomycin sulfate, sorbitol, gelatin, sodium chloride, disodium hydrogen orthophosphate, potassium chloride, potassium dihydrogen orthophosphate, water and traces of egg derived protein.

9. What is the dose and route of vaccination?

About 0.5 mL of vaccine is administered subcutaneously. The vaccine mixture is shaken gently to ensure mixing of the freeze-dried powder and sterile water, before each dose is withdrawn from the container into a syringe for injection. The injection needle should not come into contact with disinfectant or spirit (alcohol) as these may reduce the vaccine's effectiveness.

Children aged 9 months or over, adults and elderly all receive the same dose of vaccine.

A single, lifetime dose of yellow fever vaccine is sufficient for most people traveling to endemic areas. CDC's Advisory Committee on Immunization Practices advises additional booster doses for high-risk groups such as—
- Persons who received a hematopoietic stem cell transplant after receiving a dose of yellow fever vaccine and who are sufficiently immunocompetent to be safely vaccinated should be revaccinated before their next travel that puts them at risk for yellow fever virus infection.
- Persons who were infected with HIV when they received their last dose of yellow fever vaccine should receive a dose every 10 year.
- Travelers who plan to spend a prolonged period in endemic areas or those traveling to highly endemic areas such as rural West Africa during peak transmission season or an area with an ongoing outbreak.[6]

10. Is the vaccine safe, affordable and effective?

Vaccination is the single most important measure in prevention of yellow fever. The vaccine has been used for many decades and has proven to be safe having very few adverse effects following immunization (AEFI) and affordable, providing effective immunity against yellow fever within 10 days for more than 90% of the vaccinated population and within 30 days for 99% of people vaccinated. A single dose provides lifelong immunity and costs less than US$ 2.

11. Who should get the vaccine?

In countries where yellow fever occurs, the World Health Organization (WHO) recommends routine vaccination for everyone older than 9 months of age. During an epidemic outbreak, when a mass vaccination campaign is adopted, the vaccine is given to everyone over the age of 6 months (when the risk of disease is higher than an adverse events anticipated from the vaccine). It is not routinely recommended for all in rest of the world. It is basically a traveler's vaccine for majority of the nations. Yellow fever vaccine is recommended for people age 9 months or older who are traveling to or living in areas at risk for yellow fever virus transmission in Africa and South America. Proof of yellow fever vaccine is required for entry into certain countries. For some countries, there are only certain areas where there is a risk for yellow fever; for those countries, more specific information is given in the chart to guide the recommendation for vaccination. So, it is advisable to get country specific prior information before international travel.[7]

12. Is it recommended in infants?

Yes, until and unless otherwise contraindicated. It is routinely indicated in endemic areas in infants more than 9 months of age as well as traveling infants more than 9 months of age. However in epidemic situations, infants above 6 months should be vaccinated, keeping in mind the potential benefits outweigh the risks of vaccination. It is not recommended at all in infants below 6 months of age.

13. Are there more risks in vaccinating those above 60 years of age? If yes, what are other options?

Yes, people aged ≥60 years may be at increased risk for serious adverse events (serious disease or, very rarely, death) following vaccination, compared with younger persons. This is particularly true if they are receiving their first yellow fever vaccination. Travelers aged ≥60 years should discuss with their healthcare provider about the risks and benefits of the vaccine given their travel plans. In addition to considering the adverse effects of vaccine, travelers to endemic areas should protect themselves from yellow fever and other vector-borne diseases. Preventive measures include wearing clothes with long sleeves and long pants and using an effective insect repellent such as those with DEET, picaridin, IR3535, or oil of lemon eucalyptus.

14. What are the adverse effects?

Rare but serious side effects within 10 days of receiving the vaccine:
- High fever, vomiting, increased sensitivity to light, extreme tiredness, neck stiffness, seizure
- Problems with walking, breathing, speech, swallowing, vision, or eye movement, weakness or prickly feeling in your fingers or toes
- Severe pain (especially at night), or loss of bladder or bowel control. Serious side effects may be more likely in older adults >60 years of age.

Common side effects (may occur within 5–10 days after vaccination) include:
- Low fever, general ill feeling, mild headache, muscle pain, weakness, or
- Pain, swelling, or a lump where the injection was given.

15. What are the contraindications for this vaccine?

Contraindications, may be relative contraindication only, are following:
- Infants aged less than 9 months (or less than 6 months during an outbreak, where the risk of disease is higher than an adverse event from the vaccine)
- Pregnant women (unless during an outbreak)
- People with severe allergies to egg protein
- People with severe immunodeficiency
- A neurologic disorder or disease affecting the brain (or if this was a reaction to a previous vaccine)
- A bleeding or blood clotting disorder such as hemophilia
- Guillain–Barré syndrome
- An allergy to latex.

16. It is a live viral vaccine. Does one need to avoid contact with immunocompromised family members?

No. There is no evidence that people who receive yellow fever vaccine shed the vaccine virus. Therefore, there is no need to avoid people including those who are immunocompromised.

17. Does this vaccine contain thiomersal?

No, the USFDA-approved yellow fever 17D vaccine does not contain thiomersal.

18. Is it safe for reproductive age females? Any special precautions needed?

Yes, Yellow fever vaccine has been found safe in reproductive age females too. It has not been known to cause any birth defects when given to pregnant women. Even though being a live virus vaccine, it poses a theoretical risk. It has been given to many pregnant women without any apparent adverse effects on the fetus. While a 2-week delay between yellow fever vaccination and conception is probably adequate, a 1-month delay has been advocated as a more conservative approach. If a woman is inadvertently or out of necessity vaccinated during pregnancy, she is unlikely to have any problems from the vaccine and her baby is very likely to be born healthy.

19. How long is one protected after vaccination?

The World Health Organization's Weekly Epidemiological Record (WER) reveals that the WHO's Strategic Advisory Group of Experts on immunization (SAGE) has reviewed the latest evidence and concluded that a single dose of vaccination is sufficient to confer lifelong immunity against yellow fever disease.

20. Is it necessary to have a certificate of vaccination? What is the validity of this certificate?

Yes, certification is necessary. The certificate is valid after 10 days of vaccination in case of first vaccination (for booster dose, the certificate is valid with immediate effect) and up to 10 years. In absence of a valid certificate, the traveler is quarantined till the vaccine certificate becomes valid or 6 days in case of unvaccinated persons (Incubation period of natural infection) whichever is more. However in 2016, the WHO amended their guidelines to state that one dose of yellow fever vaccine provides appropriate protective immunity for life. As such, all preexisting and new Yellow Fever Vaccine Certificates are now valid for life and countries can no longer require travelers to be revaccinated or receive a booster dose in order to qualify for entry.

21. Where is this vaccine available? Does one need to go to a special clinic to get a yellow fever vaccination?

Yes. Yellow fever vaccine is regulated by International Health Regulations, so only authorized providers can administer the vaccine. Most providers of yellow fever vaccine can also give you other vaccines for travel.

22. How can one know if their destination requires yellow fever vaccination?

To find out which countries require or recommend yellow fever vaccination, check out the following resources:
1. WHO website for yellow fever—for more details on the disease and links to country-specific information
2. World Immunization Chart—for vaccination information for all countries
3. Travel Health Planner—for vaccination information that is tailored to your travel plans.

23. Is there enough stockpile of yellow fever vaccine to deal with any outbreaks? Who manages that stockpile and ensures that the world does not plunge into a crisis of scarcity of vaccine?

Yes, as a strategy the WHO keeps a stockpile of 6 million doses of yellow fever vaccine.

The stockpile is managed by the International Coordinating Group (ICG). In 1997, WHO in partnership with UNICEF, Médecins sans Frontières (MSF) and the International Federation of the Red Cross and Red Crescent Societies (IFRC) created the ICG for the *provision of vaccines* to manage emergency vaccine stockpiles for future outbreaks and coordinate the distribution of vaccines to the areas of most urgent need. ICGs have been established to provide access to cholera, meningitis and yellow fever vaccines.

REFERENCES

1. MedScape. Yellow Fever. [online] Available from: https://emedicine.medscape.com/article/232244-overview. [Last Accessed August, 2020].
2. World Health Organization. Yellow Fever. [online] Available from: https://www.who.int/immunization/monitoring_surveillance/burden/vpd/surveillance_type/passive/yellow_fever/en/. [Last Accessed August, 2020].
3. World Health Organization. Yellow fever laboratory diagnostic testing in Africa, Interim guidance. [online] Available from: http://apps.who.int/iris/bitstream/10665/246226/1/WHO-OHE-YF-LAB-16.1-eng.pdf. [Last Accessed August, 2020].
4. Frierson JG. The yellow fever vaccine: a history. Yale J Biol Med. 2010;83(2):77-85.
5. Siegrist CA. Vaccine immunology. In: Plotkin SA, Orenstein WA, Offit PA (Eds). Vaccines, 5th edition. China: Saunders; 2008. pp. 17-36.
6. CDC. Yellow Fever Vaccine Booster Doses: Recommendations of the Advisory Committee on Immunization Practices, 2015. MMWR. 2015:64(23);647-50.
7. World Health Organization. Country list: Yellow fever vaccination requirements and recommendations; malaria situation; and other vaccination requirements. [online] Available from: https://www.who.int/ith/ITH_country_list.pdf?ua=1. [Last Accessed August, 2020].

CHAPTER 37

Ebola Vaccines

Arun Wadhwa

1. What is Ebola? A new disease?

Ebola virus disease (EVD) or Ebola hemorrhagic fever (EHF) or simply Ebola is relatively a new disease. It was first appeared in 1976 in two simultaneous outbreaks—one in Nzara, South Sudan and in Yambuku village in Democratic Republic of the Congo near the Ebola river, from which the disease takes its name. The disease is fortunately limited to West Africa area.

2. Are there different kinds of Ebola disease?

The Ebola virus (EBOV) belongs to the virus family Filoviridae because it is visible as a filamentous virion on electron microscopy. It is further divided into five species depending on country of origin—(1) Zaire (EBOV), (2) Sudan (SUDV), (3) Reston (RESTV), (4) Taï Forest (TAFV), and (5) the most recent Bundibugyo (BDBV) discovered in 2007. Of these species, RESTV is the only member that has not caused reported human fatalities. The virus causes an acute, serious illness, which is often fatal, if untreated. Fatality rates range from 30% to 90% with average of 50% case fatality rate (CFR).

3. How does the disease spread?

It is thought that fruit bats are natural EBOV hosts. Ebola is introduced into the human population through close contact with the blood, secretions, organs, or other bodily fluids of infected animals such as chimpanzees, gorillas, fruit bats, monkeys, forest antelope, and porcupines. The virus then spreads from person-to-person via direct contact (through broken skin or mucous membranes) with the blood, secretions, organs, or other bodily fluids of infected people and with surfaces and materials (e.g., bedding, clothing) contaminated with these fluids. Ebola can also be spread through needlesticks and contact with objects that have been contaminated with the virus. Sexual transmission has also been reported.

4. Who is the most at risk for contracting Ebola virus disease (EVD)?

During an outbreak, those at higher risk of infection are: health workers, family members or others in close contact with infected people, mourners who have direct contact with bodies during burial rituals and people who have been in contact with, or who have eaten potentially infected animals.

5. What is the presentation of Ebola disease?

The incubation period is 2–21 days (average 8–10 days). Humans are infectious after the onset of symptoms. First symptoms are the sudden onset of fever, fatigue, muscle pain, headache, and sore throat (the dry phase). This is followed by vomiting, diarrhea (the wet phase), rash, symptoms of impaired kidney and liver function, and in some cases, both internal and external bleeding (e.g., oozing from the gums, blood in the stool). It has a very high mortality rate of 50–90%.

6. How is the diagnosis confirmed?

It can be difficult to clinically distinguish EVD from other infectious diseases such as malaria, typhoid fever, and meningitis. Laboratory findings include low white blood cell and platelet counts and elevated liver enzymes. Confirmation is made by detection of antigen or antibody by enzyme-linked immunosorbent assay (ELISA), reverse transcriptase-polymerase chain reaction (RT-PCR), or virus isolation by culture. The World Health Organization (WHO) recommends nucleic acid tests (NATs) for diagnosis and management. Rapid antigen detection tests are also used in remote settings where NATs are not readily available. These tests are recommended for screening purposes as part of surveillance activities; however, reactive tests should be confirmed with NATs. The tests are done on whole blood from live patients and oral fluid specimen collected from deceased patients or when blood collection is not possible.

7. Is there any treatment for the disease?

Like most viral infections, there is no proven treatment available. Symptomatic treatment, supportive care, and maintenance of hydration are the mainstay. However, a range of potential treatments including blood transfusions, plasma replacement therapies, immune therapies, kidney dialysis, and drug therapies are currently being evaluated.

8. It is a deadly disease. How can it be prevented?

Raising awareness for Ebola infection and protective measures can help reduce incidence and transmission. Risk reduction methods should focus on preventing wild animals to human transmission and then human-to-human transmission. Vaccination remains a viable alternative to achieve this goal.

9. Is there a vaccine for the Ebola virus disease?

An investigational vaccine called recombinant vesicular stomatitis virus-Zaire Ebola virus (rVSV-ZEBOV), which has shown to be safe and protective against the Zaire strain of the Ebola virus, is recommended by the Strategic Advisory Group of Experts (SAGE) on Immunization for use in Ebola outbreaks caused by the Zaire strain of the virus. It was approved by the United States Food and Drug Administration (USFDA) in December 2019. Ervebo (MSD) is a live attenuated vaccine and is administered as a single-dose injection. rVSV-ZEBOV was developed by the Public Health Agency of Canada. The vaccine consists of a harmless VSV, which is an animal virus that causes flu-like illness in humans. The VSV has been genetically engineered to contain a protein from the ZEBOV, so that it can provoke immune response to the EBOV. rVSV-ZEBOV vaccine has been proved to be highly protective against EBOV in a major trial in Guinea. Among the 5,837 people who received the vaccine, no Ebola cases were recorded 10 days or more after vaccination. In comparison, there were 23 cases 10 days or more after vaccination among those who did not receive the vaccine. A ring vaccination protocol was chosen for the trial, where some of the rings are vaccinated shortly after a case is detected, and other rings are vaccinated after a delay of 3 weeks.

10. Has this vaccine been used before? Is it safe?

This vaccine, although not commercially licensed, is being used under "expanded access" or what is also known as "compassionate use" in the ongoing Ebola outbreak in North Kivu. This vaccine was also used in the Ebola outbreak in Ecuador in May-July 2018. In 2015, the vaccine was given to >16,000 volunteers involved in several studies in Africa, Europe, and the United States where it was found to be safe and protective against the Ebola virus.

To assess safety, people who received the vaccine were observed for 30 minutes after vaccination and at repeated home visits up to 12 weeks later. Approximately, half reported mild symptoms soon after vaccination including headache, fatigue, and muscle pain but recovered within days without long-term effects. Two serious adverse events were judged to be related to vaccination (a febrile reaction and one anaphylaxis) and one was judged to be possibly related (influenza-like illness). All three recovered without any long-term effects.

11. Why is the vaccine not given to everyone in the Ebola outbreak area?

Although several studies have shown that the vaccine is safe and protective against the Ebola virus, more scientific research is needed before the vaccine can be licensed. The vaccine is, therefore, being used on compassionate basis, to protect persons at highest risk of the Ebola outbreak, under a "ring vaccination" strategy, which is similar to the approach used to eradicate smallpox.

12. What is this ring vaccination strategy? How is it done?

A ring vaccination tracks the epidemic, recruiting individuals at raised risk of infection due to their connection to a patient confirmed with the virus.

Contacts are defined as individuals who, in the last 21 days, lived in the same household, were visited by the patient after they developed symptoms or visited the patient, or were in close physical contact with the patient's body, body fluids, linen, or clothes. The ring is not necessarily a contiguous geographic area but captures a social network of individuals and locations that may include dwellings or workplaces further afield, where the index patient spent time while symptomatic or the households of individuals who had contact with the patient during the illness or after his or her death. Children above 1 year are included, but pregnant ladies are excluded. Experience suggests that each ring may be composed of an average of 150 persons. Participation in this "expanded access" or "compassionate use" of the Ebola vaccine is entirely free and voluntary.

The SAGE recommends vaccination of healthcare workers and frontline workers who may be in contact with Ebola patients.

13. What are the adverse effects and how will it be dealt with?

In the Ebola vaccine study in Guinea in 2015, most adverse effects were typically mild. Vaccinated individuals most commonly reported headache, fatigue, muscle pain, and mild fever. All persons vaccinated will be advised to contact the vaccination team and they will also be visited at home by trained teams to assess their well-being till 2 weeks after vaccination.

14. Are there any vaccines in the pipeline?

Being a highly lethal disease, conventional trials to study efficacy by exposure of humans to the pathogen after immunization are not ethical in this case. For such situations, the FDA has established the "animal efficacy rule" allowing licensure to be approved on the basis of animal model studies that replicate human disease, combined with evidence of safety and a potentially potent immune response from humans given the vaccine. Thus, the studies on vaccine efficacy have largely focused on animal models. Rhesus monkey undergoes a disease that resembles infections in humans whereas guinea pig and mice undergo changes that are different than humans.

Ebola being an enveloped virus, it was suggested that an effective vaccine should induce both cellular and humoral immune responses. The most common approach to elicit such a response is through live attenuated vaccines, but the lethality of the virus made this option untenable because of potential risk of incomplete attenuation. This limitation was finally overcome by gene-based vaccination approaches.

ClinicalTrials.gov, a global registry of trials involving human subjects, lists several Ebola vaccine trials in progress. Ebola Zaire was the strain of the virus that was responsible for the 2014 outbreak; accordingly, all of the vaccine candidates being advanced are designed to prevent that strain. If these vaccines work for Ebola Zaire, it is very likely that the same principles can be applied to the other strains.

A front-running vaccine candidate is a GlaxoSmithKline (GSK) chimpanzee adenovirus vector vaccine. Monovalent (EBOV) and bivalent (EBOV + SUDV) vaccines are being tried.

A vaccine candidate originating from Thomas Jefferson University's Vaccine Center may advance to clinical trials in humans. This vaccine delivers Ebola antigens with an inactivated rabies virus vector. Versions of the vaccine, which have also delivered both Ebola Zaire and Ebola Sudan antigens as well as Marburg virus antigens, have been tested in macaques.

Johnson and Johnson (J & J) in association with Bavarian Nordic has a heterologous prime-boost Ebola vaccine in development. This two-phase strategy starts with direct exposure to deoxyribonucleic acid (DNA) (the "prime") followed by offering the same or similar antigen in a virus that does not replicate well in human tissue ("the boost"). The first dose of the vaccine uses a DNA vaccine called Modified Vaccinia Ankara-Bavarian Nordic (MVA-BN) EBOV that primes the immune system to make Ebola Zaire and Ebola Sudan surface proteins; the boost vaccine Ad26-EBOV (derived from human adenovirus serotype 26 based on AdVac technology from Crucell Holland BV) is based on a recombinant adenovirus vector that delivers an Ebola Zaire surface protein.

Novavax, a biotech company in the US, has developed a recombinant protein Ebola vaccine candidate based on the Guinea 2014 EBOV strain. Their glycoprotein (GP) nanoparticle EBOV GP vaccine uses recombinant technology. A recombinant protein is a protein whose code is carried by recombinant DNA. In animal studies, a useful immune response was induced and was found to be enhanced 10- to a 100-fold by the company's "Matrix-M" immunologic adjuvant and had initiated a phase I clinical trial in Australia. The lipid nanoparticle (LNP)-encapsulated small interfering ribonucleic acids (siRNAs) are able to protect 100% of rhesus monkeys against lethal challenge when treatment was initiated at 3 days postexposure while animals were viremic and clinically ill. The top line phase I human trial results showed that the adjuvanted Ebola GP vaccine was highly immunogenic in humans also.

An additional vaccine candidate, a recombinant adenovirus (rAd) type 5 vector-based Ebola vaccine that contains glycoproteins of the 2014 strain, has been tested in the Jiangsu Province of China. In 2017, the China Food and Drug Administration (CFDA) announced approval of another Ebola vaccine based on VSV. Their findings were consistent with previous tests on rVSV-ZEBOV in Africa and Europe and so the vaccine was licensed in China.

The Russian Federal Ministry of Health is developing a recombinant influenza Ebola vaccine, GamEvac-Combi. The recombinant influenza candidate is proceeding to phase III trial.

15. Are there any other methods of vaccine delivery also being tried?

On November 5, 2014, the *Houston Chronicle* reported that a research team at the University of Texas—Austin was developing a nasal spray Ebola vaccine, which the team had been working on for 7 years. The team reported that in the nonhuman primate (NHP) studies it conducted, the vaccine had more efficacy when delivered via nasal spray than by injection.

Vaxart Inc., a company focused on developing oral recombinant vaccines, is developing a vaccine technology in the form of a temperature-stable tablet which may offer advantages such as reduced cold chain requirement and rapid and scalable manufacturing.

16. How long will the protection last? Will regular boosters be required?

The durability of EBV vaccine-induced protective immune response is best achieved by long-term follow-up or challenging NHPs after a long delay after vaccination. Human volunteers immunized with DNA vaccines demonstrated both cellular and humoral responses 52 weeks after vaccination. After an rAd boost, the titers were maintained for >2 years (J & J vaccine). A single injection of ChAd3 provided 50% protection after 10 months in NHPs (GSK vaccine). A booster with MVA 2 months after ChAd3 injection increased the durability to 100% protection during 10 months including memory T-cell responses. In persistent immunity for the VSV-EBOV (MSD), the only FDA licensed vaccine remains to be determined since data has not been reported regarding long-term protection in NHPs or human vaccinees.

17. Is the vaccine recommended for routine use in high-risk areas?

The EBV vaccine will be primarily indicated in populations identified as high risk for exposure such as hunters, healthcare workers, and family members of people who have EVD, but the trials have reached a very slow pace as the number of infected people has drastically reduced since the control of outbreak in 2015.

With the modern ease of international travel, exposure of infected individuals in high density population can result in catastrophic outbreaks. Efforts are needed to develop an emergency healthcare response system within endemic areas and healthcare mobilization in future outbreaks. GAVI, the Vaccine Alliance has provided US$5 million to Merck toward the future procurement of the vaccine once it is approved, prequalified, and recommended by the WHO. As part of this agreement, Merck committed to ensure that 300,000 doses of the vaccine are available for emergency use.

SUGGESTED READING

1. Centers for Disease Control and Prevention (CDC). (2019). Years of Ebola Virus Disease Outbreaks. [online] Available from: https://www.cdc.gov/vhf/ebola/history/chronology.html?CDC_AA_refVal=https%3A%2F%2Fwww.cdc.gov%2Fvhf%2Febola%2Foutbreaks%2Fhistory%2Fchronology.html. [Last accessed June, 2020].
2. Henao-Restrepo AM, Camacho A, Longini IM, Watson CH, Edmunds WJ, Egger M, et al. Efficacy and effectiveness of an rVSV-vectored vaccine in preventing Ebola virus disease: final results from the Guinea ring vaccination, open-label, cluster-randomised trial (Ebola Ça Suffit!). Lancet. 2017;389:505-18.

3. Pavot V. Ebola virus vaccines: Where do we stand? Clin Immunol. 2016;173:44-9.
4. Ploquin A, Leigh K, Sullivan NJ. Ebola vaccines. In: Plotkin SA, Orenstein WA, Offit PA, Edwards KM (Eds). Vaccines, 7th edition. New York: Elsevier; 2018. pp. 276-87.
5. World Health Organization (WHO). (2016). WHO Essential Medicines and Health Products: Annual Report. [online] Available from: https://www.who.int/medicines/publications/annual-reports/WHO_EMP_Report_2016_Online.pdf?ua=1. [Last accessed June, 2020].
6. World Health Organization (WHO). (2020). Ebola virus disease. [online] Available from: https://www.who.int/news-room/fact-sheets/detail/ebola-virus-disease. [Last accessed June, 2020].

SECTION 3

Vaccines in the Pipeline

38. **Respiratory Syncytial Virus Vaccines**
    M Surendranath
39. **Newer Tuberculosis Vaccines**
    Sangeeta Sharma
40. **Coronavirus Disease 2019 Vaccines**
    Arun Wadhwa
41. **Human Immunodeficiency Virus Vaccines**
    Dipti Agarwal
42. **Cytomegalovirus Vaccines**
    Unmesh A Upadhyaya
43. **Enteroviral Vaccines (EV71)**
    Piyali Bhattacharya
44. **Diarrheal Disease Vaccines other than Rotavirus**
    Shalabh Agarwal
45. **Hepatitis E Vaccines**
    Dipti Agarwal
46. **Hepatitis C Vaccines**
    Abhay K Shah, Aashay A Shah
47. **Zika Virus Vaccines**
    M Surendranath
48. **Chikungunya Vaccines**
    Sachidanand Kamath, Geeta MG

CHAPTER 38

Respiratory Syncytial Virus Vaccines

M Surendranath

1. What is burden of respiratory syncytial virus (RSV) disease?

Respiratory syncytial virus is the most important cause of viral acute lower respiratory infection (ALRI) in infants and young children all over the world. It can affect all age groups including those above 65 years of age. Highest incidence is seen in infants aged < 3 months of age and mortality is also highest among this age group. By the age of 2 years all the children will be affected with RSV. Natural infection will provide limited protection against reinfection. Disease transmission mainly occurs in winter in temperate areas but in tropical countries, it may occur round the year. Globally it is estimated that 33.1 million new episodes of RSV-ALRI occur and leading to 3.2 million hospital admissions and 118,200 deaths in under 5 years aged children. In 2017, the World Health Organization (WHO) estimated that 23% of 2.6 million annual neonatal deaths were due to vaccine preventable infectious diseases and RSV-ALRI prevention is a strategic priority in this age group. In India, various hospital-based studies revealed that RSV detection vary from 5% to 54% per year. Studies using molecular techniques have shown 15–22% per year. In a study conducted by AIIMS, New Delhi, 17% of hospitalized children with ALRI are positive for RSV by centrifugation enhanced culture and RSV is a major pathogen, about 26%, in children with bronchiolitis. In community-based studies from Ballabgarh near Delhi, the incidence rates of RSV infection were 234/1,000 child years (Broor et al.) and 420/1,000 child years (Krishnan et al.). Incidence of RSV is three times greater for preterm infants and 45% of hospitalizations occur in < 6 months of age.

2. What is molecular epidemiology of RSV in India?

Both group A and B RSV have been reported from India. Different genotypes of group A GA2, GA5, NA1, ON1 and group B GB2 SAB4 and BA are reported.

3. What are the risk factors of RSV infection?

Preterm birth, chronic lung disease, congenital heart disease, cystic fibrosis, immunocompromised such as HIV and malignancy, Down's syndrome, neuromuscular disease and very young infants <6 months of age.

4. What are the RSV vaccine strategies?

Depending on incidence of RSV infection, there are two age groups to be targeted:
1. 0–6 months
2. 6–24 months

For the prevention of the RSV infection in infants younger than 6 months, two strategies can be adopted one is maternal immunization which will help for transplacental transfer of antibodies to the new-born and other strategy is protecting the infant with vaccine such as RSV neutralizing monoclonal antibodies.

The RSV disease burden in 6–24 months age group is associated with enhanced vaccine disease in children immunized with formalin killed RSV vaccine in USA in 1960. RSV vaccine development started shortly after first identification virus in humans in 1957. Concerns of enhanced respiratory disease following vaccination with formalin killed RSV vaccine in 1960 has complicated the design and testing of RSV vaccines. Most of the live attenuated RSV vaccines could not maintain balance between safety and immunogenicity. NIH, Serum Institute India, GSK, Novavax, Johnson and Johnson and AstraZenica are developing vaccines, but still they are in phase I/II and preclinical stage. Currently, there is no RSV vaccine licensed even after 60 years of first detection of virus.

5. What are the licensed RSV intervention products?

Only two products are licensed for prevention of RSV infection for seasonal prophylaxis of preterm infants:
1. RSV-IVIG (Respigam)
2. Palivizumab-RSV mAB (Synagis)

The RSV-IVIG was prepared from donors selected with high titers of RSV neutralizing antibody. It was discontinued in October 2003 because cost and logistic difficulties of its use.

Palivizumab is a humanized monoclonal antibody (IgG 1k) developed by Medimmune USA. The US Food and Drug Administration (USFDA) has licensed this product in 1998. It is recommended for high-risk infants once a month during RSV season administered as intramuscular injection as a dose of 15 mg/kg of Synagis. It has resulted in 55% reduction in hospital admissions for RSV illness compared to placebo. Average cost of treatment per season ranged from $3321 to $12,568 per preterm infant.

The American Academy of Pediatrics (AAP) recommendations for monthly prophylaxis with palivizumab are:
- In the first year of life, palivizumab prophylaxis is recommended for infants born before 29 weeks, 0 days' gestation.
- Palivizumab prophylaxis is not recommended for otherwise healthy infants born at or after 29 weeks, 0 days' gestation.

- In the first year of life, palivizumab prophylaxis is recommended for preterm infants with CLD of prematurity, defined as birth at <32 weeks, 0 days' gestation and a requirement for >21% oxygen for at least 28 days after birth.
- Clinicians may administer palivizumab prophylaxis in the first year of life to certain infants with hemodynamically significant heart disease.
- Clinicians may administer up to a maximum of 5 monthly doses of palivizumab (15 mg/kg per dose) during the RSV season to infants who qualify for prophylaxis in the first year of life. Qualifying infants born during the RSV season may require fewer doses. For example, infants born in January would receive their last dose in March.
- Palivizumab prophylaxis is not recommended in the second year of life except for children who required at least 28 days of supplemental oxygen after birth and who continue to require medical intervention (supplemental oxygen, chronic corticosteroid, or diuretic therapy).
- Monthly prophylaxis should be discontinued in any child who experiences a breakthrough RSV hospitalization.
- Children with pulmonary abnormality or neuromuscular disease that impairs the ability to clear secretions from the upper airways may be considered for prophylaxis in the first year of life.
- Children younger than 24 months who will be profoundly immunocompromised during the RSV season may be considered for prophylaxis.
- Insufficient data are available to recommend palivizumab prophylaxis for children with cystic fibrosis or Down's syndrome.
- The burden of RSV disease and costs associated with transport from remote locations may result in a broader use of palivizumab for RSV prevention in Alaska Native populations and possibly in selected other American Indian populations.
- Palivizumab prophylaxis is not recommended for prevention of health-care-associated RSV disease.

The other new generation mAB motavizumab and suptavumab are not approved by USFDA.

6. What are the developments regarding future RSV vaccines?

Due to huge burden of disease, the vaccine industry is relentlessly continuing the research to bring new vaccine. Till 2019, there are 13 vaccine candidates in phase I, 4 candidates in phase II, 1 candidate has completed phase III trials. The candidates include mAbs and vaccines using four different approaches, particle based, live attenuated and chimeric, subunit, and vector based **(Table 1)**.

Out of these RSV F vaccine (ResVax) for maternal immunization and MED18897 RSV mAb are in phase III trials.

TABLE 1: Snapshot of respiratory syncytial virus (RSV) vaccines.

	Preclinical	Phase I	Phase II	Phase III	Market approved
Live attenuated	• Codagenix, LID/NIAID/NIH (RSV) • LID/NIAID/NIH (RSV) • LID/NIAID/NIH (PIV-3/RSV)	• Intrvac (RSV- ΔG) • Pontificia Universidad Catolica de Chile (BCG/RSV) • Sanofi, LID/NIAID/NIH (RSV276, RSV ΔNS2, Δ1313/ I1314L, RSV6120/ΔNS2/1030s) • Meissa Vaccines (RSV) • SIIPL, St. Jude Hospital (SeV/ RSV) pediatric use			
Whole-inactivated	Blue Willow Biologics (RSV)				
Particle based	• Fraunhoper (VLP) • Icosavax (VLP) • University of Massachusetts (VLP) • Georgia State University (VLP) • Sanofi (RSV F Nanoparticle) • Virometix (VLP)	Novavax (RSV F Nanoparticle) For pediatric use	Novavax (RSV F Nanoparticle) For elderly	Novavax (RSV F Nanopaticle) Phase III primary end point not met For maternal use	
Subunit	• Blue Willow Biologics (RSV F Protein) • Sciogen (RSV G Protein) • University of Saskatchewan (RSV F Protein) • Instituto de Salud Carlos III (RSV F Protein) • University of Georgia (RSV G Protein)	• Beijing Advaccine Biotechnology (RSV G Protein) for pediatric and elderly • Immunovaccine, VIB (DPX-RSV-SH Protein) for elderly • GlaxoSmithKline (RSV F Protein) for elderly • NIH/NIAID/VRC (RSV F Protein) for elderly and maternal use	• GlaxoSmithKline (RSV F Protein) for maternal use • Pfizer (RSV F Protein) For elderly and maternal		

Contd...

Contd...

	Preclinical	Phase I	Phase II	Phase III	Market approved
Nucleic acid	• Curevac (RNA) • Moderna (RNA)				
Recombinant vectors	• BravoVax (Adenovirus) • Vaxart (Adenovirus) for elderly		• Bravarian Nordic (MVA) for elderly • Janssen Pharmaceutical (Adenovirus) for peditric and maternal • GlaxoSmithKline (Adenovirus) for peditric use		
Immune-prophylaxis	• Aridis (Anti-F-mAb) • Gates MRI (AnTI-F-mAb) • Pontificia Universidad Catolica de Chile (Anti-F-mAb) • UCAB, mAbXience (Anti-F-mAb)		Merck (Anti-F-mAb) For pedatric use	Astragenica, Sanofi (Anti-F-mAb) For pediatric use	Astragenica, Sanofi (Anti-F-mAb, Synagis) For pediatric use

ResVax: RSV F Vaccine

Novavax, a US based biotechnology company has genetically engineered a novel F-protein antigen resulting in enhanced immunogenicity by exposing these antigenic sites. This RSV vaccine did not show any dose related adverse events in phase I safety trial. Maternal RSV vaccine adjuvanted with aluminum phosphate was evaluated in 720 child-bearing age women with various formulations and followed by first-in-pregnancy study in 50 healthy pregnant women. It was found to be safe and immunogenic with a potential to protect infant early in life through transplacental transfer of maternal antibodies. On the strength of these studies in November 2014, USFDA has granted Fast Track designation and allowed phase III study to assess the efficacy in phase III studies. For the licensure of vaccine in 2015, Novavax launched a global randomized, observer blind, placebo-controlled trial enrolling 4,636 third trimester pregnant woman in northern and southern hemisphere in 5 continents, 11 countries, and 87 sites. The trial was intended to determine the efficacy of maternal immunization with RSV F vaccine against medically significant symptomatic RSV-LRTI through 90, 120, 150, and 180 days of life of infant. Though the study did not meet the prespecified primary clinical end point, the efficacy of ResVax against the primary and two secondary end points in per protocol infants with RSV-LRTI through 90 days of life was 39% against medically significant RSV LRTI (97.5% CI, 1–64%), 44% against RSV-LRTI hospitalizations (95% CI, 20–62%); 48% against RSV-LRTI severe hypoxemia (95% CI, 8–75%). There were no safety issues but USFDA has recommended an additional phase III trial of ResVax to confirm the protection of infants born to vaccinated mother.

MED18897 RSV mAb

It is an investigational recombinant human immunoglobulin GI kappa (IgGIκ) mAb with extended half-life, which can be administered as a single shot before the season or at birth for prevention of severe RSV infection in infants. The product has exhibited potent antiviral activity against diverse panel of RSV A and B clinical isolates in preclinical in vivo and in vitro studies. In phase 2b studies, the product has been found to be safe and has efficacy of 70% (52.3–81.2). There are two multicentric phase III studies in the process in 3,000 healthy late preterm and term infants, and a double blind, palivizumab-controlled study evaluating the safety of MED18897 in 1,500 high-risk infants.

7. Explain the structure of RSV.

The detailed structure of respiratory syncytial virus is given in **Figures 1A and B**.

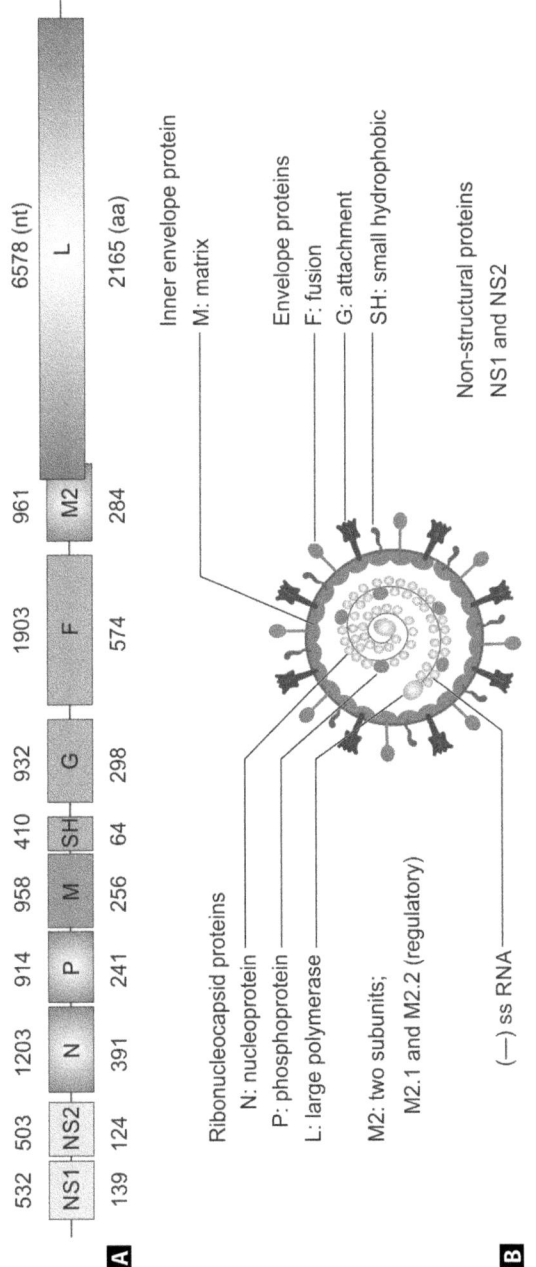

Figs. 1A and B: RSV virion genome and proteins.

SUGGESTED READING

1. Aranda SS, Polack FP. Prevention of pediatric respiratory syncytial virus lower respiratory tract illness: perspectives for the next decade. Front Immunol. 2019;10:1006.
2. Nelson CB, Broor S, Fryzek J, Wairagkar NS. Respiratory syncytial virus. In: Vashishtha VM, Kalra A (Eds). IAP Textbook of Vaccines, 2nd edition. New Delhi: Jaypee Brothers Medical Publishers (P) Ltd.; 2020. pp. 637-49.
3. Taleb SA, Al Thani AA, Al Ansari K, Yassine HM. Human respiratory syncytial virus: pathogenesis, immune responses, and current vaccine approaches. Eur J Clin Microbiol Infect Dis. 2018;37:1817-27.
4. WHO. RSV vaccine research and development. [online] Available from: https://www.who.int/immunization/research/development/ppc_rsv_vaccines/en/. [Last Accessed August, 2020].

CHAPTER 39

Newer Tuberculosis Vaccines

Sangeeta Sharma

1. Why is there a need for a new Bacillus Calmette–Guérin (BCG) vaccine?

The World Health Organization (WHO) targets of the End Tuberculosis (TB) Strategy, reiterated by the UN high level meeting in 2018 can only be achieved with a greater emphasis on prevention and treatment of latent TB infection (LTBI) and later its reactivation into active disease. Conventional BCG vaccine is the world's most widely used vaccine, in use for almost a century now, but it has important limitations. The current BCG vaccine is not very effective in preventing pulmonary tuberculosis (PTB), the most common and infectious form of the disease. Prevention of TB is much more important than cure. New effective TB vaccine can therefore be one of the best strategies to end the menace of both drug sensitive and drug resistant tuberculosis at the global level. Targeting the development of a vaccine better than BCG is thus an important goal.

2. What is the current status of the conventional BCG vaccine being used today?

Cochrane database analyses have shown that BCG vaccine being used today can only protect against dissemination and development of severe, dangerous forms of tuberculosis among children, i.e., tubercular meningitis and miliary tuberculosis. It is not very effective at preventing primary infection with *Mycobacterium tuberculosis (M.tb)* and pulmonary TB. This has an important implication for high burden countries where a huge proportion of population has LTBI. Also, in countries such as Africa, where a large proportion of people with LTBI are coinfected with HIV increases their likelihood of progression from LTBI to active TB disease.

As BCG protection wanes off in 10–15 years, it has a limited role in prevention of reinfection, reactivation and transmission during adolescence. Further, as revaccination with a second dose of the conventional BCG does not boost the immune response to a level that it can prevent reactivation/reinfection, BCG revaccination is fast losing ground and presently there are only five (5) countries in the world practicing it. Brazil stopped this practice based on their countrywide Government-funded trial.

3. What should be the characteristics of an ideal BCG Vaccine?

An ideal TB vaccine should prevent tuberculosis in all the target sub-populations, namely, Mtb-uninfected (pre-exposure) and Mtb-infected, i.e.,

LTBI, TB diseased and TB treated individuals (post-exposure). Pre-exposure strategies include both prevention of infection (POI) and prevention of disease (POD) while post-exposure strategies include prevention of progression of LTBI to active TB disease (POD); vaccination to improve treatment outcomes of TB patients (therapeutic); and vaccination to prevent recurrence of TB disease in treated patients (POR).

The greatest need is to develop a vaccine that works both before and after occurrence of infection. Further, it should be safe, not interfere with the TB diagnosis and if required, also be used as an adjunct to antitubercular chemotherapy. Mucosal delivery would be of a great help in mass immunization programs, and low cost is always a major consideration. It should also not need frequent boosters.

4. What are the challenges in development of the newer BCG vaccine?

A number of challenges have been identified and some of these are:
- Lack of good "protective markers" so that fair randomized controlled tests can be carried out to evaluate the efficacy of the candidate vaccine.
- Animal studies/models provide limited information and cannot be extrapolated on potential human vaccine candidates.
- Most human beings have already been immunized with neonatal BCG or exposed to atypical environmental mycobacteria. This interferes with the "vaccine uptake". Therefore, it may not be possible to find a clean-catch human population for the trial of a new vaccine.
- Moreover, the level of immunity cannot be increased any further in these already immunized or individuals exposed to environmental atypical mycobacteria. Thus, the new vaccine might not give the expected results in these cases.
- There have been concerns on the other hand that induction of a strong postvaccination immune response in some already infected individuals might produce immunopathology and that it would not be possible to exclude such individuals from vaccination settings.

5. What are the other non-TB usages of BCG vaccine?

The non-TB uses of BCG have been described in the following conditions:
- Leprosy
- Buruli ulcer
- As immune modulator in atopy
- As immune modulator for some types of cancers especially bladder cancer, and
- Ancylostomiasis and other helminthic infections.
- Covid19: BRACE trial is underway to assess the efficacy of BCG as an immune booster for health workers during the Covid19 epidemic. The WHO recommendation is to wait for the results of the trial before starting its use.

6. What are the main strategies for developing these newer vaccines?

The main strategies for developing new vaccines are either to boost or modify the already existing BCG or find an alternative to BCG, which are summarized here:

- Modify BCG– Ag, Cytokine, MHC-1 presentation. Recombinant and auxotrophic, e.g., VPM1002 is a recombinant urease-deficient BCG (Nieuwenhuizen et al., 2017).
- Attenuate *M.tb*–Auxotrophic. MTBVAC is a live, attenuated *M.tb* strain with two genetic deletions (phoP and fadD26) resulting in loss of virulence (Walker et al., 2010).
- Naturally attenuated/avirulent – *M. vaccae, M. microti,* etc. DAR-901 an inactivated whole-cell *M. obuense* TB vaccine originally thought to be close to *M. vaccae*.
- Subunit – natural, recombinant, synthetic.
- DNA – CpG motifs, cationic lipids, heterologous host prime boosters.
- Non-mycobacterial living vaccine vectors – *Salmonella*, vaccinia virus, adenovirus, e.g., MVA85A (Recombinant Modified Vaccinia Ankara expressing Antigen 85A), a recombinant vaccinia virus vector vaccine expressing Ag85A of M.tb; or Ad5Ag85A, attenuated serotype-5 adenovirus expressing Ag85A.

  The TB/FLU-04L, a live-attenuated influenza-A that expresses antigens Ag85A and ESAT-6.
- Vaccines with live, attenuated mycobacteria—these consist of vaccines that have been genetically modified to contain the protective antigens of the *M. tuberculosis* or an attenuated mutant strain obtained through genetic engineering. VPM1002 and MTBVAC
- Subunit vaccines (protein, DNA, recombinant natural, synthetic virus vector vaccines or recombinant protein vaccines)—capable of carrying one or more immunodominant antigen the *M. tuberculosis*, that can substitute the BCG vaccine.
    - H56:IC31, fusion protein of three mycobacterial antigens Ag85B, ESAT-6, and Rv2660c in IC31 adjuvant
    - GamTBvac, fusion protein of antigens Ag85A, ESAT6 and CFP10 with a dextran-based adjuvant
    - rBCG30, recombinant vaccine (Ag 85 B)
    - Mtb72F, recombinant vaccine that includes polyproteins, obtained by combining two antigens (Mtb32 and Mtb39)
    - ESAT6 and Ag85B, recombinant vaccine that express polyproteins.

7. What is the recent status of the clinical trials on leading new TB vaccines?

The Preferred Product Characteristics (PPC) developed by the WHO (Schrager et al., 2018) identified two target populations for the new TB vaccines: (1) infants; and (2) adolescents and adults.

Different vaccine candidates are in different phases of clinical trials.

Vaccination in Infants

MVA85A, the first TB vaccine to be tried in infants. However, phase II boost vaccination trial in South African infants with MVA85A did not add to the protective efficacy already provided by the neonatal BCG vaccination (Tameris et al., 2013).

Two live mycobacterial vaccines intended to replace BCG, namely VPM1002 and MTBVAC, have advanced to larger clinical dose defining, efficacy and safety trials in infants of TB endemic countries as prevention of *Mtb* infection (POI) and prevention of disease (POD) trials, respectively (Tameris et al., 2019).

Vaccination in Adolescents and Adults

Pre-exposure Prevention of Infection (POI) in Adolescents

Presently, two novel vaccine candidates being tested in adolescents are:
- DAR-901: Three intradermal injections of DAR-901 or saline placebo or two injections of saline placebo followed by an intradermal injection of BCG were randomized (double-blind) in HIV-negative, IGRA-negative participants with prior BCG immunization has shown to be ineffective as an immune booster (Masonou T et al., 2019)
- ID93 + GLA/SE is being tested in a phase IIa clinical trial (NCT03806686) for safety and immunogenicity as a three-dose regimen among previously BCG-vaccinated, IGRA-negative Korean healthcare workers.

Pre-exposure Prevention of Disease (POD) in Adolescents

- VPM1002 and MTBVAC are also being tested in dose-defining trials in adults in India and South Africa, in preparation for a future pre-exposure POD efficacy trial.

Post-exposure Prevention of Disease (POD) in Adults

A larger phase III trial with a wider age range and epidemiological sites, including India, is underway for M72/AS01E. This vaccine has shown good results in Mtb-infected, IGRA-positive compared to IGRA-negative adolescents and adults in its phase II trials (Day et al., 2013; Penn-Nicholson et al., 2015).

Two fusion TB vaccines having protein subunits of the three mycobacterial antigens namely H56:IC31 (Suliman et al., 2018a); and GamTBvac (Tkachuk et al., 2017) are being tested for their safety and immunogenicity in trials involving both IGRA-negative and IGRA-positive adults with prior BCG vaccination.

Some viral-vectored vaccines are in early stages of clinical trials being evaluated for alternate routes namely the intramuscular or aerosol administration of Ad5Ag85A (Jeyanathan et al., 2016); and intranasal route for TB/FLU-04L.

An inactivated preparation of M. *vaccae* has been tested, though yet to publish results, was a large randomized controlled trial using six-dose, twice weekly schedule among 10,000 Chinese adults with a positive TST followed up for TB disease for 2 years.

Prevention of Disease in High-Risk Populations

Household and close contacts: The WHO guidelines recommend TB preventive therapy for all close contacts in high TB burden countries, regardless of age or HIV status (WHO, 2020). Conducting POD efficacy trials of new TB vaccines among household and close contacts can be an attractive alternative.

HIV infection: Live mycobacterial vaccines such as BCG, VPM1002 and MTBVAC pose a risk for persons with HIV infection (Hesseling et al., 2008); and therefore inactivated mycobacterial, viral-vectored or protein-subunit candidate vaccines, including M72/AS01E, are appropriate for individuals with HIV and other immune-suppressive conditions (Thacher et al., 2014; Kumarasamy et al., 2016, 2018). Severely immune-compromised HIV-infected infants who receive BCG at birth are at risk of developing local, regional and disseminated complications of BCG disease, with an incidence of nearly 1% and higher risk of associated mortality (Hesseling et al., 2009). Recently, updated WHO guidelines make provision for BCG vaccination in stable HIV-infected children on established antiretroviral therapy, as the risk of BCG dissemination significantly declines after immune reconstitution (WHO, 2020).

Prevention of Recurrence (POR)

A POR approach aims at reducing post-treatment disease recurrence or relapse in the form of reactivation or reinfection with a new *Mtb* infection.

Three protein-subunit candidate TB vaccines have entered clinical trials in TB patients. ID93 + GLA-SE has been tested in a two- or three-dose regimen among 60 drug-sensitive culture-negative pulmonary TB patients, in preparation for larger POR efficacy trials in South African population.

The H56:IC31 is currently being tested in South Africa and Tanzania for safety and efficacy as a two-dose regimen given to 900 HIV-negative successfully treated sputum smear-negative drug-sensitive pulmonary TB patients, who are vaccinated at the end of and followed for 12 months for TB recurrence.

The M72/AS01E and VPM1002 are also being tested in multicenter, randomized, placebo-controlled trials among 2,000 successfully treated pulmonary TB patients in India and will be followed up for 12 months for TB recurrence (Van Der Meeren et al., 2018).

Therapeutic Vaccination

Therapeutic vaccination is given during the course of treatment to improve the treatment outcomes including morbidity, mortality and to reduce the risk of TB recurrence (POR). However, safety risk includes the Koch phenomenon.

Meta-analysis of 25 studies involving 2,281 Chinese MDR-TB patients (Weng et al., 2016) and a larger meta-analysis of more than 4,000 DS- and DR-TB patients in 54 studies, 6 conducted in countries, have also reported faster sputum smear conversion and radiographic improvement in *M. vaccae* recipients (Yang et al., 2011). A multidose regimen of heat-killed *M. indicus pranii (M.ip)*, previously known as *Mycobacterium w*, has also been tested on 890 retreatment pulmonary TB patients in a randomized, double-blind, placebo-controlled trial in India (Sharma et al., 2017). The inactivated liposomal formulation of fragmented *M.tb* vaccine candidate RUTI (Nell et al., 2014), is planned to enter a double-blind, placebo-controlled trial for safety and immunogenicity in 27 DR-TB patients after 3–4 months of successful intensive phase treatment.

Thus, new vaccines are required to complement the available and in-pipeline drugs and diagnostics, effective at preventing not only primary and post-exposure latent infection and disease but also reactivation and reinfection respectively. In an optimistic scenario, i.e., assuming that atleast one of the second generation candidates successfully completes phase III (efficacy) evaluation, licensure of a new TB vaccines is not anticipated till then. Until that time, extensive resources are needed to conduct reliable clinical trials. As is with other vaccines in development, particular efforts in the areas of financing, production capacity logistics, etc., must be made to ensure that once a new and effective TB vaccine is available, it can be implemented rapidly to achieve high coverage rates.

SUGGESTED READING

1. ClinicalTrials. BCG Vaccination to Protect Healthcare Workers Against COVID-19 (BRACE). [online] Available from: https://clinicaltrials.gov/ct2/show/NCT04327206. [Last Accessed August, 2020].
2. Dockrell HM, Smith SG. What have we learnt about BCG vaccination in the last 20 years? Front Immunol. 2017;8:1134.
3. Masonou T, Hokey DA, Lahey T, Halliday A, Berrocal-Almanza LC, Wieland-Alter WF, et al. CD4+ T cell cytokine responses to the DAR-901 booster vaccine in BCG-primed adults: a randomized, placebo-controlled trial. PLoS One. 2019;14(5):e0217091.
4. Nemes E, Geldenhuys H, Rozot V, Rutkowski KT, Ratangee F, Bilek N, et al. Prevention of *M. tuberculosis* infection with H4:IC31 vaccine or BCG revaccination. N Engl J Med. 2018;379:138-49.
5. Nieuwenhuizen NE, Kulkarni PS, Shaligram U, Cotton MF, Rentsch CA, Eisele B, et al. The recombinant Bacille Calmette–Guérin vaccine VPM1002: ready for clinical efficacy testing. Front Immunol. 2017;8:1147.
6. Schrager LK, Vekemens J, Drager N, Lewinsohn DM, Olesen OF. The status of tuberculosis vaccine development. Lancet Inf Dis. 2020;20(3):e28-e37.
7. Sharma S. Tuberculosis vaccines. In: Vashishtha VM, Kalra A (Eds). IAP Textbook of Vaccines, 2nd edition. New Delhi: Jaypee Brothers Medical Publishers (P); 2020. pp. 187-93.
8. von Reyn CF, Lahey T, Arbeit RD, Landry B, Kailani L, Adams LV, et al. Safety and immunogenicity of an inactivated whole cell tuberculosis vaccine booster in

adults primed with BCG: a randomized, controlled trial of DAR-901. PLoS One. 2017;12e0175215.
9. WHO. Bacille Calmette-Guérin (BCG) vaccination and COVID-19: WHO position paper. Wkly Epidemiol Rec. 2020.
10. World Health Organization. WHO preferred product characteristics for therapeutic vaccines to improve tuberculosis treatment outcomes. Geneva: World Health Organization; 2019.
11. World Health Organization. Global TB Report 2019. Geneva: Switzerland; 2019.
12. Yang XY, Chen QF, Li YP, Wu SM. *Mycobacterium vaccae* as adjuvant therapy to anti-tuberculosis chemotherapy in never-treated tuberculosis patients: a meta-analysis. PLoS One. 2011;6e23826.

CHAPTER 40

Coronavirus Disease 2019 Vaccines

Arun Wadhwa

1. What exactly is coronavirus?

Coronaviruses are so named because of the crown-like spikes on their surface. There are four main subgroupings of coronaviruses known as alpha, beta, gamma, and delta. Human coronaviruses were first identified in the mid-1960s. There are many types of human coronaviruses including some that commonly cause mild upper respiratory tract illnesses. The seven coronaviruses that can infect people are: (1) 229E (alpha), (2) NL63 (alpha), (3) OC43 (beta), (4) HKU1 (beta), (5) severe acute respiratory syndrome coronavirus (SARS-CoV) (beta), (6) Middle East respiratory syndrome coronavirus (MERS-CoV) (beta), and (7) SARS-CoV-2 (beta). A novel coronavirus is a new coronavirus that has not been previously identified.

2. What is coronavirus disease 2019 (COVID-19)?

Coronaviruses usually infect animals but sometimes viruses that infect animals can evolve and infect people and become a new human coronavirus. Three recent examples of this are: (1) SARS-CoV, (2) MERS-CoV, and (3) 2019-nCoV. On February 11, 2020, the World Health Organization announced an official name for the disease as coronavirus disease 2019, abbreviated as COVID-19. In COVID-19, "CO" stands for "corona", "VI" stands for "virus", and "D" stands for "disease". Formerly, this disease was referred to as "2019 novel coronavirus" or "2019-nCoV".

A diagnosis with coronavirus 229E, NL63, OC43, or HKU1 is not the same as a COVID-19 diagnosis. Patients with COVID-19 will be evaluated and cared for differently than patients with a common coronavirus diagnosis. The first case of the 2019–2020 coronavirus pandemic in India was reported on 30th January, 2020, originating from China.

3. How is it different from other coronaviruses?

Coronavirus disease 2019 is the infectious disease caused by the most recently discovered coronavirus. This new virus and disease were unknown before the outbreak began in Wuhan, China in December 2019. The virus that causes COVID-19 and the one that caused the outbreak of SARS in 2003 are related to each other genetically, but the diseases they cause are quite different.

SARS was more deadly, but much less infectious than COVID-19. There have been no outbreaks of SARS anywhere in the world since 2003.

4. How does it spread?

People can catch COVID-19 from others who have the virus. The disease can spread from person-to-person through small droplets from the nose or mouth which are spread when a person with COVID-19 coughs or exhales. These droplets land on objects and surfaces around the person. Other people then catch COVID-19 by touching these objects or surfaces, then touching their eyes, nose, or mouth. People can also catch COVID-19 if they breathe in droplets from a person with COVID-19 who coughs out or exhales droplets. This is why, it is important to stay >1 m (3 feet) away from a person who is sick. Studies to date suggest that the virus that causes COVID-19 is mainly transmitted through contact with respiratory droplets rather than through the air.

How long any respiratory virus survives will depend on a number of factors; for example, what surface the virus is on, whether it is exposed to sunlight, differences in temperature and humidity, and exposure to cleaning products. Under most circumstances, the amount of infectious virus on any contaminated surfaces is likely to have decreased significantly by 24 hours and even more so by 48 hours.

The risk of catching COVID-19 from someone with no symptoms at all is very low. However, many people with COVID-19 experience only mild symptoms. This is particularly true at the early stages of the disease. It is, therefore, possible to catch COVID-19 from someone who has, for example, just a mild cough and does not feel ill.

The risk of catching COVID-19 from the feces of an infected person also appears to be low. While initial investigations suggest that the virus may be present in feces in some cases, spread through this route is not a main feature of the outbreak. Because this is a risk, however, it is another reason to clean hands regularly, after using the washroom and before eating.

5. What are the signs and symptoms?

The incubation period of the disease is 5–14 days. Some patients may have no symptoms or mild nonspecific symptoms. The most common symptoms of COVID-19 are a new continuous cough and/or high temperature. Some people may also experience muscle aches, tiredness, difficulty in breathing, and shortness of breath.

6. How is it diagnosed?

Laboratory testing for the respiratory COVID-19 includes methods that detect the presence of virus and those that detect antibodies produced in response to infection.

The presence of viruses in samples is confirmed by reverse transcriptase-polymerase chain reaction (RT-PCR), which detects the coronavirus ribonucleic acid (RNA). This test is specific and is designed to only detect the RNA of the SARS-CoV-2 virus. It is used to confirm very recent or active infections. The sample is taken from nasopharynx and oropharynx and the results are available in 2 days **(Table 1)**. Nasopharyngeal swabs can also be tested for antigen and the result is available in 30 minutes.

Detection of antibodies (serology) can be used both for diagnosis and population surveillance. Antibody tests show how many people have had the disease, including those whose symptoms were minor. An accurate mortality rate of the disease and the level of herd immunity can be determined from the results of this test **(Table 2)**.

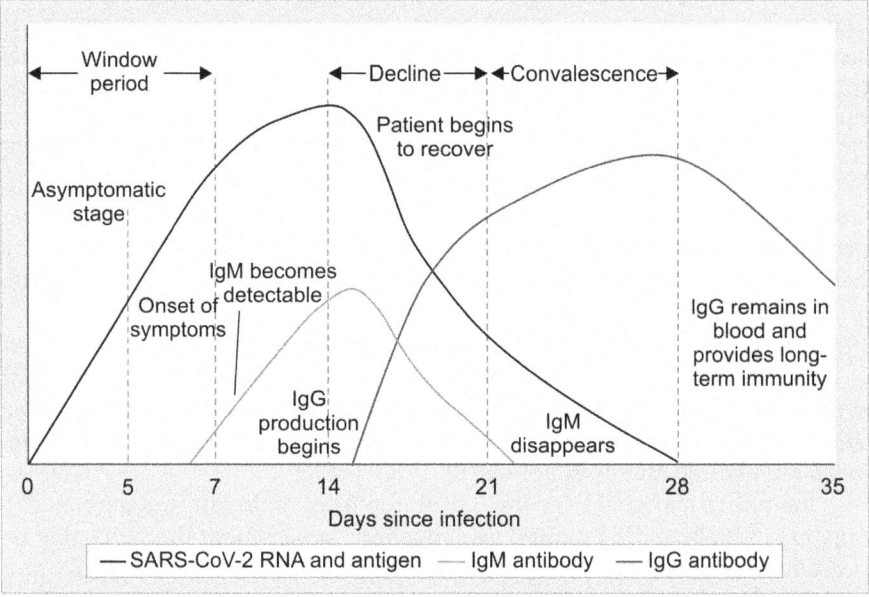

TABLE 1: Interpretation of Covid laboratory results.

Test results			
PCR	IgM	IgG	*Clinical significance*
+	−	−	Patient may be in the window period of infection
+	+	−	Patient may be in the early stage of infection
+	+	+	Patient is in the active phase of infection
+	−	+	Patient may be in the late or recurrent stage of infection
−	+	−	Patient may be in the early stage of infection. PCR result may be false-negative
−	−	+	Patient may have had a past infection and recovered
−	+	+	Patient may be in the recovery stage of an infection or the PCR result may be false-negative

(IgG: immunoglobulin G; IgM: immunoglobulin M; PCR: polymerase chain reaction; RNA: ribonucleic acid; SARS-CoV-2: severe acute respiratory syndrome coronavirus 2)

TABLE 2: Diagnostic test sensitivity in the days after symptom onset.

SARS-CoV-2	Days after symptom onset		
	1–7	8–14	15–39
RNA by RT-PCR	67%	54%	45%
Total antibody	38%	90%	100%
IgM	29%	73%	94%
IgG	19%	54%	80%

(IgG: immunoglobulin G; IgM: immunoglobulin M; RNA: ribonucleic acid; RT-PCR: reverse transcriptase-polymerase chain reaction; SARS-CoV-2: severe acute respiratory syndrome coronavirus 2)

Source: Adapted from Zhao J, Yuan Q, Wang H, Liu W, Liao X, Su Y, et al. Antibody responses to SARS-CoV-2 in patients of novel coronavirus disease 2019. Clin Infect Dis. 2020. [Online ahead of print].

A test, which uses a monoclonal antibody which specifically binds to the nucleocapsid protein (N protein) of the novel coronavirus, is being developed in Taiwan, with the hope that it can provide results in 15–20 minutes just like a rapid influenza test.

A chest radiograph shows signs of bilateral pneumonia. CT findings may be present even before symptom onset. Typical features on CT include bilateral multilobar ground-glass opacities with a peripheral, asymmetric, and posterior distribution. Subpleural dominance, crazy paving, and consolidation develop as the disease evolves.

The Food and Drug Administration (FDA) has approved a test that uses isothermal nucleic acid amplification technology instead of PCR. This method can deliver positive results in as little as 5 minutes and negative results in 13 minutes.

7. What is the treatment of the disease?

Like all viral infections, the treatment is mainly symptomatic. Paracetamol, hydration, oxygenation, and sometimes ventilation may be required. A number of combinations of anti-malaria, anti-Swine flu, and anti-human immunodeficiency virus (HIV) drugs are being investigated. People with serious illness should be hospitalized. Most patients recover thanks to supportive care.

8. What can be done for prevention?

To date, there is no vaccine and no specific antiviral medicine to prevent or treat COVID-19.

The most effective ways to protect yourself and others against COVID-19 are to frequently clean your hands, using appropriate face covers and masks, and maintain a distance of at least 1 m (3 feet) from people who are coughing or sneezing.

9. What are the vaccines being tried?

Like the SARS coronavirus, SARS-CoV-2 is believed to have originated from bats before infecting one or more mammal species sold in Wuhan animal markets. Both coronaviruses bind to similar angiotensin-converting enzyme 2 (ACE2) receptors found in the human lung and SARS-CoV-2 exhibits approximately 89% nucleotide similarly to SARS-like coronaviruses (genus beta coronavirus) found in Chinese bats. On this basis, the shaping of potential SARS-CoV-2 vaccine strategies are built on those advanced previously for SARS.

Whole virus vaccines: Inactivated whole virus and live attenuated vaccines represent a classic strategy for viral vaccinations. A major advantage of whole virus vaccines is their inherent immunogenicity and ability to stimulate toll-like receptors. These vaccines usually take 10–15 years from concept to production. Here, we have a little head start as they have been tested on animals during SARS outbreak. Live virus vaccines, however, require extensive additional testing to confirm their safety. This is especially an issue for coronavirus vaccines, given the findings of increased immunopotentiation like eosinophil infiltrates and increased infectivity after a challenge dose.

Johnson and Johnson is embarking on COVID-19 vaccines, similar to their Ebola vaccine platform. They are employing AdVac® adenoviral vector and manufacturing in their PER.C6® cell line technology. Researchers at the University of Hong Kong have developed a live influenza vaccine that expresses SARS-CoV-2 proteins. Codagenix has developed a technology called "codon deoptimization" to make versions of viruses and viral therapies that are rendered relatively harmless by replacing more virulent pathogens with milder strains.

Subunit vaccines: Subunit vaccines for both SARS coronaviruses rely on eliciting an immune response against the S-spike protein to prevent its docking with the host ACE2 receptor. Under funding from the Coalition for Epidemic Preparedness (CEPI), the University of Queensland is synthesizing viral surface proteins, to present them more easily to the immune system. Another company, Novavax, has developed and produced adjuvanted full length spike nanoparticles that have shown better immunogenic response in mice. Clover Biopharmaceuticals is developing a subunit vaccine consisted of a trimerized SARS-CoV-2 S-protein using their patented Trimer-Tag® technology. They have already used this technology to develop vaccines for HIV, respiratory syncytial virus (RSV), and flu which have proved effective in various animal models. A consortium led by Texas Children's Hospital Center for Vaccine Development has developed and tested a subunit vaccine comprised of only the receptor-binding domain (RBD) of the SARS-CoV S-protein. When formulated on alum, the SARS-CoV RBD vaccine elicits high levels of protective immunity on the homologous virus challenge. An advantage of the RBD-based vaccine is its ability to minimize host immunopotentiation.

Nucleic acid vaccines: Several major biotech companies have advanced nucleic acid vaccine platforms for COVID-19. These could be deoxyribonucleic acid (DNA), RNA, or mRNA based. The concept of immunizing with DNA began with promising results in mice in 1993 showing protective immunity against influenza, but for decades, these findings have not translated to similar findings in humans. More recently, new modifications and formulations have improved nucleic acid performance in humans, with an expectation that this approach might eventually lead to the first licensed human nucleic acid vaccine. Inovio Pharmaceuticals is one company developing a DNA vaccine.

10. Why are messenger ribonucleic acid (mRNA) vaccines being preferred?

Ribonucleic acid vaccines work by introducing an mRNA sequence (the molecule which tells cells what to build) which is coded for a disease-specific antigen. Once produced within the body, the antigen is recognized by the immune system and produces antibodies to fight the real thing. RNA vaccines are faster and cheaper to produce than traditional vaccines and are also safer for the patient, as they are not produced using infectious elements. Production of RNA vaccines is laboratory based and the process could be standardized and scaled, allowing quick responses to large outbreaks and epidemics. There is still a lot of work to be done before mRNA vaccines can become standard treatments.

11. What are the types of messenger ribonucleic acid (mRNA) vaccines?

The mRNA vaccines can be of three types: (1) Nonreplicating mRNA—the simplest type of RNA vaccine, an mRNA strand is packaged and delivered to the body, where it is taken up by the body's cells to make the antigen, (2) In vivo self-replicating mRNA—the pathogen-mRNA strand is packaged with additional RNA strands that ensure it will be copied once the vaccine is inside a cell. This means that greater quantities of the antigen are made from a smaller amount of vaccine, helping to ensure a more robust immune response, and (3) In vitro dendritic cell nonreplicating mRNA vaccine. Dendritic cells are immune cells that can present antigens on their cell surface to other types of immune cells to help stimulate an immune response. These cells are extracted from the patient's blood, transfected with the RNA vaccine, and then given back to the patient to stimulate an immune reaction.

12. Messenger ribonucleic acid (mRNA) is a new concept. Will it work?

The current work with mRNA has been mainly in infectious diseases and cancer. The mRNA vaccines have been experimented for diseases like Ebola and Zika, but no mRNA vaccine has been licensed yet. There are many challenges. Being nuclear material, they may elicit an unintended immune reaction. Delivering the vaccine effectively to cells is challenging since free RNA in the body is quickly broken down. Many RNA vaccines, like conventional vaccines, need to be frozen or refrigerated. Work is ongoing to overcome these problems.

13. Which vaccines have started human trials? What is the current status of development of severe acute respiratory syndrome coronavirus 2 (SARS-CoV-2) vaccines?

Currently, there are around 216 vaccine candidates in various stages of development and 10 of them are already in phase III trial stage. Many different vaccine platforms have emerged, both the traditional technology like recombinant inactivated protein to novel approaches like nucleic acid-based vaccines are on the anvil. This multipronged approach is quite understandable and justified considering the uncertainty over the success of all the candidates, the unprecedented fast-tracking of vaccine development, and the enormous global requirement of the licensed product that cannot be met by a few traditional vaccine manufacturers. Each of these vaccine platforms has got distinct characteristics, "pros and cons", and is in different stages of development.

Eventhough there are >130 candidate vaccines shortlisted currently, there is no specific vaccine available against SARS-CoV-2 virus. 10 of these vaccines have reached the phase III human clinical trial stage. However, the timing for widespread availability of safe and effective vaccines remains unknown. Of the 10, five are being tested by the Chinese companies. They include an inactivated alum-adjuvanted vaccine, *PiCoVacc by Sinovac*, a nonreplicating viral vector, adenovirus type 5 vector (Ad5-nCoV) vaccine by *CanSino Biologics Inc.* in collaboration with the Beijing Institute of Biotechnology, another inactivated Vero cell-derived vaccine by the *Wuhan Institute of Biological Products*, and two other inactivated vaccines by Sinopharm (China) in collaboration with other Chinese institutes. The *AstraZeneca* with University of Oxford in the UK is also testing another nonreplicating viral vector (adenovirus), ChAdOx1 nCoV-19 vaccine. It recently announced the start of a phase II/III trial of the vaccine in about 30,000 adult volunteers with other late-stage trials due to begin in several countries around the world. The US companies are testing two nucleic acid-based vaccines. *Moderna Inc.* has completed a phase I trial of its mRNA-1273 vaccine with the National Institute of Allergy and Infectious Diseases while *Inovio Pharmaceuticals*, Pennsylvania has also begun testing its DNA platform vaccine. The third vaccine developed by the US is protein subunit vaccine called NVX-CoV2373 which is being tested by *Novavax (USA)* that is currently in phase I/II trial (combined phase). Another vaccine, termed as BNT162 and includes four vaccine candidates, each represent different mRNA formats and target antigens, is being developed by the German biotech company *BioNTech* and *Pfizer*.

14. Are Indian companies also involved?

AstraZeneca has entered into an agreement with the Serum Institute of India (SII), among other worldwide vaccine manufacturers, to produce the vaccine currently under trial at the University of Oxford on a mass scale, if successful.

Zydus vaccines India has also two vaccine candidates based on plasmid DNA and a measles-based virus replicating factor vaccine.

Bharat Biotech along with FluGen has begun the development and testing of a nasal vaccine against COVID-19 called CoroFlu. It will be built on the backbone of FluGen's flu vaccine candidate known as M2SR. M2SR is a self-limiting version of the influenza virus that induces an immune response against the flu. The company has also received DGCI approval to test its inactivated vaccine Covaxin. It is an indigenous vaccine that is being developed in collaboration with ICMR's National Institute of Virology (NIV), Pune.

15. When is the earliest that we can expect a vaccine?

As of Oct 2020, most barring 10 of the vaccines are in early stage. Even if they succeed and emergency clearances given, it will not be before 18 months that a vaccine will be commercially available. Any human coronavirus (HCoV) vaccine introduced it will be first given to frontline healthcare professionals (HCPs), paramedics, elderly population, people with high-risk conditions, and then the general population.

16. What are the future prospects of CoV vaccine?

The vaccines under testing now may not be required by the time their commercial production takes place, but the vaccine should be ready, produced, and stockpiled for later use. The aim should be to produce a universal coronavirus vaccine to guard against future epidemics and endemics.

17. Any role of Bacillus Calmette-Guérin (BCG) till we have a specific vaccine?

Although not a coronavirus vaccine but has been in news as it has been shown to increase general immunity against viruses. Until we have a specific coronavirus vaccine, it can be considered to protect high-risk individuals. The correlation between universal BCG vaccination and the protection against COVID-19 suggests that BCG might confer protection against the current strain of coronavirus. BCG vaccination has been shown to produce positive "heterologous" or nonspecific immune effects leading to improved response against other nonmycobacterial pathogens like herpes, influenza, and coronavirus. BCG-vaccinated mice infected with the vaccinia virus were protected by increased interferon-γ (IFN-γ) production from CD4+ cells. This phenomenon was named as "trained immunity" and is proposed to be caused by metabolic and epigenetic changes leading to promotion of genetic regions encoding for proinflammatory cytokines. However, randomized controlled trials using BCG are required to determine the speed and effectiveness of the immune response.

18. Many studies have pointed toward protective role of Bacillus Calmette-Guérin (BCG) vaccines against incidence and severity of coronavirus disease 2019 (COVID-19) in countries that are using BCG vaccine in their National Immunization Program. What is the level of evidence? What is the current World Health Organization (WHO) stand on this issue?

TABLE 3: Impact of BCG vaccinations on the development of COVID-19.

Researcher	Type of study	Publication	Conclusion	Reference/Source
Miller A et al.	Ecological	Preprint	BCG might show long-lasting protection against COVID-19	Miller A, Reandelar MJ, Fasciglione K, Roumenova V, Li Y, Otazu GH. (2020). Correlation between universal BCG vaccination policy and reduced morbidity and mortality for COVID1-9: an epidemiological study. [online] Available from: https://www.medrxiv.org/content/10.1101/2020.03.24.20042937v1. [Last accessed June, 2020].
Berg MK et al.	Ecological	Preprint	Countries with BCG vaccinations show a significantly slower growth rate of COVID-19	Berg MK, Yu Q, Salvador CE, Melani I, Kitayama S. (2020). Mandated Bacillus Calmette-Guérin (BCG) vaccination predicts flattened curves for the spread of COVID-19. [online] Available from: https://www.medrxiv.org/content/10.1101/2020.04.05.20054163v6. [Last accessed June, 2020].
Dayal D and Gupta S	Ecological	Preprint	Universal BCG vaccination has a protective effect on the course of COVID-19	Dayal D, Gupta S. (2020). Connecting BCG vaccination and COVID-19: Additional data. [online] Available from: https://www.medrxiv.org/content/10.1101/2020.04.07.20053272v2. [Last accessed June, 2020].
Hegarty Y et al.	Ecological	Preprint	Lower levels of COVID-19-related cases and deaths rates in countries with BCG vaccination	Hegarty Y, Zafirakis H, Kamat AM, Dinardo A. (2020). BCG vaccination may be protective against COVID-19. [online] Available from: https://www.researchgate.net/publication/340224580_BCG_vaccination_may_be_protective_against_Covid-19. [Last accessed June, 2020].
Li Y et al.	Ecological	Preprint	No significant difference in COVID-19 growth rate and severity between countries with or without BCG	Li Y, Zhao S, Zhuang Z, Cao P, Yang L, He D. (2020). The correlation between BCG immunization coverage and the severity of COVID-19. [online] Available from: https://papers.ssrn.com/sol3/papers.cfm?abstract_id=3568954. [Last accessed June, 2020].

Contd...

Contd...

Researcher	Type of study	Publication	Conclusion	Reference/Source
Sala G and Miyakawa T	Ecological	Preprint	Number of total cases and deaths are significantly associated with the country's BCG policy	Sala G, Chakraborti R, Ota A, Miyakawa T. (2020). Association of BCG vaccination policy and tuberculosis burden with incidence and mortality of COVID-19. [online] Available from: https://www.medrxiv.org/content/10.1101/2020.03.30.20048165v3. [Last accessed June, 2020].
Shet A et al.	Ecological	Preprint	COVID-19-related mortality among countries with BCG policy is lower	Shet A, Ray D, Malavige N, Santosham M, Bar-Zeev N. (2020). Differential COVID-19-attributable mortality and BCG vaccine use in countries. [online] Available from: https://www.medrxiv.org/content/10.1101/2020.04.01.20049478v1. [Last accessed June, 2020].
Curtis N et al.	Commentary	Peer-reviewed journal article	BCG vaccine may provide protection to bridge the gap before a specific vaccine is developed	Curtis N, Sparrow A, Ghebreyesus TA, Netea MG. Considering BCG vaccination to reduce the impact of COVID-19. Lancet. 2020;395:1545-6.
O'Neill LAJ and Netea MG	Commentary	Peer-reviewed journal article	RCTs are needed to provide the highest quality proof	O'Neill LAJ, Netea MG. BCG-induced trained immunity: can it offer protection against COVID-19? Nat Rev Immunol. 2020;20:335-7.
Hamiel U, Kozer E, Youngster I	Large population-based cohort study	Peer-reviewed journal article	The study does not support the idea that BCG vaccination in childhood has a protective effect against COVID-19 in adulthood	Hamiel U, Kozer E, Youngster I. SARS-CoV-2 rates in BCG-vaccinated and unvaccinated young adults. JAMA. 2020;323:2340-1.

(BCG: Bacillus Calmette-Guérin; COVID-19: coronavirus disease 2019; RCTs: randomized controlled trials)

According to some nonpeer reviewed reports, the countries using BCG vaccine in their National Immunization Program are somewhat protected from severe adverse impact of the disease **(Table 3)**. However, most of these preliminary reports are basically anecdotal, ecological studies. They cannot confirm a "cause-effect" relationship of the vaccine with the disease. Recently, the WHO has issued a statement that there is no evidence of BCG-induced protection against SARS-CoV-2 infection. Few countries like Netherland, Australia, UK, and Germany have started BCG trials among healthcare workers to assess its protective effects, if any. The Indian Council of Medical Research (ICMR) is also conducting trials in this regard.

19. Are there any trials to confirm this? Is it the same Bacillus Calmette-Guérin (BCG) what we use now?

A new vaccine, BCG VPM1002, currently undergoing phase III trial for tuberculosis, will be the one being tested for COVID-19. It will be given to doctors, nurses, and elderly in Netherlands, Australia, UK, Germany, and India. If found beneficial, VPM1002 can be manufactured using state-of-the-art manufacturing methods which would make millions of doses available in a very short time.

SUGGESTED READING

1. Clover Biopharmaceuticals. (2020). Clover initiates development of recombinant subunit-trimer vaccine for Wuhan coronavirus (2019-nCoV). [online] Available from: https://pipelinereview.com/index.php/2020012873644/Vaccines/Clover-Initiates-Development-of-Recombinant-Subunit-Trimer-Vaccine-for-Wuhan-Coronavirus-2019-nCoV.html. [Last accessed June, 2020].
2. Hoffmann M, Kleine-Weber H, Krüger N, Müller M, Drosten C, Pöhlmann S. (2020). The novel coronavirus 2019 (2019-nCoV) uses the SARS-coronavirus receptor ACE2 and the cellular protease TMPRSS2 for entry into target cells. [online] Available from: https://www.biorxiv.org/content/10.1101/2020.01.31.929042v1.full. [Last accessed June, 2020].
3. Huang C, Wang Y, Li X, Ren L, Zhao J, Hu Y, et al. (2020). Clinical features of patients infected with 2019 novel coronavirus in Wuhan, China. [online] Available from: https://www.thelancet.com/journals/lancet/article/PIIS0140-6736(20)30183-5/fulltext. [Last accessed June, 2020].
4. Jiang S, Bottazzi ME, Du L, Lustigman S, Tseng CT, Curti E, et al. Roadmap to developing a recombinant coronavirus S-protein receptor-binding domain vaccine for severe acute respiratory syndrome. Expert Rev Vaccines. 2012;11:1405-13.
5. Li Q, Guan X, Wu P, Wang X, Zhou L, Tong Y, et al. Early transmission dynamics in Wuhan, China, of novel coronavirus-infected pneumonia. N Engl J Med. 2020;382:1199-207.
6. University of Cambridge. (2020). RNA vaccines: an introduction. [online] Available from: https://www.phgfoundation.org/briefing/rna-vaccines. [Last accessed June, 2020].
7. World Health Organization (WHO). (2020). DRAFT landscape of COVID-19 candidate vaccines. [online] Available from: https://www.who.int/blueprint/

priority-diseases/key-action/novel-coronavirus-landscape-ncov.pdf?ua=1. [Last accessed June, 2020].
8. World Health Organization (WHO). (2020). WHO Director-General's remarks at the media briefing on 2019-nCoV on 11 February 2020. [online] Available from: https://www.who.int/dg/speeches/detail/who-director-general-s-remarks-at-the-media-briefing-on-2019-ncov-on-11-february-2020. [Last accessed June, 2020].
9. Wu F, Zhao S, Yu B, Chen YM, Wang W, Hu Y, et al. (2020). Complete genome characterisation of a novel coronavirus associated with severe human respiratory disease in Wuhan, China. [online] Available from: https://www.biorxiv.org/content/10.1101/2020.01.24.919183v2. [Last accessed June, 2020].

CHAPTER 41

Human Immunodeficiency Virus Vaccines

Dipti Agarwal

1. What is the biology of HIV virus?

Human immunodeficiency viruses 1 (HIV-1) is an enveloped RNA virus, a lentivirus belonging to the Retroviridae family. The virus was isolated and subsequently identified as the etiologic agent of AIDS in 1983. The viral genome, consisting of two copies of a single-stranded RNA, codes for structural (Gag, Pol, and Env), regulatory (Tat and Rev), and accessory proteins (Vpu, Vpr, Vif, and Nef) **(Fig. 1)**. As in other enveloped viruses, binding of the virus to cell-surface receptors is mediated by the envelope glycoproteins, which play a critical role in initiating the viral infection.

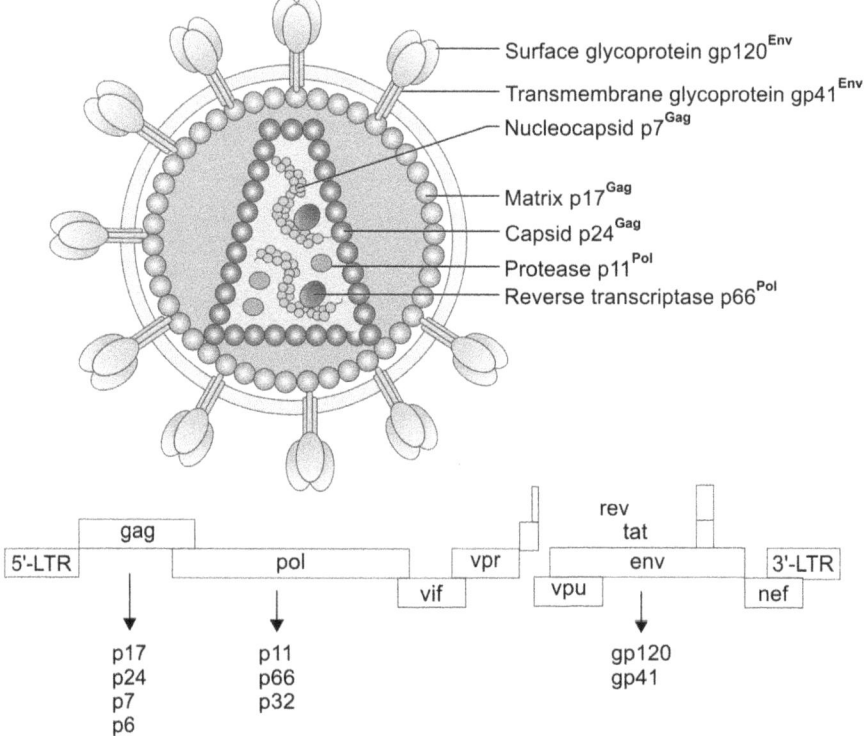

Fig. 1: Human immunodeficiency virus type 1 (HIV-1) genome and virion.

2. What is the need to have an HIV vaccine?

HIV/AIDS is the world's leading infectious disease worldwide. It has been estimated that more than 37.9 million people are living with HIV/AIDS, with about 1.7 million children less than 15 years in 2018. Nearly 32 million people have died from AIDS related illness since the start of the epidemic (end 2018). The extent of prevalence and fatality, therefore, warrants a necessity of the vaccine.

3. Is there any natural protective antibody for the virus?

Broadly neutralizing antibodies or bNAbs have been demonstrated to be naturally produced in some people infected with HIV but have not succeeded in overcoming the virus. Various studies involving neutralizing antibodies in HIV-1 infected individuals can provide information about the response that can help vaccines to be developed to elicit immune responses. Antibodies have been found to bind the CD4-binding region of gp120, gp140 and gp41. It has been shown that these antibodies neutralize the virus by blocking cell receptors. It has been demonstrated that antibodies binding to membrane proximal external region (MPER) of gp41 can prevent virus from fusing with cell and hence can play role in prevention of infection.

4. Is there any passive immunity against HIV?

Passive immunization involves use of intravenous infusions of bNAbs to prevent occurrence of HIV infection. These antibodies have been shown to protect primates. These results suggest that inducing bNAbs by vaccination should provide protection to humans. There are at present no such vaccines which could elicit antibody response. Lack of immunogen is major hindrance in development of such vaccine. Studies are underway to develop antigen-vaccine that can stimulate immune responses and form bNAbs. Studies on immune prophylaxis are also being carried which involves injecting a vector containing bNAbs genes to produce antibodies that may prevent occurrence of HIV infection.

5. Do we already have a vaccine or any possibility to have one in future?

A vaccine should be able to prevent replication of HIV virus and prevent spread of the infection. It should be able to develop both durable cellular and humoral immunity. Currently, none is available but it is possible to have one as the virus is limited to a human host with no known animal reservoir, it is not highly infectious, and natural infection generates both antibody and T-cell responses (body's innate defense mechanisms, which can be instigated/augmented by vaccine).

6. What are the reasons for not having one till now?

Human immunodeficiency virus has many characteristics that make vaccine development difficult: subclinical cases and a carrier state, a long-term

infection process, a nonspecific acute clinical disease, significant antigenic variation, viral DNA integration into the host genome, transmission through infected cells, and destruction or alteration of immunoregulatory cell function. Some of the reasons are as follows:
- High variability of the virus epitopes, the lack of durable immune correlates of protection.
- Viral antigens induce expansion of CD4 T helper cells, which results in increase in B-cells and plasma cells along with IgG hypersecretion resulting in dysregulated antibody production.
- Classic vaccines mimic natural immunity against reinfection generally seen in individuals recovered from infection; till date, there are no study supporting development of an immune responses in a person infected with HIV infection.
- Most vaccines protect against disease, not against infection; HIV infection may remain latent for a long-period before causing AIDS.
- Most effective vaccines are whole-killed or live-attenuated organisms; killed HIV-1 does not retain antigenicity and the use of a live retrovirus vaccine raises safety issues.
- Most vaccines protect against infections through mucosal surfaces of the respiratory or gastrointestinal tract; the great majority of HIV infection is through the genital tract.
- Limitations with the existing animal models and logistical problems associated with the conduct of multiple clinical trials.

7. What is the progress in the development of HIV vaccine?

Many clinical trials of HIV vaccine have been conducted. The first trial was conducted in 1987 at National Institutes of Health. However, most of the trials have reached Phase I/II and six trials have reached clinical efficacy Phase III/IIb. Multiple vaccine concepts and vaccination strategies have been tested, including DNA vaccines, subunit vaccines, live vectored recombinant vaccines, and various prime-boost vaccine combinations. The six trials are summarized here:

1. VAX004 trial was conducted between 1998 and 2003. Although it reached Phase III but did not demonstrate efficacy.
2. VAX003 trial was conducted during same period and it also aimed at humoral immunity and was not successful.
3. STEP trial reached Phase IIb and was conducted between 2004 and 2007. It was intended to see development of cellular response.
4. Phambili trial was stopped at Phase IIb stage after the results of STEP trial as this trial also aimed at cellular response.
5. RV144 trial was conducted between 2003 and 2009. This trial was aimed at humoral and cellular response. It was conducted using canary Pox vaccine and it demonstrated 31.2% efficacy in preventing infection.
6. HVTN505 trial was conducted between 2009 and 2015. It was prematurely stopped. It used DNA capsid and aimed to develop humoral as well as cellular response.

The Thai vaccine trial (RV144) was the major breakthrough; for the first time ever, it revealed that vaccine combination demonstrated a modest efficacy in preventing infection in humans.

8. Give more details about Thai HIV vaccine trial.

The HIV vaccine trial, also known as RV144, was the largest HIV vaccine study ever conducted in humans and involved more than 16,000 volunteers in Thailand. RV144 evaluated the safety and efficacy of a prime-boost combination of two vaccine components given in sequence The trial tested a "prime-boost" combination of two vaccines: (1) ALVAC HIV vaccine (the prime), and (2) AIDSVAX B/E vaccine (the boost). Harmless virus was used as a vector to deliver HIV genes and the boost contained a protein found on the HIV surface. The vaccine combination was based on HIV strains that are found commonly in Thailand. Results of the trial show that this (ALVAC-HIV and AIDSVAX B/E) vaccine regimen may reduce the risk of HIV infection in a community-based population. The regimen was found to be safe and demonstrated an efficacy of 31.2% in preventing HIV infection. The trial showed modest success and provided guideline for further clinical research for HIV vaccines. However, the vaccination did not alter the CD4 count or the viral load. The trial guided researchers to identify the factors that protected some of the recipients from HIV infection. Those participants of RV144 trial who produced high levels of immunoglobulin G were found to bind to part of the envelope V1V2 and were protected against virus. Whereas those vaccines with high levels of envelope-binding antibody belonging to the IgA family appeared to have less protection from the virus.

9. How ethical are HIV vaccine trials?

Prevention trials are complex in nature — you are enrolling people at risk of HIV who are HIV-negative. But overall, today's trials are conducted incredibly well. UNAIDS and the World Health Organization have come up with good guidance on conducting clinical trials.

10. What are the innovations in vaccine development?

New strategies examining heterologous vector prime-boost, universal inserts, replicating vectors, and novel protein or adjuvant immunogens are being explored to induce T-cell and antibody responses. HIV vaccine development requires innovative ideas and a sustained long-term commitment of scientists, governments, and the community. Innovations in vaccine development have included the following:
- *Protein subunit:* Vaccine using envelop protein such as gp160, gp120 and gp140 have been developed. They can produce neutralizing antibody and activate CD4 T-cells but do not develop CD8 response.
- *Adjuvants:* AIDSVAX B/B' vaccine (VaxGen), employed recombinant gp120 envelope proteins, and a primary clade B isolate (GNE8), with

alum salts as adjuvant, showed good safety and immunogenicity in Phase I and II trials.
- *Virus-like particles (VLPs):* They combine a viral vector with the desired antigen. However, recent trials based on VLPs have not been encouraging. AVX101, a VEEV replicon-based vaccine with promising results are in preclinical stage.
- *Live recombinant vaccines:* They involve use of a viral vector with required genes to be introduced into the host cell. The most used viral vectors are poxviruses.
- *DNA vaccines:* They involve use of non-living, non-replicating, non-transmissible plasmids, which are taken up by host cells. They encode proteins expressed by host tissues which can promote antigenic presentation. However, these vaccines have been shown to induce low immunogenicity, due a low DNA uptake.
- *Lipoidal biocarriers:* They improve bioavailability, delay elimination. CAF01, a liposomal system has been shown to build strong humoral and T helper response. Virosomes are reconstituted viral envelop lipid bilayers that function as antigen carriers. Both T helper and CD8 cells are developed in response to it. Antibody production is also stimulated by the virosomes.

11. What is mucosal immunity?

Mucosal immunity will help protecting against entry of virus and hence provide protection against systemic infection also. In rhesus monkeys, administration of oral inactivated vaccine was found to be effective in inducing vaginal and rectal IgA antibody. Studies have also demonstrated mucosal CD8 responses with systemic immunization. Recently virosome in a study was given intramuscularly followed by intranasal route. This effort could be the beginning of a new class of vaccines.

12. What is the way forward for HIV vaccine development?

Since HIV-1 was identified, development of a preventive vaccine has been a major goal. An effective HIV vaccine is a global health priority. Of the various HIV vaccine trials, only Thai trial has showed modest protection in human clinical trial **(Table 1)**.

National Institute of Allergy and Infectious Diseases (NIAID) and its partners have continued to conduct further trials based on modest success of Thai vaccine trial. Numerous investigational vaccines are at different stages of development. Researchers are developing novel prime-boost regimens that elicit strong, long-lasting protective immune responses. The Pox-Protein Public-Private Partnership, or P5, have been working to build on the modest success of RV144. Results from HVTN 702, a vaccine efficacy trial in South Africa are to come by the end of the year 2020. Two investigational vaccines based on "mosaic" immunogens—vaccine components comprising elements from multiple HIV subtype are also being developed so as to provide immune protection against the wide variety of global HIV strains.

TABLE 1: HIV clinical trials, rationale design and outcome.

Study	Regimen	Participants	Aim	Outcome
VAX004 (United States, Netherlands)	rgp120 B/B	MSM, high-risk women	bnAbs	No prevention of HIV infection
VAX003 (Thailand)	rgp120 B/E	Drug users	bnAbs	No prevention of HIV infection
Step/JVTN502 (USA)	rAd5 HIV-1 gag/pol/nef B	MSM, high-risk women	CD8 + T-cells	Increased infection risk
Phambili/HVTN503 (South Africa)	rAd5 HIV-1 gag/pol/nef B	Heterosexual men, women	CD8 + T-cells	Increased infection risk
HVTN505	*DNA/rAd5	MSM, trangender women	Ab and T-cells	No infection risk, no efficacy
RV144 (Thailand)	*ALVAC-HIV/AIDSVAX B/F gp 120 in alum	High-risk men and women	Ab and T-cells	31.2% vaccine efficacy

(r: recombinant; MSM: men who have sex with men; bnAbs: broadly neutralizing antibodies; *: prime-boost regimen)

Source: Trovato M, D'Apice L, Prisco A, De Berardinis P. HIV vaccination: a roadmap among advancements and concerns. Int J Mol Sci. 2018;19(4):1241.

In 2017, NIAID started large clinical trial to assess safety and efficacy of vaccine against HIV in women in southern Africa. The trial is called Imbokodo or HVTN 705/HPX2008. In 2019, NIAID and partners have started complementary phase III HIV vaccine trial to assess an investigational vaccine regimen for safety and efficacy among men who have sex with men and transgender people. The trial is called HPX3002/HVTN 706 or Mosaico, is taking place at multiple clinical research sites in North America, South America and Europe.

SUGGESTED READING

1. Fast PE, Kaleebu P. HIV vaccines: current status worldwide and in Africa. AIDS 2010;24(Suppl)4:S50-60.
2. Kim JH, Rerks-Ngarm S, Excler JL, Michael NL. HIV vaccines: lessons learned and the way forward. Curr Opin HIV AIDS. 2010;5(5):428-34.
3. Lema D, Garcia A, De Sanctis JB. HIV Vaccines: a brief overview. Scand J Immunol. 2014;80(1):1-11.
4. National Institute of Health. (2020). An Empirical Approach to HIV Vaccine Development. [online] Available from: http://www.niaid.nih.gov/emperical. [Last Accessed August, 2020].
5. Rerks-Ngarm S, Pitisuttithum P, Nitayaphan S, Kaewkungwal J, Chiu J, Paris R, et al. Vaccination with ALVAC and AIDSVAX to prevent HIV-1 infection in Thailand. N Engl J Med. 2009;361(23):2209-20.
6. Trovato M, D'Apice L, Prisco A, De Berardinis P. HIV vaccination: a roadmap among advancements and concerns. Int J Mol Sci. 2018;19(4):1241.

CHAPTER 42

Cytomegalovirus Vaccines

Unmesh A Upadhyaya

1. What are the key characteristics of cytomegalovirus (CMV)?

Cytomegalovirus (CMV) is a genus of viruses in the order Herpesvirales, in the family Herpesviridae, in the subfamily β-herpesvirinae. Human serves as a natural host. The virus only replicates in human cells (**Fig. 1**). Human CMV is the most studied of all CMVs. It is a large and complex virus encoding at least 200 proteins. The CMV has got the largest genome of human herpes viruses that has 235,000 base pairs.

2. What is the spectrum of diseases caused by cytomegalovirus (CMV) in humans?

Cytomegalovirus infections are generally asymptomatic in healthy individuals but may produce an infectious mononucleosis-type illness in around 10% of older children and adults after primary infections.

Three types of infection are possible with CMV virus: primary, reactivation or reinfection, if pretransplant IgG antibodies in the recipient are also considered. The risks and severity of infection and disease are highest after primary infection and lowest after reactivation.

After *primary infection*, the virus becomes latent but in certain immunocompromised individuals, may reactivate from latency to cause disease.

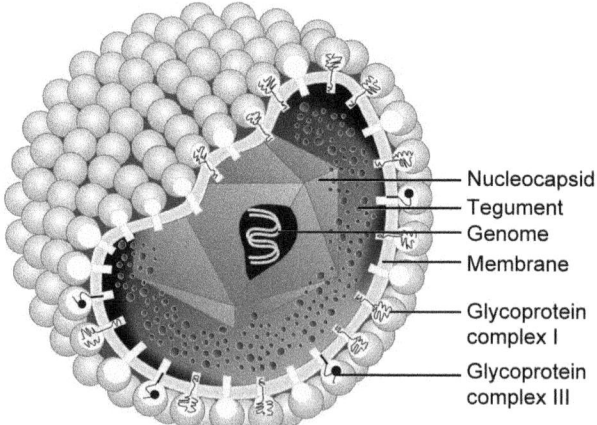

Fig. 1: A schematic representation of cytomegalovirus.

CMV can infect placental cytotrophoblasts and from there infect the fetus. It can also spread from the organs of seropositive donors to seronegative recipients.

The most common disease entity caused by CMV is *congenital infection* to fetus that results in hearing loss along with microcephaly, mental retardation, hepatosplenomegaly, and thrombocytopenic purpura. CMV infection is also suspected in contributing to arteriosclerosis and immunosenescence and may promote cancers through an oncomodulatory effect (such as glioblastoma). It may also lead to poor response to influenza vaccine in infected individuals.

3. Does cytomegalovirus (CMV) infection pose a significant disease burden?

Prevalence of congenital CMV infection is much higher in developing low- and middle-income countries (LMICs). In India and Nigeria, prevalence of congenital CMV infection ranges from 1% to 2% of annual live births that translate into huge numbers. In India, approximately 270,000–540,000 infants would be born annually with congenital CMV infection.

Cytomegalovirus infection is the most common infection after transplants of solid organs as well as hematogenous stem cell. In hematopoietic stem cell transplants (HSCTs), CMV reactivation in seropositive recipients occurs in 70–80%.

4. Why do we need vaccines against cytomegalovirus (CMV) infection?

There is a significant public health impact of congenital CMV infection as stated above. The diseases caused by the CMV result in substantial cost to society, however, this aspect is not yet fully explored. According to one estimate, the congenital CMV infections may cost approximately $1.9 billion to the US healthcare system annually. Despite the availability of a partially effective antiviral therapy, development of a CMV vaccine is the most promising strategy for addressing the burden of congenital CMV.

5. Which is the age group of people most affected by the cytomegalovirus (CMV) infection?

Cytomegalovirus can infect people of all age groups. According to the Centers for Disease Control and Prevention (CDC), over half of the adults have been infected with CMV by the age of 40 years and at least one in three children have already been infected by the age of 5 years. The CMV infection can cause health issues for those with a weakened immune system, including transplant recipient. CMV also causes congenital neonatal infection.

6. What are the objectives and goals of cytomegalovirus (CMV) vaccination?

It is important to distinguish the various situations in which a CMV vaccine would be useful. The most obvious is to immunize a seronegative woman against primary CMV infection. However, it is known that seropositive women may also be reinfected by CMV. A key question is whether the risk to the fetus is as great during reinfection as in the situation of primary infection. The results of several studies argue that the risk of fetal infection is considerably lower if the mother is seropositive, or in other words, immunity strongly protects against intrauterine infection. Nevertheless, as seropositive women sometimes do transmit CMV to their fetuses, an open question is whether their immunization can add to protection.

The CMV vaccines may have multiple indications. Broadly, the main objectives of a CMV vaccine would be the following:
- To prevent congenital infection in infants of seronegative women, and if possible seropositive women.
- To prevent CMV infection in transplant recipients:
  - Seronegative solid organ transplant (SOT) recipients at high risk of primary infection
  - Seropositive bone marrow transplant patients at high risk of reactivation.

7. Who should be the key target groups to vaccinate with a cytomegalovirus (CMV) vaccine?

Once licensed, a CMV vaccine could be given to girls at the age of puberty, women contemplating pregnancy, and even universally to toddlers in order to reduce their excretion of CMV and resultant contact exposure of their mothers. Apart from young women and adolescents, immunocompromised individuals particularly transplant recipients, who are at high risk for the disease should be targeted for CMV immunization **(Box 1)**. Considering the probable role of CMV infection in the pathogenesis of different conditions such as atherosclerosis, autoimmune diseases, immunosenescence and malignancies, impact on clinical course of sepsis, burn, and trauma, and immune responses to influenza vaccination, a case of universal vaccination of all individuals can be contemplated.

8. What should be the optimal timing for administration of a cytomegalovirus (CMV) vaccine?

The aim of the CMV vaccine is to prevent congenital infections that may depend on the age dependent seroprevalence in the population being vaccinated. If we vaccinate toddlers and young children, it will give strong indirect protection to women, many of whom are infected by their first child

---

BOX 1: Probable first targets for cytomegalovirus vaccination.
- Girls 11–13 years of age [association with human papillomavirus (HPV), tetanus, diphtheria, and pertussis (Tdap), meningococcal conjugate vaccines (MCV4)]
- Seronegative women of childbearing age
- All infants, to reduce viral circulation
- Solid organ transplant recipients
- Hematogenous stem cell transplant recipients.

during subsequent pregnancy. If the duration of vaccine induced immunity is long, then CMV vaccine can be given to preadolescents at the same age with HPV vaccine.

9. **What are the important cytomegalovirus (CMV) encoded proteins targeted the development of a CMV vaccine?**
- *gB glycoprotein*: gB glycoprotein is included in most of the studies as a vaccine and generates neutralizing antibodies. Antibodies to gB prevent entry into fibroblasts. The gB has boosted antibodies in seronegative as well seropositive women. The gB is also reducing CMV disease in recipients of SOTs.
- *Pentamer protein complex (gH, gL, and UL128-131)*: Pentamer generates most of the neutralizing antibodies in humans and prevent entry of CMV into epithelial cells. Studies done in Italy concluded that the immune response most closely correlated with prevention of transmission of CMV from infected seronegative pregnant women to their fetuses was antibody to pentamer.
- *pp65*: pp65 is the most important inductor of cytotoxic T-lymphocyte immune response.
- *IE 1/2* (immediate-early antigen) are also included in some vaccines for strong T-cell immune response.

10. **What is the status of cytomegalovirus (CMV) vaccine development?**

As of today, there is no licensed vaccine available. However, both live attenuated and inactivated CMV vaccines are under various stages of development **(Box 2 and Table 1)**.

11. **What are the key live attenuated vaccines in development?**

Two vaccine strains were attenuated starting with viruses that had been isolated for laboratory work **(Box 2)**.
- *AD169*: Elicited CMV-specific antibodies in seronegative vaccine recipients. However, significant injection-site and systemic reactogenicity limited its further development.
- *Towne vaccine*: Towne strain elicited both humoral and cellular immune responses in the vaccinees. Recipients of kidney transplants who were administered the Towne attenuated strain virus were shown to be highly protected against serious CMV disease and rejection of the graft. Protection against infection, however, was not statistically significant. The Towne vaccine could protect humans against a challenge with unattenuated CMV, but naturally acquired immunity protected against a higher dose challenge than did the vaccine. Moreover, the Towne strain failed to prevent natural acquisition of CMV by women exposed to children in daycare. Stanley A Plotkin developed this strain.
- *Recombinants with wild virus (Towne-Toledo chimera vaccines)*: An attempt was made to increase the immunogenicity of the Towne

BOX 2: Cytomegalovirus candidate vaccines evaluated in clinical trials.

- Live attenuated and disabled virus vaccines:
  - AD169 vaccine
  - Towne vaccine (± rhIL12)
  - Towne/Toledo chimera vaccines
  - V160–001 replication-defective vaccine
- Inactivated, subunit vaccines:
  - Glycoprotein B (CHO cell expression) MF59 (Sanofi)/AS01 (GSK) adjuvants
  - PADRE-pp65-CMV and Tet-pp65-CMV fusion peptide vaccines ± CpG DNA adjuvant
  - eVLP gB vaccine (HEK cells) ± alum adjuvant
  - Glycoprotein B/canarypox vector
  - pp65 (UL83)/canarypox vector
  - gB/pp65/IE1 trivalent DNA vaccine; gB/pp65 bivalent DNA vaccine
  - gB/pp65/IE1 alphavirus replicon trivalent vaccine
  - gB/pp65 LCMV bivalent vectored vaccine.

(CMV: cytomegalovirus; CpG: cytosine phosphate guanine; CTL: cytotoxic T lymphocyte cell; HCMV: human cytomegalovirus; IE1: immediate-early antigen 1; IL: interleukin; LCMV: lymphocytic choriomeningitis virus; PC: pentameric complex; rhIL: recombinant human interleukin)

TABLE 1: Candidate cytomegalovirus vaccines, targets, and their developers in various stages of development.

Developer/Sponsor	Types of vaccine	Stage of development	Target
Merck	Live, replication-defective	Phase II	Cong
Sanofi	gB, pentamer subunit	Phase I–II	Cong
City of Hope	pp65 subunit, adjuvant	Phase I	Txp
City of Hope	MVA presenting pp65, IE1, IE2	Phase II	Txp
GSK	gB, pentamer subunit, adjuvant	Preclinical	Cong
Hookipa	LCMV Vector gB, p65	Phase I	Txp
Variations Bio	gB	Phase I	Cong
Moderna	gB, pentamer RNA	Phase I	Cong
Serum Institute of India	Dense bodies	Preclinical	Cong
Queensland Institute	gB, pp65, p50 polypeptide with TLR-9 adjuvant	Preclinical	Cong
Pfizer	?	Preclinical	Cong
Astellas	DNA	Failure	Txp

(Cong: congenital; IE: immediate-early antigen; LCMV: lymphocytic choriomeningitis virus; TLR: toll-like receptor; Txp: transplant)

attenuated virus by making recombinants with the Toledo low passage "wild" CMV. Four recombinants were tested in small numbers of humans and one turned out to be suitably immunogenic. This chimeric vaccine has got reasonable safety profile with no evidence for latency or viral shedding in CMV-seropositive subjects. However, there is no efficacy data available and further studies are not being pursued.

- *Replication-defective virus vaccine*: Another approach adopted later was development of a replication-defective virus that in principle combines safety with immunogenicity. This candidate is made in cell culture using a CMV with two proteins rendered potentially unstable by chemical combination but stabilized by a chemical called Shld 1. On injection into humans in the absence of Shld 1, the virus cannot form infectious particles but does express immunogenic proteins. In phase 1 trials, the replication-defective virus gave good immune responses. This concept allows inclusion of pentameric complex in the candidate and T-cell mediated immunity is provided.
- *Vectored vaccines*: Several vaccine candidates are based on vectored genes of CMV, in particular gB and the tegument phosphoprotein 65 (pp65) (*see* **Fig. 1**). Immunogenicity has been demonstrated, and safety in some cases. In principle, they should be protective in transplant patients and perhaps in seronegative normal subjects. One such vectored vaccine with canarypox vector and glycoprotein B was developed by Sanofi Pasteur. This vector vaccine has shown favorable safety profile and a "prime-boost" effect upon combined administration with Towne strain. However, the suboptimal immunogenicity is still a limitation.

12. What are different inactivated cytomegalovirus (CMV) vaccines under development?

- *Glycoprotein B (gB) vaccine with adjuvants (MF59 & ASO1)*: The subunit vaccines employing surface protein of CMV called glycoprotein B or gB is one of the most promising strategies for a future CMV vaccine. Both GSK and Sanofi are developing gB-based subunit vaccines with adjuvants. When combined with the MF59 oil-in-water adjuvant, good levels of neutralizing antibodies were produced in humans after three injections over a 6-month period with a 0-1-6 month schedule.
  Additionally, when the subunit gB protein was combined with the AS01 adjuvant that stimulates toll-like receptor (TLR) 4, higher and more prolonged levels of anti-gB antibodies were elicited in humans, but that adjuvanted vaccine was never tested for efficacy.
- *Soluble pentameric vaccines*: The pentameric complex of proteins were present on the surface of CMV and that this structure, consisting of glycoprotein H (gH), glycoprotein L (gL), and the products of genes UL128, 130, and 131, elicited far more neutralizing antibodies than gB. A pentameric vaccine elicits CMV neutralizing antibodies at titers 1,000-fold higher than in convalescent sera. Studies done in Italy demonstrated that in pregnant women infected by CMV, a rapid response to the pentameric complex was associated with protection against transmission to the fetus.
- *Other inactivated candidate vaccines*: They include DNA plasmids, self-replicating RNA, peptides, virus-like particles (eVLP), and dense bodies (*see* **Box 2 and Table 1**). DNA plasmids coding for pp65 and gB have shown efficacy in transplant recipients. Although early studies of DNA

plasmids looked promising, later studies did not, possibly because they did not induce cellular responses. In addition, an eVLP with gB on the surface has shown high induction of neutralizing antibodies in animals. The pp65-derived peptides combined with a tetanus toxin epitope have been found immunogenic in man, and so-called "dense bodies" harvested from cell cultures of CMV, contain all of the viral antigens needed for an effective vaccine. Serum Institute of India was also developing a CMV vaccine with dense bodies.

13. What are the challenges to develop an effective cytomegalovirus (CMV) vaccine?

Reinfection with new strain or reactivation of latent infection may lead to severe CMV disease. These observations complicate CMV vaccine design and suggest that:
- For full protection, a CMV vaccine may need to stimulate immune response superior to natural immunity response.
- There may be a strong rationale for vaccinating seropositive individuals with goal of increasing immunity and preventing infections. Thus, major question is how to prevent human CMV infection of seronegative women during pregnancy and also possible seropositive women. More research is needed to augment immunity against CMV by vaccination in seropositive women. There is no known absolute immune correlate of protection for CMV vaccine.

14. Which candidate vaccines are in the most advanced stage of development at present?

- *Merck*: The Merck candidate is a replication-defective virus vaccine (V160), which becomes defective by coupling of two genes of the virus with an inhibitory chemical, the effect of which is neutralized by placing another chemical called Shld 1 in cell cultures producing the virus. This vaccine is currently in phase II.
- *Sanofi (Canarypox vector based)*: Sanofi vaccine consists of the gB glycoprotein, pentameric protein, MF59 oil in water adjuvant and antibodies against which it appears to correlate with protection against transmission from mother to fetus. This vaccine is currently in phase II.
- *City Hope CMV PepVax*: It is peptide vaccine, which prevents human cytomegalovirus (HCMV) disease in transplant patient and is now in phase III.
- *Moderna (mRNA-1647)*: This vaccine produces an immune response against pentamer and gB antigens to prevent CMV infection. This vaccine has currently completed phase II.
- *City of Hope Triplex vaccine*: It is a viral vector vaccine. Three types of antigens are used; pp65, IE-1-exone-4, and IE2-exone-5. This vaccine is in phase II currently (*see* **Table 1**).

15. What are the unanswered questions about prevention of cytomegalovirus (CMV)?

- Whether infection in seropositive can be prevented by induction of antibodies or cellular responses?
- If T-cell responses are needed to prevent infection in seronegative women?
- Can protective responses prolong over the age of childbearing?

SUGGESTED READING

1. Bernstein DI, Munoz FM, Callahan ST, Rupp R, Wootton SH, Edwards KM, et al. Safety and efficacy of a cytomegalovirus glycoprotein B (gB) vaccine in adolescent girls: a randomized clinical trial. Vaccine. 2016;34(3):313-9.
2. Cannon MJ, Schmid DS, Hyde TB. Review of cytomegalovirus seroprevalence and demographic characteristics associated with infection. Rev Med Virol. 2010;20(4):202-13.
3. Diamond DJ, La Rosa C, Chiuppesi F, Contreras H, Dadwal S, Wussow F, et al. A fifty-year odyssey: prospects for a cytomegalovirus vaccine in transplant and congenital infection. Expert Rev Vaccines. 2018;17(10):889-911.
4. Griffiths PD, Stanton A, McCarrell E, Smith C, Osman M, Harber M, et al. Cytomegalovirus glycoprotein-B vaccine with MF59 adjuvant in transplant recipients: a phase 2 randomised placebo-controlled trial. Lancet. 2011;377(9773):1256-63.
5. Lilleri D, Gerna G. Maternal immune correlates of protection from human cytomegalovirus transmission to the fetus after primary infection in pregnancy. Rev Med Virol. 2017;27(2).
6. Lilleri D, Kabanova A, Revello MG, Percivalle E, Sarasini A, Genini E, et al. Fetal human cytomegalovirus transmission correlates with delayed maternal antibodies to gH/gL/pUL128-130-131 complex during primary infection. PLoS One. 2013;8(3):e59863.
7. Manicklal S, Emery VC, Lazzarotto T, Boppana SB, Gupta RK. The "silent" global burden of congenital cytomegalovirus. Clin Microbiol Rev. 2013;26(1):86-102.
8. Pass RF, Zhang C, Evans A, Simpson T, Andrews W, Huang ML, et al. Vaccine prevention of maternal cytomegalovirus infection. N Engl J Med. 2009;360(12):1191-9.
9. Plotkin SA, Boppana SB. Vaccination against the human cytomegalovirus. Vaccine. 2019;37(50):7437-42.
10. Plotkin SA, Vashistha VM. Cytomegalovirus vaccines. In: Vashishtha VM, Kalra A (Eds). IAP Textbook of Vaccines. New Delhi: Jaypee Brothers Medical Publishers (P) Ltd; 2020. pp. 606-16.
11. Plotkin SA, Wang D, Oualim A, Diamond DJ, Kotton CN, Mossman S, et al. The status of vaccine development against the human cytomegalovirus. J Infect Dis. 2020;221(Suppl 1):S113-22.
12. Sabbaj S, Pass RF, Goepfert PA, Pichon S. Glycoprotein B vaccine is capable of boosting both antibody and CD4 T-cell responses to cytomegalovirus in chronically infected women. J Infect Dis. 2011;203(11):1534-41.

CHAPTER 43

Enteroviral Vaccines (EV71)

Piyali Bhattacharya

1. Which disease outbreak has been caused by human enterovirus?

Enterovirus A71 (EV-A71), a positive-strand RNA virus of the family *Picornaviridae*, has caused large outbreaks of hand-foot-mouth disease (HFMD) in the Asia-Pacific region in recent years.[1] It is noteworthy that Coxsackie virus A16 (CV-A16) also causes similar disease.

2. What are the clinical signs and symptoms of HFMD?

Hand-foot-mouth disease is a contagious disease common in children less than 5 years of age. Older children and adults may also suffer from HFMD. It is usually a mild self-limiting disease. Fever, sore throat, irritability and loss of appetite are the presenting symptoms of HFMD **(Figs. 1A to C)**.

However, many children present with painful mouth sores and red flat spots or blisters on the palms and soles giving it the name *hand-foot-mouth disease*. These rashes can also be found over the knees, elbows, buttocks and genital areas.

3. What are the complications of EV-A71 infections?

Children under 5 years old are susceptible to the most severe forms of EV-A71-associated neurological complications, including aseptic meningitis, brainstem and/or cerebellar encephalitis, myocarditis, acute flaccid paralysis, and rapid fatal pulmonary edema and hemorrhage.[2]

4. What is the available treatment for HFMD?

There is no specific treatment modality available as of now. Symptomatic treatment with antipyretics and adequate hydration are advised to relieve fever and maintain adequate hydration.

However, an inactivated whole virus vaccine for EV-A71 has completed human clinical trial and is available for prevention of HFMD.

5. Which countries have established vaccination for Enterovirus?

Three Chinese companies have licensed inactivated EV-A71 vaccines, all of which have demonstrated good efficacy for preventing EV-A71-associated

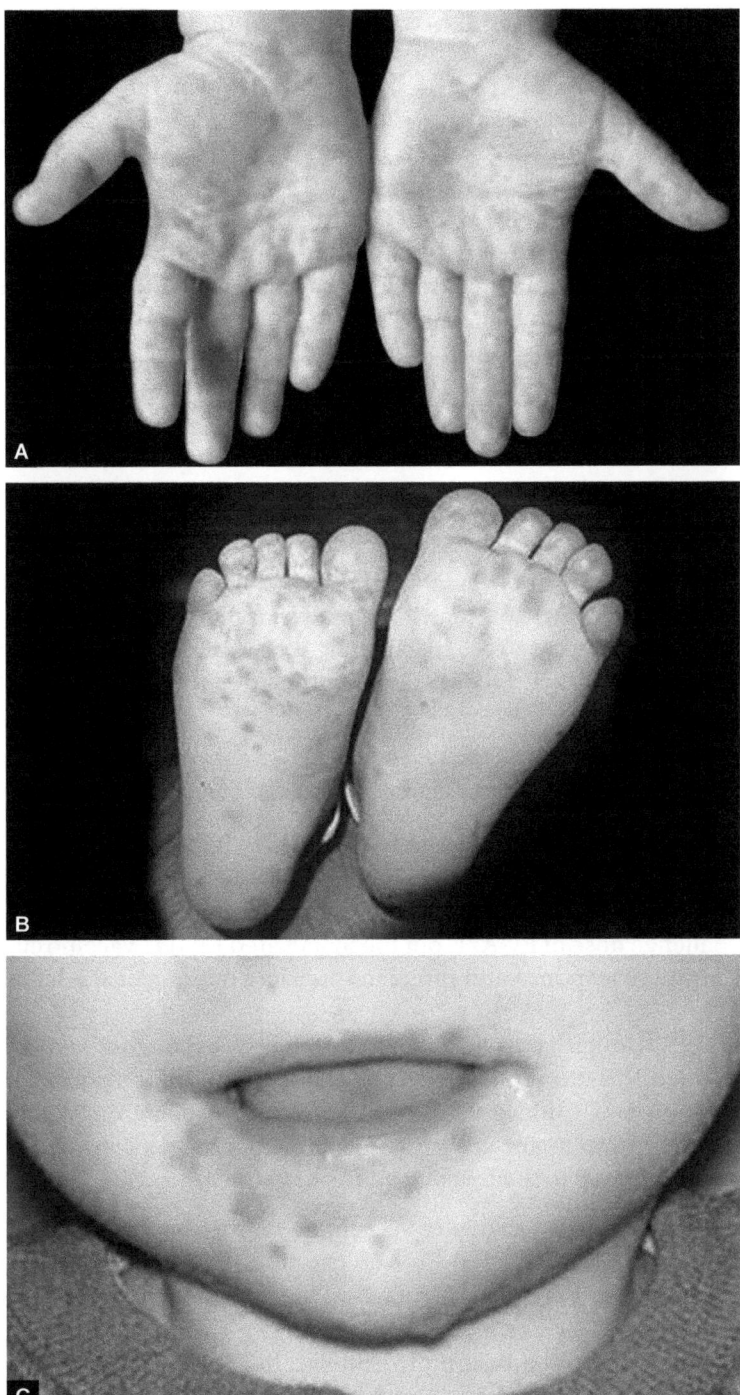

Figs. 1A to C: Hand-foot-mouth disease (HFMD) in children. Note the maculopapular spots or blisters on the palms (A), soles and face (around mouth) giving it the name hand-foot-mouth disease (B and C).

disease in clinical trials. However, real-world performance of EV-A71 vaccine has not been evaluated.

Inactivated whole EV-A71 vaccines are available in Taiwan, China, and Singapore. Beijing Vigoo Biological Co., Ltd. (Vigoo), Sinovac Biotech Co., Ltd. (Sinovac), and the Chinese Academy of Medical Sciences (CAMS) completed EV-A71 vaccine phase III clinical trials in 2013.

License for their administration was approved by China's FDA in 2015.[3,4]

Two organizations of Taiwan, Enimmune Corp. and Medigen Vaccinology Corp., continue to evaluate the safety and immunogenicity of the E59 strain EV-A71 vaccine in phase II clinical trials.

Medigen Vaccinology Corp., Taiwan, initiated a phase III clinical trial (ClinicalTrials.gov number, NCT03865238) in 2019, which is expected to be completed in 2022.

6. What are the different approaches used for the development of an EV-A71 vaccine?

Development of a vaccine would be the most effective approach to prevent EV-A71 infection. Many approaches for developing EV-A71 vaccines have been tried over the years, e.g., inactivating the whole virus, live-attenuated virus, virus-like particles (VLPs), recombinant subunits, and synthetic peptides.

7. What various types of vaccines are under consideration?

Recombinant VP1 vaccine: Research groups adopted various strategies to express EV-A71 VP1, a structural protein of EV-A71 that exhibited strong antigenicity. The VP1 subunit vaccine did protect suckling mice against a lower challenge dose of EV-A71, but the inactivated EV-A71 vaccine elicited a greater immune response and protected suckling mice against a lethal dose of EV-A71.

The VP1 protein has also been developed as an antigen for oral vaccine. Such VP1-expressing vaccines elicited immune responses by oral immunization and could protect newborn mice against EV-A71 infection. However, the recombinant VP1 protein exhibited a lower protective efficacy in mice as compared to the inactivated EV-A71 virus.[5]

Synthetic peptide vaccines: Synthetic peptides have also been tested as an alternative strategy to develop EV-A71 vaccines. The majority of research related to antigen peptides has focused on mapping EV-A71 structural proteins (VP1, VP2, VP3, and VP4).

Xu et al. generated a fusion protein with hepatitis B virus core protein (HBc) and VP2 epitope corresponding to amino acids 141–155 of VP2, named HBc-VP2 (aa141–155), which induced cross-neutralizing EV-A71 antibodies, and the anti-sera from HBc-VP2 (aa141–155) immunized mice protected newborn mice from EV-A71 infection.[6]

VLP-based vaccines: VLPs or virus-like particles, lack the viral genome and cannot replicate but still elicit innate and adaptive immunity in the host. Therefore, VLPs are thought to be associated with greater safety. Such technology has already been applied for vaccines such as hepatitis B virus and human papillomavirus (HPV), and could also be a suitable choice for EV-A71 vaccine.

Chimeric VLPs, including adenovirus or varicella-zoster virus-based VLPs induced an EV-A71-specific immune response and neutralization antibodies in vaccinated mice, and exhibited protective efficacy against EV-A71 infection.[7]

Live-attenuated vaccines: The realization of the advantages of long-lasting immunity and cost-effectiveness with the polio Sabin vaccine pointed to the possibility of an EV-A71 live-attenuated vaccine. Five cynomolgus monkeys were inoculated with EV-A71 (S1-3′) intravenously, followed by a challenge of lethal dose of EV-A71. Efficient immune response with neutralization activity against EV-A71 (BrCr-TR) (subgenotype A) and other subgenotypes was demonstrated. However, the inoculated monkeys had tremors and the virus was isolated from the lumbar spinal cord post-inoculation. Hence, safety of live-attenuated vaccine remains a concern.

A combination of codon deoptimization and synthetic virus production by Tsai et al. found that a virus with a deoptimized VP1 codon, and a high-fidelity virus with nucleotide substitution showed less virulence in a mouse model.[8,9]

Mucosal vaccines: There have been few studies focused on development of a mucosal vaccine for EV-A71 conceptualized on the fact that administration of a vaccine on the mucosal surface confers good immunity, e.g., oral polio, rotavirus, cholera, typhoid vaccines and intranasal influenza vaccine. Such vaccines induce effective mucosal and systematic immunity, and being needle-free are more acceptable for infants and young children.[9] However, the safety issue of live-attenuated vaccine remains a concern.

These EV-A71 vaccines are still at the preclinical stage of research and validation. Challenges include finding means of effective ways of breaching the epithelial barrier and the quantity of vaccine that would be required for mucosal immunization.

8. What is the protection conferred by inactivated EV-A71 vaccine?

Several studies have been conducted to determine the protection conferred by EV-A71 Vaccine. The following studies seem to be relevant:
- A randomized, double-blind, placebo-controlled phase 3 trial involving 12,000 healthy children 6-71 months of age was conducted in China. Two doses of an inactivated EV-A71 vaccine or placebo were administered intramuscularly, with a 4-week interval between doses. Children were monitored for up to 11 months.[10] The seroconversion rate was 100% 4 weeks after the two vaccinations, with a geometric mean titer of 170.6.

- Over the course of two epidemic seasons, the vaccine efficacy was 97.4% [95% confidence interval (CI) 92.9-99.0] according to the intention-to-treat analysis and 97.3% (95% CI, 92.6-99.0) according to the per-protocol analysis.
- Another test—negative case-control study in China between February 15, 2017 and February 15, 2018 enrolled 1,803 children between age 6 and 71 months with hand, foot, and mouth disease. Children who received 2 doses of vaccine were considered fully vaccinated; children who received 1 dose were considered partially vaccinated, and children who received no EV-A71 vaccine were said to be unvaccinated before hospitalization.
- The overall vaccine effectiveness was estimated to be 85.4% (95% CI, 53.2-95.4) for fully vaccinated children and 63.1% (95% CI, 13.1-84.3) for partially vaccinated children.
- Estimates of vaccine efficacy were directly proportionate to increasing age. The vaccine efficacy for full vaccination was estimated to be 91.1% in children aged 24-71 months but only 78.0% in children aged 6-23 months. Similarly, vaccine effectiveness for partial vaccination was 77.9% in children aged 24-71 months and 40.8% in children aged 6 to 23 months.[11]
- A total of 2,184 HFMD patients aged 5 years and less, from health facilities in Beijing were enrolled in a test-negative design case-control study to estimate vaccine effectiveness (VE); 24 were severe, and 2,160 were mild. For severe cases, two-dose VE estimate was 100% (95% CI: -68.1%, 100%). For mild cases, 1-dose and 2-dose adjusted VE estimates were 69.8% and 83.7%, respectively. Two-dose VE estimates varied by less than 4 percentage points regardless of control group definition.[12,13]

9. What are the adverse effects of EV-A71 vaccine?

Adverse events, such as fever (which occurred in 41.6% of the participants who received vaccine vs. 35.2% of those who received placebo), were significantly more common in the week after vaccination among children who received the vaccine than among those who received placebo.

REFERENCES

1. Huang PN, Shih SR. Update on enterovirus 71 infection. Curr OpinVirol. 2014;5:98-104.
2. McMinn PC. An overview of the evolution of enterovirus 71 and its clinical and public health significance. FEMS Microbiol Rev. 2002;26(1):91-107.
3. Mao Q, Wang Y, Bian L, Xu M, Liang Z. EV-A71 vaccine licensure: a first step for multivalent enterovirus vaccine to control HFMD and other severe diseases. Emerg Microbes Infect. 2016;5(7):e75.
4. Mao QY, Wang Y, Bian L, Xu M, Liang Z. EV71 vaccine, a new tool to control outbreaks of hand, foot and mouth disease (HFMD). Expert Rev Vaccines. 2016;15(5):599-606.
5. Zhu FC, Meng FY, Li JX, Li XL, Mao QY, Tao H, et al. Efficacy, safety, and immunology of an inactivated alum-adjuvant enterovirus 71 vaccine in children

in China: a multicentre, randomised, double-blind, placebo-controlled, phase 3 trial. Lancet. 2013;381(9882):2024-32.
6. Meng T, Kolpe AB, Kiener TK, Chow VT, Kwang J. Display of VP1 on the surface of baculovirus and its immunogenicity against heterologous human enterovirus 71 strains in mice. PLoS One. 2011;6(7):e21757.
7. Huo C, Yang J, Lei L, Qiao L, Xin J, Pan Z. Hepatitis B virus core particles containing multiple epitopes confer protection against enterovirus 71 and coxsackie virus A16 infection in mice. Vaccine. 2017;35(52):7322-30.
8. Yan Q, Wu L, Chen L, Qin Y, Pan Z, Chen M. Vesicular stomatitis virus-based vaccines expressing EV71 virus-like particles elicit strong immune responses and protect newborn mice from lethal challenges. Vaccine. 2016; 34(35):4196-204.
9. Tsai YH, Huang SW, Hsieh WS, Cheng CK, Chang CF, Wang YF, et al. Enterovirus A71 containing codon-deoptimized VP1 and high-fidelity polymerase as next-generation vaccine candidate. J Virol. 2019;93(13):1-5.
10. Miquel-Clopes A, Bentley EG, Stewart JP, Carding SR. Mucosal vaccines and technology. Clin Exp Immunol. 2019;196(2):205-14.
11. Li R, Liu L, Mo Z, Wang X, Xia J, Liang Z, et al. An inactivated enterovirus 71 vaccine in healthy children. N Engl J Med. 2014;370(9):829-37.
12. Li Y, Zhou Y, Cheng Y, Wu P, Zhou C, Cui P, et al. Effectiveness of EV-A71 vaccination in prevention of paediatric hand, foot, and mouth disease associated with EV-A71 virus infection requiring hospitalisation in Henan, China, 2017-18: a test-negative case-control study. Lancet Child Adolesc Health. 2019;10(3): 697-704.
13. Wang X, An Z, Huo D, Jia L, Li J, Yang Y, et al. Enterovirus A71 vaccine effectiveness in preventing enterovirus A71 infection among medically-attended hand, foot, and mouth disease cases, Beijing, China. Hum Vaccin Immunother. 2019;15(5):1183-90.

CHAPTER 44

Diarrheal Disease Vaccines other than Rotavirus

Shalabh Agarwal

1. How much is the disease burden of diarrheal diseases in children?

Diarrheal disease is the second leading cause of death in children under 5-year-old and is responsible for killing around 525,000 children every year **(Box 1)**. Global death toll from diarrheal diseases is about 1.7–2.5 million deaths/year ranking third among all causes of infectious diseases and most of them occur in children <3 years (under-five). Overall, the highest death rates in sub-Saharan Africa and South Asia, where rates typically range from 50 to 150 per 100,000 **(Fig. 1)**.

2. What is the estimated burden of diarrheal deaths and disease in India?

India bears about 13% of this global burden. Total diarrheal deaths in India among children aged 0–6 years were estimated to be 158,209 and proportionate mortality due to diarrhea in this age-group was 9.1%. Average estimated incidence of diarrhea in children aged 0–6 years was 1.71 and 1.09 episodes/person/year in rural and urban areas.

3. What are the infective agents which cause acute diarrhea in children besides rotavirus?

Diverse bacterial and viral agents give rise to acute diarrhea in children. Among the principal bacterial agents are *Vibrio cholerae*, a variety of *Salmonella* species including *S. typhi*, the agents of *Shigellosis, Campylobacter jejuni*, and wide variety of *E. coli*. Less commonly includes *Staphylococcus aureus, Clostridium perfringens, difficile, Klebsiella*, etc. Viruses other than

---

BOX 1: Childhood diarrhea: Key facts

- Diarrheal disease is the second leading cause of death in children under five years old. It is both preventable and treatable
- Each year diarrhea kills around 525,000 children under-five
- A significant proportion of diarrheal disease can be prevented through safe drinking-water and adequate sanitation and hygiene
- Globally, there are nearly 1.7 billion cases of childhood diarrheal disease every year
- Diarrhea is a leading cause of malnutrition in children under five years old

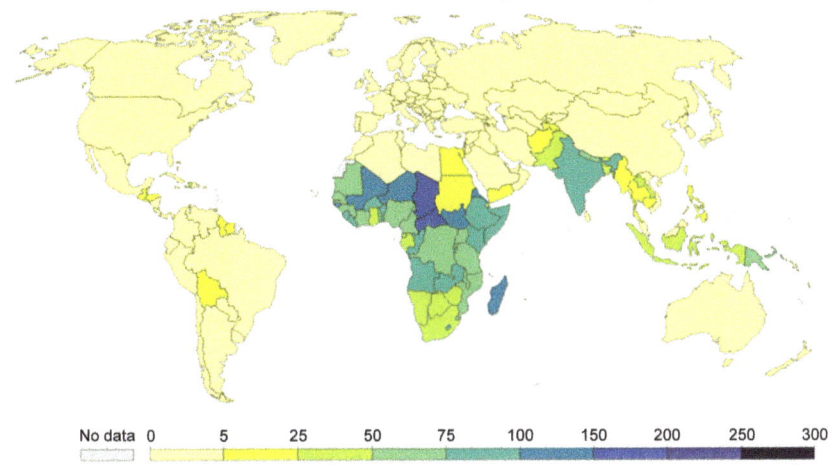

Fig. 1: Global death rates from diarrheal diseases in 2017.

Source: Institute for Health Metrics and Evaluation (IHME). (2017). Findings from the Global Burden of Disease Study 2017. [online] Available from: http://www.healthdata.org/sites/default/files/files/policy_report/2019/GBD_2017_Booklet.pdf. [Last accessed September, 2020].

rotavirus which cause diarrhea include enteric adenovirus, astroviruses, and caliciviruses (Norwalk) and various protozoa including *Giardia*, *Cyclospora*, *Cryptosporidium* species (e.g., *Giardia lamblia*, *Cryptosporidium parvum*), and *Entamoeba histolytica*. Most of the travelers' diarrhea is of bacterial etiology, caused principally by *enterotoxigenic Escherichia coli* (ETEC), *Shigella*, *Campylobacter*, and *Salmonella* species.

4. What are vaccine options available for various infective agents causing diarrhea?

Besides Rota, vaccine, which is effective against diarrhea, is cholera vaccine. Various vaccines, which are in pipeline, are against calicivirus, *Campylobacter jejuni*, ETEC, and *Shigella*.

5. How common are diarrheal episodes in children due to calicivirus infections?

Calicivirus (Norwalk virus) is considered to be the second most common cause of acute viral gastroenteritis in children after rotavirus. It has an incidence of about 12% in <5-year age group with severe diarrhea. The outbreaks are very common in winters and are commonly known as "stomach flu". It is a significant problem in both high- and low-income countries. About 1 million hospitalizations and >2 lacs deaths are estimated by noroviruses/year in <5 years age group. The usual presentation is acute gastroenteritis with vomiting, abdominal cramps, diarrhea, and fever.

6. What are the vaccine options available currently against calicivirus? What are the future prospects?

Currently, no vaccines are available against calicivirus. However, norvovirus (NoV)-derived virus-like particles (VLPs) produced in a baculoviral system are morphologically and antigenically similar to native virions, are an attractive option as an oral immunogen.

The safety and immunogenicity of the VLPs were evaluated in a phase I trial on healthy human volunteers who received 250 µg VLP oral doses in bicarbonate buffer. All volunteers showed a more than four-fold increase in IgG1 and IgA antibody titers. Same VLPs were used as a test antigen to determine the immune response by feeding 150 g doses of transgenic potatoes to healthy adult volunteers. It is not known if the modest antibody titer obtained would be protective against infection.

The newer vaccine under development is in preclinical phase. It includes NoV VLP-rotavirus protein combination vaccine, NoV VLP GII4, and enterovirus 71. This is a trivalent vaccine which has shown promise and may be available in countries where mortality and morbidity is attributed to both. The limitation of the above vaccine is the vast enterovirus genogroups that are evolving and variability in strains in different geographical region.

7. How common is diarrhea in children due to *Campylobacter jejuni*?

Campylobacter jejuni ranks as one the common bacterial causes of diarrhea in children. It is estimated to be present in 5–20% of isolates according to the Centers for Disease Control and Prevention (CDC). It also represents the second most common cause of traveler's diarrhea after ETEC. It is common in early age group and is largely foodborne. It has been linked with subsequent development of Guillain–Barre syndrome (GBS) which usually develops 2–3 weeks after the initial illness.

8. What are the vaccine prospects against *Campylobacter jejuni*?

No licensed vaccine is available at the moment. Though a candidate vaccine consisting of heat and formalin killed whole bacteria combined with LT (heat-labile enterotoxin of *E. coli*) as a mucosal adjuvant has been developed by the Navy Medical Research Institute, USA and is shown to provide 87% protection against intestinal colonization in a small number of volunteers. Current studies have focused on the use of flagellin or flagella–secreted protein FspA1 to be administered by the nasal route.

A new conjugate vaccine containing capsule polysaccharides from two strains of *Campylobacter jejuni* is also under evaluation.

An oral live multivalent vaccine expressing antigens from *Campylobacter, Shigella,* and ETEC is also currently being developed as a traveler's diarrhea vaccine.

9. How does *Escherichia coli* various strain contribute to diarrheal diseases in children?

Various types of *E. coli* can cause diarrhea like enteropathogenic *E. coli* (EPEC), enterohemorrhagic *E. coli* (EHEC), enterotoxigenic *E. coli* (ETEC), enteroinvasive *E. coli* (EIEC), etc. The clinical picture varies according to the strain and varies from watery diarrhea to hemolytic uremic syndrome (HUS). ETEC strains are the major cause of infantile diarrhea in developing countries and in travelers visiting these countries. The cause of transmission is contaminated food and water. Children <2 years are at maximum risk.

The infections due to ETEC decrease with increasing age, which suggest that these infections are of immunizing nature and may be an effective prevention strategy.

10. What are the vaccines in line against enterotoxigenic *Escherichia coli* (ETEC)?

Infection with ETEC is a major contributor to diarrheal illness in children in low- and middle-income countries and travelers to these areas. There is an ongoing effort to develop vaccines against ETEC, and the most reliable immune correlate of protection against ETEC is the small intestinal secretory IgA response that targets ETEC-specific virulence factors.

Various vaccines against *E. coli* are currently under development. They include:

Killed oral vaccine—enterotoxigenic *E. coli* vaccine (ETVAX)/double-mutant heat-labile enterotoxin (dm LT) is the most advanced ETEC candidate in clinical development. The first generation has shown efficacy against travelers' diarrhea. Second-generation oral ETEC vaccine ETVAX was evaluated in Bangladeshi volunteers. It was found to be safe and IgA responses against each of the primary antigens. The promising results in adults supported testing ETVAX in descending age group of children.

Oral killed whole cell (WC)/recombinant B subunit (Rbs) cholera vaccine was found to prevent the risk of episodes of traveler's diarrhea due to ETEC by 30–40%. However, the protection lasted for few months only.

ETEC fimbrial tip adhesin vaccine (FTA):

Adhesin-based vaccine—the ETEC fimbrial tip adhesin-based vaccine (FTA) is the most advanced subunit approach for ETEC. Intradermal immunization with the FTA vaccine was found capable of inducing both specific IgG and IgA memory B-cells to both antigens.

Multiepitope fusion vaccine—this is another subunit vaccine to ETEC. The studies till now suggest that it can be useful for developing a broadly protective anti-adhesin vaccine against ETEC.

Other live attenuated vaccines—the Center for Vaccine Development, University of Maryland (USA) developed a strategy to use live attenuated *Shigella* vectors for expression of ETEC fimbrial and LT antigen so that there can be protection against both *Shigella* and ETEC. Spi-VEC oral live attenuated typhoid vaccine was also used as a vector for delivery of

ETEC antigens. AVANT has developed the Peru 15 pCTB live attenuated oral cholera vaccine effective against both V cholera and ETEC diarrheas.

Other ETEC vaccine approaches—a combination of fimbrial antigen CS6 and LT was tried using transcutaneous immunization patch. A phase II randomized, double-blind, placebo-controlled study has been conducted and good protection rates were observed against moderate to severe diarrhea by administering two LT patches given 2-3 weeks apart.

11. How important is to prevent *Shigella* infection in children?

About 120 million cases are reported worldwide suffering from shigellosis induced dysentery and majority of them are in developing countries in children <5 years. About 1.1 million people are estimated to die from shigellosis every year and 60% of them occur in children <5 years. That is why, it is so important to have an effective vaccine against this. Shigellosis can be transmitted through fecal-oral route via contaminated food and water or through contact. Houseflies can also transmit infection. The disease is characterized by general malaise, abdominal cramps, and bloody, mucopurulent stools. Complications can be peritonitis, septicemia and hemolytic uremic syndrome (HUS) with renal failure.

Shigella sonnei, S. flexneri, and *S. dysenteriae* are the three major species responsible for bacillary dysentery. These species are further subdivided into subtypes on the basis of antigen specificity of the O-polysaccharide portion of their lipopolysaccharides (LPS). *S. flexneri* has 14 serotypes and subtypes, is endemic in developing countries and is most frequently isolated species worldwide. *S. sonnei* is the most common organism in developed countries. *S. dysenteriae* is the cause of epidemic dysentery.

12. What are the vaccine options available against shigellosis?

No vaccine is widely available to prevent shigellosis. Most *Shigella* vaccine candidates include O-SP (O-specific polysaccharide) antigen. The use of this antigen associated with LPS is based on observation that immunity is serotype specific.

The polysaccharide conjugate and live attenuated vaccines, which are being developed aim on the most frequently isolated *E. flexneri* 2a and *S. sonnei* and S d 1.

Polysaccharide conjugate vaccines—they were produced from purified *Shigella* LPS from the relevant serotypes. These were found to be 75% efficacious. Phase II and III trials were recently completed in Israel. The use of synthetic oligosaccharides that mimic the O-antigen protective epitopes offers promise for an improved and cheaper future generation of conjugate *Shigella* vaccines.

Live attenuated vaccines—problem in preparing candidate live attenuated shigellosis vaccine is that under attenuation that can cause excessive reactogenicity of the vaccine and overattenuation leads to insufficient immunogenicity. Numerous approaches at attenuating by various techniques have been met with difficulty to achieve the right balance between the robust immunogenicity, optimal colonization and shedding patterns and clinical tolerance of the attenuated strains so as to develop a multivalent vaccine to cover a spectrum of *Shigella* species. As an alternative strategy, several groups have attempted to express *Shigella* O-antigens in well tolerated live vectors as *E. coli* or attenuated *S. typhi*.

Other candidate Shigella vaccines—a formalin-inactivated *S. sonnei* vaccine (SsWC) was developed as an oral, killed, whole-cell vaccine at the Johns Hopkins University in Baltimore, USA and recently conducted phase I trials. Similarly, Antex (USA) is developing a *Shigella* inactivated whole cell vaccine as well as an oral travelers' diarrhea vaccine (Activax TM) containing antigens from *Campylobacter*, *Shigella*, and ETEC.

Novel antigen candidate vaccines—the vaccine development approach by GSK Vaccines Institute for Global Health (GVGH) is based on generalized modules for membrane antigens (GMMA). GVGH has developed a monovalent *S. sonnei* vaccine as a first step in the development of a broadly protective multivalent vaccine including GMMA with O-Ag from different Shigella serotypes. Phase I clinical trials were well-tolerated.

Subunit candidate vaccine—Shigella vaccine has been recently developed by the Indian Council of Medical Research-National Institute of Cholera and Enteric Diseases (ICMR-NICED), a leading ICMR institute in the form of heat treated/formalin killed vaccines as well as next-generation vaccines including Omp A nanoformulation and outer membrane vesicles (OMVs) to address the need for *Shigella* infection.

SUGGESTED READING

1. Balasubramanian S, Dhanalakshmi K, Sumanth A. Vaccines against diarrheal diseases. In: Vashishtha VM, Kalra A (Eds). IAP Textbook of Vaccines. New Delhi: Jaypee Brothers Medical Publishers (P) Ltd; 2000. pp. 567-81.
2. Dougan G, Huett A, Clare S. Vaccines against human enteric bacterial pathogens. Br Med Bull. 2002;62:113-23.
3. Girard MP, Steele D, Chaignat CL, Kieny MP. A review of vaccine research and development: human enteric infections. Vaccine. 2006;24(15):2732-50.
4. Holmgren J, Czerkinsky C. Mucosal immunity and vaccines. Nat Med. 2005;11:S45-53.
5. Lakshminarayanan S, Jayalakshmy R. Diarrheal diseases among children in India: Current scenario and future perspectives. J Nat Sci Biol Med. 2015;6(1):24-8.
6. Lawan A, Jesse FFA, Idris UH, Odhah MN, Arsalan M, Muhammad NA, et al. Mucosal and systemic responses of immunogenic vaccines candidates against enteric Escherichia coli infections in ruminants: a review. Microb Pathog. 2018;117:175-83.
7. Parashar UD, Bresee JS, Glass RI. The global burden of diarrhoeal disease in children. Bull World Health Organ. 2003;81(4):236.
8. Riaz S, Steinsland H, Hanevik K. Human mucosal IgA immune responses against enterotoxigenic *Escherichia coli*. Pathogens. 2020;9(9):E714.
9. World Health Organization. (2017). Diarrhoeal disease. [online]. Available from: https://www.who.int/news-room/fact-sheets/detail/diarrhoeal-disease#:~:text=Each%20year%20diarrhoea%20kills%20around,childhood%20diarrhoeal%20disease%20every%20year. [Last Accessed September, 2020].

CHAPTER 45

Hepatitis E Vaccines

Dipti Agarwal

1. What is the prevalence of hepatitis E infection globally?

World Health Organization (WHO) estimates that over 2 billion people are infected with hepatitis E virus (HEV) worldwide resulting in 70,000 deaths in a year. The infection can occur as outbreaks and also as sporadic cases. HEV infection is prevalent in Indian subcontinent, Middle East, South East Asia and Mexico. Outbreaks of infection have been seen in many countries in Africa, Asia, and North America in recent years. During the past decade (2009–2019), six outbreaks of hepatitis E, have been reported in African countries. The most recent outbreak occurred in Namibia in 2017.

2. What are the clinical manifestations of the disease?

Hepatitis E is the most common cause of acute hepatitis worldwide. The clinical manifestations are similar to acute hepatitis A. Chronic hepatitis E occurs in immunosuppressed patients. It commonly affects 15–34 years age group and is a major health problem in pregnant women with high mortality.

3. How is the infection transmitted to humans?

Hepatitis E virus (HEV) is primarily transmitted through fecal-oral route. Consumption of uncooked animal meat can result in spread of infection. Perinatal transmission occurs and can lead to poor fetal outcome. Transmission by blood transfusion is also known to occur.

4. Is there any natural immunity against HEV?

Hepatitis E virus infection on recovery may show the presence of specific IgG antibodies against viral capsid protein. The duration of anti-HEV IgG and the protection conferred by naturally acquired antibodies and whether these antibodies protect individual from reinfection is not clear.

5. Which vaccines are currently recommended against HEV infection?

Till date, three VLP-based hepatitis E vaccines (p495-, p239-, and p179-based vaccine) have been tested in various clinical trials. Recombinant 239

Hepatitis E vaccine (Hecolin®) manufactured by Xiamen Innovax Biolabs, have been licensed for use in China since 2011.

6. Vaccine is recommended for which individuals?

Vaccine is recommended for individuals at high risk of HEV infection, such as pregnant women, travelers to endemic areas and those working in animal husbandry.

7. What is the dose and schedule of the vaccine?

0.5 mL vaccine is given intramuscularly. The schedule consists of 3 doses which are given at 0, 1 and 6 months. It is available as a single dose prefilled syringe and is not recommended to be used as multidose vial.

8. What are the components of HEV?

One dose of the HEV 239 vaccine contains 30 µg of purified recombinant HEV antigen along with sodium chloride, disodium hydrogen phosphate, potassium dihydrogen phosphate, 0.8 mg aluminum hydroxide and 25 µg thiomersal. The vaccine is supplied as a suspension in a prefilled syringe.

9. What are appropriate storage conditions for the vaccine?

The vaccine can be stored for 36 months at 2–8°C in cool and dry conditions. The vaccine should not be exposed to sunlight. At room temperatures the vaccine can be kept for 2 months. The vaccine does not have a vaccine vial monitor to guide for changes in temperature.

10. What is immunogenicity conferred by vaccine?

The vaccine has been shown to be highly immunogenic in subjects receiving 3 doses given in a 0, 1 and 6 month schedule. Antibody responses after vaccination were also found to be comparable in HBsAg-positive individuals, regardless of their baseline anti-HEV status. The antibody response of the vaccine has not been studied in children aged <16 years and in elderly > 65 years of age. The immunogenicity of the vaccine has not been studied in certain conditions such as chronic liver disease. Different routes of giving vaccine and using 0, 1 and 2 months schedule has not been assessed for immunogenicity.

11. What is the efficacy of the vaccine?

Overall efficacy of recombinant HEV vaccine after 2 doses of vaccine is around 85.2% and after 3 doses, the efficacy is found to be 88.7%. Although HEV vaccine has been tested against genotype 4 but the vaccine has been shown to be effective against genotype 1. There is some evidence, which shows that neutralizing monoclonal antibody binds to capsid peptides from all 4 HEV genotypes with similar affinity, suggesting effectiveness of vaccine against all the HEV genotypes. Efficacy of the vaccine for post-exposure prophylaxis or in outbreaks has not been evaluated. There is insufficient evidence of efficacy of vaccine against HEV-infected pregnant women, in children (<16 years of age), persons aged >65 years, or in immunosuppressed persons. There is no study of vaccine against subclinical hepatitis E vaccine.

12. What is the duration of protection of the vaccine?

The anti-HEV antibodies induced by the vaccine are detected up to 4.5 years after administration of three immunization doses over 6 months in 87% recipients. However, it needs to be studied further whether long duration of protection may require booster dose.

13. What are the adverse effects of the vaccine?

Some minor side effects of the recombinant HEV 239 vaccine have been reported such as pain, swelling and itching at the injection site. No serious adverse event for the vaccine has been reported in any studies. The Global Advisory Committee on Vaccine Safety (GACVS) has also started use of the vaccine based on the safety data on the clinical trials conducted on healthy subjects. However, there are no safety data in children <16 years, those aged >65 years, and in immunocompromised subjects. Vaccine safety in pregnant women and its effect on fetus has also not been evaluated.

14. What are HEV ORF genome and their role in the formation of vaccine?

The HEV genome is a 7.2-kb mRNA-like molecule. It has three well-defined open reading frames (ORFs) in all the genotypes of HEV. ORF1 encodes a polyprotein, which forms multiple non-structural proteins, including methyltransferase, putative papain-like cysteine protease, RNA helicase and RNA-dependent RNA polymerase that are required for virus replication.

The ORF2 encodes the capsid protein. The N-terminals encoded by ORF2 are responsible for the packaging of the viral RNA genome. Genetic analysis of ORF2 has demonstrated over 85% similarity among genotypes 1–4 HEV strains that infect humans. The HEV capsid proteins have the potential to form vaccines as it results in the formation of neutralizing antibodies. Hence, ORF2 has been considered to be a good vaccine candidate and has led to the development of recombinant HEV capsid proteins as subunit vaccines.

The ORF3 resembles ORF2 and is involved in the release of virus from the host cells. Another protein was recently identified to stimulate the replication of genotype 1 by a newly discovered ORF4 genome.

15. What are virus-like particles or VLPs?

A recombinant virus-like particle (VLP) based antigen is an ideal candidate in vaccine formulation due to its high immunogenicity and desirable safety performance. The VLPs are subviral particles made up of three definitive domains: S (S, aa 129-319), middle (M, aa 320-455), and protruding (P, aa 456-606) domain. S domain forms the viral shell. M domain is responsible for the formation of symmetries of the HEV capsid. P domain forms the protrusions of the viral shell. The presence of virion-like epitopes on the surface of VLPs is the structural basis to elicit protective antibody against the viral infection.

16. Are there any combination vaccine of HEV?

As both hepatitis A and E have fecal-oral transmission, few studies were conducted in mice which have demonstrated that combining vaccine of HAV and HEV can induce neutralizing antibodies against both HAV and HEV effectively. Other combinations with rotavirus, norovirus, astrovirus are also being studied. Both norovirus and HEV have similar surface protrusions of the viral capsids can induce protective antibodies against the infections. Fusion gene fragment of HEV capsid protein and hepatitis B surface antigen were linked with synthetic glycine and has demonstrated potential role in hepatitis B/HEV bivalent vaccine.

17. Can the vaccine be given orally?

Oral vaccine may be an efficient approach for HEV vaccine. It has been shown that vaccines delivered to the mucosal interface result in development of secretory IgA. Vaccine antigens can be incorporated into many edible species. Studies conducted in primates demonstrated that serum IgG and fecal IgA was found after oral intake of 10 mg purified HEV-VLP isolates. Chloroplast has been shown to have high levels of transgene expression. HEV-ORF2 protein has been used with leaves and fresh fruits in few studies. Further research is needed on the development of plant-derived hepatitis E oral vaccine.

18. Why expression of vaccine in prokaryotes is required?

The inability to form HEV in culture system makes it impossible to develop live or inactivated vaccines. *Escherichia coli* is the most commonly used expression system. There has been significant progress in developing recombinant vaccines based on the ORF2 viral capsid protein. VLPs are nanoparticles that form particulate antigen and present as key epitopes on the particle surface needed for the development of VLP-based vaccine.

19. What is the current status of the vaccine?

Presently vaccine based on HEV 239, a truncated protein (aa 368-606 of ORF2) expressed in *E. coli,* has been licensed for use in China and is found to be effective against hepatitis E disease in 16-65 year-old healthy subjects. However, there is no data on safety and efficacy profile of this vaccine in pediatric population, elderly subjects, pregnant women, patients with underlying chronic liver disease and immunocompromised subjects. The WHO issued a recommendation in 2018 to provide guidance to national regulatory authorities and manufacturers to assure the quality, safety and efficacy of recombinant hepatitis E vaccines. There is limited data on the degree of cross-protection the vaccine may confer against other genotypes of HEV. Due to lack of adequate data, the WHO has not made any recommendation on the universal use of this vaccine as yet. However, individual countries may decide on use of the vaccine based on the epidemiological studies in their region. There is insufficient information on the efficacy of schedules with <3 doses or with 0, 1, 2 schedule and on the need for booster doses.

20. What are the recent advances in HEV 239 vaccine?

The HEV 239 recombinant vaccine is a major breakthrough in protection against hepatitis E vaccine. However, complete understanding of HEV vaccine still remains limited. Recent studies have shown that pORF3 could serve as a new target of vaccine against quasi-enveloped HEV particles. Such a vaccine might serve as a booster shot for the current pORF2-based subunit vaccine to ultimately provide better protection than from the pORF2 vaccine alone. Using these new strategies, it is hopeful that the next generation of HEV vaccines will have wider usage.

SUGGESTED READING

1. Shah A, Agarwal D. Hepatitis E vaccines. In: IAP Textbook of Vaccines, 2nd edition. New Delhi: Jaypee Brothers Medical Publishers (P) Ltd.; 2019. pp. 600-6.
2. WHO. (2015). Hepatitis E position paper. [online] Available from: https://www.who.int/policy/hepatitis. [Last Accessed August, 2020].
3. WHO. (2019). GRADE Table 01a. Efficacy of hepatitis E vaccination in immunocompetent individuals against hepatitis E disease. Available from: http://www.who.int/immunisation/policy/position_papers/hepe_grad_efficacy_virus_infection?pdf>ua=1. [Last Accessed August, 2020].
4. WHO. (2019). GRADE Table 03a. Duration of protection against hepatitis E virus infection following primary immunization with hepatitis E vaccine in immunocompetent individuals. Available from: http://www.who.int/immunisation/policy/position_papers/hepe_grad_efficacy_virus_infection?pdf>ua=1. [Last Accessed August, 2020].

CHAPTER 46

Hepatitis C Vaccines

Abhay K Shah, Aashay A Shah

1. What is the importance of hepatitis C (HC) infection?

Hepatitis C is still considered as an important public health problem since its first identification in 1989. It is a common cause of chronic liver disease. Hepatitis C virus (HCV) persists in up to 85% of infected individuals as a chronic infection characterized by liver infiltration of inflammatory cells that can lead to fibrosis. Chronic hepatitis C infection significantly increases the risk of developing cirrhosis and hepatocellular carcinoma. As per the estimate, 3% of the world population is chronically infected with HCV and it accounts for 20% of cases of acute hepatitis and 70% of cases of chronic hepatitis. The mean time of appearance of chronic hepatitis, cirrhosis and hepatocellular carcinoma is 10, 20 and 30 years, respectively after HCV infection.

2. What is the epidemiology of HCV infection?

Chronic HCV infection occurs worldwide with the highest prevalence in Africa and Asia. The prevalence of HCV infection averages 3% of the world population, with peaks of 5.2% in Africa, 3.55% in Asia, while in the USA and Oceania it is 1.9% and in Europe 1.75%. Approximately 185 million people or 2.5% of the world's population are currently infected with hepatitis C virus (HCV), and there are 3–4 million new infections each year. A total of 60–80% of infections will develop into chronic disease resulting in 350,000–500,000 deaths annually due to HCV-related conditions.

There were an estimated 1.75 million new cases worldwide in 2015. The World Health Organization aims for a 90% reduction in new HCV infections by 2030.

3. Describe HC virus morphology.

Hepatitis C virus is a small (55–65 nm in size), enveloped, positive-sense single-stranded ribonucleic acid (RNA) virus of the family Flaviviridae, which includes the flaviviruses and pestiviruses. There are at least six HCV genotypes and more than 50 subtypes. The virion contains a positive single-stranded RNA genome of 9.5 kb. The viral genome encodes a large single polyprotein of about 3,000 amino acids (aa), and is cleaved into three structural proteins (core, E1, and E2), and seven nonstructural proteins (p7, NS2, NS3, NS4A,

NS4B, NS5A, and NS5B). The HCV structural proteins comprise the core protein and two envelope glycoprotein, E1 and E2. The E1 and E2 proteins are thought to be associated with viral fusion and entry in the host cells by endocytosis and are the primary targets of humoral immune responses. The non-structural proteins, including proteases (NS2/3 and NS3), helicase (an enzyme that unwinds double-stranded nucleic acid; NS3), and RNA-dependent RNA polymerase (NS5B), perform various functions essential for the viral life cycle.

4. How many genotypes of HCV are identified? What is its importance?

Based on genetic differences between HCV isolates, the HCV species is classified into six genotypes (1-6) with several subtypes within each genotype (represented by lower-cased letters). Subtypes are further broken down into quasispecies based on their genetic diversity. Subtypes 1a and 1b are found worldwide and cause 60% of all cases. Infection with one genotype does not protect against other one and infections with more than one genotype do coexist. The importance of HCV genotype lies in its geographical distribution and treatment response to pegylated interferon (PEG-IFN) and ribavirin. Unfortunately, along with genotype 4 viruses, genotype 1 is the least sensitive to standard-of-care therapy, a combination of PEG-IFN alpha and ribavirin.

5. How HCV enters our body?

Hepatitis C virus enters a susceptible host either directly, through needle inoculation or transfusion of contaminated blood products, or inadvertently, through breakage of a percutaneous barrier (as exemplified by sexual or perinatal transmission).

6. What is the natural history of HCV infection?

Following primary (acute) infection with HCV, a significant proportion of people will spontaneously eradicate the infection. Approximately 25% of individuals acutely infected with HCV are able to eliminate the virus spontaneously while the rest develop persistent infection and chronic liver disease, including fibrosis, cirrhosis, and hepatocellular carcinoma

After infection, HCV RNA appears in the plasma within a few days and usually shows a peak within the first few months. HCV induces hepatic damage both by a direct cytopathic effect on hepatocytes and by immune-mediated mechanisms. The inflammatory processes leading to initial liver injury, which is assessed by serum elevation of the liver specific alanine aminotransferase (ALT) enzyme, generally occurs within 1-3 months. If infection is not resolved within the first 6-12 months, patients generally remain chronically infected for life. Between 15% and 50% of acute hepatitis C infections spontaneously resolve, whereas 50-85% of infected individuals develop chronic infection. Up to 20% of chronically infected HCV patients may develop progressive liver damage leading to end-stage disease, usually over a period of 20–30 years, although some patients progress faster.

7. Which are the risk factors for development of diseases following HCV infection?

Risk factors for disease include the male sex, alcohol use, coinfection with human immunodeficiency virus (HIV) or hepatitis B virus (HBV), obesity, age during infection (younger people have a slower course of disease) and iron levels in the liver. Hepatocellular carcinoma occurs in approximately 2.5% of these cases. There is no direct correlation between quantity of HCV RNA and liver damage indicating immune mediated process for liver damage.

8. Which are the challenges for HC vaccine development?

One of the major challenges facing the development of a vaccine for HCV is the high degree of genetic diversity that is exhibited by the virus, estimated to be 10-fold higher than that seen in HIV. Another barrier to HCV vaccine development is the lack of in vitro systems and immunocompetent small animal models that facilitate determining whether vaccination induces protective immunity. These problems are further complicated by lack of a convenient infectious tissue culture system for testing neutralizing antibodies or passage of attenuated viral strains. In addition, the only infectious animal model is the chimpanzee, an endangered species that is difficult to study; in addition, the course of HCV infection in the chimpanzee is not necessarily representative of that in humans. There are number of other challenges associated with vaccine development.

- There is high rate of mutation in the hypervariable region of the envelope proteins. The hypervariable region is a major site of antienvelope antibody response and contains a principal neutralization epitope.
- Antibody responses to the envelope proteins develop slowly and achieve only modest titers during primary infection. Hence, neutralizing antibodies may emerge too late to prevent chronic infection.
- In addition, antienvelope antibodies tend to be short-lived, disappearing gradually after viral clearance.
- Immunologic correlates of protection and disease progression have not been clearly defined.

9. Which are the approaches considered for HC vaccines development?

Vaccines with T-cell Response
Two vaccines designed to prevent infection solely by eliciting T-cell–mediated immunity have been tested in phase I (safety and immunogenicity) trials in human volunteers not at risk for HCV infection. A prototype vaccine with the HCV core protein and ISCOMATRIX adjuvant was assessed for its ability to induce T-cell responses in healthy individuals not at risk for HCV infection. Although the vaccine was generally well-tolerated, CD8þ T-cell responses were detected in only 2 of the 8 participants receiving the highest dose.

The second vaccine tested in healthy volunteers and designed to elicit T-cell responses is the foundation of the only candidate vaccine to have advanced to a trial in at-risk subjects. This vaccine is composed of a replication defective chimpanzee adenovirus (ChAd) vector encoding NS3, NS4, and NS5 proteins.

Peptide Vaccines
A vaccine candidate being developed for both prophylaxis and therapy uses synthetic peptides derived from the core, NS3, and NS4 proteins as they are known to stimulate both cytotoxic and helper T-cells. The results from two clinical trials in healthy volunteers showed that response was correlated with higher peptide doses and the use of adjuvants (poly l-arginine). However, the strength of the responses was very weak when compared to viral vector and VLP systems and there is no information on long-term memory responses.

Vaccines with Humoral Immune Response
Clearance of HCV infection is associated with the early development of serum antibodies capable of blocking infection by multiple heterologous HCV strains. Antibodies with these characteristics are called broadly neutralizing antibodies (bNAbs). The targets of the NAb response against HCV are the viral envelope glycoproteins, E1 and E2. E1 and E2 are membrane-anchored proteins that are believed to form a heterodimer on the surface of viral particles. Hypervariable region 1 (HVR1), a 27-amino acid region at the N-terminus of E2, is an immunodominant epitope that evolves rapidly under antibody pressure. Characterization of these bNAbs has helped to identify epitopes that could be incorporated into a vaccine.

Prophylactic B- and T-cell Combined Vaccines
Next-generation vaccines against HCV will likely combine both T-cell and antibody-based approaches into one single vaccine. B-cell vaccines that contain recombinant protein or peptide from E1 and/or E2 may have to be combined with a T-cell vaccine and heterologously expressed. A vaccine containing both B-cell and T-cell epitopes are also useful for this purpose. Three such vaccines are tested in chimpanzees, out of which two are based on strains of vaccinia virus and a third on a VPL.

Another option is for the vaccine to contain both B- and T-cell epitopes. Three vaccines that contain both B- and T-cell HCV epitopes have been tested in the chimpanzee. Two are based on strains of vaccinia virus and a third on a VLP.

10. What are various vaccines under development?

Vaccines based on Adjuvanted Recombinant HCV Proteins
A vaccine consisting of the recombinant gpE1/gpE2 heterodimer in combination with an oil/water microemulsified adjuvant has been tested extensively for efficacy in the chimpanzee model. 30–40 µg of the immunizing subunits were administered intramuscularly on months 0, 1, and 6, approximately. A challenge with a homologous viral strain was given

intravenously 2–3 weeks after the 3rd immunization. Five out of seven animals receiving the vaccine were completely protected against HCV infection, as evidenced by negativity in both serological tests and real-time polymerase chain reaction (RT-PCR) assays for viral RNA for the duration of the follow-up period (> 1 year). Importantly, the two chimpanzees that became infected after challenge eventually resolved the acute infection and did not progress to chronic infection, whereas most control animals (seven out of ten) became chronically infected following viral challenge. Completely protected animals were the highest responders to the vaccine in terms of titers of total anti-gpE1/gpE2 antibodies measured in enzyme immunoassay (EIA) formats. Complete protection was later correlated with antibodies that block the binding of recombinant gpE2 to the HCV receptor component CD81, whereas it did not correlate with antibody titers to the N-terminal hypervariable region of gpE2 (E2HVR1).

This study provided the first supporting data for the feasibility of developing a vaccine against HCV because it indicated the capability of recombinant envelope glycoprotein immunization either to elicit sterilizing immunity or to prevent the progression to chronic infection following an acute, transient infection after viral challenge. The study has now been extended to address the key question of whether the vaccine is able to protect against experimental challenge with a heterologous 1a viral strain.

In addition, expression of a C-gpE1-gpE2 gene cassette in insect cells has been reported to result in the generation of 40–60 nm virus-like particles (VLPs) within cytoplasmic cisternae. After partial purification, these VLPs appear to be immunogenic in small animals and may be considered an interesting tool for the design of a vaccine for humans, if sufficient yields and purity can be attained.

Because the E2HVR1 region of gpE2 has been shown to possess viral neutralizing epitopes and to be highly mutable, attempts have been made to select a cross-reacting version using phage display of mimotopes. Such mimotopes or consensus E2HVR1 peptides may be valuable components of an HCV vaccine. To specifically investigate the effectiveness of this approach, a consensus E2HVR1 peptide sequence has been fused to the B subunit of cholera toxin and expressed in plants by transduction with tobacco mosaic virus vector. Intranasal administration of crude extracts in experimental mice effectively generated cross-reactive E2HVR1 antibodies capable of capturing virions.

Preclinical evaluation of gpE1/gpE2 adjuvanted with MF59C.1 (an oil-in-water emulsion) in human volunteers generated low-to-moderate Ab responses alongside a clear T-helper 1 response in nearly all participants. NAbs as well as proliferative CD4 T-cell responses against gpE1/gpE2 was cross-reactive and targeted multiple epitopes.

HCV Core Protein and ISCOMATRIX Adjuvant
(HCV Core ISCOMATRIX Vaccine)
The recombinant form of the viral nucleocapsid C protein has also been investigated as a possible vaccine component, because it has been shown

to be the target of HCV-specific CD4+ and CD8+ T-cell responses that are associated with the recovery from acute infection and with an asymptomatic course of chronic infection. Another important reason is that C protein is the most conserved HCV polypeptide and contains CD4+ and CD8+ epitopes highly conserved among the different genotypes. This makes C protein a valuable candidate for the generation of cross-reactive immunity against different HCV strains. Finally, the recombinant C protein has been shown to self-assemble into particles which are highly immunogenic in animal models and induce CD4+ T-cell priming and high anti-C antibody titers.

The use of the ISCOM adjuvant in combination with the recombinant C protein also allowed an effective priming of CD8+ CTL responses in rhesus macaques. This approach represents a promising option for the development of an HCV vaccine capable of priming cross-reactive HCV-specific T-cell responses. One such approach using a "polyepitope" vaccine would consist of the use of a consecutive sequence of conserved HCV T-cell epitopes in the form of a recombinant polypeptide or DNA vaccine. The immune response in this case would be directed against multiple, highly conserved epitopes that can be presented by diverse human major histocompatibility class (MHC) class I and class II molecules thus optimizing the generation of strong, cross-reactive immunity.

A prototype vaccine having HCV core protein and ISCOMATRIX adjuvant (HCV Core ISCOMATRIX vaccine), ISCOMATRIX vaccines, have been shown to induce CD4(+) and CD8(+) T-cell responses to a range of antigens in both animal models and in human studies.

Additionally, ISCOMATRIX vaccines have been shown to be safe and generally well-tolerated in several clinical trials. The phase I placebo-controlled, dose escalation clinical study was designed to evaluate the safety, tolerability and immunogenicity of the HCV core ISCOMATRIX vaccine in healthy individuals. The 30 subjects received three immunizations of HCV core ISCOMATRIX vaccines or placebo vaccine on days 0, 28 and 56. The HCV core ISCOMATRIX vaccines contained 5, 20 or 50 μg HCV core protein with 120 μg ISCOMATRIX adjuvant. The adverse events reported were generally mild to moderate in severity, of short duration and self-limiting. The most common adverse events were injection site reactions such as pain and redness as well as myalgia. Antibody responses were detected in all but one of the participants receiving the HCV core ISCOMATRIX vaccine and there was no indication of a dose response. CD8(+) T-cell responses were only detected in two of the eight participants receiving the highest dose. T-cell cytokines were detected in 7 of the 8 participants in the highest dose group. The results of this study support the further evaluation of this prototype HCV core ISCOMATRIX vaccine in HCV infected subjects.

Other strategies include the fusion of recombinant HCV proteins with bacterial pore-forming toxoids in order to generate both CD4+ and CD8+ mediated cellular immune responses. The detoxified bacterial toxoids have the ability to induce pore-mediated endocytosis in antigen-presenting cells, thus resulting in the effective presentation of both toxoid-derived and HCV-derived epitopes in association with class I and class II MHC molecules.

Vaccines based on HCV DNA

Deoxyribonucleic acid-based vaccines have several theoretical advantages including the ease and cost of manufacture and the gene-mediated synthesis in vivo of native and possibly complex protein structures that would otherwise be difficult to produce. In addition, they have good stability and the ready ability to employ multiple genes to elicit broad immune responses. One distinctive feature of DNA-based vaccines is their ability to stimulate significant MHC class I-restricted CTL responses via de novo endogenous protein synthesis in the cytosol. The disadvantages of this approach include a weaker potency as compared with other vaccine formulations, as well as safety issues related to the potential of exogenous DNA to integrate into the host genome, thereby increasing the risks of mutagenesis and carcinogenesis. In the chimpanzee model, only one small DNA vaccine study has been reported so far. DNA was administered using a bio-injector into the quadriceps on weeks 0, 9, and 23, followed by experimental challenge with homologous monoclonal virus, 3 weeks later. Importantly, both vaccinees resolved their acute infections quickly, whereas the control, unvaccinated animal became chronically infected following viral challenge. Although humoral and cellular immune responses to the vaccine were observed in only one animal out of two, both vaccinated animals displayed lower viral titers following challenge and developed hepatitis earlier as compared to control animals, as a result of the primed immunity.

An important parameter to be considered in DNA-based vaccination strategies is the method of vaccine delivery. It has been observed that administration of a gpE2 DNA vaccine by gene gun, in which DNA is administered intraepithelially on gold microparticles, resulted in anti-gpE2 titers that were 100 times higher than those following intramuscular injection by needle. This increase in vaccine potency translates to the need for a lower dose of DNA vaccine in human immunization, thus reducing safety concerns around the integration frequency. Other methods to improve the potency of DNA vaccines include the application of an electric field at the site of DNA injection, with a procedure called "in vivo electroporation". In the case of a gpE2 DNA vaccine, electroporation led to a 10-fold increase in gpE2 protein expression levels and in subsequent gpE2-specific immune responses. The latter also included the generation of cross-reactive anti-E2HVR1 antibodies that were not obtained without electroporation. In addition, a significant increase in gpE2-specific CD4+ T helper and CD8+ CTL responses was observed with this strategy.

Another promising method of vaccine delivery is represented by the formulation of DNA into microparticles, which enhances uptake by antigen-presenting dendritic cells with a corresponding increase in antigen presentation and priming of specific immune responses. Lipid formulations of DNA, which have also been reported to improve transfection efficiency in vivo as well as uptake by dendritic cells, are now part of an immunization regimen for rhesus macaques against simian-human immunodeficiency virus (SHIV) challenge that could be extended to vaccination against HCV and other infectious diseases.

ChronVac-C is a DNA-based vaccine using plasmids expressing HCV proteins NS3 and 4a made by Tripep AB (Stockholm, Sweden). This is coadministered intramuscularly with electroporation (EP) as a delivery system. EP consists of a number of short electrical pulses, which are said to be painful but short lived. EP has been shown to enhance cellular responses probably through creation of pores in the cell membranes of target cells that enhance vaccine delivery. Additionally the damage to the cell membranes is thought to enhance a local inflammatory response at the site of vaccination. A phase I clinical trial in 12 treatment naïve, genotype-1 HCV infected patients, with low viral load (<800,000 IU/mL) is currently underway. Interim results suggest that 4/6 showed a decline in viral load of >0.5 logs with a concomitant increase in T-cell reactivity in three of these patients. DNA vaccines are able to induce strong cytotoxic T-cell responses. Moreover, their production is feasible, inexpensive, and they are safe in animals and humans.

HCV Vaccines Delivered by Vectors
The use of a defective or attenuated viral or bacterial vector to deliver vaccines can offer improved immunogenicity as a result of a wide tropism of the vector, including that of antigen-presenting cells, as well as being able to stimulate innate immune responses which in turn stimulate adaptive immune responses to the encoded vaccine antigens. Furthermore, the use of a vector that is already used as a vaccine itself offers a potential advantage with respect to safety, manufacturing, and distribution issues.

This vaccine is aimed at priming HCV-specific CD4 and CD8 T-cells, using an adenovirus-based vector approach and focusing on the virus NS (NS3-NS4A-NS4B- NS5A-NS5B) proteins. Adenoviral vectors serotype 6 (Ad6) and 24 (Ad24) carrying genes coding for the HCV NS proteins (genotype 1b) were used as prime followed by a plasmid DNA boost. This regimen elicited HCV-specific and multispecific CD4+ and CD8+ T-cells in four of the five vaccines. Following a delayed experimental challenge with a heterologous 1a strain, these four animals showed a clear amelioration of acute viremia and hepatitis followed by eradication of viremia.

Subsequent testing in healthy human volunteers using human Ad6 priming and chimpanzee adenovirus 3 (ChAd3) boost. However, boosting was not as robust with heterologous adenovirus as it was later found to be with modified vaccinia Ankara (MVA), so the vaccine was advanced to HCV at-risk subjects with ChAd3 prime and MVA boost, both expressing NS3–5. This latest regimen was tested in healthy human volunteers and demonstrated optimal priming and boosting with the generation of high frequencies of polyfunctional, broad HCV-specific memory CD4 and CD8 T-cells. The ChAd3-NS prime and MVA-NS boost strategy is being evaluated in a staged phase I/II study, under way in Baltimore, San Francisco, and New Mexico. Vaccine responses were primed with the ChAd3-NS at a dose previously found to be well-tolerated and immunogenic in healthy volunteers, followed by boosting 8 weeks later with MVA-NS. The primary endpoint of this study is to prevent HCV persistence in HCV naïve populations of PWID at high risk for infection. Phase I of the trial was completed with safety signal and immunogenicity parameters supporting advancement, and enrollment in phase II of the trial began in 2013.

Other vector approaches to HCV vaccination are less developed till date but includes the use of an attenuated rabies viral vector into which the HCV gpE1-gpE2-p7 gene cassette was inserted. Recombinant defective adenoviruses expressing the HCV C-gpE1-gpE2 gene cassette have also been shown to prime HCV-specific CTLs in mice immunized intramuscularly, although the induction of anti-gpE1/gpE2 antibodies required further immunization with purified gpE1/gpE2 glycoproteins.

Recombinant canarypox viruses expressing an HCV gene cassette containing C-gpE1-gpE2-p7-NS2-NS3 were shown to induce HCV-specific humoral and cellular immune responses in mice, although the most effective immunization regimen required an initial priming with a plasmid DNA expressing the HCV genes and a subsequent boost with the recombinant canarypox virus.

Attenuated *Salmonella typhimurium* transformed with a plasmid expressing the HCV NS3 gene has been recently investigated in the human leukocyte antigen (HLA)-A2. One transgenic mouse model for its capability to induce NS3-specific CTLs. The results of the study indicated that the bacterium-based immunization was effective by oral administration and the resulting CTL responses persisted for at least 10 months.

11. What is the status of different vaccine candidates?

These are given in **Tables 1 and 2**.

TABLE 1: Current hepatitis C virus vaccine development strategies.

Main target	Stage	Immunogen	Vaccine regimen induced immune response	Potential improvements
T-cells	Phase II	NS3–NS5 Chimpanzee adenovirus 3 priming + modified vaccinia Ankara boost	• Polyfunctional CD4 and CD8 T-cells • No antibodies (Abs)	• More potent vectors (e.g., CMV) • Invariant chain combination (enhanced Ag presentation) • Combination with recombinant proteins • Combination with immune check point blockade (for direct-acting antiviral-treated subjects
Antibodies	Phase I	gpE1/gpE2 Recombinant gpE1/ gpE2 + adjuvant (MF59C.1	Broadly neutralizing antibodies Some CD4 T-cells	• Better adjuvants • Better CD8 T-cell response inducers • Combination with nonstructural proteins

Source: Adapted from Shoukry NH. Hepatitis C vaccines, antibodies, and T-cells. Front Immunol. 2018;9:1480.

TABLE 2: Prophylactic and therapeutic vaccine candidates.

Prophylactic vaccine candidates	Efficacy	Stage
Recombinant gpE1/gpE2 in oil/water adjuvants	Protects chimpanzees against chronic infection	Phase I clinical trials
Recombinant gpE1 in alum	Prime humoral and cellular immune responses in humans	Phase I/II clinical trials
Recombinant VLPs containing C, gpE1 and gpE2	Highly immunogenic in mice and baboons	Preclinical
DNA encoding gpE1/gpE2 in polylactide coglycolide particle	Substantial increase in anti-gpE1/gpE2 antibody titer in mice compared with naked DNA	Preclinical
DNA prime and protein boost (using C, gpE1, gpE2 and NS3)	Protection or amelioration in chimp challenge model	Preclinical
DNA prime and canarypox boost (encoding all HCV genes)	Broad Th1 cellular immune responses in mice	Preclinical
Vaccinia virus expressing all HCV genes (A Prince; personal communication)	Chimpanzee challenge studies in progress	Preclinical
Defective alpha-viral particles expressing gpE1/gpE2 and NS genes	Mouse studies in progress	Preclinical
Modified vaccinia Ankara expressing gpE1/gpE2	Induces Th1 response in HLA A2.1 mice	Preclinical
Semliki forest virus expressing NS3	Induces NS3-specific CTLs in mice	Preclinical
Detective ovine at adenovirus expressing NS3	Strong Th1 cellular response in mice	Preclinical
Immunotherapeutic Vaccine Candidates		
Alum-adjuvanted gpE1 glycoprotein	Boosts humoral and cellular immune responses to gpE1 in HCV patients. May ameliorate hepatitis	Phase I/II patient trials
Adjuvanted peptide cocktails (A von Gabain, intercell, personal communication)	Designed to boost CD4+ and CD8+ responses to conserved T-cell epitopes using novel adjuvant	Phase II patient trials
Oil/water-adjuvanted gpE1/gpE2 proteins	Prophylactic efficacy in chimpanzees. Boosts anti-gpE1/gpE2	Phase Ib patient trials
ISCOMATRIX®-adjuvanted core protein	Primes Th1-type CD4+ and CD8+ CTL responses in macaques and uninfected humans to conserved epitopes within core antigen	Phase Ib patient trials

Contd...

Contd...

ISCOMATRIX®-adjuvanted NS3-NS4-NS5-C polyprotein (MH, unpublished data)	Primes broad Th1-type CD4+ and CD8+ CTL responses in chimpanzees which have reduced viremia and hepatitis, after challenge with heterologous HCV	Preclinical
Prime with recombinant adenovirus and boost with electroporated DNA (expressing HCV NS3, 4, and 5) (A Nicosia, personal communication)	Primes broad CD4+ and CD8+ T-cells chimpanzee challenge studies in progress	Preclinical
Heat-killed yeast expressing C and NS372	Primes specific CD4+ and CD8+ T-cells in mice	Preclinical

(VLPs: virus-like particles; DNA: deoxyribonucleic acid; HCV: hepatitis C virus; HLA: human leukocyte antigen; CTL: cytotoxic T lymphocyte)

12. What is therapeutic HCV vaccine? What is its importance?

A vaccine that prevents and treats HCV infection is urgently required. A therapeutic vaccine would also be an invaluable adjunct to current treatment options for HCV. Today's gold-standard treatment for HCV consists of pegylated-interferon and ribavirin. But the current medical therapy for chronic hepatitis C eradicates the virus in a minority of patients and it is associated with high cost and serious side effects. The current cure rates using this treatment are 45% for genotype-1 and -4 infections, 70% for genotype-3 and 80% for genotype-2. Once cirrhosis is established, a cure is less likely still and liver transplantation may be the only option. There is, therefore, a pressing need to develop vaccination strategies aimed at preventing and possibly eradicating HCV infection.

SUGGESTED READING

1. Abdelwahab KS, Ahmed Said ZN. Status of hepatitis C virus vaccination: recent update. World J Gastroenterol. 2016;22(2):862-73.
2. Bailey JR, Barnes E, Cox AL. Approaches, progress, and challenges to hepatitis C vaccine. Develop Gastroenterol. 2019;156:418-30.
3. Drane D, Maraskovsky E, Gibson R, Mitchell S, Barnden M, Moskwa A, et al. Priming of CD4þ and CD8þ T-cell responses using a HCV core ISCOMATRIX vaccine: a phase I study in healthy volunteers. Hum Vaccin. 2009;5:151-7.
4. Dunlop JI, Owsianka AM, Cowton VM, Patel AM. Current and future prophylactic vaccines for hepatitis C virus vaccine. Deve Ther. 2015;5:31-44.
5. Ebeling F. Epidemiology of the hepatitis C virus. Vox Sang. 1998;74:143-6.
6. Ghasemi F, Ghayour-Mobarhan M, Gouklani F,4 Meshkat Z. Development of preventive vaccines for hepatitis C virus E1/E2 Protein. Iran J Pathol. 2018(Spring);13(2):113-24.
7. Patel K, Muir AJ, McHutchinson JG. Diagnosis and treatment of chronic hepatitis infection. BMJ. 2006;332:1013-7.

8. Plotkin SA, Orenstein W, Offit PA, Edwards KM. Plotkin's Textbook of Vaccinology. Amsterdam: Elsevier; 2017.
9. Seeff LB. Natural history of chronic hepatitis. Hepatology. 2002;36:S35-46.
10. Sene D, Limal N, Cacoub P. Hepatitis C virus-associated extrahepatic manifestations: a review. Metab Brain Dis. 2004;19:357-81.
11. Shah AK. Hepatitis C vaccine. In: Vashishtha VM (Ed). IAP Textbook of Vaccines, 2nd edition. New Delhi: Jaypee Brothers Medical Publishers (P) Ltd.; 2020.
12. Shepard CW, Finelli L, Alter MJ. Global epidemiology of hepatitis C virus infection. Lancet Infect Dis. 2005;5(9):558-67.
13. Shoukry NH. Hepatitis C vaccines, antibodies, And T-cells. Front Immunol. 2018;9:1480.
14. Swadling L, Capone S, Antrobus RD, Brown A, Richardson R, Newell EW, et al. A human vaccine strategy based on chimpanzee adenoviral and MVA vectors that primes, boosts, and sustains functional HCV-specific T-cell memory. Sci Transl Med. 2014;6:261ra153.
15. World Health Organization. Hepatitis C. Weekly Epidemiol Rec. 1997;72:65-72.

CHAPTER 47

Zika Virus Vaccines

M Surendranath

1. What is the epidemiology of Zika virus infection?

Zika fever is caused by Zika virus (ZIKV), an arthropod born virus (arbovirus). The Zika virus is a member of the Flavivirus genus, family Flaviviridae. It is related to dengue, yellow fever, West Nile and Japanese encephalitis viruses, which belong to Flaviviridae family.

Zika virus was discovered in 1947 in a Rhesus macaque in Zika forest in Uganda. It was isolated from monkey in 1952. Virus isolated from human in Nigeria in 1954. Confirmed cases of Zika fever are rare till 2007. In 2007, major epidemic occurred in Yap Island, Micronesia. More recently epidemics have occurred in Polynesia, Easter Island, the Cook Islands and Caledonia. A large outbreak occurred in 2015 in Brazil. Since April 2015, a large ongoing outbreak of Zika virus spread across much of South and Central America and the Caribbean. According to CDC, Brazilian authorities reported more than 200,000 cases are identified and 3,500 microcephaly cases between October 2015 and January 2016. Some of the affected infants had severe microcephaly and some died.

Despite the large outbreaks in 2015–2016, subsequent years have been relatively quiet in terms of ZIKV. In the United States and US territories, there were over 41,000 cases in 2016, fewer than 1,200 cases in 2017, and only 220 cases in 2018 **(Fig. 1)**.

2. What is incidence of Zika virus infection in India?

Three cases were reported in India from Ahmedabad, Gujarat in 2017 and another case from Krishnagiri district of Tamil Nadu. One case of Zika virus infection in a 78-year-old woman was reported from Jaipur on September 21st, 2018. Following that, National Centre for Disease Control (NCBC) reported 157 cases including 63 pregnant women, which was confirmed by RT-PCR. To-date no cases of microcephaly or congenital Zika syndrome are reported on follow-up of infected pregnant women. Government of India is maintaining 34 laboratories to detect Zika virus infection in febrile illness patients. These laboratories are developed as a part of National Zika Action plan. Despite the presence of agent, susceptible host, and ideal tropical climate, the presence is lower in India. With this outbreak, India has shifted to WHO category.

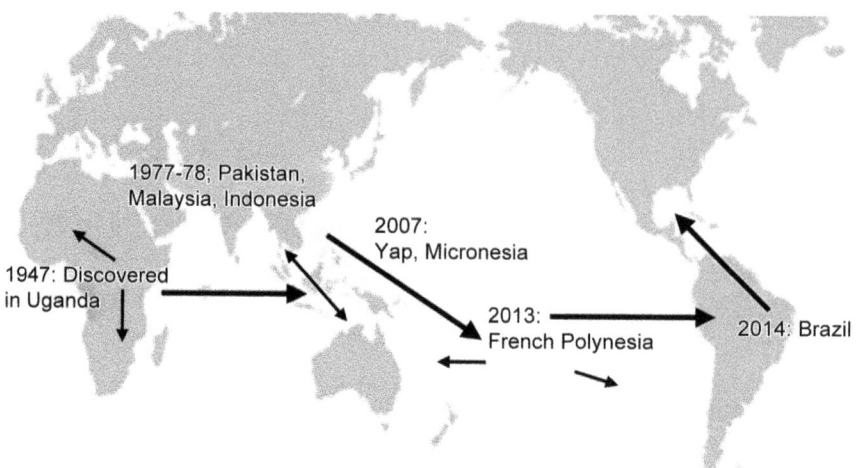

Fig. 1: Outbreak and migration areas of Zika virus infection.

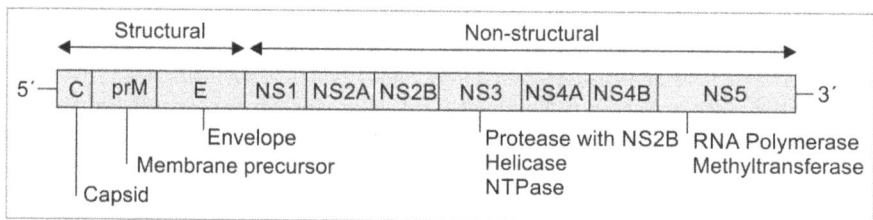

Fig. 2: The structure of Zika virus (ZIKV) genome and its encoded proteins.

3. What is structure of Zika virus?

Zika is an emerging, mosquito-borne, enveloped, nonsegmented, 10-kilobase, single-stranded, positive-sense RNA Flavivirus of global significance. Three main genetic lineages of ZIKV [2 from Africa (African I and African II lineages) and 1 from Asia] have been identified. Genetic analyses indicate that its geographic circulation was limited to the areas around Africa and Asia by the 2000s; ZIKV then evolved into 2 distinct lineages with differential pathogenesis—African (i.e., African I lineage) and Asian.

The Zika genome is analogous to that of other Flaviviridae RNA viruses (i.e., yellow fever, Japanese encephalitis, West Nile, tick-borne encephalitis, and dengue type 1-4 viruses) and encodes for three major structural proteins [i.e., prM, capsid (C), and E (a primary target of neutralizing antibody development)] and seven nonstructural proteins (i.e., NS1, NS2A, NS2B, NS3, NS4A, NS4B, and NS5) **(Fig. 2)**. Notably, the nonstructural NS5 protein is implicated in RNA synthesis and viral replication. Importantly, the proteins documented to have significance in terms of immune response include nonstructural protein NS5 that has been shown to suppress type I IFN signaling through STAT2-mediated degradation in the ZIKV-infected host. During viral shedding, prM is cleaved by furin protein to generate mature infectious virions. Zika virus E protein is the main surface protein that participates in host cell receptor attachment and virus lipid bilayer fusion, while the nonstructural NS1 through NS5 proteins are engaged in virus propagation. Robust adaptive immune responses to ZIKV E, NS1, NS3, NS4B, and NS5 proteins such as production of neutralizing antibodies and T-cell responses have been detected in animal models of ZIKV infection, which indicates that vaccination may protect against ZIKV disease.

4. How the Zika virus infection transmitted?

Zika is spread mostly by the bite of an infected *Aedes* species mosquito (*Aedes aegypti* and *Aedes albopictus*). Fetus may be affected by infected pregnant mother, through sex and may be through blood transfusion, but not confirmed.

5. What are the clinical features of Zika virus infections?

Eighty percent of Zika virus infections are asymptomatic and 20% have mild symptoms. Incubation period is 3-10 days. Most common symptoms are fever, rash, headache, joint pains, red eyes, and muscular pain. Symptoms can last for several days to a week. Symptoms are mild. Very rarely, it results in death. One infection can give protection against further infections. Guillain-Barré syndrome is increasingly reported with Zika fever. Zika infection in pregnancy can affect the fetus. Zika associated birth defects are selected structural anomalies of brain or eyes and may be present at birth or detected from birth to age of 2 years. Microcephaly at birth, with or without low birth weight. Brain anomalies may be intracranial calcification, lissencephaly, pachygyria, schizencephaly, gray matter heterotopia, corpus callosum abnormalities, cerebellar abnormalities, porencephaly, hydranencephaly, ventriculomegaly, and hydrocephaly. Congenital eye anomalies such as micro- or anophthalmia, coloboma, cataract, intraocular calcifications, chorioretinal anomalies involving macula, optic nerve atrophy can occur. Neurodevelopmental abnormalities, hearing abnormalities, congenital contractures, seizures are also reported. Zika virus infection of mother during pregnancy causes congenital Zika syndrome.

6. What are the vaccines under the research for Zika virus?

At least two scenarios can be envisaged for a ZIKV vaccine for which WHO SAGE advised on immunization strategies; these are outbreak response and routine/endemic transmission use. Vaccine development started in the second half of 2015. First reports of phase I clinical evaluation of vaccine candidates have been published in late 2017. Over 45 vaccine candidates have been evaluated in the discovery phase, over 25 are in nonclinical development, and 9 are in clinical evaluation. Four types of vaccines have been in phase I clinical trials **(Table 1)**:
1. *DNA vaccine*: Vaccine works by creating a plasmid that encodes the genes for virus envelop proteins. DNA vaccine consists of prM + E viral proteins. Once the plasmid enters the nucleus of target cell, the host cell will start producing the viral proteins, which will induce immune response.

TABLE 1: Ongoing trials: Zika virus vaccine.

Vaccine	Adjuvant	Developer	Regimen (weeks/route)	Phase	Clinical trial
GLS-5700 Synthetic ZIKV prM/E	None	Inovio and GeneOne Life Sciences	1, 2 mg/ID 2 mg/ID	I	NCT02809443 NCT02887482
VRC-ZKADNA085-00-VP	None	NIH/VRC	0 + 8, 0 + 12, 0 + 4 + 8, 0 + 4 + 20 4 mg/IM/both arms	I	NCT02840487
VRC-ZKADNA090-00-VP ZIKV wt prM/E	None	NIH/VRC	0 + 4 + 8 4 mg/IM Needle vs, PharmaJet	I	NCT02996461
VRC-ZKADNA090-00-VP ZIKA wt prM/E	None	NIH/VRC	0 + 4 + 8 4 mg vs, 8 mg/IM/both arms, PharmaJet	II	NCT03110770
Inactivated ZIKV MRB766	Aluminum	Bharat Biotech	0 + 30 days 2.5 vs, 5 mg vs, 10 mg	I	CTRI/2017/05/008539
Inactivated ZIKV (VLA 1601)	Aluminum	Valneva (+ Emergent Biosolutions)	0 + 1 vs, 0 + 4 3 vs, 6 antigen units	I	NCT03425149
Zika-purified inactivated vaccine (ZPIV)	Aluminum	WRAIR	0, 0+1, 0+2, 0+4, 5 mg/IM 0+4, 2.5 vs, 5 vs, 10 mg/IM 0+4, 5 mg/IM (±YF ± ixario) ZPIV booster at 1 year (Puerto Rico) 0+4, 5 mg/IM	I	NCT02937233 NCT02952833 NCT03008122 NCT02963909
Inactivated ZIKV (TAK-426)	Aluminum	Takeda	0 + 4, 2 vs, 5 vs, 10 mg/IM	I	NCT03343626
Live measles virus-Zika (MV-Zika)	None	Themis	Low vs, high dose 0 vs, 0+4	I/II	NCT02996890
Messenger RNA (mRNA)	none	Valera/Moderna	mRNA-1325	I/II	NCT03014089

Source: Barrett, A.D.T. Current status of Zika vaccine development: Zika vaccines advance into clinical evaluation. NPJ vaccines. 2018;3:4.

The US National Institute of Allergy and Infectious Diseases (NIAID) is developing the vaccine which now is in phase II trials.

Tebas et al. published results of phase I clinical trials studies of prM+ E consensus DNA vaccine in Zika naïve subjects who received three doses (at 0, 4, and 12 weeks) of either 1 mg or 2 mg by intradermal route. About 62% had neutralizing titers 2 weeks after third dose of vaccine. Gaudinski et al. reported two phase I trials using two prM + E DNA vaccines VRC 5288 consisting of ZIKV prM + E (French Polynesian strain) with carboxy-terminal 98 amino acids from Japanese encephalitis virus that encodes the stem-anchor region while VRC 5283 consists of only ZIKV prM+E sequence. Best results were obtained with VRC 5283.

2. *Modified RNA vaccine*: Viral RNA sequence is used as a vaccine. Unlike DNA vaccine, these vaccines can produce as soon as they enter the cell without penetrating the nucleus. Two candidate-modified RNA vaccines are currently undergoing phase I trials. Vaccine generated by Richner et al. consists of lipid-encapsulated nanoparticle (mRNA LNP) given by intramuscular route containing modified mRNA encoding the prM/E genes that are expressed in the cells to produce virus-like particles. Second one is generated by Pardi et al. and consists of mRNA LNP based on Zika virus RNA of a French Polynesian isolate from 2013.

3. *Purified formalin inactivated vaccine (PIV)*: A purified inactivated Zika vaccine (ZPIV) developed by Walter Reed Army Institute of Research (WRAIR) based similar approach used for developing Japanese encephalitis and dengue vaccines. In phase I trial, when used as two-dose schedule with 4 weeks apart, 92% of subjects showed seroconversion measured as neutralization titers >10 and 77% showing neutralization titers >100 and GMT of 173 at 4 weeks after second dose. Modjarrad K et al. reported results of phase I clinical trials of aPIV with aluminum as adjuvant based on a PIV with aluminum as adjuvanted based on Puerto Rican strain of ZIKV.

4. *Live-attenuated Zika virus*: The experimental vaccine, known as rZIKV/D4Δ30-713, was developed by scientists of NIAID laboratory of viral diseases. The laboratory used genetic engineering techniques to create a chimeric virus, made by combining genes from multiple viruses. The chimeric virus consists of dengue virus type 4 backbone that expresses Zika virus surface proteins. The vaccine is being evaluated in phase I clinical trial initiated in August 2018. Another live-attenuated vaccine is currently in phase III clinical trial in Brazil. Future research is aiming to create a combination dengue and Zika vaccine. MV-ZIKA is live-attenuated viral vectored vaccine used measles virus Schwarz strain as backbone into which nucleotide sequence encoding Zika virus structural protein prM and E were inserted. Phase 1 clinical trial is going on.

5. A vaccine is designed to protect against multiple mosquito-borne diseases, including Zika. AGS-v is designed to trigger an immune response to mosquito salivary proteins rather than specific virus or parasite carried by mosquito. The vaccine contains four synthetic

proteins from mosquito salivary glands. The proteins are designed to induce antibodies in a vaccinated individual and to cause a modified allergic response that can prevent infection when a person is bitten by a disease-carrying mosquito. This vaccine is in phase I clinical trial.
6. Another investigational vaccine is a genetically engineered version of vesicular stomatitis virus of cattle.
7. *Therapeutic vaccination*: Monoclonal antibodies developed against Zika virus have been used as prophylactic vaccine against ZIKV viremia and have a potential to prevent maternal–fetal transmission. Passive administration of human mAbs provides a potentially important approach for short-term protective immunity especially for pregnant women or can give protection till the immune response of active immunization develops.

7. **What are the challenges of developing Zika virus vaccine?**
- Antibody-mediated immune enhancement of dengue virus infection needs to be avoided where other Flavivirus infections are present. The vaccine must elicit protective immunity irrespective of previous dengue infection. It is not yet clear to what extent the preexisting immunity to other Flavivirus influences the Zika vaccine immune responses.
- Vaccine should be safe for all age groups and protect all age groups against Zika virus infection.
- Vaccine should be able to transfer protective antibodies to fetus and neonate.
- Vaccine should not cause neurological side effects such as Guillain-Barré syndrome.
- Till date no correlates of protection established.
- Clinical efficacy is very difficult to assess when 80% infections are asymptomatic.

SUGGESTED READING
1. Centre for Disease Control and Prevention. Zika Virus. [online] Available from: https://www.cdc.gov/zika/index.html. [Last Accessed August, 2020].
2. Poland GA, Ovsyannikova IG, Kennedy RB. Zika vaccine development: current status. Mayo Clin Proc. 2019;94(12):2572-86.
3. Song BH, Yun SI, Woolley M, Lee YM. Zika virus: history, epidemiology, transmission, and clinical presentation. J Neuroimmunol. 2017;308:50-64.
4. Vashishtha VM. IAP Textbook of Vaccines 2020. New Delhi: Jaypee Brothers Medical Publishers (P) Ltd,; 2020. pp. 632-7.
5. WHO. Zika Epidemiology Update (July 2019). [online] Available from: https://www.who.int/emergencies/diseases/zika/epidemiology-update/en/. [Last Accessed August, 2020].
6. World Health Organization. Zika virus infection: India. [online] Available from: https://www.who.int/emergencies/diseases/zika/india-november-2018/en/. [Last Accessed August, 2020].
7. ZikaVirusNet.com. Zika virus. [online] Available from: zikavirusnet.com. [Last Accessed August, 2020].

CHAPTER 48

Chikungunya Vaccines

Sachidanand Kamath, Geeta MG

1. What are the key characteristics of Chikungunya virus (CHIKV)?

Chikungunya virus (CHIKV) is a mosquito-borne virus. It belongs to the family Togaviridae, genus Alphavirus. The virus was first isolated from human samples obtained during outbreak of febrile disease with debilitating joint pains and rash in Tanganyika Territory (now Tanzania), 1952. The word "Chikungunya" is derived from Makonde language; meaning "that which bends up". It requires BSL3 containment for laboratory storage.

Biology of Chikungunya Virus
This organism is an icosahedral virus particle, ~65 nm diameter. The external envelope comprised of trimeric spikes of 240 E1/E2 protein heterodimers embedded in lipid membrane. E1 involved in membrane fusion; E2 involved in receptor binding. Envelope surrounds icosahedral nucleocapsid comprised of single copy of RNA genome with 240 capsid proteins **(Fig. 1)**.

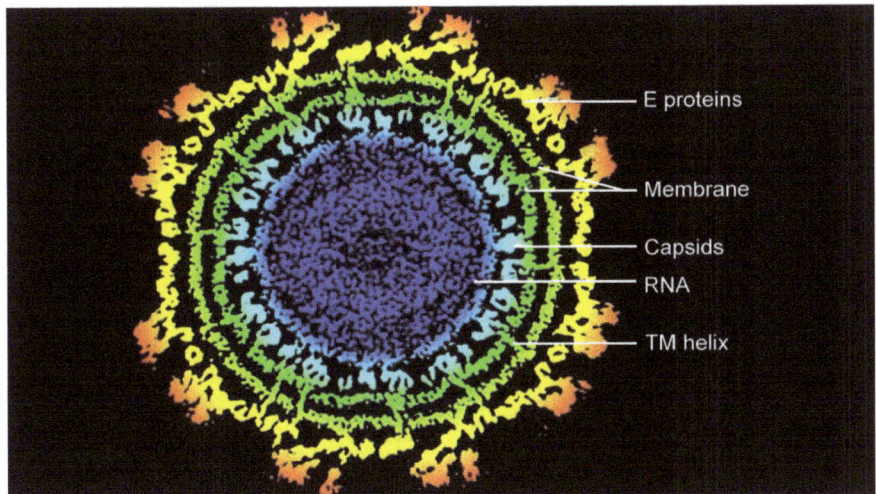

Fig. 1: Chikungunya virus (CHIKV)—virion structure.
Source: Chikungunya Vaccines Pipeline, WHO Collaborating Centre for Vaccine Research, Evaluation, and training on Emerging Infectious Diseases.

2. What is the origin and phylogenetics of Chikungunya virus?

There are three major genotypes of CHIKV: West African, East/Central/South Africa virus lineage (ECSA), and Asian along with an Indian Ocean lineage (IOL), a subtype of ECSA **(Fig. 2)**. Chikungunya virus evolved in sub-Saharan Africa in transmission cycles involving arboreal mosquitoes and wild primates. Emergence into urban transmission involving peridomestic mosquitoes has occurred repeatedly, probably for centuries. The Asian and Indian Ocean lineages have recently spread to five continents, causing millions of cases of severe and often chronic arthralgia. Based on failure since the 1950s to control dengue virus, the prospects for controlling urban CHIKV spread are poor. The arrival of an Asian strain of CHIKV in the Americas in 2013 has dramatically increased the human populations at risk.

The CHIKV-ECSA was first detected in Brazil in the municipality of Feira de Santana (FS) by mid-2014. Following that, a large number of CHIKV cases have been notified in FS, which is the second-most populous city in Bahia state, northeastern Brazil, and plays an important role on the spread to other Brazilian states due to climate conditions and the abundance of competent vectors.

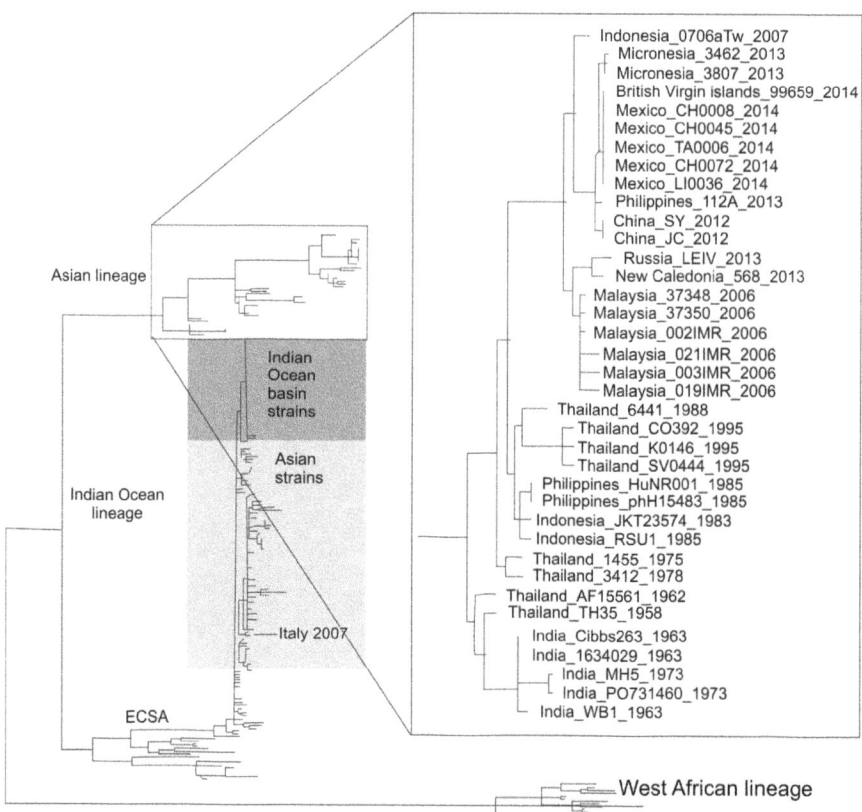

Fig. 2: Phylogenetic tree of Chikungunya virus (CHIKV).

Source: Chikungunya Vaccines Pipeline, WHO Collaborating Centre for Vaccine Research, Evaluation, and training on Emerging Infectious Diseases.

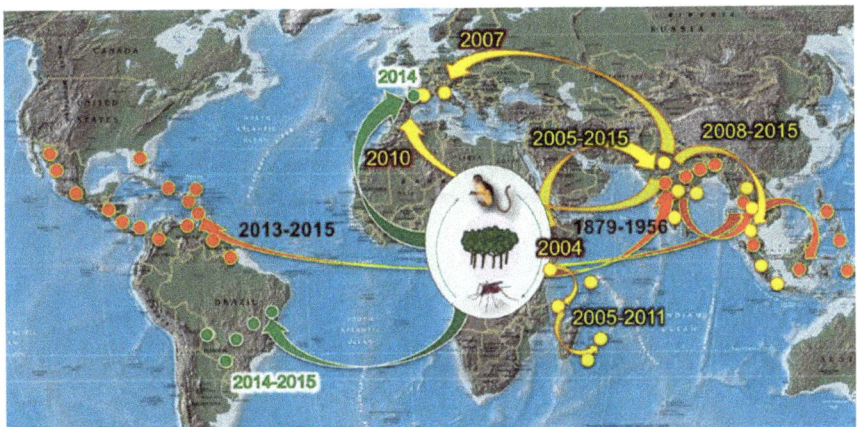

Fig. 3: Re-emergence and spread of Chikungunya virus (CHIKV) to different continents.
Source: Chikungunya Vaccines Pipeline, WHO Collaborating Centre for Vaccine Research, Evaluation, and training on Emerging Infectious Diseases.

3. Why is Chikungunya considered to be a re-emerging infection?

Chikungunya virus, an arbovirus belonging to the family Togaviridae has been receiving a lot of attention in the recent past due to the large outbreaks it has caused and the considerable morbidity and loss of productivity it has led to in several countries of Asia, Africa and in hitherto unaffected countries in Europe as well, and is considered to be a re-emerging infection **(Fig. 3)**.

4. What is the global burden of Chikungunya?

Nearly 1.3 billion people live in areas endemic for Chikungunya. The disease is prevalent in ~60 countries over the world. Numerous epidemics of Chikungunya have been reported in several countries in Southern and South East Asia. Distinct strains of Chikungunya virus within varying transmission cycles have been reported from different locations. The African variant has managed to persist over the years with frequent outbreaks due to a sylvatic cycle maintained between monkeys and wild mosquitoes. Conversely, the Asian variant causes epidemics that are maintained by an urban cycle, characterized by long interepidemic quiescence for more than 10 years or so.

The first Asian epidemic was reported in Bangkok, Thailand, in 1958, continued until 1964, and reappeared after a hiatus in the mid-1970s and declined again in 1976. Major outbreaks were also reported from northwestern and southern parts of India, Sri Lanka, Myanmar, and Thailand in the early 1960s **(Fig. 4)**. Overall, 101 countries/territories have reported CHIKV cases. Around two-thirds of all cases are located in low- and middle-income countries (LMICs). So far, around 1.66 million cases have been suspected out of which 42,721 were confirmed cases and 252 deaths in the Americas were reported till 2015 (>3/4ths of cases were in LMICs).

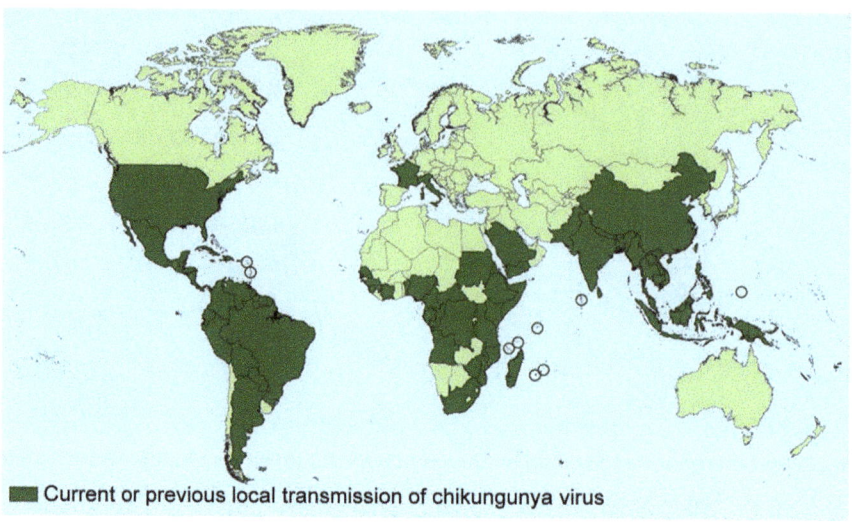

Fig. 4: Countries and territories where Chikungunya cases have been reported* (as of September 17, 2019).
*Does not include countries or territories where only imported cases have been documented.
Source: CDC. Chikungunya. [online] Available from: https://www.cdc.gov/chikungunya/pdfs/chik_world_map_09-17-19-p.pdf. [Last Accessed August, 2020].

5. What are the epidemiological features of recent outbreaks of Chikungunya in India?

Since CHIKV infections were first reported in 1952-53, the disease has spread rapidly to involve vast areas of the tropics including Africa, South East Asia and the Indian Ocean region. There was a large outbreak in the Indian Ocean islands of Reunion and Mauritius in 2005-2006, in which *Aedes albopictus* was found to be the main vector. There were more than a million cases reported from India in 2006-2007, in which the two Southern States of Kerala and Tamil Nadu were hit hardest, and *Aedes aegypti* was the main vector, except in Kerala, where *A. albopictus* was also implicated. The 2007 epidemic in Italy and 2010 epidemic in France were proof that the virus was not confined to the tropics as was previously believed. Epidemics often occur at an interval of about 10 years and often occur following the monsoon season due to the high vector density. Humans are the reservoirs of infection during epidemics. Although *Aedes aegypti* was considered the traditional vector, *A. albopictus* has assumed importance as a vector in recent epidemics, and this has been attributed to the mutation of the virus, enabling efficient transmission by *A. albopoctus*. Four strains of CHIKV have been identified including the ECSA (Eastern, Central and South African), West African, Asian, and Reunion strains.

6. What are the key clinical characteristics of the Chikungunya infection?

The incubation period of CHIKV disease is typically 3-7 days, followed by onset of clinical signs. Attack rates can be extremely high: 70-90% reported in some outbreaks. Estimates of subclinical infection rates vary but are generally low (5–25%).

Acute disease (~2–3 weeks) characterized by fever with inflammatory arthralgia/arthritis, accompanied by other nonspecific symptoms, e.g., myalgia, headache, rash. Post-acute phase (4 weeks to 3 months) occurs in ~50% of patients and involves persistent joint pain.

Chronic phase (>3 months to years) occurs in a small proportion of patients. In most cases, it involves various musculoskeletal features treatable with nonsteroidal anti-inflammatory drugs (NSAIDs), analgesics, physiotherapy; some (~5%) have chronic inflammatory rheumatism.

Atypical, severe presentations reported in ~0.5–5% of cases, including encephalopathy, encephalitis, myocarditis, hepatitis. Fatal outcomes associated with CHIKV infection have been described in recent epidemics (CFR <1% in most). Most severe/fatal cases associated with other underlying morbidity. Mother to neonate transmission frequent if viremic at delivery and associated with high rates (>50%) of clinical disease in neonates with severe presentation.

7. Who are at risk for severe symptoms?

The disease is especially severe, and often results in encephalopathy, in newborns whose mothers are in the viremic phase, and in old age, including in those with underlying conditions. Dermatological manifestations include transient maculopapular rash, photosensitivity with hyperpigmentation and exfoliative dermatitis. Ophthalmological involvement may occur and includes transient anterior uveitis, optic neuritis and retrobulbar neuritis.

8. What are the laboratory diagnostic features of Chikungunya?

Diagnosis is confirmed by virus isolation, PCR, demonstration of IgM antibodies or a rising titer of IgG antibodies. The detection of IgM antibodies by ELISA is usually possible after 2 weeks, but may take up to 6 weeks. A four-fold rise in IgG titers repeated after 2–4 weeks is diagnostic. Leukopenia with lymphocytosis and a raised CRP and ESR are usually seen, though thrombocytopenia is uncommon. A positive rheumatoid factor may be detected in a few patients either in the acute phase or later.

9. What are the WHO criteria for diagnosis of Chikungunya fever?

Clinical criteria: Acute onset of fever >38.5°C and severe arthralgia/arthritis not explained by other medical conditions.

Epidemiological criteria: Residing or having visited epidemic areas, having reported transmission within 15 days prior to the onset of symptoms.

Laboratory criteria: At least one of the following tests in the acute phase:
- Virus isolation
- Presence of viral RNA by RT-PCR

- Presence of virus specific IgM antibodies in single serum sample collected in acute or convalescent stage
- Four-fold increase in IgG values in samples collected at least 3 weeks apart.

10. What are the WHO case definitions of Chikungunya?

- *Possible case*: A patient meeting clinical criteria
- *Probable case*: A patient meeting both the clinical and epidemiological criteria
- *Confirmed case*: A patient meeting the laboratory criteria, irrespective of the clinical presentation.

It should be kept in mind that it is not necessary to do confirmatory tests in all suspected cases in an epidemic situation, where establishment of an epidemiological link will suffice.

11. Is there any specific treatment for Chikungunya fever?

Treatment is supportive including rest, adequate hydration, antipyretics and analgesics, since no effective antiviral agent is available at present. Chronic joint symptoms are treated with NSAIDs or chloroquine phosphate.

12. Why is it necessary to have a Chikungunya vaccine?

The availability of a vaccine to prevent chikungunya virus (CHIKV) infection is a felt need, considering the pandemic proportions it is likely to assume, the propensity to cause long-term morbidity in large segments of the population, and the risk of fatalities in susceptible individuals, including those at the extremes of age and with compromised immune status. Moreover, there is no specific treatment at present for the disease. CHIKV is classified as a biosafety level 3 pathogen, and the spectre of it being put to use in the gray zone of bioterrorism has been raised.

13. Which vaccines against Chikungunya are undergoing preclinical trials?

Efforts to develop Chikungunya vaccines were initiated in 1960s. Interest resurfaced from 2000 onwards with the re-emergence of the disease in several countries. Over 80 organizations are engaged in efforts to develop a Chikungunya vaccine. Around 40 candidate vaccines are in different stages of development **(Fig. 5)**.

There is no commercially available vaccine to prevent CHIKV infections at present. Inactivated vaccines, attenuated vaccines, chimeric, DNA, m-RNA, viral vectored vaccines, recombinant adenovirus, subunit protein vaccines and virus-like particle (VLP) vaccines are undergoing trials in the preclinical phase.

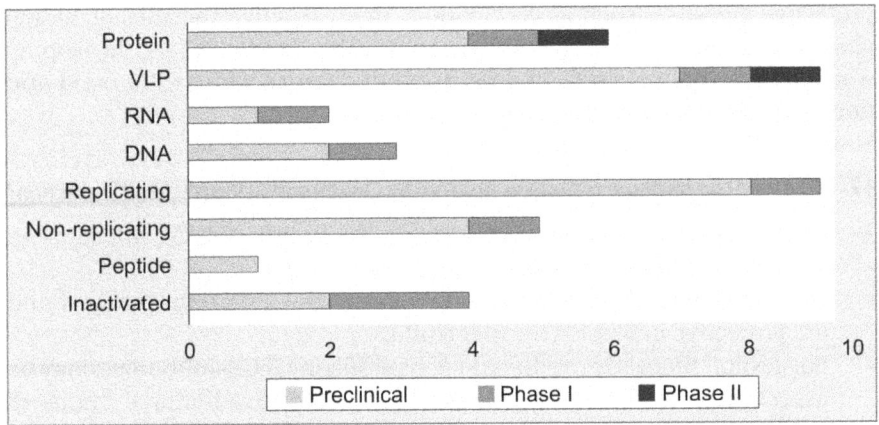

Fig. 5: Different CHIKV vaccine candidates in different stages of development.
Source: Kang G. Chikungunya Vaccines in the Pipeline, 2018. Available from: https://www.who.int/immunization/research/meetings_workshops/28_Kang_Chikungunya.pdf Accessed on September 12, 2020.

14. Is there any role for passive immunization in prevention of Chikungunya?

A study from France has demonstrated the protective efficacy of CHIKV immunoglobulins from convalescent sera in prevention of encephalopathy in mouse neonates and severely immune compromised adult mice.

15. What is the epidemiologic role of CHIKV virus-like particles?

The effectiveness of CHIKV virus-like particles induced in insect cells using recombinant baculoviruses has been demonstrated in wild type adult mouse models. VLPs lack the viral genome and are therefore not able to replicate, although they share a common structure with the wild virus. A single dose of 1 μg of the vaccine has been shown to confer protection from both viremia as well as joint involvement.

The CHIKV VLPs induced in insect cells are considered to be effective candidate vaccines in epidemic situations, since production can be rapidly scaled up to meet the increased need. Although the VLPs were produced using the ECSA strain, cross neutralization of the other CHIKV strains was demonstrated. The rapid scale up possible with the technology involved in mass production of VLPs could be an asset to the concept of pandemic preparedness.

16. What is the role of Integrated Vector Management in prevention of Chikungunya?

The strategy advocated by the WHO at present is "Integrated Vector Management" which includes environmental modification, as well as chemical and biological control strategies. This public health approach will need to be strengthened and should take precedence over individual protective measures such as vaccination. The use of live vaccines including chimeric vaccines have advantages in controlling diseases of the developing world due to the low cost involved in production as well as the rapid and durable protection they afford.

17. What are the immune responses induced by Chikungunya virus (CHIKV) infection?

- Robust IgM/IgG antibody responses following CHIKV infection in humans and animal models.
- Neutralizing antibodies primarily target E1/E2 structural proteins and are protective in passive transfer studies.
- Suggestion that early production of neutralizing IgG3 antibodies, may be associated with reduced risk of prolonged disease; additional studies of Ig subclasses and infection outcome possibly warranted.
- Cytotoxic T-cells contribute to but not necessary for virus clearance. Unclear whether CMI may contribute to immunopathology of CHIK disease.
- Natural infection results in lifelong immunity.

18. Which are the candidate vaccines for Chikungunya in development?

Animal studies are needed to demonstrate the degree of protection conferred by the inactivated vaccine since there are concerns that the antigenicity may be impaired following inactivation. The VLPs induced in insect cells, represent a safe and efficacious option for development of a vaccine for use in humans. Chimeric vaccines will need to be tested in nonhuman primate models before use in clinical trials.

A Phase I/II trial of an experimental vaccine is being conducted at three sites in the United States under the aegis of the National Institute of Allergy and Infectious Diseases (NIAID), part of the National Institutes of Health. The candidate vaccine for the purpose was the result of research done at Themis Bioscience of Vienna, Austria. This is a measles vaccine virus tailored to produce CHIKV proteins in vivo. A similar Phase II trial is also underway in Europe **(Table 1)**.

19. What is the current status of a Chikungunya vaccine in India?

In India, Bharat Biotech, a Hyderabad-based company, has an inactivated vaccine against CHIKV in the pipeline, and preclinical trials are on. There are thus adequate grounds to be reasonably certain that a safe and efficacious vaccine against CHIKV infections will become available in not too distant future.

20. What are the challenges in developing a CHIKV vaccine?

Regulatory challenges: Requirement of a classical Phase III trial for proof of vaccine efficacy and licensure is having a very long timelines and is also

TABLE 1: Current CHIK vaccine candidates in different stages of development.

Entity	Vaccine type	Preclinic	Phase I	Phase II	Phase III
Valneva/Karolinska Institute	Live, attenuated (CHIKV-Δ5nsp 3)	X			
Takeda/UTMB	Live, attenuated (CHIK/IRES)	X			
Arbovax/NC state University	Live, attenuated (transmembrane deletion)	X			
UTMB	Live, attenuated chimeric (various alphavirus backbones)	X			
Themis Bioscience/ Pasteur Institute	Live, vectored (measles virus)		X	2016	
Profectus/Yale/ UTMB	Live, vectored (VSVΔG-CHIKV)	X	2016?		
Karolinska Institute/ CSIC Madrid	Live, vectored (MVA-CHIKV E1E26KE3)	X			
University Wisconsin/Takeda	Live, vectored (MVA-CHIKV E3E3)	X			
NIAID	Virus-like particle (mammalian cells)		X	2015-16	
TI Pharma/ Wageningen University	Virus-like particel (insect cells)	X			
Merck	Virus-like particle (insect cells)	X			
Bharat Biotech	Inactivated (various strains, various methods)	X	2016?		
Indian Immunological	Inactivated (formalin-treated 181/25 from US army)	X	2016?		
DRDE, India	Inactivated (fromalin treated Indian 2006 isolate	X			
Nanotherapeutics inc. (from baxter)	Inactivated	X			
Medigen	DNA (plasmid-launched 181/25 live attenuated)	X			
DRDE, India	Recombinant subunit (E. coli expressed E1/E2)	X			
National Inst. Virology, India	Recombinant subunit (E. coli expressed E2)	X			

Source: Chikungunya Vaccines Pipeline, WHO - Initiative for Vaccine Research & WHO Collaborating Centre for Vaccine Research, Evaluation, and training on Emerging Infectious Diseases.

very expensive to do. Regulatory timelines in endemic countries are long and these are lengthened even further for candidates requiring additional permissions, e.g., separate committees for candidates that are genetically modified (GMOs). Some candidates based on newer technologies (e.g., mRNA vaccines) may have small safety databases and may have additional requirements, e.g., insect cell substrates.

Other challenges: Many endemic countries for CHIKV have poor surveillance systems with no active surveillance. Chikungunya can be confused with other febrile illnesses; exact incidence rates are hard to predict/interpret. Further, there is low funding since many governments do not consider it a serious disease. Furthermore, the size and duration of the epidemics is uncertain, there is low awareness of the disease, and countries have many other competing priorities such as Zika, Dengue, etc.

SUGGESTED READING

1. Chhabra M, Mittal V, Bhattacharya D, Rana U, Lal S. Chikungunya fever: a re-emerging viral infection. Indian J Med Microbiol. 2008;26:5-12.
2. Couderc T, Khandoudi N, Grandadam M, Visse C, Gangneux N, Bagot S, et al. Prophylaxis and therapy for Chikungunya virus infection. J Infect Dis. 2009;200(4):516-23.
3. Gao S, Song S, Zhang L. Recent progress in vaccine development against chikungunya virus. Front Microbiol. 2019;10:2881.
4. Kumar NP, Sabesan S, Krishnamoorthy K, Jambulingam P. Detection of Chikungunya virus in wild populations of Aedes albopictus in Kerala State, India. Vector Borne Zoonotic Dis. 2012;12(10):907-11.
5. Metz SW, Gardner J, Geertsema C, Le TT, Goh L. Vlak JM, et al. Effective chikungunya virus-like particle vaccine produced in insect cells. PLoS Negl Trop Dis. 2013;7(3): e2124.
6. Sun S, Xiang Y, Akahata W, Holdaway H, Pal P, Zhang X, et al. Structural analyses at pseudo atomic resolution of Chikungunya virus and antibodies show mechanisms of neutralization. Elife. 2013;2:e00435.
7. WHO. Guidelines on clinical management of chikungunya fever. Regional Office for South East Asia. New Delhi: WHO; 2008.

SECTION 4

Novel Vaccine Strategies

49. **Deoxyribonucleic Acid Vaccines**
    Sumit Mehndiratta
50. **Chimeric Vaccines**
    Puneet Kumar
51. **Therapeutic Vaccines**
    Ajay Kalra, Srinivas G Kasi, Premashish Mazumdar
52. **Newer Adjuvants Vaccines**
    Puneet Kumar, Sanjay Niranjan

CHAPTER 49

Deoxyribonucleic Acid Vaccines

Sumit Mehndiratta

1. What do you mean by deoxyribonucleic acid (DNA) vaccines?

Deoxyribonucleic acid (DNA) vaccines are a novel technology that use genetically engineered, naked DNA that encodes the protein and bears the antigens of the pathogenic organism. This antigen encoded by the plasmid introduced into host can induce humoral or cell-mediated response against the organism (viruses, bacteria, etc.). These are also termed as *third-generation vaccines* or *genetic vaccines*.

2. How are these deoxyribonucleic acid (DNA) vaccines different from conventional vaccines?

In conventional vaccines, the antigen is exogenously administered, but in DNA vaccines, there is endogenous synthesis of the antigen against which immune response is elicited.

3. What is the basic structure and components of deoxyribonucleic acid (DNA) plasmid?

As described, the DNA vaccines are composed of genetically modified, purified closed-circular plasmid DNA that were originally derived from bacteria or nonreplicating viral vectors which encode viral antigens. The DNA plasmid, or vector, needs certain regulatory genetic elements, which are essential for the intracellular expression of the gene encoding the antigens of pathogen. Essentially, the expression plasmid is composed of two parts: (1) the antigen expression unit and (2) the production unit.

The antigen expression unit has a site for the origin of replication for plasmid propagation, transcriptional promoter, enhancer (to augment gene expression), immunogenic gene, and ribonucleic acid (RNA)-processing elements (polyadenylation signal and intron element). The production unit comprises bacterial sequences, which are necessary for the amplification and selection of the plasmid **(Fig. 1)**.

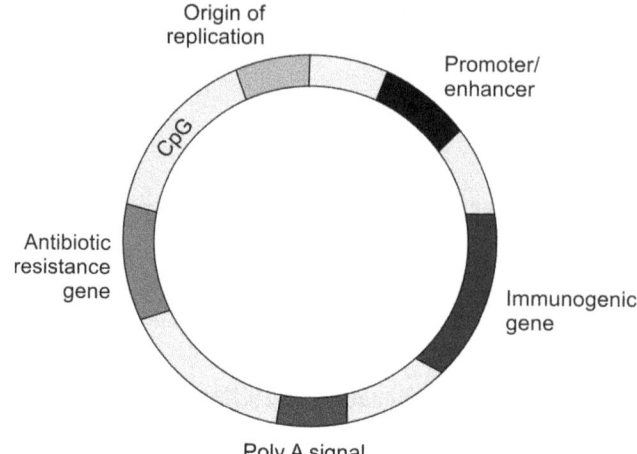

Fig. 1: Schematic representation of deoxyribonucleic acid (DNA) vaccine plasmid.

4. What is the mechanism of action of these vaccines?

Research and advances in genetics have shown that naked DNA can be safely used to sustain high levels of antigen expression in cells. Moreover, it is stable and easy to produce. The basic concept of a DNA vaccine is that after inoculation in the host, the DNA component is expressed in vivo. It creates antigenic protein that primes the host immune system to elicit a protective response analogous to an infection with real antigen. This way, a DNA vaccine mimics a natural infection by the pathogen.

This process utilizes the technology of genetic engineering. The genes encoding the antigen of choice of the infectious agent are inserted into a bacterial plasmid, which are then amplified in the bacteria. These are then recovered with a high degree of purity. Subsequently, the plasmid, along with necessary regulatory elements to express the antigens, is injected into the host. The antigen of the pathogen is then expressed in the host cell. This leads to stimulation of the immune system of the host and the production of TCD8+ and TCD4+ cells as well as immune B cells. The DNA plasmid, which had been inoculated, remains in transfected cells of the host throughout the life of that cell and continually produces the antigen of the pathogen **(Fig. 2)**.

5. How the potency of deoxyribonucleic acid (DNA) vaccines can be enhanced?

Deoxyribonucleic acid vaccines are poorly immunogenic per se because the DNA lacks cell-type specificity. Also, the DNA lacks the intrinsic ability to amplify or spread to surrounding cells in vivo. There is a poor uptake of plasmids by host cells, which result in a suboptimal response. To overcome these limitations, significant progress has been made over the years to increase their efficacy. These newer vaccines are also referred as the "second generation of DNA vaccines".

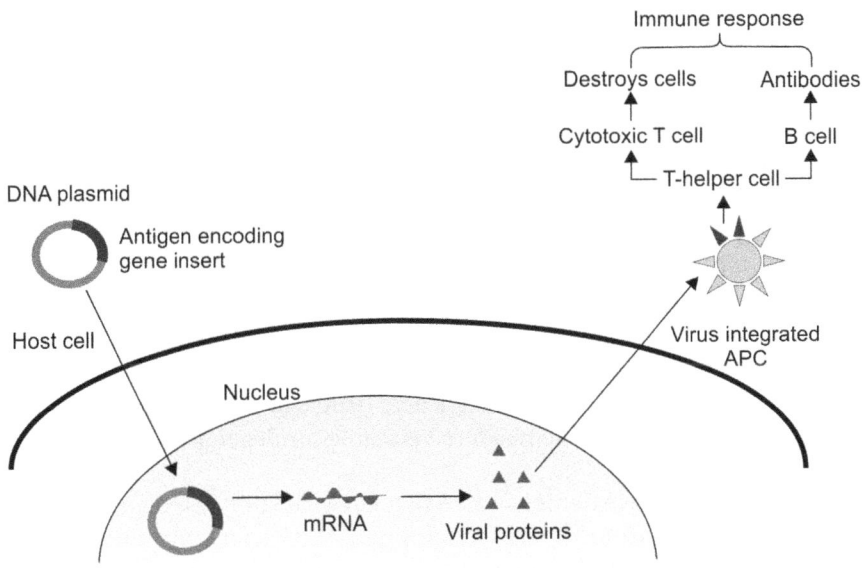

Fig. 2: Schematic model: mechanism of action of DNA vaccine.
(APC: antigen-presenting cell; DNA: deoxyribonucleic acid; mRNA: messenger ribonucleic acid)

Various strategies have been employed to achieve this purpose. These include the use of newer delivery systems, alteration the route of administration, enhancement of antigen presentation to band T-cells, and modification of the properties of antigen-presenting cells. The use of genetic and molecular adjuvants and immunostimulatory signals, coadministration of cytokine genes, augmenting antigen-presenting cell and T-cell interaction, blockage of immune checkpoints, etc., are some of the other modalities, which have been used in research trials.

Saline injection and gene gun delivery have been used to deliver DNA vaccines in studies. A standard hypodermic syringe is used in the former and the mode is either intramuscular or intradermal while the latter involves the use of compressed helium to ballistically accelerate the entry of plasmid DNA into target cells. Other methods that have been studied are aerosol instillation and topical application. It has been found that intradermal injections are superior to subcutaneous or intramuscular injections. Electroporation is technique used to assist intramuscular injections where muscle fibers have been temporarily damaged using myotoxins.

The plasmid DNA has its own immunostimulatory activity. It has sequences known as *CpG motifs* that are recognized by the human immune system as foreign. Hence, the plasmid itself stimulates the production of nonspecific cytokines that increase the specific immune response directed against the encoded antigen.

6. What is the potential of deoxyribonucleic acid (DNA) vaccines against severe acute respiratory syndrome coronavirus 2 (SARS-CoV-2) responsible for coronavirus disease 2019 (COVID-19)?

World is currently battling the pandemic of coronavirus disease 2019 (COVID-19). Presently, no curative therapy is available. So, a lot of research is underway to develop a vaccine against severe acute respiratory syndrome coronavirus 2 (SARS-CoV-2). The etiological agent SARS-CoV-2 belongs to family of coronaviruses. *Coronavirus* is named after their crown-like appearance under the electron microscope caused by the surface transmembrane spike class I fusion (S) glycoprotein. Different technology platforms based on nonreplicating viral vectors, peptides, recombinant proteins, DNA, messenger ribonucleic acid (mRNA), live attenuated viruses, and inactivated viruses are considered suitable for development of suitable vaccine.

Previous trials have demonstrated that DNA vaccine-based approach for SARS and Middle East respiratory syndrome (MERS) can induce production of neutralizing antibody responses and provide protection against these pathogens. DNA vaccines have inherent advantage of accelerated developmental timeline and rapid production of large doses and it is one of the most suitable approaches to develop a candidate vaccine.

Severe acute respiratory syndrome coronavirus 2 has a single-stranded positive-sense 30+ Kb RNA genome. One frame of this genome encodes the spike protein (S protein). These glycoproteins promote entry into host cells and are the main target of antibodies. The immunogenic epitopes, which encode spike glycoprotein, have been identified. These are then used as candidate for production of DNA vaccines.

Multiple candidate vaccines including DNA vaccines are under various phases of clinical trials. As per dated World Health Organization (WHO) (draft 7th July, 2020), four DNA plasmid vaccines are listed in clinical evaluation stage.

1. INO-4800 *(DNA plasmid encoding S protein)*, *Inovio Pharmaceuticals* (NCT04336410 and NCT04447781). In this vaccine trial, DNA sequence encoding SARS-CoV-2 immunoglobulin E (IgE) spike has been used to produce immune response. The phase II trials are scheduled to begin soon.
2. Deoxyribonucleic acid plasmid vaccine, *Cadila Healthcare Limited*. Phase I/II (not yet recruiting) (CTRI/2020/07/026352).
3. Deoxyribonucleic acid vaccine (GX-19), *Genexine Consortium*. Phase I (NCT04445389).
4. Deoxyribonucleic acid plasmid vaccine + Adjuvant, *Osaka University/ AnGes/Takara Bio*. Phase I https://www.clinicaltrials.jp/cti-user/trial/Show.jsp (JapicCTI-205328).

Multiple other DNA vaccines are under preclinical evaluation stage. The research and available data regarding vaccines against SARS-CoV-2 are rapidly evolving.

7. What are the advantages of these vaccines?

Deoxyribonucleic acid vaccines have following advantages over conventional vaccines:
- Deoxyribonucleic acid vaccines generate an immune response that is precise and specific because the host is inoculated with plasmid encoding for a particular antigen only.
- There is in vivo expression of antigen, which is subjected to the same processes of glycosylation and posttranslational modification, as the antigen derived via natural infection with the pathogen.
- These vaccines induce both cell-mediated and humoral immune responses. The antigen presentation is by both class I and II major histocompatibility complex (MHC) molecules. The humoral immune response generated in response to a DNA vaccine is qualitatively better than that of a conventional vaccine.
- The immunogenicity persists for a long duration of time. When introduced into a nondividing tissue such as muscle, there is long-term production of the antigenic protein in the host. Thus, booster doses of vaccine may not be required to sustain immunity.
- These vaccines are relatively inexpensive to develop and produce as compared to conventional vaccines.
- Deoxyribonucleic acid vaccines are safer and more stable than conventional vaccines.
- The production and development of these vaccines is relatively easier.
- There are logistic benefits such as the ease of storage and transportation and minimal requirement of cold chain and handling.
- A mixture of plasmids can be used to produce a more broad-spectrum vaccine. Multiple variants of an antigen can be inserted into a single plasmid, thus enhancing the protective spectrum. This is beneficial in the development of vaccines against pathogens like influenza which has several strains.
- There is no risk of reversion to a pathogenic form as is seen with use of live attenuated vaccines.

8. What are the disadvantages of these vaccines?

Deoxyribonucleic acid vaccines have a number of limitations and disadvantages as well:
- The use of these vaccines is limited to protein antigens only. Hence, they cannot be used for nonprotein-based antigens like bacterial polysaccharides.
- They may have relatively lower immunogenicity than inactivated vaccines.
- There is a possible risk of inducing antibody production against DNA (anti-DNA antibody or autoimmunity).
- They may induce immunological tolerance by antigens expressed inside the host due to the persistent expression of a foreign antigen, which is not seen with conventional vaccines.

- The successful induction of an immune response by a DNA vaccine is dependent on a variety of factors, which may be disease specific. These are type of antigen, route and method of inoculation, adjuvant used, etc. Therefore, different strategies need to be explored in order to obtain the desired effects against a specific pathogen.
- There is a risk of atypical processing and inappropriate expression of antigens of the pathogenic organism.
- There is risk of integration of the plasmid containing the foreign genetic sequence into crucial genes [e.g., tumor suppressor genes like p53, retinoblastoma (Rb), etc.] in the host genome, resulting in the loss of their function. Consequently, it may lead to malignant transformation of the cells.
- There is a potential risk of affecting genes that control cell growth.

9. What is the potential use of these vaccines in cancer immune therapeutics?

Deoxyribonucleic acid vaccination has a huge potential and is a promising new therapeutic modality in treatment of various malignancies. The tumor antigens can be either:

- *Mutational antigens*, which are also called *tumor-specific antig*ens (derived from mutated self-proteins not be present in normal cells) like Bcr-Abl, p53, etc.
- *Tumor-associated antigens* (nonmutated proteins overexpressed or aberrantly expressed in malignant cells) like MAGE-1, Gp100, alpha-fetoprotein, Her2/neu, etc.

These antigens in the vaccine can be used to produce an immune response in the host, which would specifically target the antigens that play a central role in the initiation, progression, and metastasis of tumors.

Initial trials of DNA vaccines were carried out using nonmutated tumor antigens, but they failed to generate a good immune response due to immune tolerance in the host. However, there are certain neoantigens which are formed due to tumor specific DNA alterations which are exclusively expressed in cancer tissue. These neoantigens can be identified by the process of exon sequencing the tumor tissue, which is then compared to data from normal tissue. The mutations are then identified. The antigens that are recognized by MHC I or II are then selected using prediction algorithms. Their ability to stimulate a humoral response is validated using in vitro and in vivo studies. One of the major hurdles is the time needed to manufacture such a personalized vaccine.

Another approach is the development of polyepitope DNA vaccines. These have a significant advantage that, while production, several antigens can be simultaneously delivered in the same gene sequence to be inserted. This induces a broad-spectrum response to multiple antigens (with both immune-dominant and unconventional epitopes). DNA vaccines have also been shown to have synergistic effects with other conventional modalities of cancer treatment.

10. What is the prospect of use of these vaccines against allergic disorders?

The incidence of allergic diseases has been on a rise over the past years. The search for preventive therapies includes the exploration of the potential of DNA vaccines in the prevention and treatment of allergic disorders. Allergen-specific immunotherapy is a novel approach for allergic disorders. DNA vaccines are known to induce Th1 cell and T-regulatory response with production of interferon-γ (IFN-γ) which balances and thus counteracts the Th2-mediated allergic manifestations in the host.

It is known that, in predisposed individuals, the manifestations of allergic response are due to the production of IgE in the host after contact with the allergen. Allergen-specific immunotherapy utilizes the host's own immune system to produce allergen-specific blocking immunoglobulin G (IgG). These blocking IgG antibodies prevent the binding of IgE to the allergens and the subsequent cascade of allergic inflammatory response induced by IgE-allergen immune complexes. It also potentially modulates allergen-specific cellular responses by a variety of mechanisms. Currently, vaccines trials are underway for disorders like rhinoconjunctivitis, atopic dermatitis, and asthma.

11. What are the guidelines to assure quality and safety of these vaccines?

The draft of guiding principles for evaluation of quality, safety, and efficacy of DNA vaccines for human use is available at https://www.who.int/biologicals/DNA_vaccines_R_WHO.BS.2020.2380_12_May_2020.pdf.

12. Is there any licensed vaccine for any human disease based on deoxyribonucleic acid (DNA) platform?

No, presently, there are no approved DNA vaccines for use in humans. Nevertheless, some DNA-based vaccines were approved by the Food and Drug Administration (FDA) and the United States Department of Agriculture (USDA) for veterinary use, including a vaccine against West Nile virus in horses and canine melanoma.

However, DNA vaccines have been shown to induce protective immune responses to a number of pathogens including viruses, bacteria, and parasites. They have also displayed efficacy in the treatment or prevention of cancer, allergic diseases, and autoimmune diseases. Research and trials have been underway for a long time now to develop vaccines against malaria, hepatitis B, herpes simplex virus, influenza, tuberculosis, anthrax, Zika virus, human papillomavirus (HPV), certain malignancies, etc., and this field is developing at a fast pace.

The field of DNA vaccines has witnessed rapid evolution over the past few years. The details of the DNA vaccines that have been registered and are under trial can be accessed from the website https://clinicaltrials.gov database.

SUGGESTED READING

1. Amanat F, Krammer F. SARS-CoV-2 vaccines: status report. Immunity. 2020;52:583-9.
2. Aurisicchio L, Pallocca M, Ciliberto G, Palombo F. The perfect personalized cancer therapy: cancer vaccines against neoantigens. J Exp Clin Cancer Res. 2018;37:86.
3. Barouch DH. Rational design of gene-based vaccines. J Pathol. 2006;208:283-9.
4. Becker PD, Noerder M, Guzmán CA. Genetic immunization: bacteria as DNA vaccine delivery vehicles. Hum Vaccin. 2008;4:189-202.
5. Bharati K, Vrati S. DNA vaccines: Getting closer to becoming a reality. Indian J Med Res. 2013;137:1027-8.
6. Brennick CA, George MM, Corwin WL, Srivastava PK, Ebrahimi-Nik H. Neoepitopes as cancer immunotherapy targets: key challenges and opportunities. Immunotherapy. 2017;9:361-71.
7. Callaway E. The race for coronavirus vaccines: a graphical guide. Nature. 2020;580:576-7.
8. Donnelly JJ, Ulmer JB, Liu MA. DNA vaccines. Dev Biol Stand. 1998;95:43-53.
9. Donnelly JJ, Ulmer JB, Shiver JW, Liu MA. DNA vaccines. Annu Rev Immunol. 1997;15:617-48.
10. Dorofeeva Y, Shilovskiy I, Tulaeva I, Focke-Tejkl M, Flicker S, Kudlay D, et al. Past, presence, and future of allergen immunotherapy vaccines. Allergy. 2020. [Online ahead of print].
11. Ghaffarifar F. Plasmid DNA vaccines: where are we now? Drugs Today (Barc). 2018;54:315-33.
12. Hasson SS, Al-Busaidi JK, Sallam TA. The past, current and future trends in DNA vaccine immunisations. Asian Pac J Trop Biomed. 2015;5:344-53.
13. Hobernik D, Bros M. DNA vaccines—how far from clinical use? Int J Mol Sci. 2018;19:3605.
14. Isakovic A, Weiss R, Thalhamer J, Scheiblhofer S. Protective and therapeutic DNA vaccination against allergic diseases. Methods Mol Biol. 2014;1143:243-58.
15. Jahanafrooz Z, Baradaran B, Mosafer J, Hashemzaei M, Rezaei T, Mokhtarzadeh A, et al. Comparison of DNA and mRNA vaccines against cancer. Drug Discov Today. 2020;25:552-60.
16. Karimkhanilouyi S, Ghorbian S. Nucleic acid vaccines for hepatitis B and C virus. Infect Genet Evol. 2019;75:103968.
17. Keskin DB, Anandappa AJ, Sun J, Tirosh I, Mathewson ND, Li S, et al. Neoantigen vaccine generates intratumoral T cell responses in phase Ib glioblastoma trial. Nature. 2019;565:234-9.
18. Khan KH. DNA vaccines: roles against diseases. Germs. 2013;3:26-35.
19. Klinman DM, Barnhart KM, Conover J. CpG motifs as immune adjuvants. Vaccine. 1999;17:19-25.
20. Kowalczyk DW, Ertl HC. Immune responses to DNA vaccines. Cell Mol Life Sci. 1999;55:751-70.
21. Kulkarni V, Rosati M, Valentin A, Ganneru B, Singh AK, Yan J, et al. HIV-1 p24(gag) derived conserved element DNA vaccine increases the breadth of immune response in mice. PLoS One. 2013;8:e60245.
22. Lee J, Kumar SA, Jhan YY, Bishop CJ. Engineering DNA vaccines against infectious diseases. Acta Biomater. 2018;80:31-47.
23. Le TT, Andreadakis Z, Kumar A, Román RG, Tollefsen S, Saville M, et al. The COVID-19 vaccine development landscape. Nat Rev Drug Discov. 2020;19:305-6.

24. Li L, Petrovsky N. Molecular adjuvants for DNA vaccines. Curr Issues Mol Biol. 2017;22:17-40.
25. Li L, Petrovsky N. Molecular mechanisms for enhanced DNA vaccine immunogenicity. Expert Rev Vaccines. 2016;15:313-29.
26. Liu MA. A comparison of plasmid DNA and mRNA as vaccine technologies. Vaccines (Basel). 2019;7:37.
27. Liu MA. DNA vaccines: an historical perspective and view to the future. Immunol. Rev. 2011;239:62-84.
28. Liu MA. DNA vaccines: a review. J Intern Med. 2003;253:402-10.
29. Lopes A, Vandermeulen G, Préat V. Cancer DNA vaccines: current preclinical and clinical developments and future perspectives. J Exp Clin Cancer Res. 2019;38:146.
30. Marć MA, Domínguez-Álvarez E, Gamazo C. Nucleic acid vaccination strategies against 33 infectious diseases. Expert Opin Drug Deliv. 2015;12:1851-65.
31. Myhr AI. DNA vaccines: regulatory considerations and safety aspects. Curr Issues Mol Biol. 2017;22:79-88.
32. Pierini S, Perales-Linares R, Uribe-Herranz M, Pol JG, Zitvogel L, Kroemer G, et al. Trial watch: DNA-based vaccines for oncological indications. Oncoimmunology. 2017;6:e1398878.
33. Plotkin SA, Plotkin SL. The development of vaccines: how the past led to the future. Nat Rev Microbiol. 2011;9:889-93.
34. Porter KR, Raviprakash K. DNA vaccine delivery and improved immunogenicity. Curr Issues Mol Biol. 2017;22:129-38.
35. Ribeiro AM, Souza AC, Amaral AC, Vasconcelos NM, Jeronimo MS, Carneiro FP, et al. Nanobiotechnological approaches to delivery of DNA vaccine against fungal infection. J Biomed Nanotechnol. 2013;9:221-30.
36. Sahin U, Tureci O. Personalized vaccines for cancer immunotherapy. Science. 2018;359:1355-60.
37. Santos S, Ramírez M, Miranda E, Reyes N, Martínez O, Acosta-Santiago M, et al. Enhancement of immune responses by guanosine-based particles in DNA plasmid formulations against infectious diseases. J Immunol Res. 2019;2019:3409371.
38. Scheiblhofer S, Thalhamer J, Weiss R. DNA and mRNA vaccination against allergies. Pediatr Allergy Immunol. 2018;29:679-88.
39. Smith TR, Patel A, Ramos S, Elwood D, Zhu X, Yan J, et al. Immunogenicity of a DNA vaccine candidate for COVID-19. Nat Commun. 2020;11:2601.
40. Soltani S, Farahani A, Dastranj M, Momenifar N, Mohajeri P, Emamie AD. DNA vaccine: methods and mechanisms. Adv Hum Biol. 2018;8:132-9.
41. Srivastava IK, Liu MA. Gene vaccines. Ann Intern Med. 2003;138:550-9.
42. Stevenson FK, Rosenberg W. DNA vaccination: a potential weapon against infection and cancer. Vox Sang. 2001;80:12-8.
43. Tregoning JS, Kinnear E. Using plasmids as DNA vaccines for infectious diseases. Microbiol Spectr. 2014;2:101128.
44. Tsen SW, Paik AH, Hung CF. Enhancing DNA vaccine potency by modifying the properties of antigen-presenting cells. Expert Rev Vaccines. 2007;6:227-39.
45. Valenta R, Karaulov A, Niederberger V, Gattinger P, van Hage M, Flicker S, et al. Molecular aspects of allergens and allergy. Adv Immunol. 2018;138:195-256.
46. Webster RG, Robinson HL. DNA vaccines: a review of developments. BioDrugs. 1997;8:273-92.
47. Weeratna RD, McCluskie MJ, Xu Y, Davis HL. CpG DNA induces stronger immune responses with less toxicity than other adjuvants. Vaccine. 2000;18:1755-62.

48. Williams JA. Vector design for improved DNA vaccine efficacy, safety, and production. Vaccines (Basel). 2013;1:225-49.
49. World Health Organization (WHO). (2019). DNA vaccines. [online] Available from: https://www.who.int/biologicals/areas/vaccines/dna/en/. [Last accessed July, 2020].
50. World Health Organization (WHO). (2020). Draft landscape of COVID-19 candidate vaccines. [online] Available from: https://www.who.int/publications/m/item/draft-landscape-of-covid-19-candidate-vaccines. [Last accessed July, 2020].
51. Yu J, Tostanoski LH, Peter L, Mercado NB, McMahan K, Mahrokhian SH, et al. DNA vaccine protection against SARS-CoV-2 in rhesus macaques. Science. 2020. [Online ahead of print].

CHAPTER 50

Chimeric Vaccines

Puneet Kumar

1. What are chimeric vaccines?

Chimeric vaccines are an emerging class of genetically engineered vaccines, developed using a *chimeric gene*. A chimeric gene is an artificial gene constructed by juxtaposition of fragments of unrelated genes or other deoxyribonucleic acid (DNA) segments, which may themselves have been altered.

2. How are chimeric vaccines different from live vector vaccines and deoxyribonucleic acid (DNA) vaccines?

All the three (live vector vaccines, DNA vaccines, and chimeric vaccines) are different types of genetic engineered/recombinant vaccines. Live vector vaccines are those that are engineered by incorporation of a pathogen's antigenic peptides into a harmless carrier virus or a bacterium. DNA vaccines, in contrast, consist of a DNA plasmid that encodes a viral gene that can be expressed inside of the animal to be immunized. Chimeric vaccines, on the other hand, are produced by substituting genes from target pathogen for similar genes, in a safe, but closely related organism. For example, yellow fever (YF) vaccine virus is used and some of its genes are substituted by similar genes of another flavivirus: Japanese encephalitis virus (JEV) and resultant chimeric virus is developed into an effective vaccine against JE.

3. How does this technology help in developing better vaccines?

This technology has been used in at least five different ways to develop new, better vaccines:
1. A well-known, safe, and effective vaccine virus is used as a vector to carry genes of a lesser immunogenic virus, so as to improve the efficacy of vaccine against latter. For example, a chimeric virus (ChimeriVax-JE virus) has been constructed using YF 17D vaccine virus with heterologous genes from JEV. ChimeriVax-JE virus has been used to develop a very effective vaccine against JE.
2. This technology has also been used to develop chimeric genes that express epitopes of more than one antigen of the same pathogen, in cases where there is antigenic variability. For example, factor H-binding protein

(fHbp) is a novel meningococcal vaccine candidate, but one limitation of fHbp as a vaccine candidate is antigenic variability, since antibodies to fHbp in the variant 1 (v.1) antigenic group do not protect against strains expressing v.2 or v.3 proteins and vice versa. Hence, recombinant chimeric protein has been developed that expressed epitopes from all three variant groups. This approach can be helpful in development of vaccines against severe acute respiratory syndrome coronavirus 2 (SARS-CoV-2), by developing chimeric genes that express various immunogenic epitopes of one or more key proteins of the virus: Spike (S), membrane (M), nucleocapsid (N) proteins, and envelop (E).

3. Chimerization has also been used to achieve attenuation of live vaccine candidates as in tetravalent dengue vaccine.
4. Vectors for vector-based vaccines have also been engineered using chimerization, so as to overcome the problem of preexisting antivector immunity in these vaccines.
5. Chimerization, as a technology, has also been used to study to track antigen-specific immune responses, to assess their protective capacity, and address other questions related to immune response to a specific pathogen. This ultimately helps in development of better, "targeted" vaccines.

4. What are the agents against which chimeric vaccines are being developed?

Most of the work on chimeric vaccines has been done on using YF 17D vaccine virus to develop effective vaccines against other medically important flaviviruses like JE, dengue fever, West Nile fever (WNV), and tickborne fever.

For *JE*, a chimeric was constructed in 1999 by replacing the genes encoding two structural proteins (prM and E) of yellow fever 17D virus with the corresponding genes of an attenuated strain of JEV, SA14-14-2. Since the prM and E proteins contain antigens conferring protective humoral and cellular immunity, the immune response to vaccination with progeny virus (named ChimeriVax-JE virus) is directed principally at JE. It has been demonstrated to be genetically stable and is able to induce a rapid humoral immune response and to protect against a very severe, direct intracerebral JE virus challenge in mice and nonhuman primates. It appears safer (lower neurovirulence) than yellow fever 17D vaccine, but has a similar profile of immunogenicity and protective efficacy. ChimeriVax-JE, now known as JE-CV or IMOJEV® and manufactured by Acambis/Sanofi-Aventis, has proven safe, immunogenic, and effective in a number of human trials. Most of initial trials involved adult volunteers, but now has been tested in both adults and children >9 months of age. This vaccine has recently obtained marketing authorization in some countries in Southeast Asia and Australia. It has an indication as a one-dose vaccine and booster requirements remain to be determined. Another chimeric vaccine against JE is being developed using a new type of flavivirus vaccine, a pseudoinfectious virus (RepliVAX WN) that prevents WNV-induced disease. A chimeric RepliVAX (RepliVAX JE) has been developed by replacing the WNV prM/E genes with those of JEV. The initial prototype RepliVAX JE failed, but was genetically modified further to develop a second-generation RepliVAX (RepliVAX JE.2). RepliVAX JE.2 elicited neutralizing antibodies in both mice and hamsters and provided 100% protection from a lethal challenge with JEV or WNV, respectively. RepliVAX JE.2 has been further improved by replacing WNV nonstructural 1 (*NS1*) gene in RepliVAX JE with that of JEV (producing TripliVAX JE). This has elicited higher anti-E immunity and displayed better efficacy in mice than RepliVAX JE in initial trials. Furthermore, TripliVAX JE displayed reduced immune interference caused by preexisting anti-NS1 immunity.

For *dengue virus (DENV)*, using conventional technologies for development of vaccine is fraught with numerous challenges: absence of an animal model, need to develop a live attenuated vaccine, existence of four antigenically distinct serotypes with the resulting risk of competition between vaccine strains, immunologic risks related to antibody-dependent enhancement that has been hypothesized to be the cause of severe forms of the illness, absence of a well-defined correlate of protection and preexisting vaccine, and complexity associated with industrial production of a tetravalent vaccine. To overcome some of these problems, researchers have used an approach identical to that of ChimeriVax-JE virus vaccine to construct chimeric virus ChimeriVax-D2. This vaccine was licensed in 2015 (Dengvaxia® by Sanofi Pasteur, Lyon, France), but it was found that the vaccine performance was dependent on serostatus. It was found to be highly efficacious and safe in seropositive people (i.e., those who already had suffered from the infection at least once). However, in seronegative vaccinees, approximately 3 years after vaccination, the vaccine increased the risk of developing severe dengue when the individual experiences a natural dengue infection. Hence, the World Health Organization (WHO) recommends this vaccine only in seropositive individuals.

Other strategies that have been tried for construction of better dengue vaccine are:
- Using recombinant DENVs and achieving attenuation by antigenic chimerization between two related dengue viruses (DENV-DENV Chimera, Inviragen).
    - Using Dengue 2 PDK-53 virus as a chimeric carrier (DENVax vaccine being developed by Takeda). The difference from Dengvaxia is the presence of NS proteins due to the DENV2 backbone. The conserved NS proteins within the dengue backbone may well be required to generate T-cell-mediated responses to dengue infection and antibodies against NS1 are associated with cross-protective humoral immune responses. The vaccine efficacy is currently being tested in approximately 20,000 recipients in phase III trials in Asia and Latin America.
- Using DENV4 containing a 30-nucleotide 32 noncoding region (NCR) deletion.
- Another candidate vaccine consists of three full-length DENV serotypes attenuated by one or more deletions in the 3' untranslated region with

DEN1Δ30, DEN2Δ30, and DEN4Δ30 while the fourth component is a chimeric virus in which the prM and E proteins of DENV2 replace those of DENV4 in the DEN4Δ30 background. This vaccine was developed by the US National Institutes of Health (NIH) and done well in phase I and phase II clinical trials and is currently under phase III trials in Brazil.
- Using RepliVAX technology to produce a dengue vaccine by replacing the prM/E genes of RepliVAX WN (a WNV RepliVAX) with the same genes of dengue virus type 2 (DENV2). Here also, the initial prototype RepliVAX D2 failed, but was genetically engineered to develop a second-generation RepliVAX D2 (designated RepliVAX D2.2) and subsequent results have been promising.

For *meningococcal disease*, fHbp is a novel target for vaccine development. It is a principal antigen in a multicomponent meningococcal vaccine recently licensed in Europe (4CMenB vaccine: Bexsero®) for prevention of serogroup B diseases. The protein specifically binds human complement factor H (fH), which downregulates complement activation on the bacterial surface and enables the organism to evade host defenses. Anti-fHbp antibodies can bind to meningococci and elicit complement-mediated bactericidal activity directly. The antibodies also can block binding of the human complement downregulator, fH. However, one limitation of fHbp as a vaccine candidate is antigenic variability, since antibodies to fHbp in the variant 1 (v.1) antigenic group do not protect against strains expressing v.2 or v.3 proteins and vice versa. Further research on fHbp molecule has given lot of information on the locations of the fHbp epitopes important for eliciting bactericidal antibodies. It has been found that one epitope expressed by nearly all v.1 proteins mapped to the B domain while epitopes expressed by fHbp v.2 or v.3 mapped to the C domain. Thus, a chimeric fHbp molecule has been engineered that contains the A domain (which is conserved across all variant groups), a portion of the B domain of a v.1 protein, and the carboxyl-terminal portion of the B domain and the C domain of a v.2 protein. The resulting recombinant chimeric proteins expressed epitopes from all three variant groups. In mice, the chimeric vaccines elicited serum antibodies with bactericidal activity against a panel of genetically diverse strains expressing fHbp v.1, v.2, or v.3. The data demonstrate the feasibility of preparing a meningococcal vaccine from a single recombinant protein that elicits broad bactericidal activity, including group B strains. Work is underway to design a second-generation chimeric fHbp that may elicit higher antibody responses than the first-generation chimeric vaccine. More than 610 fHbp amino acid sequence variants have been identified and efforts are underway to find out the best one for vaccine development. Another strategy being tried is construction of mutants of *Neisseria meningitidis* that express chimeric fHbp, which can be used to prepare native outer membrane vesicle (OMV) vaccines that may elicit higher and broader anti-fHbp bactericidal antibody responses than the recombinant chimeric fHbp vaccines.

For *Leishmaniasis* also, a chimeric therapeutic vaccine is being developed using three recombinant leishmanial antigens (LeIF, LmSTI-1, and TSA) in the form of a fusion protein combined with monophosphoryl lipid A in squalene oil as adjuvant. Other vaccine candidates have utilized other chimeric proteins like polyprotein KSAC (a fusion protein composed of KMP-11, SMT, A2, and cysteine peptidase B), murine and human major histocompatibility complex (MHC) class I- and II-specific epitopes from four proteins (LiHyp1, LiHyp6, LiHyV, and HRF) to develop the vaccine. All these candidates are in early phase of development.

For *influenza virus*, hepatitis B virus core virus-like particles (VLPs) produced in *Escherichia coli*, have been used that display extracellular domain of a universal protein of influenza viruses, the M2 protein on its surface. This M2-HBcAg VLP vaccine candidate of Sanofi Pasteur (Lyon, France) has entered clinical trials and has been shown to be safe and immunogenic. Other researchers have used major antigenic component in influenza, hemagglutinin (HA) to construct phenotypically mixed, chimeric influenza vaccines and many such candidates are under phase I clinical trials.

For *human immunodeficiency virus (HIV)*, *p17/p24*: Ty VLP produced by British Biotech Pharmaceuticals Ltd. (Oxford, UK) comprises a fusion protein of PL that spontaneously assembled into VLPs (Ty VLPs) in yeast and a gag component of the HIV isolate IIIB. It has been tested for both prophylactic (phase I and phase II trials) and therapeutic vaccination.

Coronaviruses: At least one of the candidate vaccine for *SARS-CoV-2* is also utilizing this technology of chimerization. The candidate vaccine by the International AIDS Vaccine Initiative (IAVI)/Merck is using replication-competent VSV chimeric virus technology (VSVΔG) delivering the SARS-CoV-2 spike (S) glycoprotein and is in preclinical phase of development. Similar approach is being used to develop vaccine against Middle East respiratory syndrome coronavirus (MERS-CoV). A chimeric, spherical VLP (sVLP) vaccine expressing receptor binding domain (RBD) of MERS-CoV has been shown to induce specific antibody and cellular immune responses in mice, preventing pseudotyped MERS-CoV entry into susceptible cells.

This technology is being tried to develop vaccines against many other infections like malaria, Chikungunya fever, cytomegalovirus and foot-and-mouth disease, and DNA vaccines/therapeutic vaccines for even noninfective conditions like *Alzheimer's disease* and *malignancies* like B-cell lymphoma, multiple myeloma and even dental caries, hypertension, and nicotine addiction.

SUGGESTED READING

1. Beernink PT, Shaughnessy J, Pajon R, Braga EM, Ram S, Granoff DM. The effect of human factor H on immunogenicity of meningococcal native outer membrane vesicle vaccines with over-expressed factor H binding protein. PLoS Pathog. 2012;8:e1002688.
2. Bernstein DI, Guptill J, Naficy A, Nachbagauer R, Berlanda-Scorza F, Feser J, et al. Immunogenicity of chimeric haemagglutinin-based, universal influenza virus vaccine candidates: interim results of a randomised, placebo-controlled, phase 1 clinical trial. Lancet Infect Dis. 2020;20:80-91.

3. Children's Hospital Oakland Research Institute. (2014). Towards improved meningococcal vaccines. [online] Available from: http://www.chori.org/Principal_Investigators/Granoff_Dan_M/Downloadables/TowardsImprovedMeningococcal.pdf. [Last accessed August, 2020].
4. Chokephaibulkit K, Sirivichayakul C, Thisyakorn U, Sabcharoen A, Pancharoen C, Bouckenooghe A, et al. Safety and immunogenicity of a single administration of live-attenuated Japanese encephalitis vaccine in previously primed 2- to 5-year-olds and naive 12- to 24-month-olds: multicenter randomized controlled trial. Pediatr Infect Dis J. 2010;29:1111-7.
5. Cockburn I. Chimeric parasites as tools to study Plasmodium immunology and assess malaria vaccines. Methods Mil Biol. 2013;923:465-79.
6. De Brito RCF, Cardoso JMO, Reis LES, Vieira JF, Mathias FAS, Roatt BM, et al. Peptide vaccines for leishmaniasis. Front Immunol. 2018;9:1043.
7. Erasmus JH, Auguste AJ, Kaelber JT, Luo H, Rossi SL, Fenton K, et al. A chikungunya fever vaccine utilizing an insect-specific virus platform. Nat Med. 2017;23:192-9.
8. Farlex W. (2014). The Free Dictionary by Farlex. [online] Available from: http://medical-dictionary/thefreedictionary.com/chimeric + gene. [Last Accessed August, 2020].
9. Frøyland M, Ruffini PA, Thompson KM, Gedde-Dahl T, Fredriksen AB, Bogen B. Targeted idiotype-fusion DNA vaccines for human multiple myeloma: preclinical testing. Eur J Haematol. 2011;86:385-95.
10. Gall J, Kass-Eisler A, Leinwand L, Falck-Pedersen E. Adenovirus type 5 and 7 capsid chimera: fiber replacement alters receptor tropism without affecting primary immune neutralization epitopes. J Virol. 1996;70:2116-123.
11. Gall JG, Crystal RG, Falck-Pedersen E. Construction and characterization of hexonchimeric adenoviruses: specification of adenoviral serotype. J Virol. 1998;72:10260-4.
12. Giuntini S, Beernink PT, Reason DC, Granoff DM. Monoclonal antibodies to meningococcal factor H binding protein with overlapping epitopes and discordant functional activity. PLoS One. 2012;7:e34272.
13. Guo L, Lu X, Kang SM, Chen C, Compans RW, Yao Q. Enhancement of mucosal immune responses by chimeric influenza HA/SHIV virus-like particles. Virology. 2003;313:502-13.
14. Guriakhoo F, Zhang ZX, Chambers TJ, Delagrave S, Arroyo J, Barrett AD, et al. Immunogenicity, genetic stability, and protective efficacy of a recombinant, chimeric yellow fever-Japanese encephalitis virus (ChimeriVax-JE) as a live, attenuated vaccine candidate against Japanese encephalitis. Virology. 1999;257:363-72.
15. Halstead SB, Thomas SJ. New Japanese encephalitis vaccines: alternatives to production in mouse brain. Expert Rev Vaccines. 2011;10:355-64.
16. Huang CY, Butrapet S, Tsuchiya KR, Bhamarapravati N, Gubler DJ, Kinney RM. Dengue 2 PDK-53 virus as a chimeric carrier for tetravalent dengue vaccine development. J Virol. 2003;77:11436-47.
17. Ishikawa T, Wang G, Widman DG, Infante E, Winkelmann ER, Bourne N, et al. Enhancing the utility of a prM/E-expressing chimeric vaccine for Japanese encephalitis by addition of the JEV NS1 gene. Vaccine. 2011;29:7444-55.
18. Ishikawa T, Widman DG, Bourne N, Konishi E, Mason PW. Construction and evaluation of a chimeric pseudoinfectious virus vaccine to prevent Japanese encephalitis. Vaccine. 2008;26:2772-81.

19. Konar M, Granoff DM, Beernink PT. Importance of inhibition of binding of complement factor H for serum bactericidal antibody responses to meningococcal factor H-binding protein vaccines. J Infect Dis. 2013;208:627-36.
20. Kosalaraksa P. (2014). Antibody Response of a Boosted Japanese Encephalitis Chimeric Virus Vaccine (JE-CV) in Children. [online] Available from: http://www.clinicaltrials.gov/ct2/show/NCT01954810. [Last accessed August, 2020].
21. Kotecha A, Perez-Martin E, Harvey Y, Zhang F, Ilca SL, Fry EE, et al. Chimeric O1K foot-and-mouth disease virus with SAT2 outer capsid as an FMD vaccine candidate. Sci Rep. 2018;8:13654.
22. Marin-Mogollon C, van Pul FJA, Miyazaki S, Imai T, Ramesar J, Salman AM, et al. Chimeric *Plasmodium falciparum* parasites expressing *Plasmodium vivax* circumsporozoite protein fail to produce salivary gland sporozoites. Malar J. 2018;17:288.
23. Martin NG, Snape MD. A multicomponent serogroup B meningococcal vaccine is licensed for use in Europe: what do we know, and what are we yet to learn? Expert Rev Vaccines. 2013;12:837-58.
24. McArthur MA, Holbrook MR. Japanese encephalitis vaccines. J Bioterror Biodef. 2011;S1:2.
25. Monath TP, Guirakhoo F, Nichols R, Yoksan S, Schrader R, Murphy C, et al. Chimeric live, attenuated vaccine against Japanese encephalitis (ChimeriVax-JE): phase 2 clinical trials for safety and immunogenicity, effect of vaccine dose and schedule, and memory response to challenge with inactivated Japanese encephalitis antigen. J Infect Dis. 2003;188:1213-30.
26. Monath TP, McCarthy K, Bedford P, Johnson CT, Nichols R, Yoksan S, et al. Clinical proof of principle for ChimeriVax: recombinant live, attenuated vaccines against flavivirus infections. Vaccine. 2002;20:1004-18.
27. Monath TP, Soike K, Levenbook I, Zhang ZX, Arroyo J, Delagrave S, et al. Recombinant, chimaeric live, attenuated vaccine (ChimeriVax) incorporating the envelope genes of Japanese encephalitis (SA14-14-2) virus and the capsid and nonstructural genes of yellow fever (17D) virus is safe, immunogenic and protective in non-human primates. Vaccine. 1999;17:1869-82.
28. Ophorst OJA, Kostense S, Goudsmit J, De Swart RL, Verhaagh S, Zakhartchouk A, et al. An adenoviral type 5 vector carrying a type 35 fiber as a vaccine vehicle: DC targeting, cross neutralization, and immunogenicity. Vaccine. 2004;22:3035-44.
29. Osorio JE, Brewoo JN, Silengo SJ, Arguello J, Moldovan IR, Tary-Lehmann M, et al. Efficacy of a tetravalent chimeric dengue vaccine (DENVax) in Cynomolgus macaques. Am Trop Med Hyg. 2011;84:978-87.
30. Peele AK, Srihansa T, Krupanidhi S, Ayyagari VS, Venkateswarulu TC. Design of multi-epitope vaccine candidate against SARS-CoV-2: a in-silico study. J Biomol Struct Dyn. 2020:1-9.
31. Roldão A, Mellado MC, Castilho LR, Carrondo MJ, Alves PM. Virus-like particles in vaccine development. Expert Rev Vaccines. 2010;9:1149-76.
32. Sanofi Pasteur Inc. (2014). Long-term Follow-up of Immunogenicity of a Single Dose of Japanese Encephalitis Chimeric Virus Vaccine (JE-CV) in Toddlers. [online] Available from: http://www.clinicaltrials.gov/ct2/show/NCT01001988. [Last accessed August, 2020].
33. Sun W, McCroskery S, Liu WC, Leist SR, Liu Y, Albrecht RA, et al. A Newcastle disease virus (NDV) expressing membrane-anchored spike as a cost-effective inactivated SARS-CoV-2 vaccine. bioRxiv. 2020;2020.

34. Timmerman JM, Singh G, Hermanson G, Hobart P, Czerwinski DK, Taidi B, et al. Immunogenicity of a plasmid DNA vaccine encoding chimeric idiotype in patients with B-cell lymphoma. Cancer Res. 2002;62:5845-52.
35. Wang C, Zheng X, Gai W, Wong G, Wang H, Jin H, et al. Novel chimeric virus-like particles vaccine displaying MERS-CoV receptor-binding domain induce specific humoral and cellular immune response in mice. Antiviral Res. 2017;140:55-61.
36. Wilder-Smith A. Dengue vaccine development: status and future. Entwicklung von Impfstoffen gegen Dengue: aktueller Stand und Zukunft. Bundesgesundheitsblatt Gesundheitsforschung Gesundheitsschutz. 2020;63:40-4.
37. World Health Organization (WHO). (2014). Japanese Encephalitis. [online] Available from: http://www.who.int/vaccine_research/development/japanese_encephalitis/en/. [Lat Accessed August, 2020].
38. World Health Organization (WHO). (2020). Draft landscape of COVID-19 candidate vaccines. [online] Available from: https://www.who.int/publications/m/item/draft-landscape-of-covid-19-candidate-vaccines. [Last Accessed August, 2020].
39. Yang H, Yan Z, Zhang Z, Realivazquez A, Ma B, Liu Y. Anti-caries vaccine based on clinical cold-adapted influenza vaccine: a promising alternative for scientific and public-health protection against dental caries. Med Hypotheses. 2019;126:42-5.
40. Yao Q. Enhancement of mucosal immune responses by chimeric influenza HA/SHIV virus-like particles. Res Initiat Treat Action. 2003;8:20-1.
41. Yao Q. Th cell-independent immune responses to chimeric hemagglutinin/simian human immunodeficiency virus-like particles vaccine. J Immunol. 2004;173:1951-8.
42. Yu YZ, Wang S, Bai JY, Zhao M, Chen A, Wang WB, et al. Effective DNA epitope chimeric vaccines for Alzheimer's disease using a toxin-derived carrier protein as a molecular adjuvant. Clin Imunol. 2013;149:11-24.

CHAPTER 51

Therapeutic Vaccines

Ajay Kalra, Srinivas G Kasi, Premashish Mazumdar

1. What is a therapeutic vaccine?

Generally, vaccines are administered to healthy individuals to protect against a specific infection. An antigen or its equivalent is administered to stimulate the recipient's immune system to respond and results in immunity to subsequent infection with the same pathogen.

Therapeutic vaccines, on the other hand, are administered to individuals who are already diseased, with the aim of stimulating the suppressed immune system of the recipient, to mount a response against the pathogen causing the chronic infection. The scope of therapeutic vaccines includes cancers, allergies, neurological diseases, addictions and other noncommunicable diseases.

2. What type of diseases would therapeutic vaccines be most likely to be effective against?

While the thrust of research has been toward therapeutic cancer vaccines, the scope of therapeutic vaccines includes chronic infections (Hep B, Hep C, HPV, HIV, *H. pylori*, CMV, etc.), allergies, autoimmune conditions, neurological diseases, addictions and other noncommunicable diseases.

3. Why has the development of therapeutic cancer vaccines met with very limited success?

Immune suppression in the tumor microenvironment has been implicated as a major factor for the limited success of cancer vaccines. The immunosuppressive factors include T-cell anergy, programmed cell death, the presence of immunosuppressive immune cell types and secretion of soluble immunosuppressive factors.

4. What are tumor antigens?

Tumor antigens are antigens found predominantly in cancer tissues. Tumor specific T lymphocytes can mount an immune response against these tumor antigens, when presented by antigen-presenting cells (APCs).

Initially tumor antigens were broadly classified into two categories: (1) *tumor-specific antigens* (TSA), which are present only on tumor cells and not on any other cell; and (2) *tumor-associated antigens (TAA)*, which are present on some tumor cells and also some normal cells.

However, many antigens thought to be tumor-specific may be present on some normal cells as well.

The modern classification of tumor antigens is based on their molecular structure and source.
- Products of mutated oncogenes and tumor suppressor genes: β-catenin, BRCA1/2
- Products of other mutated genes
  - Overexpressed or aberrantly expressed cellular proteins: BING-4, CyclinB[1]
  - Tumor antigens produced by oncogenic viruses: HPV E6, E7
  - Oncofetal antigens: CEA
  - Altered cell surface glycolipids and glycoproteins: MUC1
  - Cell type-specific differentiation antigens: MUC1, PSA.

5. What are the platforms being studied for therapeutic cancer vaccines?

The platforms being studied are:
- Tumor cell vaccines, also called whole cell vaccines. These consist of cancer cells removed during surgery and then injected into the patient. Tumor cell vaccines may be either autologous, where cells are taken from the patient's own tumor, or allogeneic, where cells are taken from other patients' tumors.
- Antigen vaccines use TSA, rather than the whole tumor cells.
- Dendritic cell vaccines use dendritic cells, which are special cells that breakdown the antigens on cancer cells into smaller pieces and thereby help the T-cells identify them. Similar to autologous cell vaccines, dendritic cells used in therapeutic vaccines must be specifically prepared in the lab for each individual patient.
- Anti-idiotype vaccines use anti-idiotype antibodies that look like cancer-specific antigens. They trick the body into attacking both the anti-idiotypes and the antigens that exist in the cancer cells.
- DNA vaccines use small pieces of DNA that, when injected into the body, instruct cells to keep making certain antigens. The more antigens are produced, the more T-cells the immune system makes to fight them off.
- Vector-based vaccines make use of certain viruses, bacteria, or yeast cells to stimulate the immune system. These organisms are modified to ensure that they cannot cause disease, and they are used to carry the tumor-specific antigens into the body. The vaccine used in the MEL11 study, a phase II study exploring a new treatment approach to advanced-stage melanoma, is a vector-based vaccine.

6. What are neoantigens?

Non-synonymous mutations in the tumor cell genome gives rise to neoantigens. They are highly immunogenic and have a higher affinity toward

MHC, and are not affected by central immunological tolerance. Neoantigens are highly individual-specific and usually do not involve known oncogenes. Hence, identification of neoantigens is critical for tumor vaccine therapy. Several clinical trials have shown that neoantigens can be recognized by CD8+ and CD4+ T cells in tumor tissue, and thus trigger an anti-tumor immune response in vivo.

7. What are the therapeutic cancer vaccines in current usage?

In April 2010, the USFDA approved the first cancer treatment vaccine. This vaccine (*Sipuleucel-T Provenge*, manufactured by Dendreon), is approved for use in castration resistant metastatic prostate cancer. It is designed to stimulate an immune response to prostatic acid phosphatase (PAP), an antigen present on most prostate cancers. In a clinical trial, sipuleucel-T increased the survival of men with a certain type of metastatic prostate cancer by about 4 months. Unlike some other cancer treatment vaccines under development, sipuleucel-T is customized to each patient. The vaccine is created by isolating immune system cells called antigen-presenting cells (APCs) from a patient's blood through a procedure called leukapheresis. The APCs are sent to Dendreon, where they are cultured with a protein called PAP-GM-CSF. This protein consists of PAP linked to another protein called granulocyte-macrophage colony-stimulating factor (GM-CSF). The latter protein stimulates the immune system and enhances antigen presentation. APC cells cultured with PAP-GM-CSF constitute the active component of sipuleucel-T. Each patient's cells are returned to the patient's treating physician and infused into the patient. Patients receive three treatments, usually 2 weeks apart, with each round of treatment requiring the same manufacturing process. Although the precise mechanism of action of sipuleucel-T is not known, it appears that the APCs that have taken up PAP-GM-CSF stimulate T-cells of the immune system to kill tumor cells that express PAP.

The US biotech Antigenics has won Russian approval to market *Oncophage* to treat kidney cancer. This product has not received USFDA approval.

Intravesical BCG is approved for treatment and prophylaxis of urothelial carcinoma in situ of the urinary bladder and for prophylaxis of primary or recurrent stage Ta and/or T1 urothelial carcinoma following transurethral resection. In a meta-analysis, intravesical BCG showed a 27% reduction in the risk of disease progression [hazard ratio (HR) 0.73; $p \leq 0.001$].

The IMLYGIC, also known as T-VEC, is a genetically modified oncolytic viral therapy approved by the FDA in 2015 for the treatment of advanced melanoma. It is a genetically modified, live, attenuated herpesvirus that encodes for GM-CSF. Upon subcutaneous or intralesional injection, in patients with recurrent melanoma, local tumoricidal effect is seen through viral replication and cell lysis. The GM-CSF produced enhanced T-cell priming by APCs that present tumor antigens released during viral-mediated tumor lysis. Tumor-antigen–loaded DCs migrate systemically and effect a distant immune response, although responses in injected tumor are superior to those of distant metastases.

8. What are the developments in therapeutic cancer vaccines?

Several promising therapeutic vaccines have completed phase III trials, with negative results. The current trend is to employ vaccines in combination with other therapeutic approaches, which include chemotherapy, radiotherapy (RT), endocrine therapy, small-molecule inhibitors, cytokines, or immune checkpoint inhibitors (ICI).

Of the 118 cancer vaccines that have completed phase III trials, 27 have been withdrawn/terminated, 55 have completed phase III trails and the remaining are active.

Most of these trials are using vaccines in combination with other cancer treatment modalities.

These include vaccines against breast cancer, gliomas, pancreatic cancers, prostate cancers and chordomas. None have entered clinical usage.

9. What is the current status of therapeutic vaccines for use in autoimmune diseases?

Autoimmune diseases are conditions wherein the body mounts an immunological response against self-antigens. This results from loss of immunotolerance. The current treatment modalities involve use of monoclonal antibodies which have several drawbacks.

The proinflammatory response to self-antigens closely resembles normal protective immune responses to viruses and intracellular pathogens, involving Th1 cells, IFN. The goal of therapeutic vaccines against autoimmune diseases involves shifting the immune response to a Th2 type, IL-4 and IL-10 mediated or T regulatory cell, which induce an anti-inflammatory response.

Various platforms are being investigated. These include DNA vaccines, whole autoreactive T cells, dendritic cell vaccines and B cell based immunogenic vaccines.

Antigens targeted for vaccines include AB_1, Tau (Alzheimer's disease), alpha-synuclein (Parkinson's disease), IL-1B (T2 DM0), IFN-gamma (SLE), TNF-alpha (RA, Crohn's disease, psoriasis).

10. What is the status of vaccines for multiple sclerosis?

Glatiramer acetate (Copaxone), a peptide that resembles myelin basic protein (MBP), has been licensed by USFDA for the management of multiple sclerosis.

Tovaxin, an autologous T-cell vaccine, BHT-3009, a DNA-based vaccine coding for MBP and NeuroVax, have not had encouraging results from phase II/III trials.

11. What is the status of vaccines for rheumatoid arthritis?

Modalities studied include whole T-cell vaccine and TCR peptide vaccine, anti-TNF-α vaccine, DNA vaccine and DC vaccines.

Administration of Rheumavax, an autologous modified dendritic cells (DC) pulsed with a mixture of four citrullinated peptide antigens (cit-vimentin), in a phase I trial, resulted in reduction in anti-cyclic citrullinated peptide (CCP) antibody titers and induction of a tolerogenic T-cell profile.

In a phase I trial of DEN-181, a nanoparticulate liposome formulation that encapsulates autoantigenic peptide and NF-kB inhibitor, 1,25 dihydroxycholecalciferol (calcitriol), to target DCs, the vaccine was found to be safe and modulated antigen-specific T cells in RA patients of appropriate HLA type.

12. What is the status of therapeutic vaccines for type I diabetes mellitus?

Peptide vaccines, glutamic acid dehydrogenase (GAD65) and GAD65 plus alum adjuvant, called Diamyd, failed to show any significant reduction in insulin requirements to maintain blood sugar levels.

DiaPep277, a 24 amino-acid peptide derived from human heat-shock protein 6, has been demonstrated to modulate immunological attack on β-cells in the NOD mouse model of type 1 diabetes and also activates regulatory T-cells by interacting with their toll-like receptor. Following encouraging results in phase II trials, the planned phase III trial has been held back for logistic reasons.

13. What are the other conditions for which therapeutic vaccines are being investigated?

These include atherosclerosis, obesity, addictions, Alzheimer's disease, hypertension and a host of other conditions.

14. What is the basic immunopathology in persistent viral infections?

Control and elimination of persistent viruses such as hepatitis, herpes or papilloma viruses requires multispecific and polyfunctional effector T cell responses directed against continuously expressed viral antigens. Humoral immune response, additionally, aims to lower viral antigen load and to limit virus spread. Persistent viremia is partially due to exhaustion of antiviral T cells. T-cell expression of programmed death 1 (PD-1), cytotoxic T lymphocyte antigen 4 (CTLA-4), and interleukin 10 (IL-10), have been reported to be potential factors of establishing immune suppression and viral persistence. Blocking these negative signaling pathways could restore the host immune system, enabling it to respond to further stimulation.

15. Which are the persistent infections for which vaccines are in development?

Hepatitis B, hepatitis C, HPV, HSV, CMV, HIV, *H. pylori*, TB, malaria.

16. Which are the therapeutic vaccines most likely to enter clinical usage in the near future?

Trials of therapeutic vaccines are currently underway for some diseases and are most likely to come in the near future as discussed here:

Human Papillomavirus:

A therapeutic vaccine could help women who are already infected with HPV. Therefore, medical researchers are also investigating therapeutic vaccines for use as an adjunct to standard therapies. Such a vaccine could:
- Help prevent low-grade disease from progressing
- Cause existing lesions to regress
- Control the spread of metastatic cancer, and/or
- Prevent recurrence of cervical cancer after treatment.

Therapeutic vaccines elicit cellular immune response leading to the elimination of infected and malignant cells expressing viral proteins. In general, these vaccines focus on the main HPV oncogenes, E6 and E7. Since expression of E6 and E7 is required for promoting the growth of cervical cancer cells (and cells within warts), it is hoped that immune responses against the two oncogenes might eradicate established tumors.

Two therapeutic vaccines are in clinical trials:
1. MVA E2 is a recombinant vaccinia viral vaccine. MVA E2 [composed of modified vaccinia virus Ankara (MVA)] expressing the E2 gene of bovine papillomavirus.
   In a phase I/II trial, therapeutic vaccination with MVA E2 proved to be very effective in stimulating the immune system against papillomavirus, and in generating regression of flat condyloma lesions in men.
2. VGX-3100, (HPV16 E6/E7, HPV18 E6/E7 DNA Vaccine), which consists of plasmids pGX3001 and pGX3002, entered a phase III clinical trial called REVEAL-1 for the treatment of HPV-induced high-grade squamous intraepithelial lesions.

Hepatitis C Virus Infection:

The rationale for hepatitis C therapeutic vaccine are many:
- Patients with insufficient immune control progress toward chronic hepatitis C.
- Specific T-cell responses and IFN-α are generally absent in patients who progress; nonspecific T cells cause inflammation and fibrosis.
- Redirection of immune response to control chronic hepatitis C could halt or reverse liver fibrosis progression.
- Immune responses against the E1 envelope protein especially are weak (antibodies) or absent (T-cells), therefore the E1 envelope is a prime candidate. Development of poly-epitope vaccine has the potential advantages of targeting all patient segments and lower costs.

The following therapeutic vaccines are in human trials:
- Intercell AG (IC41): HCV peptide cocktail with polyarginine is phase II trials in combination with Peg-IFN-α.
- Globe Immune (GI-5005) expressing core-NS3 fusion protein is in phase II trials, in combination with Peg-IFN-α.

- Tripep (ChronVac-C): DNA-based vaccination with NS3/4A-expressing plasmid is in phase Ib trials.
- CIGB-230, which is a mixture of plasmid expressing HCV structural antigens with a recombinant HCV core protein, is in phase Ib trials.
- Transgene (TG4040), which is a modified vaccinia Ankara (MVA) virus expressing NS proteins (NS3-NS5B) is in phase II trials, in combination with Peg-IFN-α.

Human Immunodeficiency Virus Infection:
Current treatment of symptomatic HIV infection is the use of HAART. But antiretroviral therapy (ART) can arrest HIV replication and halt progression to AIDS, but ART cannot eradicate HIV from viral reservoirs. This is the gap that therapeutic vaccines aim to fill. Moreover, recent studies have shown that a combination of ART and therapeutic vaccines may result in a better outcome.

The goal of therapeutic vaccination is to change the host immune response either by redirecting the host immune response towards highly conserved HIV sequences that are shared among diverse viruses or to broaden the host immune response to recognize a wide array of escape variants.

Various platforms being investigated are protein/subunit vaccines, pulsed dendritic cells vaccine, viral vector vaccines and nucleic acid vaccines.

A number of such vaccines are currently being developed and in various phases of trials as given in **Table 1**. Clinical trials of therapeutic vaccines generally recruit volunteers with CD4 counts >250 cells/mm³, and most studies require a CD4 count >350 cells/mm³. Lower CD4 counts may render the subjects unable to mount an adequate immune response. Most trials require that therapeutic vaccine recipients continue taking antiretroviral drugs during the study.

TABLE 1: Therapeutic vaccines pipeline 2019.

Trial	Description	Phase
DNA.HTI + MVA.HTI	DNA + modified vaccinia Ankara strain vector vaccines	I
MAG-pDNA + rVSVIN HIV-1 Gag	DNA + viral vector vaccines, ATI	I
MVA.tHIVconsv3 ± MVA.tHIVconsv4	MVA.tHIVconsv3 ± MVA.tHIVconsv4	I
DC-HIV04: a1DC + inactivated whole autologous HIV, a1DC + conserved HIV peptides	DC Vaccine	I
Ad26.Mos4.HIV + MVA-Mosaic or clade C gp140 + mosaic gp140	Adenovirus and modified vaccinia Ankara strain vectors encoding mosaic HIV antigens + Env protein boosts	I
PENNVAX-GP or INO-6145 + IL-12 DNA adjuvant (INO-9012)	DNA vaccine + DNA adjuvant	I/II
p24CE1/2 + p55^gag conserved-element DNA vaccines	DNA vaccine	I/II

Some interesting and promising candidate vaccines are:
- LFn-p24C, a detoxified anthrax-derived polypeptide fused to the subtype C HIV gag protein p24, native HIV-1 Tat protein, was well-tolerated and HIV-specific responses were associated with increases in CD4 counts following immunizations.
- Vacc-4x, is a combination of four synthetic peptides sequences within the highly conserved HIV core protein p24. This candidate vaccine is undergoing additional, phase IIa trials to assess the effect of the therapeutic vaccination on viral load compared with placebo. In a phase II randomized double-blind placebo controlled trial with this vaccine was found to be safe and immunogenic, and elicited a threefold reduction of viral load.
- DCs were obtained by leukapheresis and pulsed with Gag, Env, and Pol peptides and influenza A matrix peptide. Immunization with this vaccine resulted in significantly increased frequency of HIV-1 peptide-specific IFN-γ–positive cells.

17. Will therapeutic vaccines be able to cure the disease targeted?

Probably not. If therapeutic vaccines are effective, they may be able to help keep the diseases under control. However, most researchers do not think therapeutic vaccines will be able to completely eliminate infection because the viruses hide in certain cells of the body where it can last for decades. The primary benefit might be in better controlling the disease progressions, preventing relapses and decreasing the exposure to the standard therapeutic drugs with concomitant decrease in their side effects.

SUGGESTED READING

1. Abbot A. Therapeutic HIV vaccines show promise. Nature. 2010;466:539.
2. Angelov DN, Waibel S, Guntinas LO. Therapeutic vaccine for acute and chronic motor neuron diseases: implications for amyotrophic lateral sclerosis. PNAS. 2003:100 (Suppl 8); 4790-5.
3. DeMaria PJ, Bilusic M. Cancer vaccines. Hematol Oncol Clin N Am. 2019;33: 199-214.
4. Fujirebio. Hepatitis C therapeutic vaccine. [online] Available from: www.innogenetics.com. [Last Accessed August, 2020].
5. Jochmus I, Schäfer K, Faath S, Müller M, Gissmann L. Chimeric virus-like particles of the human papillomavirus type 16 (HPV 16) as a prophylactic and therapeutic vaccine. Arch Med Res. 1999;30(4):269-74.
6. Klade CS, Wedemeyer H, Berq T. Therapeutic vaccination of chronic hepatitis C nonresponder patients with the peptide vaccine IC41. Gastroenterology. 2008;134(5):1385-95.
7. Li J, Bao M, Ge J, Ren S, Zhou T, Qi F, et al. Research progress of therapeutic vaccines for treating chronic hepatitis B. Hum Vaccin Immunother. 2017;13(5):986-97.
8. Lowe DB, Shearer MH, Jumper CA, Zhou E, Kennedy RC. Plasmid DNA as Prophylactic and Therapeutic vaccines for Cancer and Infectious Diseases. Plasmids: Current Research and Future Trends. Poole: Caister Academic Press; 2008.

9. Philips C. FDA approves first therapeutic cancer vaccine. NCI Can Bull. 2010;7:9.
10. Sela M, Hilleman MR. Therapeutic vaccines: realities of today and hopes for tomorrow. PNAS. 2004:101(Suppl 2);14559.
11. Sela M, Mozes E. Therapeutic vaccines in autoimmunity. PNAS. 2004:101(Suppl 2);14586-92.
12. Tindle R. Human papillomavirus vaccines for cervical cancer. Curr Opin Immun. 1996;8(5):643-50.
13. Treatment Action Group. Pipeline Report 2019: Research Toward a Cure and Immune-Based Therapies. [online] Available from: https://www.treatmentactiongroup.org/wp-content/uploads/2019/09/pipeline_research_toward_cure_2019.pdf. [Last Accessed August, 2020].
14. Vandepapelière P. Therapeutic vaccination against chronic viral infections. Lancet Infect Dis. 2002;2(6):353-67.
15. Whitacre DC, Peters CJ, Sureau C, Nio K, Li F, Su L, et al. Designing a therapeutic hepatitis B vaccine to circumvent immune tolerance. Hum Vaccin Immunother. 2020;16(2):251-68,
16. Yang A, Farmer E, Wu TC, Hung C. Perspectives for therapeutic HPV vaccine development. J Biomed Sci. 2016;23:75-9.

CHAPTER 52

Newer Adjuvants Vaccines

Puneet Kumar, Sanjay Niranjan

1. What are adjuvants?

Adjuvants, in context of vaccines, are formulations that increase and/or modulate immune response to an antigen in vivo as per the need. The word "adjuvant" is derived from Latin word "adjuvare" which means, "to help".

2. What are the functions of an adjuvant?

Live vaccines carry necessary immune-stimulating signals themselves, so adjuvants are not required for them. When pathogen is processed to an inactivated antigen, to subunit, or to recombinant proteins, they lose some of immune-stimulating property of pathogen and adjuvants are then required for potentiation of the immunogen.

Classically, adjuvants were added to the vaccine formulations just to increase the immune response (antibody titer) to the antigen. These adjuvants were developed using empirical methods, thus, these are not optimal for many of the challenges in vaccination today. However, with advancements in immunology and allied fields, adjuvants are being developed and used to perform various other *specific* functions, so as to *optimize/fine-tune* immune response as per the need:

- Increase immunogenicity (seroconversion rate) in populations with reduced responsiveness because of age (in young infants/preterm babies and the elderly), disease, or therapeutic interventions. For example, an adjuvant, MF59, enhances the response of influenza vaccine in elderly
- To help induce robust mucosal immune response
- Facilitate the use of smaller doses of antigen, thus making the vaccine production faster and more cost-effective
- Provide a strong priming response, so reduce number of doses of a vaccine and/or obviate need of boosters that simplifies logistics and improves patient compliance
- Increase the breadth of immune response to enable cross-protection and increase duration of immune response
- *Accelerate* immune response that may be of critical importance in certain situations like vaccination in response to outbreak, bioterrorist attack, etc.

- To achieve qualitative alteration of the immune response. Newer adjuvants are increasingly developed to help induce functionally appropriate types of immune response (e.g., Th1 versus Th2 cell, CD8$^+$ versus CD4$^+$ T-cells, and specific antibody isotypes), as per the requirement. For example, for vaccines against chronic infections [e.g., human immunodeficiency virus (HIV), hepatitis C virus (HCV), tuberculosis (TB), and herpes simplex virus (HSV)], intracellular pathogens, and malignancies, cellular immune responses are more important than humoral immune response. Further, specific adjuvants may also increase the generation of memory, especially T-cell memory and alter the breadth, specificity, or affinity of the response, as per the need.

3. What are the features of an ideal adjuvant?

Ideal adjuvant should be stable with long shelf-life, biodegradable, cheap to produce, not induce immune responses against themselves, and promote an appropriate immune response (i.e., cellular or humoral immunity depending on requirements for protection).

4. What are their mechanisms of action?

Adjuvants act through one or more of many modes of action including the delivery of antigen, recruitment of specific immune cells to the site of immunization, activation of these cells to create an inflammatory microenvironment, and maturation of antigen-presenting cells (APCs) for enhancement of antigen uptake and antigen presentation in secondary lymphoid tissues.

Particulate adjuvants [e.g., emulsions, microparticles, immunestimulating complexes (ISCOMs), and liposomes] act by increasing the antigen availability and uptake by immune cells. Antigen-carrying vehicles (like liposomes and microfluidized squalene or squalane emulsions) target antigens to APCs, including dendritic cells (DCs), follicular dendritic cells (FDCs), and B lymphocytes. They also activate innate immunity pathways in vivo, thus generating an immunocompetent environment at injection site. Modern adjuvant formulations contain small molecules with immunomodulating properties. These immunostimulatory adjuvants are derived predominantly from pathogens and often represent pathogen-associated molecular patterns [e.g., lipopolysaccharide (LPS), monophosphoryl lipid A (MPL), and cytosine-phosphate-guanine (CpG) DNA], which activate cells of the innate immune system. Thus, cytokine cascades are triggered. The cytokines elicit cell-mediated immune responses and the formation of antibodies of protective isotypes, such as immunoglobulin G1 (IgG1). Antibodies of these isotypes activate complement and collaborate with antibody-dependent effector cells in protective immune responses.

Some adjuvants like chitosan-adjuvate nanoparticles act by preventing degradation of the antigen, thus potentiating its immunogenicity. This is in contrast to classical aluminum salt adjuvants, which in fact can destabilize certain protein antigens.

Although aluminum-containing adjuvants are one of the oldest and the most widely used adjuvants, their mechanism of action is still not fully delineated. It was only in 2008 that it was realized that alum adjuvant triggers an ancient pathway of innate recognition of crystals in monocytes and triggers them to become immunogenic DCs, nature's adjuvant. It is also clear now that adjuvants trigger the stromal cells at the site of injection, leading to the necessary chemokines that attract the innate immune cells to the site of injection.

The discovery of toll-like receptor (TLR) family in 1996, followed by identification of its key role in initiating an adaptive immune response (the first necessary step to lasting immunity), was a milestone in understanding and development of adjuvants. The discovery that TLR4 functioned as an LPS-sensing receptor explained the mechanism of action of TLR-agonist molecules.

With increasing insight of various mechanisms of actions of new/emerging adjuvants, adjuvants are now classified into five major types depending on their principle mechanism of action:
1. Immunomodulation (modification of cytokine networks)
2. Presentation (maintenance of antigen confirmation)
3. Cytotoxic T-lymphocytes (CTLs) induction
4. Targeting specific cells
5. Depot generation.

Of course, an adjuvant can have multiple modes of action and a vaccine can have more than one adjuvant for desired immunogenicity.

5. With advances in molecular biology and genetic engineering, we have more and more specific antigens. Do we still need new or better adjuvants?

Yes, and in fact, the need of better adjuvants is even more! Newer vaccines are based on highly purified antigens, better reactogenicity, and safety profile than some of the early whole-pathogen vaccines. However, the purity of these subunit antigens and the absence of the self-adjuvanting immunomodulatory components associated with attenuated or killed vaccines often result in *weaker* immunogenicity. Thus, with these vaccines, novel adjuvant formulations need to be developed that can use the interplay between innate and adaptive immune systems and the central role played by APC to *enhance* the immune response. In fact, adjuvants can now be "designed" to *optimize* immune response as per the need. For example, T-cell immunity can be triggered if the vaccine is against intracellular pathogen or cancer. In addition, new adjuvants may also allow vaccines to be delivered mucosally. Currently, adjuvants are selected on the basis of the route of administration and the type of immune response (antibody, cell-mediated, or mucosal immunity) that is desired for a particular vaccine. In fact, the choice of adjuvant or immune-enhancer determines whether the immune response is effective, ineffective, or damaging. Vaccine design has therefore now become more tailored and emerging vaccines are based on the use of innovative adjuvants combined with careful antigen selection. This, in turn, has opened up the potential of extending the field of vaccinology to develop better prophylactic and *therapeutic* vaccines against chronic infectious [e.g., HSV, HIV, HCV, hepatitis B virus (HBV), human papillomavirus (HPV), or *Helicobacter pylori*] and even *noninfectious diseases* such as malignancies, tumors (e.g., melanoma, breast, or colon cancer), Alzheimer disease, multiple sclerosis, insulin-dependent diabetes, rheumatoid arthritis, allergy, and other immune-mediated disorders.

6. **What are the different approaches that are currently being tried to develop newer adjuvants?**

- Developing efficient and safe adjuvants for use in human vaccines remain both a challenge and a necessity. The development of vaccine adjuvants for human use has been one of the slowest processes in the history of medicine. This is because of a number of knowledge gaps, the most important of which is the complexity involved in designing adjuvants that are both potent and well-tolerated. Alum adjuvants, consisting of aluminum salts, first described in the 1920s, were the only licensed adjuvants till late 1990s. Despite decades of research and hundreds of preclinical candidates, even today only a handful of adjuvants are approved for human use (e.g., aluminum salts, microfluidized squalene-in-water emulsion MF59®, and MPL). MF59 was developed in 1990s and has been shown to increase in antibody levels in the elderly, but no significant difference in younger individuals when compared to unadjuvanted vaccine. Thus, it is being used in a seasonal influenza vaccine (Fluad®) licensed for use in elderly since 1997. MF59 has also been shown to be superior to alum in inducing antibody responses to hepatitis B vaccine in baboons and humans. It is also being tested currently as a part of Aflunov® (an investigational prepandemic influenza vaccine) and two H1N1 pandemic vaccines (Focetria® and Celtura®). Both MF59 and AS03 create a transient and local immunocompetent environment following injection. They promote cytokine and chemokine productions, and recruitment of cells to injection site. The activated antigen-loaded APCs migrate to draining lymph nodes where APCs could prime naive CD4+ T-cells. The chemokine-driven immune cell recruitment is the key characteristic of the mechanism for both MF59 and AS03 **(Fig. 1)**.
- Recent advances in our understanding of innate immunity have led to the identification of immune pathways and adjuvant formulations more suitable for clinical advancement. Ligands of the innate recognition systems thus emerge as new adjuvants for vaccine design whereas manipulation of the signaling pathways offers new avenues for fine-tuning immune responses and optimizing immunotherapies.

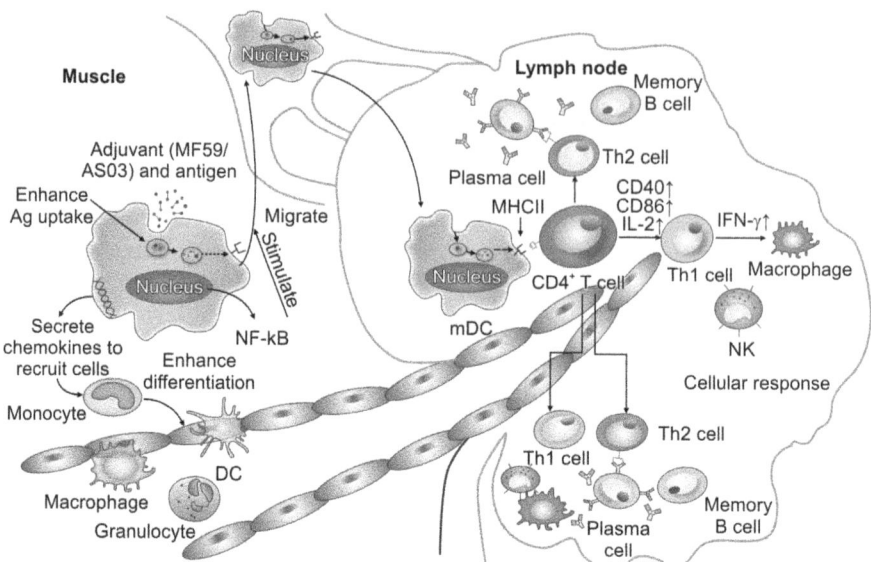

Fig. 1: Models for the activation mechanism of newer adjuvants, MF59 and AS03.

- Many adjuvants appear to be ligands for TLRs. TLRs are a family of conserved pattern recognition receptors that recognize specific microbial patterns and allow the cell to distinguish between self and nonself materials. The very property of the TLRs to link innate and adaptive immunity offers a novel prospect to develop vaccines engaging TLR signaling. Thus, *TLR agonists* are being developed as adjuvants and are showing promise as vaccine adjuvants and even as stand-alone products capable of eliciting nonspecific protection against a wide range of infectious pathogens. However, recent evidence suggests that some adjuvants activate the innate immune system in a TLR-independent manner possibly through other pattern recognition receptors and signaling machinery. In particular, newly identified intracellular retinoic acid-inducible gene (RIG)-like receptors, nucleotide oligomerization domain (NOD)-like receptors, or even as yet unknown recognition machinery for the adjuvant may regulate TLR-independent vaccine immunogenicity. By understanding more about TLR-dependent and TLR-independent innate immune activation, we would be able to devise novel adjuvants and thus control the consequent adaptive immune responses to vaccine. TLR4 and TLR9 agonists are being extensively studied.
- Toll-like receptor 4 (TLR4) agonists are species specific and animal studies may not work for humans. LPS and less toxic MPL are major TLR4 agonists and they activate two intracellular signaling pathways myeloid differentiation factor 88 (MyD88) and TIR-domain-containing adapter-inducing interferon-beta (TRIF) which act by stimulating kinases leading to nuclear factor kB-dependent proinflammatory responses (MyD88) or

type 1 interferon responses (TRIF). As MPL is isolated from *Salmonella minnesota* (*S. minnesota*) (gram-negative bacterium), synthetic version is being tried to reduce hurdles in production. Synthetic RC 529 is designed alternative to *S. minnesota* MPL (in hepatitis B vaccine in Argentina) while glucopyranosyl lipid adjuvant (GLA) is synthetic MPL of *Escherichia coli* form of LPS (being studied on TB and influenza vaccines). EB6020 is another synthetic one in phase I trial. On the other hand, a Brazilian manufacturer is trying to produce MPL from LPS extracted as side product of *Bordetella pertussis* whole-cell vaccine manufacturing process (to enhance immunity of influenza vaccine). Hepta-acyl sulfonyl sucrose is another one under development. However, seeing human diversity, one cannot say all recipients will respond equally to a given TLR4 agonist molecule or a combination of them will work. Formulation activity depends on ratio of lipid to agonist and how agonist is combined with liposomes. In Cervarix®, MPL is combined with aluminum salts jointly named AS04. MPL is the most widely used TLR 4 agonist.
- Toll-like receptor 9 (TLR9) agonist unmethylated CpG found in bacterial DNA is powerful adjuvant and activates innate immune system by interactions with intracellular TLR9. Response differs between species. CpG motifs trigger B-cell activation and induce production of Th1 and proinflammatory cytokines interleukin-1 (IL-1), IL-6, IL-18, tumor necrosis factor-α (TNF-α), and interferon gamma. In some cases, they can redirect Th2 responses to Th1. CpG is being considered for malaria vaccine, pneumococcal conjugate vaccine (PCV), hepatitis B vaccines, and in HIV-infected patients. CpG oligodeoxynucleotides are also promising mucosal adjuvants.
- It is known that particulate adjuvants, like mineral salts, oil-in-water emulsions, and microparticles, do not activate DCs directly, but their mechanism of action is poorly characterized. In the last few years, it has been revealed that particulate adjuvants induce chemokine production in accessory cells like macrophages, monocytes, and granulocytes, leading to cell recruitment at injection site followed by the differentiation of monocytes into activated DCs. The *NLRP3 inflammasome complex* is one of the molecular targets of particulate adjuvants and it is required for alum adjuvanticity. Thus, it is another pathway that can be exploited for development of better adjuvants.
- Some *heat shock proteins (HSPs)* like HSP70 and Gp96, in addition to maintaining cell homeostasis under physiological and stress conditions, are potent inducers of immunity. They activate DCs partly through TLRs, activate natural killer cells, increase presentation of antigens to effector cells, and augment T-cell and humoral immune responses against the peptides bound to HSPs, but not against HSPs per se. Thus, they are highly effective carrier molecules for cross-presentation. Moreover, they have peptide-independent immunomodulatory capacity also. Their roles in priming multiple host defense pathways are being exploited in adjuvant development for vaccines against cancer and infectious diseases. The antigenic peptide in the vaccine is complexed with either tissue derived

or recombinant HSPs in vitro to generate HSP-peptide complexes as peptide-specific vaccine.

A synthetic glycolipid α-*galactosylceramide* (α-GalCer) represents a new class of immune stimulators and vaccine adjuvants that activate type I natural killer T (NKT) cells to swiftly release cytokines and to exert helper functions for acquired immune responses. This is specially being tried in anticancer and antiviral vaccines with encouraging results. β-*mannosylceramide* is another novel adjuvant in this category.

Saponins, also among newer adjuvants, are triterpenoid molecules with a complex sugar backbone extracted from plants. South American tree *Quillaja saponaria Molina* (Quil-A) extract is being used in veterinary vaccines since the 1970s, but was too reactogenic for humans. Plant sources from India and China are also being researched. Mechanism of action of Quil-A saponins is related to its affinity to cholesterol and it forms a complex creating pores in the cholesterol-containing membranes. This affinity of saponins for cholesterol led to two adjuvants for human use: (1) ISCOMs and (2) AS01.

Immune-stimulating complexes are complexes of partially purified saponins from Quil-A, combined with cholesterol that form less reactogenic porous particles 50–60 nm size. ISCOMs and their simpler formulations—ISCOMATRIX and ISCOPREP (which can be simply mixed with the antigen) combine the advantages of a particulate carrier system with the presence of an in-built adjuvant (Quil-A) and consequently have been found to be more immunogenic, while removing hemolytic activity of the saponin, producing less toxicity. ISCOMs and ISCOMATRIX vaccines have now been shown to induce strong antigen-specific cellular or humoral immune responses to a broad range of antigens of viral, bacterial, parasite origin, or tumor in a number of animal species including nonhuman primates and humans. AS01 is a combination of QS21 (a pure form isolated from Quil-A), liposomes (contains cholesterol), and MPL (TLR4 agonist). AS02 formulation shows higher CD4T-cell response to malaria antigen and QS21 in its pure form is being used as an adjuvant to cancer vaccines and for herpes zoster vaccine.

Biodegradable micro- or nanoparticles that have been extensively studied and used as carrier or delivery systems for various medications are now being tried as vaccine-delivery systems. In these formulations, antigen can either be entrapped or adsorbed to the surface of the particles. These can act as depot from which the encapsulated antigen is gradually released. Additionally, the polymeric particles may offer protection to encapsulate the antigens delivered and facilitate uptake by M-cells in the mucosa-associated lymphoid tissue (MALT), thus serving as a vehicle for mucosal immunization. Thus, these delivery systems act as adjuvants for vaccine. Polyelectrolytes—polyoxidonium and poly[di(carboxylatophenoxy)phosphazene] (PCPP) have shown adjuvant property. Also, polycations (polyarginine, chitosan, and cationic lipids) have adjuvant activity. Cation adjuvant CAF01 is composed of dimethyldioctadecylammonium (DDA) and trehalose-6, 6-dibehenate (TDB)—a synthetic analog of Mycobacterium cord factor. CAF01 was originally developed as a cell-mediated immunity (CMI)-promoting adjuvant for subunit vaccine against TB and is now known to enhance both CMI and humoral responses.

Similarly, *nonbiodegradable nanoparticles*, like gold, latex, silica, and polystyrene, have also been used as vaccine delivery/adjuvant systems either alone or in combination with other strategies like electroporation. *Virosomes, virus-like particles (VLPs),* and *virus vectors* are another group of vaccine delivery systems being explored as adjuvants in modern vaccine formulations (*vide infra, Q. 8*).

Most conventional adjuvants are poorly defined, complex substances that fail to meet the stringent criteria for safety and efficacy desired in new generation vaccines. Adjuvants for newer vaccines need to be more focused and safer. Modern adjuvant formulation is often *composed of multiple adjuvants,* which can potentially act synergistically and are specifically adapted to each target and to the relevant correlate(s) of protection. Such "second-generation adjuvant systems" are already in use with licensed vaccines like Cervarix® (vaccine against HPV) and Fendrix® (new hepatitis B vaccine) and in development for the new upcoming vaccines against malaria and genital herpes. The prepandemic vaccines also use new generation of adjuvanted systems.

One emerging class of newer adjuvants is *carbohydrate-based adjuvants*. *γ-inulin* is a carbohydrate derived from the plant roots of the *Compositae* family. It is a potent adjuvant inducing humoral and cellular immunity without the toxicity. γ-inulin can be combined with a variety of other adjuvant components, e.g., aluminum hydroxide, to produce a range of adjuvants with varying degree of Th1 and Th2 activity. They principally stimulate the innate immune system through their ability to activate the alternative complement pathway that has proven ability to induce both cellular and humoral immunity. Thus, they use a "natural" mechanism and the biochemical basis of their action is well-understood in general terms. With their excellent tolerability, long shelf-life, low cost, and easy manufacture, they offer great potential for use in a broad range of prophylactic and therapeutic vaccines. Based on successful animal studies in a broad range of species, human trials are about to get underway to validate the use of inulin-based adjuvants in prophylactic vaccines against hepatitis B, malaria, and other pathogens. If such trials are successful, then it is possible that inulin-derived adjuvants might 1 day replace alum as the adjuvant of choice in most human prophylactic vaccines. Other carbohydrates that have been studied as adjuvants are glucans, dextrans, lentinans, glucomannans, galactomannans, and acemannan.

It is known that parasitic infections can alter host immune responses. Among parasitic infections, helminth infection often leads to systemic immune suppression or anergy, allowing their long-term survival in the host and restricting pathology. Thus, persons who are chronically infected with helminths have lesser incidence of allergies and autoimmune diseases. Helminth infection or helminth extracts drive $CD4^+$ T-helper (Th) cell responses toward Th2 type and activate APCs such that these cells express an anti-inflammatory phenotype. Among the myriad molecules present on or secreted by helminth parasites, *glycans* have been shown to be the key in inducing Th2-type and anti-inflammatory immune responses. New insights into these pathways could be useful to antagonize suppression and hence boost vaccine efficacy or to optimize suppression induced by helminth-derived molecules and control inflammatory diseases. There is another adjuvant under development that is derived from a helminth. It is called *activation-associated protein-1 (ASP-1)* and is derived from a helminth, *Onchocerca volvulus*. It has potent adjuvant activity and, unlike alum adjuvant, is able to induce both Th1- and Th2-associated humoral responses and Th1 cellular responses. Thus, it can be further developed as a promising adjuvant for subunit-based and inactivated vaccines.

Among the newer approaches is to design "mucosal adjuvant" that can induce maximal protective mucosal immunity to the antigen (*vide infra*, Q. 7).

Another emerging approach is to use "cellular adjuvants". For example, recent research has shed light on pivotal role of DCs in the initiation and regulation of the immune response. Subsequent preclinical studies and pilot clinical trials have provided some evidence on the potential advantages of using DCs as cellular adjuvants. Current research efforts are focused on the definition of optimal protocols for DC-based therapies in patients.

Recent advances in basic immunology have revealed central role of cytokines in linking the innate and adaptive immunity through their action on DCs. Thus, *cytokines* are being increasingly used as adjuvants, especially for therapeutic vaccines against chronic infections and cancer vaccines. The initial results have been encouraging.

7. What are mucosal adjuvants?

Oral polio vaccine, oral rotavirus vaccine, and nasal live influenza vaccine easily achieve desired immune response through mucosa due to live virus. Nonlive antigens are poorly immunogenic through mucosal route and adjuvants are being tried to enhance it.

A large proportion of pathogens either invades through or cause disease at mucosal surfaces. This can be prevented by induction of immunity in the common mucosal immune system (CMIS), which interconnects inductive tissues, including Peyer's patches (PPs) and nasopharyngeal-associated lymphoreticular tissue (NALT) and effector tissues of the intestinal and respiratory tracts. However, mucosal vaccines have to overcome several formidable barriers in the form of significant dilution and dispersion, competition with a myriad of various live replicating bacteria, viruses, inert food, and dust particles, enzymatic degradation, and low pH before reaching the target immune cells. Thus, vaccination through mucosal membranes requires potent adjuvants to enhance immunogenicity as well as delivery systems to decrease the rate of dilution and degradation and to target the vaccine to the site of immune function.

When vaccine antigen is administered together with mucosal adjuvant, antigen-specific Th1 and Th2 cells, CTLs, and immunoglobulin A (IgA) B-cell responses are effectively induced by oral or nasal routes via the CMIS. In the early stages of induction of mucosal immune response, the uptake of orally or nasally administered antigens is achieved through a unique set of antigen-sampling cells, M-cells located in follicle-associated epithelium (FAE) of inductive sites. After successful uptake, the antigens are immediately processed and presented by the underlying DCs. Elucidation of the molecular/cellular characteristics of M-cells and mucosal DCs is very likely to facilitate the design of a new generation of effective mucosal adjuvants and of a vaccine delivery vehicle that maximizes the use of the CMIS.

Numerous such candidate adjuvants have been studied: *mutants of heat-labile enterotoxin from Escherichia coli*, mutants of *cholera toxin from Vibrio cholerae*, a chimeric protein formed by genetic combination of mutant cholera toxin A subunit and heat-labile toxin B subunit, another chimeric protein combining enzymatically active *CTA1* gene from whole cholera toxin to a gene encoding a synthetic analog of *Staphylococcus aureus* protein A (with a high affinity toward B cells), MPL (derived from the LPS of *Salmonella minnesota*, a gram-negative bacteria), N-acetylmuramyl-L-alanyl-D-isoglutamine (*muramyl dipeptide*) derived from cell wall of mycobacteria, proteosomes (multimolecular preparations of meningococcal outer membrane protein), CpG motif-containing DNA, saponins like QS-21, cytokines like interleukin IL-1, IL-12 chemoattractant lymphotactin, regulated upon activation, normal T-cell expressed, and secreted (RANTES) and defensins, and recently, nanoparticles.

Even though these are potent mucosal adjuvants, their toxicity outweighs the advantages. For example, dmLT, dmLT (R192G), and LTK63 have not found to be safe for nasal route. Hence, mutations have been introduced to reduce their toxicity. CTA1-DD is currently in development of influenza nasal vaccine and a double mutant dmLT [oral/sublingual against enterotoxigenic *Escherichia coli* (ETEC)] is currently being investigated.

8. **What are virosomes, virus-like particles, and virus vectors? What are their advantages over other conventional adjuvants?**

A virosome is a drug or vaccine delivery mechanism consisting of unilamellar phospholipid bilayer vesicle incorporating virus-derived proteins to allow the virosomes to fuse with target cells. Virosomes are not able to replicate, but are pure fusion-active vesicles. They are approximately 150 nm in diameter, at least 100 times smaller than the particles in aluminum-adjuvanted vaccines (*see* **Fig. 1**).

Virosome technology has been used to induce immunity to a variety of antigens without the adverse reactions associated with other adjuvants. The novelty of this biodegradable delivery system lies in the natural presentation of antigens and the stimulation of a specific immune response, induced by the active targeting of antigens to immunocompetent cells. Virosomes have been shown to elicit both cell-mediated and humoral immune responses.

Virosome technology has been most advanced in influenza and hepatitis A, in association with protein or peptides, but it is rapidly being used for other antigens as well. A potential advantage of this technology is to take advantage of the physical properties of virosomes in terms of uptake by APCs, as well as the chemical composition, and compatibility with adjuvant molecules derived from lipid A. Some vaccines like Epaxal® (for hepatitis A) and Invivac® (for influenza) are already licensed in some countries.

Virus-like particles are essentially noninfective virus consisting of self-assembled viral envelope proteins without accompanying the genetic material. They maintain a morphology and cell-penetrating ability similar to infective viral particles and can stimulate both cellular and humoral immunity. The first licensed recombinant HBV vaccines, Recombivan® and Energin-B®, were composed of the viral small envelope protein, which upon expression in yeast formed 22 nm VLPs. While effective, these had relatively low immunogenicity (85–90%). They were further improved upon and a potential third-generation hepatitis B vaccine, Bio-Hep-B®, is a VLP-based vaccine with 100% immunogenicity and is licensed in Israel. Gardasil®, the currently available HPV vaccine, is a VLP-based vaccine. Most recently, this approach is being tried to develop vaccine against human bocavirus (HBoV), a recently identified pathogen with a worldwide distribution that is closely related to pediatric acute respiratory infection and gastroenteritis.

Viral-vectored vaccines consist of a nonreplicating virus that contains some defined genetic material from the pathogen to which immunity is desired. Advantages of viral-vectored vaccines include their ease of manufacture, good immune response, and potential for mucosal immunization. The most common viruses used for this purpose are adenovirus and modified vaccinia virus Ankara (MVA), although other viruses like proxyviruses, measles virus, vesicular stomatitis virus, HSV, and alphavirus are also being studied.

9. What are the limitations of adjuvants?

To be successful, the adjuvants being developed need to overcome some crucial limitations like problems related to stability, bioavailability, and cost. Not only stability of the adjuvant, but stability of the antigen and its epitope configuration need to be considered, since addition of protein antigen to the adjuvant formulation or vice versa can impact the epitopes of the antigen. The adverse effects related to the adjuvant per se can affect the overall safety profile of the vaccine formulation. Potential increase in immune toxicity from improved immunogenicity provided by vaccine adjuvants is also of concern. Furthermore, since each adjuvant generates a characteristic immune response (e.g., Th1 or Th2 bias), there is no "universal" adjuvant for all vaccine formulations. Also seeing human diversity, one cannot say all recipients will respond equally to a given adjuvant. No adjuvant so far has ability to induce functional $CD8^+$ T-cells to a level comparable to that of live viral vaccines. Therefore, there is a need to develop adjuvants capable of inducing $CD8^+$ T-cell responses. Development of better adjuvants must not be overlooked because vaccines are formed by a combination of antigens and adjuvants.

SUGGESTED READING

1. Adjuvanted hepatitis B vaccine: new drug. Patients with renal failure: similar response rate but fewer boosters needed. Prescrire Int. 2008;17(98):234-6.
2. Agger EM, Rosenkrands I, Hansen J, Brahimi K, Vandahl BS, Aagaard C, et al. Cationic liposomes formulated with synthetic mycobacterial cordfactor (CAF01): a versatile adjuvant for vaccines with different immunological requirements. PLoS One. 2008;3(9):e3116.
3. Ansong D, Asante KP, Vekemans J, Owusu SK, Brobby NA, Dosoo D, et al. T cell responses to the RTS,S/AS01(E) and RTS,S/AS02(D) malaria candidate vaccines administered according to different schedules to Ghanaian children. PLoS One. 2011;6(4):e18891.
4. Baldrige JR, McGowan P, Evans JT, Cluff C, Mossman S, Johnson D, et al. Taking a toll on human disease: toll-like receptor 4 agonists as vaccine adjuvants and monotherapeutic agents. Expert Opin Biol Ther. 2004;4(7):1129-38.
5. Barton GM, Kagan JC. A cell biological view of toll-like receptor function: regulation through compartmentalization. Nat Rev Immunol. 2009;9(8):535-42.
6. Beran J. The importance of the second generation adjuvanted systems in "new" vaccines. Klin Mikrobiol Infekc Lek. 2008;14(1):5-12.
7. Bolhassani A, Rafati S. Heat-shock proteins as powerful weapons in vaccine development. Expert Rev Vaccines. 2008;7(8):1185-99.
8. Boyaka PN, Marinaro M, Jackson RJ, van Ginkel FW, Cormet-Boyaka E, Kirk KL, et al. Oral QS-21 requires early IL-4 help for induction of mucosal and systemic immunity. J Immunol. 2001;166(4):2283-90.
9. Boyaka PN, McGhee JR. Cytokines as adjuvants for the induction of mucosal immunity. Adv Drug Deliv Rev. 2001;51(1-3):71-9.
10. Bracci L, La Sorsa V, Belardelli F, Proietti E. Type I interferons as vaccine adjuvants against infectious diseases and cancer. Expert Rev Vaccines. 2008;7(3):373-81.
11. Burt D, Mallett C, Plante M, Zimmermann J, Torossian K, Fries L. Proteosome-adjuvanted intranasal influenza vaccines: advantages, progress and future considerations. Expert Rev Vaccines. 2011;10(3):365-75.
12. Christensen D, Agger EM, Andreasen LV, Kirby D, Andersen P, Perrie Y. Liposome-based cationic adjuvant formulations (CAF): past, present, and future. J Liposome Res. 2009;19(1):2-11.
13. Cluff CW, Baldrige JR, Stöver AG, Evans JT, Johnson DA, Lacy MJ, et al. Synthetic toll-like receptor 4 agonists stimulate innate resistance to infectious challenge. Infect Immun. 2005;73(5):3044-52.
14. Cohen J, Benns S, Vekemans J, Leach A. The malaria vaccine candidate RTS,S/AS is in phase III clinical trials. Ann Pharm Fr. 2010;68(6):370-9.
15. Cooper CL, Davis HL, Angel JB, Morris ML, Elfer SM, Seguin I, et al. CPG 7909 adjuvant improves hepatitis B virus vaccine seroprotection in antiretroviral-treated HIV-infected adults. AIDS. 2005;19(14):1473-9.
16. Cooper CL, Davis HL, Morris ML, Efler SM, Al Adhami M, Krieg AM, et al. CPG 7909, an immunostimulatory TLR9 agonist oligodeoxynucleotide, as adjuvant to Engerix-B HBV vaccine in healthy adults: a double-blind phase I/II study. J Clin Immunol. 2004;24(6):693-701.
17. Cooper PD, Turner R, McGovern J. Algammulin (gamma inulin/alum hybrid adjuvant) has greater adjuvanticity than alum for hepatitis B surface antigen in mice. Immunol Lett. 1991;27(2):131-4.
18. Cooper PD. Vaccine adjuvants based on gamma inulin. Pharm Biotechnol. 1995;6:559-80.

19. Courtney AN, Thapa P, Singh S, Wishahy AM, Zhou D, Sastry J. Intranasal but not intravenous delivery of the adjuvant α-galactosylceramide permits repeated stimulation of natural killer T cells in the lung. Eur J Immunol. 2011;41(11): 3312-22.
20. Cox JC, Coulter AR. Adjuvants—a classification and review of their modes of action. Vaccine. 1997;15(3):248-56.
21. Cunningham KA, Carey AJ, Lycke N, Timms P, Beagley KW. CTA1-DD is an effective adjuvant for targeting anti-chlamydial immunity to the murine genital mucosa. J Reprod Immunol. 2009;81(1):34-8.
22. da Hora VP, Conceição FR, Dellagostin OA, Doolan DL. Non-toxic derivatives of LT as potent adjuvants. Vaccine. 2011;29(8):1538-44.
23. de Bruijn IA, Nauta J, Gerez L, Palache AM. The virosomal influenza vaccine Invivac: immunogenicity and tolerability compared to an adjuvanted influenza vaccine (Fluad) in elderly subjects. Vaccine. 2006;24(44-46):6629-31.
24. de Gregorio E, D'Oro U, Wack A. Immunology of TLR-independent vaccine adjuvants. Curr Opin Immunol. 2009;21(3):339-45.
25. Deng ZH, Hao YX, Yao LH, Xie ZP, Gao HC, Xie LY, et al. Immunogenicity of recombinant human bocavirus-1,2 VP2 gene virus-like particles in mice. Immunology. 2014;142(1):58-66.
26. Dumais N, Patrick A, Moss RB, Davis HL, Rosenthal KL. Mucosal immunization within activated human immunodeficiency virus plus CpG oligodeoxynucleotides induces genital immune responses and protection against intravaginal challenge. J Infect Dis. 2002;186(8):1098-105.
27. Dzierzbicka K, Kolodziejczyk AM. Adjuvants—essential components of new generation vaccines. Postepy Biochem. 2006;52(2):204-11.
28. Ellis RD, Martin LB, Shaffer D, Long CA, Miura K, Fay MP, et al. Phase 1 trial of the *Plasmodium falciparum* blood stage vaccine MSP1(42)-C1/Alhydrogel with and without CPG 7909 in malaria naïve adults. PLoS One. 2010;5(1):e8787.
29. Ellis RD, Mullen GE, Pierce M, Martin RB, Miura K, Fay MP, et al. A Phase 1 study of the blood-stage malaria vaccine candidate AMA1-C1/Alhydrogel with CPG 7909, using two different formulations and dosing intervals. Vaccine. 2009;27(31): 4104-9.
30. El'shina GA, Gorbunov MA, Shervarli VI, Lonskaia NI, Pavlova LI, Khaitov RM, et al. Evaluation of the effectiveness of influenza trivalent polymer subunit vaccine "Grippol". Zh Mikrobiol Epidemiol Immunobiol. 1998;3:40-3.
31. Faveeuw C, Trottein F. Optimization of natural killer T cell-mediated immunotherapy in cancer using cell-based and nanovector vaccines. Cancer Res. 2014;74(6):1632-8.
32. Fernandez CS, Jegaskanda S, Godfrey DI, Kent SJ. In-vivo stimulation of macaque natural killer T cells with α-galactosylceramide. Clin Exp Immunol. 2013;173(3):480-92.
33. Frey S, Poland G, Percell S, Podda A. Comparison of the safety, tolerability, and immunogenicity of an MF59-adjuvanted influenza vaccine and a non-adjuvanted influenza vaccine in non-elderly adults. Vaccine. 2003;21(27-30):4234-7.
34. Garalpati S, Facci M, Polewicz M, Strom S, Babiuk LA, Mutwiri G, et al. Strategies to link innate and adaptive immunity when designing vaccine adjuvants. Vet Immunol Immunopathol. 2009;128(1-3):184-91.
35. Ghendon Y, Markushin S, Akopova I, Koptiaeva I, Krvtsov G. Chitosan as an adjuvant for polio vaccine. J Med Virol. 2011;83(5):847-52.
36. Ghendon Y, Markushin S, Krivtsov G, Akopova I. Chitosan as an adjuvant for parenterally administered inactivated influenza vaccines. Arch Virol. 2008;153(5):831-7.

37. Giuliani MM, Del Giudice G, Giannelli V, Dougan G, Douce G, Rappuoli R, et al. Mucosal adjuvanticity and immunogenicity of LTR72, a novel mutant of *Escherichia coli* heat-labile enterotoxin with partial knockout of ADP-ribosyltransferase activity. J Exp Med. 1998;187(7):1123-32.
38. Guy B, Pascal N, Françon A, Bonnin A, Gimenez S, Lafay-Vialon E, et al. Design, characterization and preclinical efficacy of a cationic lipid adjuvant for influenza split vaccine. Vaccine. 2001;19(13-14):1794-805.
39. Guy B. The perfect mix: recent progress in adjuvant research. Nat Rev Microbiol. 2007;5(7):505-17.
40. Hajjar AM, Ernst RK, Tsai JH, Wilson CB, Miller SI. Human Toll-like receptor 4 recognizes host-specific LPS modifications. Nat Immunol. 2002;3(4):354-9.
41. Harn DA, McDonald J, Atochina O, Da'dara AA. Modulation of host immune responses by helminth glycans. Immunol Rev. 2009;230(1):247-57.
42. Heath AW. Cytokines as immunological adjuvants. Pharm Biotechnol. 1995;6: 645-58.
43. He Y, Barker SJ, MacDonald AJ. Recombinant Ov-ASP-1, a Th1-biased protein adjuvant derived from the helminth *Onchocerca volvulus*, can directly bind and activate antigen-presenting cells. J Immunol. 2009;182(7):4005-16.
44. Holmgren J, Lycke N, Czerkinsky C. Cholera toxin and cholera B subunit as oral-mucosal adjuvant and antigen vector systems. Vaccine. 1993;11(12): 1179-84.
45. Huang JR, Tsai YC, Chang YJ, Wu JC, Hung JT, Lin KH, et al. α-Galactosylceramide but not phenyl-glycolipids induced NKT cell anergy and IL-33-mediated myeloid-derived suppressor cell accumulation via upregulation of egr2/3. J Immunol. 2014;192(4):1972-81.
46. Irache JM, Salman HH, Gomez S, Espuelas S, Gamazo C. Poly(anhydride) nanoparticles as adjuvants for mucosal vaccination. Front Biosci (Schol Ed). 2010;2:876-90.
47. Ishii KJ, Akira S. Toll or toll-free adjuvant path toward the optimal vaccine development. J Clin Immunol. 2007;27(4):363-71.
48. Janeway CA, Medzhitov R. Innate immune recognition. Annu Rev Immunol. 2002;20:197-216.
49. Kamijuku H, Nagata Y, Jiang X, Ichinohe T, Tashiro T, Mori K, et al. Mechanism of NKT cell activation by intranasal coadministration of alpha-galactosylceramide, which can induce cross-protection against influenza viruses. Mucosal Immunol. 2008;1(3):208-18.
50. Kemp MM, Kumar A, Mousa S, Park TJ, Ajayan P, Kubotera N, et al. Synthesis of gold and silver nanoparticles stabilized with glycosaminoglycans having distinctive biological activities. Biomacromolecules. 2009;10(3):589-95.
51. Kensil CR, Soltysik S, Wheeler DA, Wu JY. Structure/function studies on QS-21, a unique immunological adjuvant from Quillaja saponaria. Adv Exp Med Biol. 1996;404:165-72.
52. Kim D, Hung CΦ, W*u* TC, Park YM. DNA vaccine with α-galactosylceramide at prime phase enhances anti-tumor immunity after boosting with antigen-expressing dendritic cells. Vaccine. 2010;28(45):7297-305.
53. Kruit WH, Suciu S, Dreno B, Mortier L, Robert C, Chiarion-Sileni V, et al. Selection of immunostimulant AS15 for active immunization with MAGE-A3 protein: results of a randomized phase II study of the European Organisation for Research and Treatment of Cancer Melanoma Group in Metastatic Melanoma. J Clin Oncol. 2013;31(19):2413-20.
54. Kuijk LM, van Die I. Worms to the rescue: can worm glycans protect from autoimmune diseases? IUBMB Life. 2010;62(4):303-12.

55. Kumar P. Alternative vaccine delivery methods. In: Vashishtha VM (Ed). IAP Textbook of Vaccines, 1st edition. New Delhi: Jaypee Brothers Medical Publishers (P) Ltd; 2014. pp. 484-98.
56. Kundli M. New hepatitis B vaccine formulated with an improved adjuvant system. Expert Rev Vaccines. 2007;6(2):133-40.
57. Lahiri A, Das P, Chakravortty D. Engagement of TLR signaling as adjuvant: towards smarter vaccine and beyond. Vaccine. 2008;26(52):6777-83.
58. Lambrecht BN, Kool M, Willart MA, Hammad H. Mechanism of action of clinically approved adjuvants. Curr Opin Immunol. 2009;21(1):23-9.
59. Lasek W, Zagozdzon R, Jakobisiak M. Interleukin 12: still a promising candidate for tumor immunotherapy? Cancer Immunol Immunother. 2014;63(5):419-35.
60. Lell B, Agnandji S, von Glasenapp I, Haertle S, Oyakhiromen S, Issifou S, et al. A randomized trial assessing the safety and immunogenicity of AS01 and AS02 adjuvanted RTS,S malaria vaccine candidates in children in Gabon. PLoS One. 2009;4(10):e7611.
61. Li Z. In vitro reconstitution of heat shock protein-peptide complexes for generating peptide-specific vaccines against cancers and infectious diseases. Methods. 2004;32(1):25-8.
62. Lundgren A, Bourgeois L, Carlin N, Clements J, Gustafsson B, Hartford M, et al. Safety and immunogenicity of an improved oral inactivated multivalent enterotoxigenic *Escherichia coli* (ETEC) vaccine administered alone and together with dmLT adjuvant in a double-blind, randomized, placebo-controlled Phase I study. Vaccine. 2014;32(52):7077-84.
63. Lycke N. From toxin to adjuvant: the rational design of a vaccine adjuvant vector, CTA1-DD/ISCOM. Cell Microbiol. 2004;6(1):23-32.
64. Lührs P, Schmidt W, Kutil R, Buschle M, Wagner SN, Stingl G, et al. Induction of specific immune responses by polycation-based vaccines. J Immunol. 2002;169(9):5217-26.
65. MacDonald AJ, Cao L, He Y, Zhao Q, Jiang S, Lustigman S. rOv-ASP-1, a recombinant secreted protein of the helminth Onchocerca volvulus, is a potent adjuvant for inducing antibodies to ovalbumin, HIV-1 polypeptide and SARS-CoV peptide antigens. Vaccine. 2005;23(26):3446-52.
66. Mallapragada SK, Narsimhan B. Immunomodulatory biomaterials. Int J Pharm. 2008;364(2):265-71.
67. Manocha M, Pal PC, Chitralekha KT, Thomas BE, Tripathi V, Gupta SD, et al. Enhanced mucosal and systemic immune response with intranasal immunization of mice with HIV peptides entrapped in PLG microparticles in combination with Ulex Europaeus-I lectin as M cell target. Vaccine. 2005;23(48-49):5599-617.
68. Maraskovsky E, Schnurr M, Wilson NS, Robson NC, Boyle J, Drane D. Development of prophylactic and therapeutic vaccines using the ISCOMATRIX adjuvant. Immunol Cell Biol. 2009;87(5):371-6.
69. Marciani DJ. Vaccine adjuvants: role and mechanisms of action in vaccine immunogenicity. Drug Discov Today. 2003;8(20):934-43.
70. Mata-Haro V, Cekic C, Martin M, Chilton PM, Casella CR, Mitchell TC. The vaccine adjuvant monophosphoryl lipid A as a TRIF-biased agonist of TLR4. Science. 2007;316(5831):1628-32.
71. Mattarollo SR, West AC, Steegh K, Duret H, Paget C, Martin B, et al. NKT cell adjuvant-based tumor vaccine for treatment of myc oncogene-driven mouse B-cell lymphoma. Blood. 2012;120(15):3019-29.
72. Mbow ML, De Gregorio E, Valiante NM, Rappuoli R. New adjuvants for human vaccines. Curr Opin Immunol. 2010;22(3):411-6.

73. McCluskie MJ, Weeratna RD, Payette PJ, Davis HL. The potential of CpG oligodeoxynucleotides as mucosal adjuvants. Crit Rev Immunol. 2001;21(1-3):103-20.
74. McKenzie A, Watt M, Gittleson C. ISCOMATRIX vaccines: safety in human clinical studies. Hum Vaccin. 2010;6(3):10754.
75. Mohan T, Mitra D, Rao DN. Nasal delivery of PLG microparticle encapsulated defensin peptides adjuvanted gp41 antigen confers strong and long-lasting immunoprotective response against HIV-1. Immunol Res. 2014;58(1):139-53.
76. Mohan T, Sharma C, Bhat AA, Rao DN. Modulation of HIV peptide antigen specific cellular immune response by synthetic α- and β-defensin peptides. Vaccine. 2013;31(13):1707-16.
77. Mohan T, Verma P, Rao DN. Novel adjuvants & delivery vehicles for vaccines development: a road ahead. Indian J Med Res. 2013;138(5):779-95.
78. Moser C, Amacker M, Zurbriggen R. Influenza virosomes as a vaccine adjuvant and carrier system. Expert Rev Vaccines. 2011;10(4):437-46.
79. Mukherjee C, Mäkinen K, Savolainen J, Leino R. Chemistry and biology of oligovalent β-(1→2)-linked oligomannosides: new insights into carbohydrate-based adjuvants in immunotherapy. Chemistry. 2013;19(24):7961-74.
80. Mutwiri G, Gerdts V, Lopez M, Babiuk LA. Innate immunity and new adjuvants. Rev Sci Tech. 2007;26(1):147-56.
81. Nambiar JK, Ryan AA, Kong CU, Britton WJ, Triccas JA. Modulation of pulmonary DC function by vaccine-encoded GM-CSF enhances protective immunity against Mycobacterium tuberculosis infection. Eur J Immunol. 2010;40(1):153-61.
82. Norton EB, Lawson LB, Freytag LC, Clements JD. Characterization of a mutant *Escherichia coli* heat-labile toxin, LT(R192G/L211A), as a safe and effective oral adjuvant. Clin Vaccine Immunol. 2011;18(4):546-51.
83. Novartis Vaccines. (2019). MF59® Adjuvant Fact Sheet. [online] Available from: www.novartisvaccines.com/downloads/diseases-products/MF59-Adj-factsheet.pdf. [Last accessed August, 2020].
84. Pearse MJ, Drane D. ISCOMATRIX adjuvant for antigen delivery. Adv Drug Deliv Rev. 2005;57(3):465-74.
85. Peppoloni S, Ruggiero P, Cotorni M, Morandi M, Pizza M, Rappuoli R, et al. Mutants of the *Escherichia coli* heat-labile enterotoxin as safe and strong adjuvants for intranasal delivery of vaccines. Expert Rev Vaccines. 2003;2(2):285-93.
86. Petrovsky N. Novel human polysaccharide adjuvants with dual Th1 and Th2 potentiating activity. Vaccine. 2006;24(Suppl 2):S2-26-9.
87. Philbin VJ, Levy O. Developmental biology of the innate immune response: implications for neonatal and infant vaccine development. Pediatr Res. 2009;65(5 Pt 2):98R-105.
88. Pizza M, Giuliani MM, Fontana MR, Douce G, Dougan G, Rappuoli R. LTK63 and LTR72, two mucosal adjuvants ready for clinical trials. Int J Med Microbiol. 2000;290(4-5):455-61.
89. Pizza M, Giuliani MM, Fontana MR, Monaci E, Douce G, Mills KH, et al. Mucosal vaccines: nontoxic derivatives of LT and CT as mucosal adjuvants. Vaccine. 2001;19(17-19):2534-41.
90. Plotkin S, Orenstein W, Offit P. Plotkin's Vaccines, 7th edition. Philadelphia: Elsevier; 2018. pp. 61-74.
91. Qiu HN, Wong CK, Chu IM, Hu S Lam CW. Muramyl dipeptide mediated activation of human bronchial epithelial cells interacting with basophils: a novel mechanism of airway inflammation. Clin Exp Immunol. 2013;172(1):81-94.

92. Rakhmilevich AL, Imboden M, Hao Z, Macklin MD, Roberts T, Wright KM, et al. Effective particle-mediated vaccination against mouse melanoma by coadministration of plasmid DNA encoding Gp100 and granulocyte-macrophage colony-stimulating factor. Clin Cancer Res. 2001;7(4):952-61.
93. Sabbatini PJ, Ragupathi G, Hood C, Aghajanian CA, Juretzka M, Iasonos A, et al. Pilot study of a heptavalent vaccine–keyhole limpet hemocyanin conjugate plus QS21 in patients with epithelial ovarian, fallopian tube, or peritoneal cancer. Clin Cancer Res. 2007;13(14):4170-7.
94. Sablan BP, Kim DJ, Barzaga NG, Chow WC, Cho M, Ahn SH, et al. Demonstration of safety and enhanced seroprotection against hepatitis B with investigational HBsAg-1018 ISS vaccine compared to a licensed hepatitis B vaccine. Vaccine. 2012;30(16):2689-96.
95. Salgaller ML, Lodge PA. Use of cellular and cytokine adjuvants in the immunotherapy of cancer. J Surg Oncol. 1998;68(2):122-38.
96. Salman HH, Irache JM, Gamazo C. Immunoadjuvant capacity of flagellin and mannosamine-coated poly(anhydride) nanoparticles in oral vaccination. Vaccine. 2009;27(35):4784-90.
97. Sanders MT, Brown LE, Deliyannis G, Pearse MJ. ISCOM-based vaccines: the second decade. Immunol Cell Biol. 2005;83(2):119-28.
98. Santini SM, Belardelli F. Advances in the use of dendritic cells and new adjuvants for the development of therapeutic vaccines. Stem Cells. 2003;21(4):495-505.
99. Sasaki S, Sumino K, Hamajima K, Fukushima J, Ishii N, Kawamoto S, et al. Induction of systemic and mucosal immune responses to human immunodeficiency virus type 1 by a DNA vaccine formulated with QS-21 saponin adjuvant via intramuscular and intranasal routes. J Virol. 1998;72(6):4931-9.
100. Segal BH, Wang XY, Dennis CG, Youn R, Repasky EA, Manjili MH, et al. Heat shock proteins as vaccine adjuvants in infections and cancer. Drug Discov Today. 2006;11(11-12):534-40.
101. Silva DG, Cooper PD, Petrovsky N. Inulin-derived adjuvants efficiently promote both Th1 and Th2 immune responses. Immunol Cell Biol. 2004;82(6):611-6.
102. Singh M, O'Hagan DT. Recent advances in vaccine adjuvants. Pharm Res. 2002;19(6):715-28.
103. Sjölander A, Cox JC, Barr IG. ISCOMs: an adjuvant with multiple functions. J Leukoc Biol. 1998;64(6):713-23.
104. Sogaard OS, Lohse N, Harboe ZB, Offersen R, Bukh AR, Davis HL, et al. Improving the immunogenicity of pneumococcal conjugate vaccine in HIV-infected adults with a toll-like receptor 9 agonist adjuvant: a randomized, controlled trial. Clin Infect Dis. 2010;51:42-50.
105. Sominskaya I, Skrastina D, Dislers A, Vasiljev D, Mihailova M, Ose V, et al. Construction and immunological evaluation of multivalent hepatitis B virus (HBV) core virus-like particles carrying HBV and HCV epitopes. Clin Vaccine Immunol. 2010;17(6):1027-33.
106. Stephenson I, Zambon MC, Rudin A, Colegate A, Podda A, Bugarini R, et al. Phase I evaluation of intranasal trivalent inactivated influenza vaccine with nontoxigenic *Escherichia coli* enterotoxin and novel biovector as mucosal adjuvants, using adult volunteers. J Virol. 2006;80(10):4962-70.
107. Sundling C, Schön K, Mörner A, Forsell MN, Wyatt RT, Thorstensson R, et al. CTA1-DD adjuvant promotes strong immunity against human immunodeficiency virus type 1 envelope glycoproteins following mucosal immunization. J Gen Virol. 2008;89(Pt 12):2954-64.
108. Sun HX, Xie Y, Ye YP. ISCOMs and ISCOMATRIX. Vaccine. 2009;27(33):4388-401.

109. Thapa P, Zhang G, Xia C, Gelbard A, Overwijk WW, Liu C, et al. Nanoparticle formulated alpha-galactosylceramide activates NKT cells without inducing anergy. Vaccine. 2009;27(25-26):3484-8.
110. Thomas PG, Carter MR, Da'dara AA, DeSimone TM, Harn DA. A helminth glycan induces APC maturation via alternative NF-kappa B activation independent of I kappa B alpha degradation. J Immunol. 2005;175(4):2082-90.
111. Thomas PG, Harn DA. Immune biasing by helminth glycans. Cell Microbiol. 2004;6(1):13-22.
112. Tovey MG, Lallemand C, Thypronitis G. Adjuvant activity of type I interferons. Biol Chem. 2008;389(5):541-5.
113. Traquina P, Morandi M, Contorni M, Van Nest G. MF59 adjuvant enhances the antibody response to recombinant hepatitis B surface antigen vaccine in primates. J Infect Dis. 1996;174(6):1168-75.
114. Tritto E, Mosca F, De Gregorio E. Mechanism of action of licensed vaccine adjuvants. Vaccine. 2009;27(25-26):3331-4.
115. Ulrich JT, Myers KR. Monophosphoryl lipid A as an adjuvant: past experiences and new directions. Pharm Biotechnol. 1995;6:495-524.
116. Valkenburg SA, Li OT, Mak PW, Mok CK, Nicholls JM, Guan Y, et al. IL-15 adjuvanted multivalent vaccinia-based universal influenza vaccine requires CD4+ T cells for heterosubtypic protection. Proc Natl Acad Sci U S A. 2014;111(15):5676-81.
117. Van Die I, Cummings RD. Glycans modulate immune responses in helminth infections and allergy. Chem Immunol Allergy. 2006;90:91-112.
118. Van Kampen KR, Shi Z, Gao P, Zhang J, Foster KW, Chen DT, et al. Safety and immunogenicity of adenovirus-vectored nasal and epicutaneous influenza vaccines in humans. Vaccine. 2005;23(8):1029-36.
119. Van Riet E, Hartgers FC, Yazdanbakhsh M. Chronic helminth infections induce immunomodulation: consequences and mechanisms. Immunobiology. 2007;212(6):475-90.
120. Villarreal DO, Wise MC, Walters JN, Reuschel EL, Choi MJ, Obeng-Adjei N, et al. Alarmin IL-33 acts as an immunoadjuvant to enhance antigen-specific tumor immunity. Cancer Res. 2014;74(6):1789-800.
121. Vyas SP, Gupta PN. Implication of nanoparticles/microparticles in mucosal vaccine delivery. Expert Rev Vaccines. 2007;6(3):401-18.
122. Xiao W, Du L, Liang C, Guan J, Jiang S, Lustigman S, et al. Evaluation of recombinant Onchocerca volvulus activation associated protein-1 (ASP-1) as a potent Th1-biased adjuvant with a panel of protein or peptide-based antigens and commercial inactivated vaccines. Vaccine. 2008;26(39):5022-9.
123. Xu K, Xu SH, Feng X, Yu SQ, Zeng Y. IL15 DNA adjuvant enhances cellular and humoral immune responses induced by DNA and adenoviral vectors encoding HIV-1 subtype B gp160 gene. Bing Du Xue Bao. 2014;30(1):62-5.
124. Yuki Y, Kivono H. New generation of mucosal adjuvants for the induction of protective immunity. Rev Med Virol. 2003;13(5):293-310.
125. Zepp F. Principles of vaccine design—Lessons from nature. Vaccine. 2010;28 Suppl 3:C14-24.
126. Zhao HG, Huang FY, Guo JL, Tan GH. Evaluation on the immune response induced by DNA vaccine encoding MIC8 co-immunized with IL-12 genetic adjuvant against *Toxoplasma gondii* infection. Zhongguo Ji Sheng Chong Xue Yu Ji Sheng Chong Bing Za Zhi. 2013;31(4):284-9.

SECTION 5

Vaccination of Special Groups

53. **Adolescent Immunization**
    CP Bansal, Ashok K Banga
54. **Vaccination Strategies for Travelers**
    Rashna Dass Hazarika
55. **Maternal Immunization**
    Harish K Pemde, Ravitanaya Sodani
56. **Vaccines for Healthcare Professionals**
    Rashna Dass Hazarika

Adolescent Immunization

CP Bansal, Ashok K Banga

1. Why so much buzz around "adolescent immunization"?

Twenty-two percent of the country's population is of adolescents. In absolute numbers, it becomes 250,000,000, bigger than the whole population of many countries. Adolescents are the biggest and strongest resource of any country and their health represents the country's true growth potential. Unfortunately the vaccination coverage in adolescents is dismal in relation to early childhood vaccination. Immunization is the most important preventive health service that can be provided to an adolescent.

2. Adolescent vaccination is almost nonexistent in India's Universal Immunization Program. Explain.

There is lack of systematic epidemiological data defining the exact burden of various diseases in adolescent period. What we have is data for tetanus vaccine only. India has attained >99% coverage by 2017 [World Health Organization–United Nations International Children's Emergency Fund (WHO-UNICEF)].

Most Indian adolescents are expected to be either having partial or no vaccination at all since overall vaccination coverage of the vaccines given to infants and young children is low. Moreover, immunity gained in early childhood declines with time unless boosted periodically.

3. Why so much emphasis on adolescent immunization now?

Immunization of adolescents is being considered very important because:
- Adolescents need protection against certain diseases that have higher morbidity, e.g., hepatitis A, chickenpox.
- Certain diseases have higher incidence during adolescent period, e.g., mumps, meningococcal infection.
- Need of boosting the waning immune responses of certain vaccines administered during infancy or childhood (measles, pertussis, tetanus, and diphtheria).
- With increasing childhood immunization, the average age of few diseases such as diphtheria and measles has shifted upward, which makes adolescents more susceptible to these diseases.

- Adolescents are suffering more because the epidemiology of certain vaccine preventable illnesses such as hepatitis A has changed due to improving economy, better sanitation, and personal hygiene.
- To provide protection against diseases such as cervical cancer appearing during adulthood.
- Vaccination of adolescents has also become an important component of few vaccine preventable illnesses control or elimination projects such as measles elimination, rubella, and congenital rubella syndrome (CRS) control program.
- Few new diseases have also emerged as a major burden during the adolescent period, e.g., dengue.
- Some new and more efficacious vaccines against infectious diseases have become available or likely to be available (typhoid conjugate and dengue vaccines).
- New insights on some other vaccines such as human papillomavirus (HPV) and tetanus, diphtheria, and acellular pertussis (Tdap).
- Tendency of the adolescents to indulge in risk-taking activities such as substance abuse, IV drugs administration and promiscuity that exposes them to certain diseases such as hepatitis B and HPV infection.

4. Describe adolescent immunization schedule.

The Government of India has not prescribed any adolescent-specific immunization schedule so far.

Indian Academy of Pediatrics, taking the lead here, has devised an adolescent immunization schedule.

It divides the vaccines needed in three broad categories:
1. *Mandatory*: HPV and Tdap
2. *Catch-up*: Measles, mumps, and rubella (MMR), varicella, typhoid, and hepatitis B and A
3. *Vaccines given under "special circumstances"*: Influenza, Japanese encephalitis (JE), pneumococcal polysaccharide vaccine (PPSV), and rabies.

The revised Indian Academy of Pediatrics-Advisory Committee on Vaccines and Immunization Practices (IAP-ACVIP) recommendations for 2018-19 immunization for children aged 0 through 18 years.

Criteria for prioritization of adolescent vaccines are based on the:
- Severity of the disease
- Their significance to the adolescents and adults
- Burden and risk of acquiring the infection during adolescent period.

Recommendations are:

Recommended for all adolescents:
- Human papillomavirus
- Dengue
- Mumps/MMR

- Tetanus and diphtheria (Td)/Tdap
- Hepatitis A
- Typhoid
- Varicella
- Hepatitis B.

Vaccines that should be given under special circumstances:
- Meningococcal
- Pneumococcal polysaccharide vaccine
- Japanese encephalitis
- Influenza
- Rabies
- Cholera
- Yellow fever.

5. What is catch-up immunization?

Administration of vaccines at a later age, if due to any reason the vaccines have not been given at recommended age.

Following are the recommendations for individual vaccines:

Human Papillomavirus Vaccine

There is very high burden of cervical cancer in India, accounting nearly 25% of global cervical cancer deaths. In 2012, there were 123,000 new cases of cervical cancer and 67,000 deaths in India.

Routine vaccination:
- Minimum age for vaccination—9 years.
- Human papillomavirus 4 (HPV4) (Gardasil) and HPV2 (Cervarix) are licensed and available in India.
- Either HPV4 or HPV2 is recommended in a two-dose series for females 9–14 years and three-dose series from 15 to 45 years.
- Two-dose series (9–14 completed years) at 0 and 6 months.
- HPV4 can also be given for males aged 11 or 12 years but not yet licensed for use in males in India.

Catch-up vaccination: Administer the vaccine to females up to the age of 45 years, if not previously vaccinated.

Tetanus-diphtheria-acellular Pertussis and Tetanus-diphtheria Vaccines

Tetanus-diphtheria-acellular pertussis (Tdap) along with HPV vaccine is so far considered as a "mandatory" adolescent vaccine.

There is no data on the burden of pertussis in adolescents in India. Also the data on the efficacy/effectiveness of the Tdap from our country and other South Asian countries are sorely lacking.

All adolescents must take at least one dose of Tdap at 10 years or later. Key indication of Tdap would be to use it during pregnancy to protect very young infants from pertussis. Tdap vaccine can be administered regardless of the interval since the last tetanus and diphtheria toxoid containing vaccine.

Recent studies have shown that Tdap vaccine effectiveness decreases with the passage of time and protection wanes rapidly after 1–2 years.

Meningococcal Vaccine

- Recommended only for certain high-risk group of children, during outbreaks and to international travelers, including students going for studying abroad and travelers to Hajj and sub-Saharan Africa.
- Both meningococcal conjugate vaccines (Quadrivalent MenACWY-D, Menactra by Sanofi Pasteur) and polysaccharide vaccines (quadrivalent and bivalent) are licensed in India.
- A serogroup A meningococcal polysaccharide–tetanus toxoid (PsA-TT) is monovalent group A, (MenAfriVac by Serum Institute of India) is made for African countries only and is not available in India.

Conjugate vaccines are preferred over polysaccharide vaccines due to their potential for herd protection and their increased immunogenicity, particularly in children younger than 2 years of age.

Influenza Vaccine

It is recommended only for the vaccination of persons with certain high-risk conditions.

- *First time vaccination*: 6 months to below 9 years—two doses 1 month apart; 9 years and above—single dose.
- Annual revaccination with single dose.
- *Dosage [trivalent inactivated influenza vaccine (TIV)]*: Aged 6–35 months—0.25 mL; 3 years and above—0.5 mL.
- All the currently available TIVs and quadrivalent vaccines in the country contain the "Swine flu" or "A (H1N1)" antigen; no need to vaccinate separately.
- *Best time to vaccinate*: As soon as the new vaccine is released and available in the market, preferably before the onset of rainy season.

Pneumococcal Vaccines (PCV)

Pneumococcal diseases occur worldwide. Incidence varies from place to place. Children below the age of 2 years are at the highest risk. Elderly and high-risk population do need this vaccine.

Routine vaccination with PCV10 or PCV13:

- *Minimum age*: 6 weeks
- PCV13 is also licensed for the prevention of pneumococcal diseases in adults >50 years of age.

- *Primary schedule*: Three primary doses at 6, 10, and 14 weeks.
- *Those with late start of vaccination after 1 year*: Two doses of PCV10 or single dose of PCV13.

Vaccination of persons with high-risk conditions: Children aged 6 through 18 years who have anatomic or functional asplenia (including sickle-cell disease), HIV infection or an immunocompromising condition, cochlear implant or cerebrospinal fluid leak.

Pneumococcal Polysaccharide Vaccine (PPSV23)

- *Minimum age*: 2 years.
- Not recommended for routine use in healthy individuals. Recommended only for the vaccination of persons with certain high-risk conditions as mentioned above.
- Administer PPSV at least 8 weeks after the last dose of PCV13 to children.
- An additional dose of PPSV should be administered after 5 years to these children.
- Pneumococcal polysaccharide vaccine should never be used alone for prevention of pneumococcal diseases among high-risk individuals.

Hepatitis A Vaccine

Incidence of hepatitis A virus (HAV) infection in India is reducing and has resulted in pushing up the average age of infection. This has increased the proportion of infections that results in severe disease during adolescents and adults. Due to their tendency of more frequent eating outside home, adolescents are more vulnerable to acquire HAV infection. Hepatitis A vaccination needs to be given a high priority for catch-up immunization of adolescents.

Administer two doses of killed vaccine at least 6 months apart or single dose of live vaccine.

Hepatitis B Vaccine

India is now in category of intermediate endemicity for hepatitis B with prevalence of 2–7% (average of 4%). Predominant mode of transmission of hepatitis B in India is horizontal. Perinatal transmission through mother to child is also significant. Adolescents are more vulnerable to get hepatitis B infection through indulgence in sexual activities. Thus, vaccination of adolescents against hepatitis B becomes imperative.

Administer a three-dose series to those not previously vaccinated.

Japanese Encephalitis Vaccine

Routine vaccination:
- Recommended only for individuals living in endemic areas till 18 years of age.

- The vaccine should be offered to the children residing in rural areas only and those planning to visit endemic areas (depending upon the duration of stay).
- Three types of new generation JE vaccines are licensed in India:
  1. Live-attenuated, cell-culture derived SA-14-14-2:
     - Minimum age—8 months
     - Two dose schedule, at 9 months and at 16–18 months
     - Not available in private market for office use
  2. Inactivated cell culture derived SA-14-14-2 (JEEV® by BE India):
     - Minimum age—1 year [United States-Food and Drug Administration (US-FDA)—2 months]
     - *Primary immunization schedule*:
       - Two doses of 0.25 mL each intramuscularly (IM) on days 0 and 28 for children aged ≥1 to ≤3 years
       - Two doses of 0.5 mL for children >3 years and adults aged ≥18 years
     - Need of boosters still undetermined
  3. Inactivated Vero cell culture-derived Kolar strain, 821564XY, JE vaccine (JENVAC® by Bharat Biotech)
     - Minimum age—1 year
     - *Primary schedule*: Two doses of 0.5 mL each IM at 4 weeks interval
     - Need of boosters still undetermined.

Catch-up vaccination: All susceptible children up to 18 years should be administered during disease outbreak/ahead of anticipated outbreak in campaigns.

Typhoid Vaccines

India and few other South-east Asian countries have very high incidence of typhoid fever. Children aged 5–15 years and adolescents are at the greatest risk of developing this disease. According to Global Burden of Disease Study, in 2016, India had 6.6 million typhoid cases (499 cases per 100,000 population) and 66,439 typhoid deaths, 56% of which were among children under 15 years of age. Incidence was quite high in 2–4 years age group also (340.1 cases per 100,000/year) in India.

With the same reasoning as for hepatitis A, adolescents are more vulnerable to catch typhoid infection also and should therefore be vaccinated on priority.

Routine vaccination:

- Both Vi-PS (polysaccharide) and Vi-PS conjugate vaccines are available.
- *Minimum ages*:
  - Vi-PS (polysaccharide) vaccines—2 years
  - Vi-PS (Typbar-TCV™)—6 months

- *Vaccination schedule*:
  - *Vi-PS vaccines:* Single dose at 2 years; revaccination every 3 years (no evidence of hyporesponsiveness on repeated revaccination so far)
  - *Vi-PS conjugate (Typbar-TCV™):* Single dose at 9–12 months and a booster during 2nd year of life.

  Booster dose not needed when first dose was given after the age of 2 years.

Catch-up vaccination: Recommended throughout the adolescent period, i.e., 18 years.

Measles, Mumps, and Rubella Vaccine

Routine vaccination:
- Minimum age—9 months
- Administer the first dose of MMR vaccine at the age of 9 months and 2nd at 15 months.

Mumps vaccine: Available as combination only with measles and rubella as measles-mumps-rubella (MMR) and not stand alone.

The highest incidence of mumps in India is seen in children above 5 years of age, mostly in the adolescent age group. There is a considerable waning of immunity following mumps vaccination. Since the first dose of MMR is now offered before 12 months of age when a robust immune response may not be elicited, the need for additional doses becomes all the most important. Whether the third dose of the vaccine is given to adolescents is a debatable issue. At least, a single-dose of mumps/MMR is a must for every adolescent irrespective of their past vaccination status.

Government replacing MMR with MR in national programs is thus a debatable issue and IAP was not in favor of neglecting "mumps" vaccination at almost the same cost and efforts.

Varicella Vaccine

The varicella disease is far more severe ailment with greater morbidity and mortality in adolescents and adults than in early childhood. Furthermore, this infection during pregnancy may have serious health hazards for the fetus and newborn infant.

Routine vaccination: Two doses at 15 months and 3 months apart.

Catch-up immunization:
- For children up to 13 years without evidence of immunity, administer two doses at 12 weeks interval.
- For any age >13 years, the minimum interval between two doses is 4–8 weeks.

Dengue Vaccine

Dengue is the fastest spreading viral infection in the world and is therefore, the top concern for India and entire South-East Asia (SEA) region.

Though dengue affects all age groups, it is primarily a disease of adolescents and adults. Majority of dengue cases occur in the age group of 14–45 years with the highest burden seen in the 15–24 years subgroup.

Recently a live recombinant tetravalent dengue vaccine (Dengvaxia®) has been introduced and thus prevention of dengue has become possible. WHO has approved its use in the highly endemic countries where around 90% of the population may be infected with the dengue virus.

Present vaccine has certain limitations and is not yet freely available in India. Two more robust vaccines are in pipeline.

FREQUENTLY ASKED QUESTIONS

1. Can MMR and chickenpox vaccine be given at the same time?

Yes, but at different sites or as a combination vaccine, if available.

2. Do you recommend MMR or rubella vaccine to adolescent girls?

Measles-mumps-rubella is the ideal recommendation for both boys and girls. A dose of mumps containing vaccine, i.e., MMR should be given during adolescence irrespective of past vaccination history considering the fast waning of immunity against mumps and higher risk of the disease during this period.

3. Rubella vaccination certificate is insisted by temple authorities at Thiruannamalai, Tamil Nadu (India) for performance of marriage in Arunachala Eswara temple. Why is this not practiced everywhere?

Yes, it would be ideal if temple and school authorities everywhere insist on such a certificate for MMR/MR or rubella.

4. Why do American universities require MMR vaccination certificate from students coming from India?

Because measles still continues to be a problem in adolescents in some parts of the United States of America. Mumps and rubella infection, under control in the USA, if emerges in a foreign student, can cause epidemiological concern.

5. Do American universities require any other immunization certificate from adolescents of India?

Yes, some universities insist on complete immunization certificate since birth, but some insist for varicella, hepatitis A, and typhoid.

6. What is the role of Td/Tdap in routine immunization?

The World Health Organization (WHO) now recommends Td instead of tetanus toxoid (TT) in prophylaxis of wound management and against neonatal and maternal tetanus. Td is to be repeated every 10 years. Tdap is given as a single booster at 10 years to those who can afford it.

7. **Many studies have reported efficacy of even a single dose of the HPV vaccines. Do you think there is a need for further shortening of HPV administration schedule?**

Yes, it is true. Many studies from different countries including India are underway to explore the feasibility of using a single dose of HPV vaccine in immunization schedules. This will facilitate better coverage along with lower cost. However, as of today, there is no such recommendation from any authority to use a single dose of the HPV vaccine in immunization schedule.

8. **A 12-year-old girl has received a quadrivalent HPV vaccine 6 months back. She has now moved to a place where this brand is not available. What should she do now? Can she complete her HPV schedule with a bivalent vaccine which is available there?**

Ideally, one should stick to the same brand of the vaccine. And, this is more important in case of HPV vaccination. However, one should not abandon or delay completion of the schedule, and complete the two-dose schedule with the available brand of the same.

There are limited data available on the use of different HPV vaccines in the same subject. A recent trial evaluated the immunogenicity and safety of a mixed vaccination schedule with one dose of 9vHPV and one dose of 2vHPV administered in different order versus two doses of 9vHPV vaccine. The mixed HPV vaccination schedules used were found immunogenic with an acceptable safety profile.

9. **What can be the adolescent immunization schedule card?**

Figure 1 shows IAP ACVIP immunization schedule for persons aged 7 through 18 years, 2014.

Figure 2 shows IAP recommended immunization schedule for children aged 0–18 years (with range), 2014.

10. **What are the recommendations for adolescent travelers?**

All age appropriate vaccines should be completed before travel in addition to those listed in **Table 1**.

11. **Why might some adults need vaccines?**

Some adults incorrectly assume that the vaccines they received as children will protect them for the rest of their lives. Generally this is true, except that:

- Some adults were never vaccinated as children.
- Newer vaccines were not available when some of them were children.
- Immunity can begin to fade overtime.
- As we age, we become more susceptible to serious disease caused by common infections (e.g., flu, Pneumococcus).

The Advisory Committee oh Immunization Practices (ACIP) annually reviews the recommended adult immunization schedule to ensure that the schedule reflects current recommendations for the licensed vaccines that **Figure 3** displays.

Vaccine ▼ Age ▶	7–10 years	11–12 years	13–18 years
Tdap	1 dose (if indicated)	1 dose	1 dose (if indicated)
HPV		2 doses	Complete 2/3-dose series
MMR		Complete 2-dose series	
Varicella		Complete 2-dose series	
Hepatitis B		Complete 3-dose series	
Hepatitis A		Complete 1/2-dose series	
Typhoid		1 dose every 3 years	
Influenza vaccine		One dose every year	
Japanese encephalitis vaccine		Catch-up up to 15 years	
Pneumococcal vaccine			
Meningococcal vaccine			

Legend: For all children/Pre-adolescents | For catch-up immunization | For high-risk group

Fig. 1: Indian Academy of Pediatrics–Advisory Committee on Vaccines and Immunization Practices (IAP-ACVIP) immunization schedule for persons aged 7 through 18 years, 2014 (with range)

Note: For more details please visit http://www.indianpediatrics.net/oct2014/oct-785-803.htm.

	Birth	6 weeks	10 weeks	14 weeks	6 months	9 months	12 months	13 months	15 months	16-18 months	2-3 years	4-6 years	9-14 years	15-18 years
BCG	BCG													
Hepatitis B	HB1	Hb2	Hb3	HB*4										
Polio	OPV0	IPV**1	IPV**2	IPV**3						IPV***B1				
DTwP/DTaP		DTP1	DTP2	DTP3						DTP B1		DTP B2		
HiB		HIB1	HIB2	HIB3						HIB B1				
Pneumococcal		PCV1	PCV2	PCV3					PCV B1				PCV	
Rotavirus		Rota 1	Rota 2	Rota 3****										
MMR						MMR1			MMR2			MMR3/MMRV		
Varicella									Varicella 1			Varicella 2		
Hepatitis A							Hep A1			Hep A2*****				
Typhoid					TCV^									
Influenza							Influenza (yearly)******							
Meningococcal						MCV1	MCV2				MCV			
JE							JE 1	JE 2						
Tdap													Tdap	Td
HPV##													HPV 1 and 2	HPV 1, 2, 3
Cholera									Cholera 1 and 2					

▓	Range of recommended age for all children
▓	Range of recommended age for high-risk children/area
▓	Range of recommended age for catch-up immunization
▓	Not recommended

*Fourth dose of hepatitis B permissible for combination vaccines only
**In case IPV is not available of feasible, the child should be offered bOPV (three doses). In such cases, give two fractional doses of IPV at 6 weeks and 14 weeks
*** bOPV, if IPV booster (standalone or combination) not feasible
****Third dose not required for RV1. Catch-up up to 1 year of age in UIP schedule
***** Live-attenuated hepatitis A vaccine: Single dose only
******Begin influenza vaccination after 6 months of age, about 2–4 weeks before season; give two doses at the interval of 4 weeks during first year and then single dose yearly till 5 years of age

^TCV: Typhoid conjugate vaccine, ##HPV: human papillomavirus
Meningococcal vaccine (MCV): 9 months through 23 months; two doses, at least 3 months apart; 2 years through 55 years; single dose only
Japanese encephalitis (JE): For individuals living in an endemic areas and for travelers to JE endemic areas provided their expected stay is for a minimum period of 4 weeks
HPV: Two doses at 6 months interval 9–14 years age; Three doses (at 0, 1–2 and 6 months) 15 years or older immunocompromised
Cholera vaccine: Two doses 2 weeks apart for >1 year old; For individuals living in high-endemic areas and traveling to areas where risk of transmission is very high

Fig. 2: Indian Academy of Pediatrics–Advisory Committee on Vaccines and Immunization Practices (IAP-ACVIP) recommended immunization schedule for children aged 0–18 years (with range), 2018–19.

Note: For more details please visit http://www.indianpediatrics.net/oct2014/oct-785-803.htm

(BCG: bacillus Calmette-Guérin; DTap: diphtheria, tetanus, acellular pertussis vaccine, DTwP: diphtheria, tetanus, whole cell pertussis; Hib: *Haemophilus influenzae* type b; HPV: human papillomavirus; IPV: inactivated poliovirus vaccine; MMR: measles-mumps-rubella; OPV0: oral poliovirus vaccine at birth; PCV: pneumococcal conjugate vaccine; Td: tetanus, reduced dose diphtheria toxoid; Tdap: tetanus, reduced dose diphtheria and acellular pertussis vaccine)

Source: Balasubramanian S, Shah A, Pemde HK, et al. Indian Academy of Pediatrics (IAP (Advisory committee on Vaccines and immunization practices (ACVIP) Recommended immunization schedule (2018-19) and update on immunization for children aged 0 through 18 years. Indian Pedhlatr. 2018;55(12):1066-74

TABLE 1: Vaccines for adolescent travelers.

Vaccine	Place of travel*	Dose recommended
Meningococcal vaccine	USA/UK/endemic areas Saudi Arabia and Africa#	Two doses 4–8 weeks apart
Yellow fever^	Yellow fever endemic zones**	10 days before travel
Oral cholera vaccine	Endemic area or area with an outbreak	Two doses 1 week apart
Japanese B encephalitis	Endemic areas for Japanese encephalitis. In India: North Arcot district of Tamil Nadu and neighboring districts of Andhra Pradesh; also in most parts of South, Central, Northern, and North-Eastern states; South-East Asian and East-Asian countries	Single dose (up to 15 years)
Rabies vaccine (pre-exposure prophylaxis)	For adolescents going on trekking, for children where pet dogs are present	0–7 two dose schedule (WHO)

*All the persons, including adults going to Saudi Arabia for Hajj pilgrimage are required to take one dose of oral poliovirus vaccine (OPV) in addition to quadrivalent meningococcal vaccine.
#Quadrivalent vaccine for those traveling to the United States and bivalent (A + C) or quadrivalent for those traveling to the United Kingdom.
^Mandatory for all travelers to yellow fever endemic zones as per international health regulations.
**The list of endemic countries can be obtained at http://wwwn.cdc.gov/travel/yellowBookch4-YellowFever.aspx currently available only at select government controlled centers in India.

Note: For more information on travelers vaccination, please visit http://wwwnc.cdc.gov/travel/default.aspx.

SUGGESTED READING

1. Indian Academy of Pediatrics, Advisory Committee on Vaccines and Immunization Practices (ACVIP), Vashishtha VM, Kalra A, Bose A, Choudhury P, et al. Indian Academy of Pediatrics (IAP) recommended immunization schedule for children aged 0 through 18 years, India, 2013 and updates on immunization. Indian Pediatr. 2013;50:1095-108.
2. Indian Academy of Pediatrics Committee on Immunization (IAPCOI). Consensus recommendations on immunization and IAP immunization timetable 2012. Indian Pediatr. 2012;49:549-64.
3. Recommended Adult Immunization Schedule–United States 2010. MMWR. [online] Available from: http://www.cdc.gov/mmwr/PDF/wk/mm5901-Immunization.pdf [Last accessed June, 2020].
4. Recommended Immunization Schedule for Persons Aged 7 through 18 Years—United States 2010. [online] Available from: http://www.cdc.gov/vaccines/recs/schedules/downloads/child/2010/10_7-18yrs-schedule-pr.pdf [Last accessed June, 2020].
5. Sankaranarayanan R (2013). Trial of two versus three doses of Human Papillomavirus (HPV) vaccine in India. [online] Available from: http://clinicaltrials.gov/show/NCT00923702 [Last accessed June, 2020].
6. Sankaranarayanan R. Evaluation of fewer than three doses of HPV vaccination in India, in WHO Consultation Meeting. 2013: WHO, Geneva.

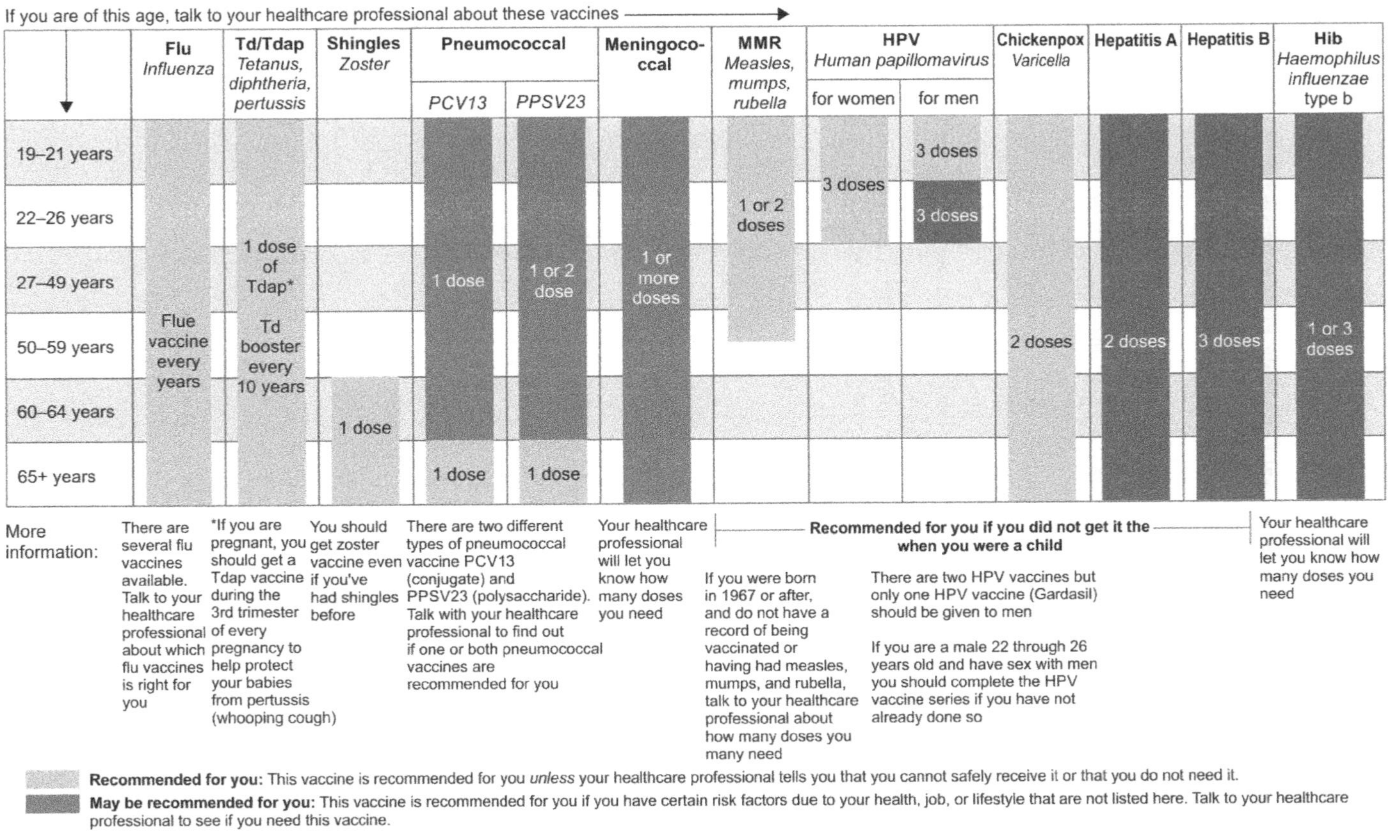

Fig. 3: Recommended adult immunization schedule by vaccine and age group—United States 2014.

7. Singhal T, Amdekar YK, Agarval RK. IAP Guidebook on Immunization, 4th edition. IAP Committee on Immunization. New Delhi, India: Jaypee Brothers Medical Publishers; 2009.
8. Vashishtha VM, Choudhury P, Bansal CP, Yewale VN, Agarwal R. IAP Guidebook on Immunization 2013-2014. Gwalior: National Publication House, Indian Academy of Pediatrics; 2014.
9. Vashishtha VM, Yewale VN, Bansal CP, Mehta PJ. IAP perspectives on measles and rubella elimination strategies. Indian Pediatr. 2014;51:719-22.
10. Vashishtha VM. Adolescent Immunization Schedule: Need for a Relook. Indian Pediatr. 2019;56(2):101-4.
11. World Health Organization (2014). Summary of the SAGE April 2014 Meeting. [online] Available from: http://www.who.int/immunization/sage/meetings/2014/april/report_summary_april_2014/en/ [Last accessed June, 2020].
12. World Health Organization (2014). WHO prequalified vaccines. [online] Available from: http://www.who.int/immunization_standards/vaccine_quality/PQ_vaccine_list_en/en/ [Last accessed June, 2020].
13. World Health Organization. WHO position paper on hepatitis A vaccines—June 2012. Wkly Epidemiol Rec. 2012;87:261-76.
14. Yamini Balya Chikitsalaya (2013). IAP Immunization time-table 2013. [online] Available from: http://www.doksaab.in/wp-content/uploads/2014/08/vaccination-chart.pdf [Last accessed June, 2020].

CHAPTER 54

Vaccination Strategies for Travelers

Rashna Dass Hazarika

1. Why is there a need to vaccinate before traveling?

During the last 50 years, the number of persons traveling across the globe has increased tremendously. It has been seen that many travelers are frequent sufferers of a number of diseases such as influenza, hepatitis A, typhoid and paratyphoid fever, and yellow fever. The latest to be added to this list are the severe acute respiratory syndrome (SARS) group of viruses and coronavirus disease 2019 (COVID-19). Till date, influenza has been assessed to have the highest attack rate at 8.9 per 100 persons-months of travel.

2. What vaccines are required for travelers?

This depends on a few factors such as what are the vaccines that the person has already received, where the person is planning to travel, and for how long the person is planning to stay.

3. Is there a specific schedule of vaccination to be followed for travelers?

No, the schedule depends on the individual person's past immunization history, the countries to be visited, the type and duration of travel, and the time interval from vaccination to travel.

4. What is the best time to vaccinate the traveler?

This depends on the vaccine and whether single or multiple doses needed. Usually for single-dose vaccines, the person should have received the vaccine *at least 2 weeks* prior to travel. It is best that the individual contemplating traveling to a different location contact the healthcare provider at least 4–8 weeks prior to travel.

5. What are the different categories of immunization before travel?

The different categories of immunization to be considered before travel are:
- Routine vaccines (to be reviewed for status of completion)
- Vaccines recommended for special destinations
- Vaccines demanded by some countries.

6. What are the routine vaccinations that must be checked for completion before traveling?

These constitute all vaccinations given as part of the national immunization schedule [Bacillus Calmette-Guérin (BCG), diphtheria, pertussis and tetanus (DPT), inactivated polio vaccine (IPV), hepatitis B, *Haemophilus influenzae* type b (Hib), pneumonia, rotavirus, measles, mumps and rubella (MMR), and human papillomavirus (HPV)].

7. What are the vaccines recommended for special destinations?

These are usually against diseases endemic for a particular place. They may include cholera, hepatitis A, Japanese encephalitis (JE), meningococcal invasive disease, typhoid fever, and rabies as outlined below in **Table 1**.

TABLE 1: Vaccines recommended for special destinations.

Vaccines	Destination
Meningococcal conjugate vaccine (ACWY)	Africa, Saudi Arabia
Yellow fever	Sub-Saharan Africa, tropical South America
Hepatitis A	Africa, Asia, Central and South America, Middle East, and Western Pacific
Rabies	Asia, Africa, Middle East, Latin America, and Caribbean
Japanese encephalitis	Asia
Typhoid fever	Asia, Africa, Caribbean, Central and South America, and Middle East
Cholera	Asia, Africa, and Haiti
Polio	Pakistan, Afghanistan, Nigeria, Ethiopia, Kenya, Somalia, and Syria

A complete list along with detailed information regarding vaccines recommendation on travelling to a particular country can be accessed at the following Centers for Disease Control and Prevention (CDC) website: https://wwwnc.cdc.gov/travel/.

8. What are the vaccines demanded by some countries before arrival?

These include polio, meningococcal and yellow fever vaccine.

9. Who should receive the tetanus, diphtheria and acellular pertussis (TdaP) vaccine?

Tetanus, diphtheria and acellular pertussis (TdaP) vaccine is indicated for those who have never received the vaccine ever and elders above 65 years, visiting relatives with infants below 1 year of age, and in those who are traveling for activities that can predispose to trauma or are traveling to areas with an outbreak of diphtheria or pertussis.

10. Is it necessary to get the measles, mumps and rubella (MMR) vaccine before travel?

Yes, it is mandatory that all unimmunized persons residing in a measles-endemic region should get two doses of a measles-containing vaccine before traveling to the Americas. Similarly, those traveling from the Americas to a measles-endemic region and born after 1957 should get two doses of a measles-containing vaccine 28 days apart and at least 14 days before travel.

11. What will be the vaccination schedule for those who have been partially immunized against measles?

Infants between 6 and 11 months should receive one dose of a measles-containing vaccine. Infants vaccinated before 1 year of age should receive two additional doses 28 days apart. All other unvaccinated children and adults should receive two doses of a measles-containing vaccine 28 days apart.

12. Do immunocompromised individuals need vaccinations before travel?

Yes, immunocompromised individuals are particularly liable to be affected by organisms such as pneumococcus, influenza, and meningococcus in addition to the other diseases likely in a normal individual.

13. Can all vaccines be administered to the immunocompromised traveler?

Yes, if there is mild immunosuppression. However, live vaccines are contraindicated in the severely immunocompromised host [i.e., those on corticosteroid therapy for >2 weeks at a dose equivalent to >20 mg/day of prednisolone, human immunodeficiency virus (HIV) infection with CD4+ cell count <200 cells/mm^3].

14. Can the yellow fever vaccine be administered to the immunocompromised traveler?

Persons with limited immunodeficiencies or asymptomatic HIV going to the yellow fever endemic region can be given the vaccine but will have to be monitored closely for any adverse effects.

15. How many doses of vaccines are required in the immunocompromised traveler?

Vaccine response may be suboptimal and so these patients will have to be evaluated by serologic testing 1 month after vaccination and if required, a dose may be repeated.

16. Which patients require vaccination against pneumococcus and meningococcus?

Patients with asplenia/hyposplenia and terminal complement defects will require to be vaccinated against pneumococcus and meningococcus with the 13-valent pneumococcal conjugate vaccine (PCV13) and 23-valent pneumococcal polysaccharide vaccine (PPSV23) and the conjugate quadrivalent meningococcal ACWY vaccine.

17. Is it safe to vaccinate pregnant women before travel?

Yes, there is no added risk of vaccinating pregnant women with the inactivated viral, bacterial vaccines, or toxoids. It is wise to vaccinate a pregnant woman with the inactivated influenza vaccine at least 2 weeks prior to travel.

18. Which vaccines are contraindicated in the pregnant woman traveler?

The rubella, yellow fever, and BCG vaccines cannot be given to the pregnant woman. If a woman is contemplating pregnancy, then she should be advised to defer the pregnancy for 28 days or more after receiving a rubella-containing vaccine.

19. Which group of people fall into traveler's visiting friends and relatives (VFRs) category?

Visiting friends and relatives (VFRs) are people who are originally from a different country residing in a high-income country and who frequently visit their home country. Examples of this group are a huge majority of Indians residing in the USA.

20. Are visiting friends and relatives (VFRs) at increased risk of certain diseases?

Yes, VFRs are at increased risk of travel-related infectious diseases such as malaria, typhoid and paratyphoid fever, tuberculosis, cholera, measles, and hepatitis A.

21. What are the current recommendations for meningococcal vaccine for travelers?

The current recommendation for meningococcal vaccine for travelers is:
- *Destination specific*:
    - Traveling to areas with current outbreaks
    - Those who are <30 years of age and traveling to sub-Saharan Africa during the dry season (December–June).
- *Special risk group*:
    - All pilgrims arriving to Saudi Arabia for purposes of Hajj and Umrah
    - Individuals with functional or anatomic asplenia, terminal complement deficiency, or any other immunosuppressing conditions
    - New entrants to college, particularly who are going to live in dormitories
    - Persons who are going to work in refugee settings.

22. Is it necessary for travelers to get the hepatitis A vaccine?

Hepatitis A remains the most common vaccine-preventable disease in travelers.
    Nonimmune travelers are at significant risk of acquiring hepatitis A infection from unclean drinking water or food.

23. From which age group should the hepatitis A vaccine be offered in travelers?

All unimmunized individuals ≥1 year of age traveling to hepatitis A endemic zones must receive a dose of the hepatitis A vaccine.

24. At what time should the hepatitis A vaccine be given for travelers?

As the hepatitis A virus has a long incubation period, a dose of the inactivated hepatitis A vaccine administered even a day before travel will be protective for all healthy individuals ≤40 years of age. However, in those >40 years or those with some form of chronic diseases such as chronic liver disease or chronic kidney disease and planning to depart to a hepatitis A endemic area in <2 weeks should receive a dose of the inactivated hepatitis A vaccine along with the immunoglobulin in a dose of 0.02 mL/kg.

25. How do we protect travelers <1 year from hepatitis A infection?

Infant travelers <1 year of age can be given the immunoglobulin before travel. This will protect them for 3–5 months.

26. What is the current recommendation for typhoid vaccine in travelers?

It is recommended that all travelers who plan to stay for >1 month in typhoid-endemic zones or in those areas with prevalence of antibiotic-resistant strains must receive the typhoid conjugate vaccine or the oral live vaccine TY21 at least a week before the travel date. However, they must be told that the vaccine is not 100% effective and that they will still need to maintain good hygiene practices.

27. Which group of travelers will require to be vaccinated against rabies?

Pre-exposure prophylaxis against rabies is recommended for:
- Travelers intending to work in areas where rabies is enzootic and rabies control programs are ineffective
- In areas where adequate and safe postexposure management is not accessible
- Travelers with extensive outdoor exposure in rural areas such as during hiking, running, bicycling, or camping. This is irrespective of the travel duration
- Areas where the rabies vaccines are in short supply.

28. How many doses of the cell culture rabies vaccines need to be administered before travel?

Two intramuscular injections of the cell culture vaccines are to be administered on day 0 and day 14 prior to travel.

29. What is the schedule for administering the cholera vaccine in travelers?

The first dose of the cholera vaccine (killed bivalent or killed whole cell) is to be administered at least 2 weeks prior to departure. For effective protection, the full course of two doses should be completed before departure.

30. Which travelers must receive the Japanese encephalitis (JE) vaccine?

The following travelers should receive the JE vaccine:
- Those who plan to spend >1 month in the endemic area, especially during the JE virus transmission season (postrainy season)
- Those who are likely to visit endemic rural or agricultural areas during the transmission season
- Short-term travelers to endemic areas during the JE virus transmission season for hiking, camping, or other outdoor activities
- Travelers to an area with an ongoing JE outbreak.

31. What are the new recommendations on use of Japanese encephalitis (JE) vaccines for the travelers going to endemic regions?

Till quite recently, the JE vaccine was only "recommended" for travelers who plan to spend a month or longer in endemic areas during the transmission season. The criterion of 1 month was arbitrary.

However, the epidemiology of JE and risk to the traveler have changed in recent times and continue to evolve. However, a recent review of JE cases globally found that at least half the cases reported were in travelers of <30 days. A report on the US international travelers through 2014 included 87 cases of JE and only 50% had visits of over 30 days. There are recent incidents from Bali and Thailand where even a short 10-day stopover with very little rural exposure, outside transmission season, resulted in JE infection.

Considering the changing epidemiology of JE and the publication of above reports, the CDC in its 2019 guidelines has strengthen the JE recommendation by recommending JE vaccine even for the travelers who visit the endemic areas for short term, also provided they visit during transmission season, visit rural places, and go for outdoor activities. For adults, vaccination schedule has been changed to 0 and 7–28 days (previously 0 and 28 days). A booster dose should be (previously may be) given for people who are the risk of re-exposure **(Box 1)**.

> **BOX 1:** Japanese encephalitis (JE) vaccine: Recommendations of the CDC Advisory Committee on Immunization Practices (ACIP).
>
> *CDC-ACIP 2019 recommendations:*
> - Should be given for travelers staying in endemic area for ≥1 month
> - JE vaccine also should be considered for shorter term (e.g., <1 month) travelers with an increased risk of JE based on planned travel duration, season, location, activities, and accommodations
> - Vaccination also should be considered for travelers to endemic areas who are uncertain of specific duration of travel, destinations, or activities (previously, it was may be considered)
> - In adults aged 18–65 years, the primary vaccination schedule is two doses administered on days 0 and 7–28 (previously, it was 0 and 28 days)
> - For adults and children, a booster dose (i.e., third dose) should be given at ≥1 year after completion of the primary IXIARO series if ongoing exposure or re-exposure to JE virus is expected (previously, it was may be given).

32. Which Japanese encephalitis (JE) vaccine to be used and at what time in a person contemplating travel to an endemic area?

Any of the available JE vaccines—live SA 14-14-2, killed SA 14-14-2, or the Vero cell-derived Kolar strain vaccines can be given. Two doses given at least 4 weeks apart and the last dose being completed a week before travel.

33. What is the current recommendation in India for the polio vaccine in travelers?

As per Government of India guidelines, all persons traveling to polio-endemic areas such as Pakistan, Afghanistan, Nigeria, Ethiopia, Kenya, Somalia, and Syria will require to take a dose of oral polio vaccine (OPV) 4 weeks prior to travel irrespective of the age and vaccination status. Residents of these seven polio infected countries are required to receive a dose of OPV, regardless of age and vaccination status, at least 4 weeks prior to departure to India. A certificate of vaccination is required to be submitted while applying for a visa to visit India. This dose of OPV remains valid for a year.

34. Are there any vaccine requirements specified by Government of India for travelers coming to India from other countries?

The Government of India mandatorily requires the following:
- All persons coming from polio-endemic countries or those areas where polio is in circulation must take a single dose of OPV 4 weeks prior to their travel date
- All persons coming from yellow fever-endemic zones should have taken the yellow fever vaccine prior to visiting India.

35. What is the risk of catching Zika virus infection on my next travel destination?

It is difficult to determine the risk of Zika in other countries. Zika frequently causes only mild symptoms and people with Zika might not go to the doctor.

If they go to a doctor, the doctor might not test for Zika or report cases to the government. A lack of reported cases does not mean a lack of risk. The CDC considers any country that has ever had Zika cases to have possible risk, but they cannot say how high or low that risk is.

The CDC now recommends pregnant women and couples trying to become pregnant within the next 3 months. First talk to their healthcare providers and carefully consider the risks and possible consequences of Zika infection before traveling to areas that report past or current spread of Zika but no current outbreak **(Fig. 1)**. Pregnant women avoid mosquito bites and sexual exposure during travel. If partner travels, avoid sex or use condoms for remainder of pregnancy. Women planning to conceive may wish to delay pregnancy.

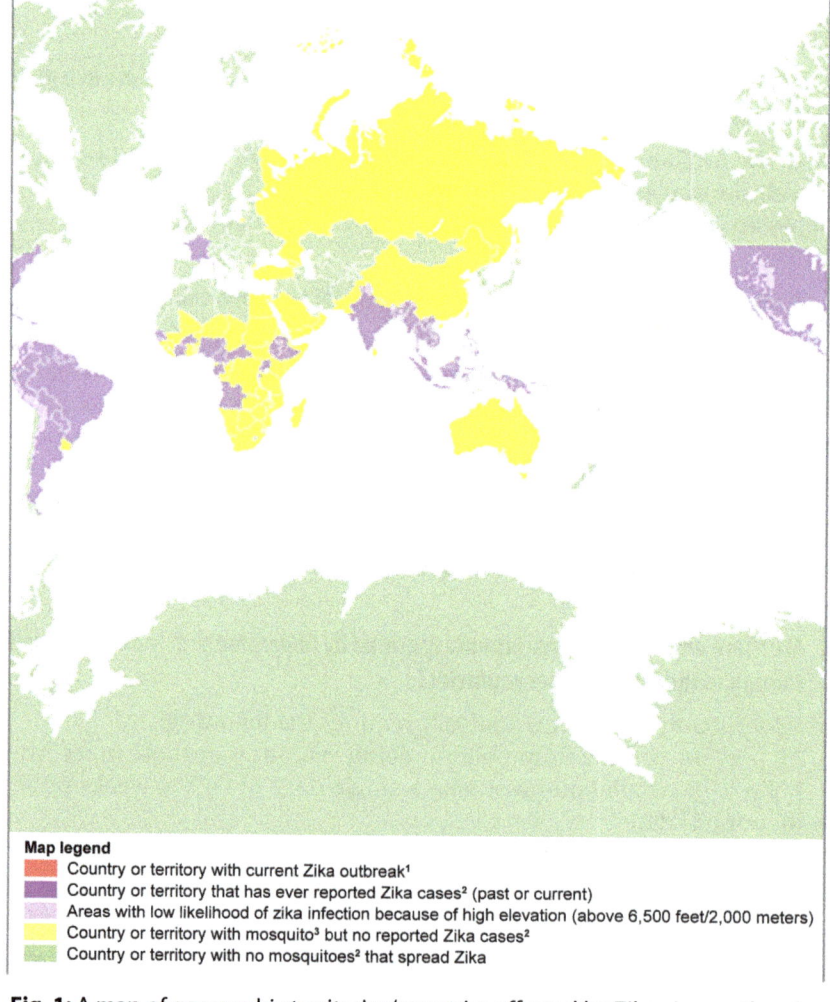

Fig. 1: A map of geographic territories/countries affected by Zika virus outbreaks.
[1-3] Refer for details to CDC Zika map at: https://wwwnc.cdc.gov/travel/page/zika-information

The CDC continues to recommend that pregnant women not travel to areas where a Zika outbreak is occurring.

SUGGESTED READING

1. Centers for Disease Control and Prevention (CDC). (2019). Travelers' Health Most Frequently Asked Questions. [online] Available from https://wwwnc.cdc.gov/travel/page/faq. [Last accessed September 2020].
2. Guidelines of Ministry of Health & Family Welfare, Govt of India. https://main.mohfw.gov.in/sites/default/files/08285260748Requirement.pdf.
3. Hills SL, Walter EB, Atmar RL, Fischer M, ACIP Japanese Encephalitis Vaccine Work Group. Japanese Encephalitis Vaccine: Recommendations of the Advisory Committee on Immunization Practices. MMWR Recomm Rep. 2019;68(2):1-33.
4. World Health Organization (WHO). (2019). Travel advice/vaccines. [online] Available from https://www.who.int/travel-advice/vaccines. [Last accessed September 2020].

CHAPTER 55

Maternal Immunization

Harish K Pemde, Ravitanaya Sodani

1. Why maternal vaccines are important?

Several infections with serious consequences for the mother or fetus can be prevented by preconception and during pregnancy vaccination. Certain infections (including measles, mumps, rubella, and varicella) occurring for the first time during pregnancy can adversely affect the pregnancy outcomes with several types of afflictions of fetus. Vaccinating pregnant women to provide protection to the mother, fetus, and infant through active antibody production and transplacental antibody transfer—"two for one" protection. **Figure 1** displays the interaction and the protective role of maternal antibodies to infant. Ensuring immunity against these diseases is important before pregnancy as these vaccines are contraindicated during pregnancy.

2. Are vaccines safe during pregnancy?

Certain vaccines are safe and recommended for women before, during, and after pregnancy to help keep them and their babies healthy. The antibodies mothers develop in response to these vaccines not only protect them, but also cross the placenta and help protect their babies from serious diseases early

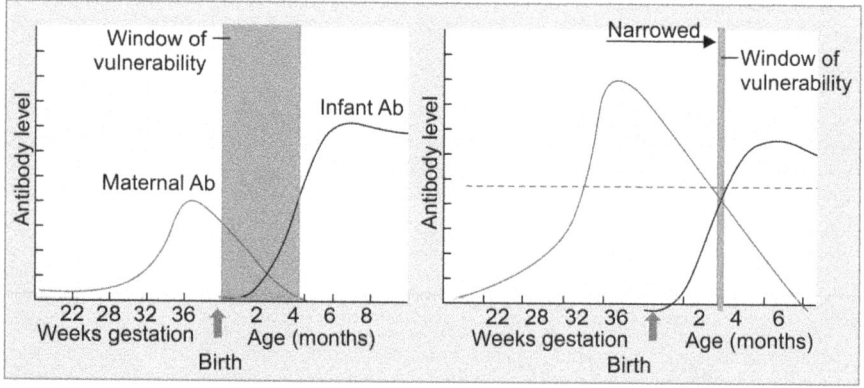

Fig. 1: Interaction of maternal and infant antibodies: How maternal antibodies narrow down the "window of vulnerability".

in life. It is important to remember that only few vaccines can be given during pregnancy. Most vaccines are contraindicated during pregnancy hence pregnancy should be ruled out before giving such vaccines to the women of child-bearing age.

3. What are the routine immunizations recommended to all pregnant women during pregnancy?

Immunizations that are routinely recommended for all pregnant women: tetanus, diphtheria, acellular pertussis (Td or Tdap) vaccine, and influenza vaccine. These immunizations have a good safety profile in pregnancy, can provide passive protection to the newborn, and are not associated with miscarriage. New maternal vaccines are under development, and there is a need to determine how to integrate these vaccines into existing platforms utilizing a life-course approach. **Box 1** and **Table 1** display the different vaccines recommended for maternal vaccination globally.

4. What factors determine placental transfer of antibodies to developing fetus and newborn?

Transplacental passage of antibodies depends on maternal antibody concentration, antibody type (significant amounts of IgG are transported but not IgM, IgA, or IgE), IgG subtype (IgG1 is preferentially transported), and gestational age. Fetal IgG concentration is much lower than maternal concentration in the first half of pregnancy, but increases to 50% of maternal levels at 28–32 weeks of gestation, equals maternal levels by 36 weeks, and often exceeds maternal levels at term.

The placenta remains an organ of tremendous interest and investigation. Recent evidence suggests that it plays an active role in immunologic reactions and can interact and respond to pathogens. Thus, local immunologic mechanisms mediated at the fetomaternal junction help to protect the fetus from rejection, while cytokines provide the required growth factors necessary for implantation of the fetus in the placenta. Different factors can influence the placenta's role in immunity. For example, maternal infection with HIV or malaria reduces the ability of the placenta to transport IgG through impairment of antibody Fc receptor function. By contrast, higher levels of total maternal IgG reduce transfer of antigen-specific IgG by competitively binding to placental Fc receptors.

IgG transfer across the placenta appears to vary by subtype. For example, IgG1, which is induced by protein antigens such as tetanus toxoid, is more efficiently transferred than IgG2, which is induced by polysaccharide antigens such as those in encapsulated bacteria. IgG1 and IgG3 transfer ratios rose with increasing gestational age, with IgG1 showing a peak transfer ratio at 37 weeks of pregnancy. IgG2 transfer ratios are always lower than the other IgG subclasses **(Fig. 2)**.

TABLE 1: Immunizations that may be administered before, during, and after pregnancy.

Vaccine	Before pregnancy	During pregnancy	After pregnancy	Type of vaccine
Hepatitis A	Yes, if indicated	Yes, if indicated	Yes, if indicated	Inactivated
Hepatitis B	Yes, if indicated	Yes, if indicated*	Yes, if indicated	Inactivated
Human papillomavirus (HPV)	Yes, if indicated	No, delay until after pregnancy, if indicated	Yes, if indicated	Inactivated
Influenza IIV	Yes	Yes	Yes	Inactivated
Influenza LAIV¶	Yes, if less than 50 years of age and healthy; avoid conception for 4 weeks	No	Yes, if less than 50 years of age and healthy; avoid conception for 4 weeks	Live
MMR	Yes, if indicated, avoid conception for 4 weeks	No	Yes, if indicated, give immediately postpartum if susceptible to rubella	Live
Meningococcal:				
1. Quadrivalent conjugate (MenACWY)	If indicated	If indicated	If indicated	Inactivated
2. Serogroup B (MenB)	If indicated	No, delay until after pregnancy, if indicatedᐃ	If indicated	Inactivated
Pneumococcal (Polysaccharide)	If indicated	If indicated	If indicated	Inactivated
Tdap	Yes, if indicated	Yes, vaccinate during each pregnancy ideally between 27 and 36 weeks of gestation	Yes, immediately postpartum, if not received previously	Toxoid/inactivated
Tetanus/diphtheria Td	Yes, if indicated	Yes, if indicated, Tdap preferred	Yes, if indicated	Toxoid
Varicella	Yes, if indicated, avoid conception for 4 weeks	No	Yes, if indicated, give immediately postpartum if susceptible	Live

*Conventional recombinant hepatitis B vaccines should be used during pregnancy. Administration of the adjuvanted recombinant hepatitis B vaccine is not recommended during pregnancy because of lack of safety data.
¶Confirm that LAIV is a recommended option for influenza vaccination each season.
ᐃDelay MenB until after pregnancy unless at increased risk and vaccination benefit outweighs uncertain risks.
(LAIV: live attenuated influenza vaccine; MMR: measles, mumps, and rubella vaccine)

BOX 1: Vaccines available for maternal administration under "specific situations" and "futuristic vaccines".

Vaccines available for maternal administration under specific situations:
- Hepatitis A & B
- Meningococcal disease
- Cholera
- Japanese encephalitis
- Yellow fever
- Tick-borne encephalitis

Maternal vaccines in development:
- RSV
- Group B Streptococcus (GBS)
- CMV
- Hepatitis E
- HSV

(CMV: cytomegalovirus; HSV: herpes simplex virus; RSV: respiratory syncytial virus)

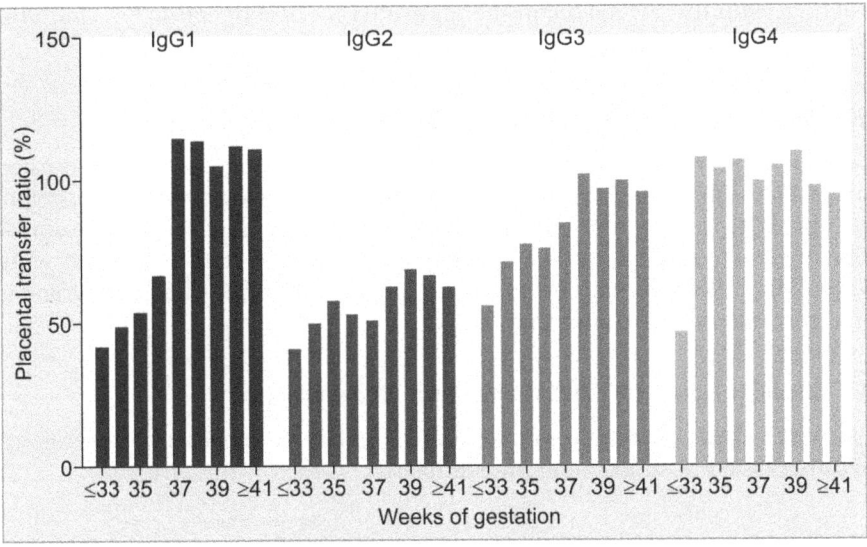

Fig. 2: Percentage of placental transfer ratios of IgG subclasses delivered to preterm and term newborns in different gestational weeks.

5. Which vaccines are contraindicated in pregnancy?

Live vaccines have the potential to infect the fetus so are contraindicated in pregnancy except yellow fever vaccine which can be given if risk of yellow fever exposure is high.

6. What is the ideal timing of maternal vaccination when passive neonatal immunity is the goal?

Vaccination between 28 and 32 weeks optimizes placental transfer of maternal antibodies.

7. If for some reason Tdap is given in early pregnancy, then should we repeat the dose later?

No, if given once in pregnancy, dose should not be repeated again.

8. Which infections are associated with greater morbidity in pregnancy state and adverse pregnancy outcomes?

Measles, mumps, rubella and varicella are vaccine preventable diseases, which are associated with severe infection in pregnancy with adverse fetal outcomes.

9. For how long pregnancy should be avoided after taking a live vaccine?

The ACIP recommends avoiding pregnancy for 28 days following each dose of a live vaccine (for varicella vaccination, the manufacturer recommends waiting 3 months; FOGSI recommends avoidance of conception for 3 months post-rubella vaccination).

10. What is the current status of HPV vaccination during pregnancy?

Human papillomavirus (HPV) vaccination is not recommended during pregnancy due to limited data on vaccine safety. However, women who inadvertently receive the HPV vaccine during pregnancy can be reassured that there is no evidence of adverse pregnancy or fetal outcomes with vaccination. Women who have not completed the series due to pregnancy may resume the series after they deliver.

11. Should one check for rubella immunity in each pregnancy?

No, once rubella immunity is documented (IgG titers) repeat rubella serology is unnecessary in subsequent pregnancies.

12. Should we repeat Tdap/Td vaccine in each pregnancy?

Yes, Tdap/Td is indicated in each pregnancy, even if the woman has a previous history of pertussis or vaccination, and even if consecutive pregnancies occur within 12 months.

13. What is the status of Td vaccine use in public sector? Is there any role of TT vaccination during pregnancy?

Government of India has recently recommended substitution of TT vaccine with Td. As of June 2018, 133 out of 194 member states have already replaced TT with Td vaccine in their routine immunization program, 61 countries are still using TT. 8 out of the 14 remaining high-risk countries for maternal and neonatal tetanus are still using TT for campaign activities **(Fig. 3)**. However, as of 2019, all campaigns will be conducted with Td vaccine.

The UNICEF and WHO have a joint target to complete replacement of TT with Td vaccine in routine immunization programs and in SIAs by January 2020. As of January 2019, UNICEF will no longer fund the supply of TT vaccine, and will only support access to Td vaccine for use in immunization programs. Further as of January 2020, all countries supplied through UNICEF, can only access Td vaccine through UNICEF procurement services. For countries, self-procuring TT vaccine, we do expect that TT vaccine will remain available on the global market. However, as a result of decreased demand through UNICEF and market evolution toward production of Td vaccine, the cost may increase, as well as the lead times required to fill orders.

14. Which is the preferred schedule for no, incomplete or unknown immunization status against tetanus and diphtheria in pregnancy?

Pregnant women who have never received three doses of a vaccine containing tetanus and diphtheria toxoids (Td) should undertake or complete the series of three vaccinations. The preferred schedule in pregnant women is at time 0, 4 weeks later, and at 6–12 months after the initial dose.

15. What is the recommendation for flu vaccine in pregnant women?

All women who are pregnant or might be pregnant during the influenza season should receive the inactivated influenza vaccine as soon as it becomes available and before onset of influenza activity in the community, regardless of their stage of pregnancy.

16. Is there any data on the effectiveness of flu vaccines during pregnancy?

There are many studies from developed countries such as Norway, Switzerland, UK, and USA that have documented effectiveness of flu vaccines during pregnancy. Few studies from developing countries have also documented benefit of flu vaccine to mothers. Four randomized controlled trials conducted in Mali, South Africa, Nepal and Bangladesh evaluated the efficacy of maternal administration of Trivalent Influenza Vaccine (TIV) against laboratory-confirmed maternal and infant infection. Efficacy rates ranged from 30% in Nepal to 63% in Bangladesh. The Nepalese trial, specifically powered to detect low birth weight as a primary outcome, showed a 15% reduction in low birth weight among newborns whose mothers had been immunized with influenza, as compared to babies born to unimmunized mothers.

17. Can we give pneumococcal vaccine in pregnancy when clinically indicated?

Pneumococcal polysaccharide vaccine can be given safely in 2nd/3rd trimester but ACIP has not published pregnancy recommendations for the pneumococcal conjugate vaccine (PCV13).

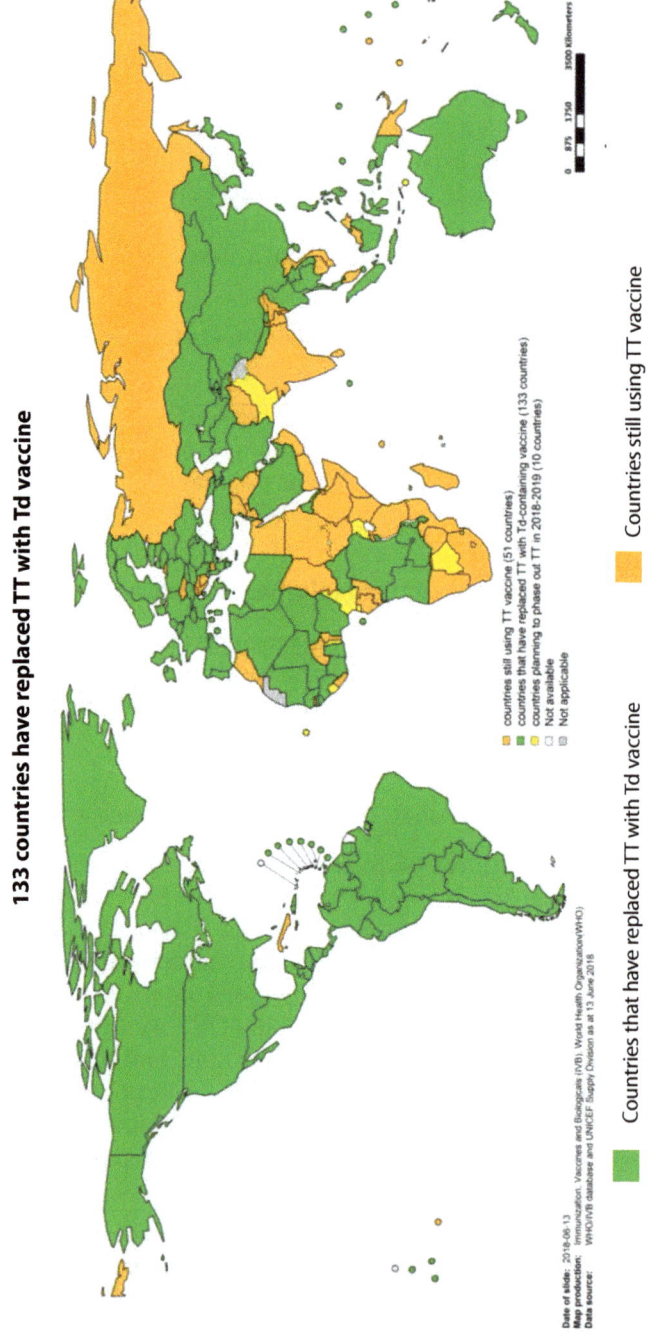

Fig. 3: Current status of global usage of TT and Td vaccines.

18. What are the indications for hepatitis B during pregnancy?

Hepatitis B vaccination during pregnancy is indicated in:
- Pregnant women who are completing an immunization series begun prior to conception.
- Unvaccinated, uninfected pregnant women (hepatitis B surface antigen negative) who are at high risk for acquiring hepatitis B virus (HBV).

19. For postexposure prophylaxis which vaccine can be given without a concern during pregnancy?

If indicated, the hepatitis A and B, tetanus, and rabies vaccines can all be given to pregnant women as part of postexposure prophylaxis management.

20. Which immunizations should be avoided during pregnancy?

Human papillomavirus, MMR, varicella, MMRV, BCG and live attenuated influenza vaccine (LAIV) should be avoided during pregnancy.

Certain travel vaccines: yellow fever, typhoid fever, and Japanese encephalitis, should generally not be given during pregnancy, unless healthcare provider determines that the benefits outweigh the risks.

21. Which vaccines contraindicated during pregnancy can be given before discharge if not given earlier?

The MMR and varicella are the two vaccines that are contraindicated during pregnancy and should be given to mother before discharge to protect a nonimmune mother and newborn.

22. Which vaccines should be given to nonimmunized postnatal mothers?

Rubella, hepatitis B, varicella, influenza, tetanus (Td/Tdap) and HPV vaccinations should be given to all nonimmunized postnatal mothers.

23. What is the recommendation for the management of dog bite during pregnancy?

There is no evidence that rabies vaccination is associated with fetal abnormalities or adverse pregnancy outcomes of any kind. Pregnancy is therefore not a contraindication to post-exposure prophylaxis if a rabies exposure has occurred. The danger of rabies after a significant exposure far outweighs any theoretical risk from administration. For patients in a continuous or frequent risk category, pre-exposure prophylaxis might also be necessary during pregnancy.

24. In what circumstances is it appropriate to administer Tdap vaccine outside 27–36 week of gestation window?

There are certain circumstances in which it is appropriate to administer the Tdap vaccine outside of the 27–36-weeks-of-gestation window. For example, in cases of wound management, a pertussis outbreak, or other extenuating circumstances, the need for protection from infection supersedes the benefit of administering the vaccine during the 27–36-weeks-of-gestation window.

25. What is the best time to administer Tdap vaccine?

Immunization of pregnant women with Tdap between 27 and 30 weeks is associated with highest umbilical cord GMCs of IgG to PT and FHA compared with immunization beyond 31 weeks **(Fig. 4)**. However, there are some reports that favor Tdap even during 2nd trimester. Early 2nd-trimester maternal Tdap immunization significantly increased neonatal antibodies. Recommending immunization from the second trimester onward would widen the immunization opportunity window and could improve seroprotection (Eberhardt CS et al., 2016).

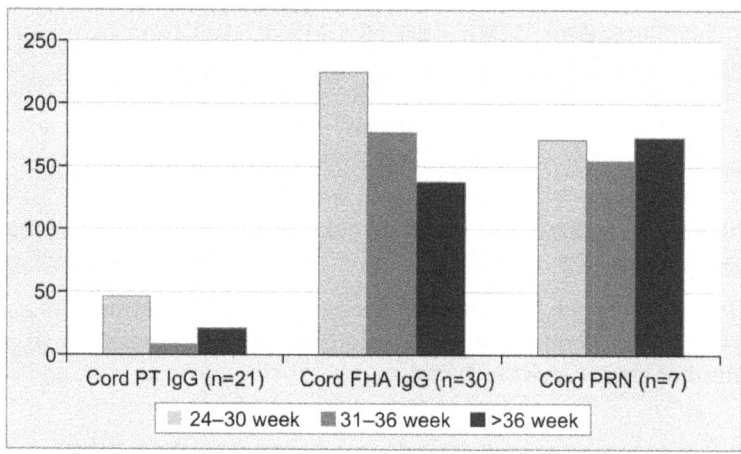

Fig. 4: Timing of maternal Tdap and cord antibodies levels.

26. Are there any effectiveness data available for use of maternal Tdap?

In one study, there was 90–93% effectiveness against pertussis infection in infants under the age of 2 months (Gkentzi D et al., 2017). In Argentina, there was a 51% relative reduction of pertussis cases in young infants whose mothers immunized against pertussis in pregnancy and who lived in states with high Tdap coverage (>50%) compared to young infants who lived in states with low coverage (<50%) of maternal pertussis immunization during pregnancy (Vizzotti C et al., 2016). There are many other recent studies that have documented effectiveness of maternal Tdap against infantile pertussis (Winter K et al., 2017; Becker-Dreps S et al., 2018).

27. What is cocooning?

Cocooning is the administration of Tdap to previously unvaccinated family members and caregivers, and women in the immediate postpartum period, in order to provide a protective cocoon of immunity around the newborn.

28. Are vaccines safe if mother is breastfeeding?

Yes. It is safe to receive routine vaccines right after giving birth, even while breastfeeding. However, yellow fever vaccine is not recommended for breastfeeding women unless travel to certain countries is unavoidable and a healthcare provider determines that the benefits of vaccination outweigh the risks.

SUGGESTED READING

1. Becker-Dreps S, Butler AM, McGrath LJ, Boggess KA, Weber DJ, Li D, et al. Effectiveness of prenatal tetanus, diphtheria, acellular pertussis vaccination in the prevention of infant pertussis in the US. Am J Prev Med. 2018;55(2):159-66.
2. Benowitz I, Esposito DB, Gracey KD, Shapiro ED, Vázquez M. Influenza vaccine given to pregnant women reduces hospitalization due to influenza in their infants. Clin Infect Dis. 2010;51:1355-61.
3. Blanchard-Rohner G, Meier S, Bel M, Combescure C, Véronique O, Samia S, et al. Influenza vaccination given at least 2 weeks before delivery to pregnant women facilitates transmission of seroprotective influenza-specific antibodies to the newborn. Pediatr Infect Dis J. 2013;32:1374-80.
4. Center for Disease Control and Prevention. Vaccines for Pregnant Women. [online] Available from: http://www.cdc.gov/vaccines/adults/rec-vac/pregnant.html. [Last Accessed August, 2020].
5. Dabrera G, Zhao H, Andrews N, Begum F, Green H, Ellis J, et al. Effectiveness of seasonal influenza vaccination during pregnancy in preventing influenza infection in infants, England, 2013/14. Euro Surveill. 2014;19:20959.
6. Eberhardt CS, Blanchard-Rohner G, Lemaître B, Boukrid M, Combescure C, Othenin-Girard V, et al. Maternal immunization earlier in pregnancy maximizes antibody transfer and expected infant seropositivity against pertussis. Clin Infect Dis. 2016;62(7):829-36.
7. Gkentzi D, Katsakiori P, Marangos M, Hsia Y, Amirthalingam G, Heath PT, et al. Maternal vaccination against pertussis: a systematic review of the recent literature. Arch Dis Child Fetal Neonatal Ed. 2017;102:F456-63.
8. Håberg SE, Trogstad L, Gunnes N, Wilcox AJ, Gjessing HK, Samuelsen SO, et al. Risk of fetal death after pandemic influenza virus infection or vaccination. N Engl J Med. 2013;368(4):333-40.
9. Kim DK, Hunter P, Advisory Committee on Immunization Practices. Recommended Adult Immunization Schedule, United States, 2019. Ann Intern Med. 2019;170:182-92.
10. Madhi SA, Cutland CL, Kuwanda L, Weinberg A, Hugo A, Jones S, et al. Influenza vaccination of pregnant women and protection of their infants. N Engl J Med. 2014;371:918-31.
11. Omer SB. Maternal immunization. N Engl J Med. 2017;376(13):1256-67.
12. Omer SB, Richards JL, Madhi SA, Tapia MD, Steinhoff MC, Aqil AR, et al. Three randomized trials of maternal influenza immunization in Mali, Nepal, and South Africa: methods and expectations. Vaccine. 2015;33:3801-12.
13. Poehling KA, Szilagyi PG, Staat MA, Snively BM, Payne DC, Bridges CB, et al. Impact of maternal immunization on influenza hospitalizations in infants. Am J Obstet Gynecol. 2011;204:S141-8.
14. Steinhoff M, Tielsch J, Katz J, Englund J, Kuypers J, Khatry S, et al. Evaluation of year-round maternal influenza immunization in tropical SE Asia: a placebo-controlled randomized trial. Open Forum Infect Dis. 2015;2(Suppl 1):1898.

15. Steinhoff MC, Omer SB, Roy E, El Arifeen S, Raqib R, Dodd C, et al. Neonatal outcomes after influenza immunization during pregnancy: a randomized controlled trial. CMAJ. 2012;184:645-53.
16. Tapia MD, Sow SO, Tamboura B, Téguété I, Pasetti MF, Kodio M, et al. Maternal immunisation with trivalent inactivated influenza vaccine for prevention of influenza in infants in Mali: a prospective, active-controlled, observer-blind, randomised phase 4 trial. Lancet Infect Dis. 2016;16:1026-35.
17. Vizzotti C, Juarez MV, Bergel E, Romanin V, Califano G, Sagradini S, et al. Impact of a maternal immunization program against pertussis in a developing country. Vaccine. 2016;34:6223-8.
18. Winter K, Nickell S, Powell M, Harriman K. Effectiveness of prenatal versus postpartum tetanus, diphtheria, and acellular pertussis vaccination in preventing infant pertussis. Clin Infect Dis. 2017;64(1):3-8.
19. Zaman K, Roy E, Arifeen SE, Rahman M, Raqib R, Wilson E, et al. Effectiveness of maternal influenza immunization in mothers and infants. N Engl J Med. 2008;359:1555-64.

CHAPTER 56

Vaccines for Healthcare Professionals

Rashna Dass Hazarika

1. Why vaccines for healthcare professionals (HCPs)?

Healthcare professionals are at the highest risk of acquiring as well as transmitting vaccine preventable diseases. Moreover, many HCPs in India are still not fully vaccinated against many of the potentially contagious diseases.

2. Do we have defined guidelines for vaccination of HCPs in India?

Though the World Health Organization (WHO), Centers for Disease Control and Prevention (CDC) and some country specific guidelines are available, they have not been fully implemented in India.

3. Which category of workers falls under HCPs?

Healthcare professionals include all paid and unpaid workers in a healthcare setup who are constantly exposed to infectious materials from patients and their aerosols or body fluids, machines and contaminated air. The best example currently is the COVID-19 risk to all HCPs.

4. What are the diseases likely to be acquired or spread by HCPs?

Based on studies in hospital settings, the most common diseases acquired or spread by HCPs are hepatitis B, influenza, measles, mumps, rubella, pertussis and varicella and now COVID 19 as well.

HEPATITIS B

5. What is the infectivity of hepatitis B?

A nonimmune individual is 100 times more likely to acquire hepatitis B virus (HBV) infection after a needle stick injury than an immune individual.

6. How long can the HBV remain stable and infective on environmental surfaces, and what determines the risk of infection?

The HBV remains stable on environmental surfaces for at least 7 days, and the risk is related to the degree of contact with the infected blood.

7. What is the schedule for HBV in those HCPs who are not immunized or in whom we are not sure about the immunization status?

These HCPs should receive a three-dose schedule at 0, 1, 6 months.

8. Do we have specific guidelines for HBV in HCPs for India?

Yes, the Government of India in June 2018 issued directives to immunize all healthcare workers with occupational exposures, and who have not received the primary series at birth.

9. For postexposure vaccination, when is the most appropriate time for testing to document immunity?

The HCPs should be tested for hepatitis B surface antibody (anti-HBS) 1–2 months after the completion of the vaccination.

10. What level of anti-HBS indicates immunity?

The vaccinee is considered to be immune if the anti-HBS level is at least 10 mIU/mL, and no further serologic testing or vaccination is recommended.

11. What should be done if anti-HBS is <10 mIU/mL?

If the anti-HBS is <10 mIU/mL, then the HCP should receive another series of HBV followed up by retesting of anti-HBS level at 1–2 months post-completion of the vaccine series.

12. When should a person be considered a nonresponder to the HBV?

A person is considered a nonresponder to the HBV if the anti-HBS titers remain < 10 mIU/mL even after two complete series of vaccination with the HBV.

13. How do we manage HCPs who are HBV nonresponders?

The HCPs who are HBV nonresponders, will need hepatitis B immunoglobulin (HBIG) for any known or probable exposure to hepatitis B infection. These persons also need to be counseled about the precautions to prevent HBV infection.

For details on postexposure management of HCP after occupational exposure to blood and body fluids, please see **Table 1**.

14. An intensivist has already received three doses of hepatitis-B vaccine, but he has never got serologic testing to know his post-vaccination status. Is it necessary to perform a post-vaccination serologic testing now?

Yes. Any HCP who is more likely to get in touch with blood or blood products or perform procedures must get his/her serologic testing done at least once. The further actions are based on their anti-HBS results.

TABLE 1: Postexposure management of healthcare personnel after occupational percutaneous and mucosal exposure to blood and body fluids, by healthcare personnel HepB vaccination and response status.

Healthcare personnel status	Postexposure testing		Postexposure prophylaxis		Postvaccination serologic testing[†]
	Source patient (HBSAg)	HCP testing (anti-HBS)	HBIG*	Vaccination	
Documented responder[§] after complete series	No action needed				
Documented nonresponder after 2 complete series	Positive/ unknown	Not indicated	HBIG × 2 separated by 1 month	—	No
	Negative	No action needed			
Response unknown after complete series	Positive/ unknown	<10 mIU/mL**	HBIG × 1	Initiate revaccination	Yes
	Negative	<10 mIU/mL	None		
	Any result	>10 mIU/mL	No action needed		
Unvaccinated/ incompletely vaccinated or vaccine refusers	Positive/ unknown	—**	HBIG × 1	Complete vaccination	Yes
	Negative	—	None	Complete vaccination	Yes

(HBsAg: hepatitis B surface antigen; anti-HBS: antibody to hepatitis B surface antigen; HBIG: hepatitis B immune globulin)

*HBIG should be administered intramuscularly as soon as possible after exposure when indicated. The effectiveness of HBIG when administered >7 days after percutaneous, mucosal, or nonintact skin exposures is unknown. HBIG dosage is 0.06 mL/kg.

[†]Should be performed 1–2 months after the last dose of the HepB vaccine series (and 6 months after administration of HBIG to avoid detection of passively administered anti-HBS) using a quantitative method that allows detection of the protective concentration of anti-HBS (>10 mIU/mL).

[§]A responder is defined as a person with anti-HBS >10 mIU/mL after 1 or more complete series of HepB vaccine.

A nonresponder is defined as a person with anti-HBS <10 mIU/mL after 2 complete series of HepB vaccine.

**HCP who have anti-HBs <10 mIU/mL, or who are unvaccinated or incompletely vaccinated, and sustain an exposure to a source patient who is HBsAg-positive or has unknown HBsAg status, should undergo baseline testing for HBV infection as soon as possible after exposure, and follow-up testing approximately 6 months later. Initial baseline tests consist of total anti-HBc; testing at approximately 6 months consists of HBsAg and total anti-HBc.

Source: Reproduced from Schillie S, Vellozzi C, Reingold A, Harris A, Haber PP, Ward JW, et al. Prevention of Hepatitis B Virus Infection in the United States: Recommendations of the Advisory Committee on Immunization Practices. MMWR. 2018;67(RR-1):18.

Flowchart 1 shows an algorithm depicting the procedure for conducting pre-exposure evaluation for healthcare personnel previously vaccinated with complete, greater than or equal to 3-dose hepatitis B vaccine series who have not had postvaccination serologic testing. Such testing should be performed

Flowchart 1: Pre-exposure evaluation for healthcare personnel previously vaccinated with complete, ≥3-dose Hep-B vaccine series who have not had postvaccination serologic testing.*

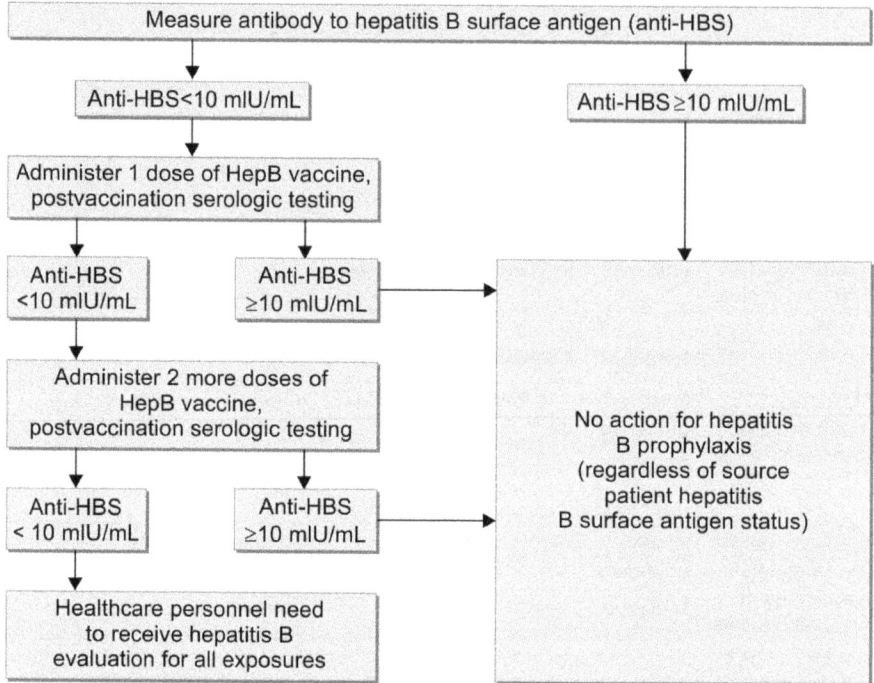

*Should be performed 1–2 months after the last dose of vaccine using a quantitative method that allows detection of the protective concentration of anti-HBS (≥10 mIU/mL) (e.g., enzyme-linked immunosorbent assay [ELISA]).

1–2 months after the last dose of vaccine using a quantitative method that allows detection of the protective concentration of anti-HBS [≥10 mIU/mL, e.g., enzyme-linked immunosorbent assay (ELISA)].

INFLUENZA

15. Why should we be concerned about influenza in HCPs?

Healthcare professionals are constantly exposed to patients with influenza in their workplace. They are not only at high risk of acquiring the disease but also of transmitting it to their coworkers and patients. One must also keep in mind that many HCPs who are above 60 years of age and with comorbid conditions such as diabetes mellitus, hypertension, cardiac illnesses, and COPD, are at increased risk of being infected by the flu virus compared to the others.

16. What are the advantages of vaccinating HCPs with the flu vaccine?

Prevent infection of self and also spread of the disease in the healthcare facilities and to the patients. Secondly giving flu vaccine to HCPs also helps in reducing the spread of infections to the vulnerable groups who cannot take the vaccine, i.e., those below 6 months of age, or are allergic to the vaccine or those who respond poorly to the vaccine (>85 years of age), or are immunocompromised.

17. What is the current recommendation for flu vaccine in HCPs?

Both the CDC and WHO recommend annual flu vaccine for all healthcare workers. Based on evidence from WHO, Indian Council of Medical Research (ICMR) and subject experts, the Government of India currently recommends vaccination of all high-risk groups with the flu vaccine. High-risk groups include HCPs, i.e., doctors, nurses, paramedics working in accident and emergency rooms, intensive care units, screening centers for detection of influenza patients during an outbreak, those involved in treatment and management of high-risk group patients in wards, laboratory personnel handling influenza containing samples, members of rapid response team who are involved in epidemiological investigations in outbreak situations, and also drivers and staff of vehicles involved in the transfer of influenza patients.

18. What are the recommended influenza vaccines currently?

Based on the WHO-based selection of strains for the southern hemisphere for 2018, ICMR currently recommends the quadrivalent vaccine for use in India containing the following strains:
- An A/Michigan/45/2015 (H1N1) pdm09-like virus
- An A/Singapore/INFIMH-16-0019 (H3N2)-like virus
- A B/Phuket/3073/2013-like virus (B/Yamagata/16/88 lineage)
- The quadrivalent influenza vaccine must contain the above three strains plus a B/Brisbane/60/2008-like virus (Victoria lineage).

The ICMR studies have shown that there is co-circulation of the Victoria and Yamagata lineages of influenza B and 50–80% of the type B samples are similar to the vaccine strain. The remaining 20–50% belong to the other lineage included in the quadrivalent vaccine.

Currently the CDC and WHO recommends that the flu vaccines in the northern hemisphere must contain the following:

A. Egg based vaccine containing:
- Influenza A/Guangdong-Maonan/SWL 1536/2019 (H1N1) pdm-09 like virus
- Influenza A/Hong Kong/2671//2019 (H3N2) like virus
- Influenza B/Washington/02/2019 (Victoria lineage) like virus
- Influenza B/Phuket/3073/2013 (Yamagata lineage) like virus

B. Cell or recombinant based vaccines containing:
- Influenza A/Hawaii/70/2019 H1N1 pdm09 like virus
- Influenza A/Hong Kong/45/2019 (H3N2) like virus
- Influenza B/Washington/02/2019 (B/Victoria lineage) like virus
- Influenza B/Phuket/3073/2013 (B/Yamagata lineage) like virus.

19. When should one use the flu vaccine in India?

The quadrivalent flu vaccine is to be taken at least 1 month prior to the influenza season.

MEASLES, MUMPS AND RUBELLA (MMR)

20. Are HCPs at more risk for measles?

Measles is a highly contagious disease with serious complications such as pneumonia and encephalitis. Most of these patients present to the emergency rooms putting the HCPs at increased risk of acquiring the disease than the normal population.

21. What are the current guidelines when an HCP gets exposed to a measles patient?

As per CDC, once contact occurs, then the person should be evaluated for measles antibodies if resources allow. However, if the immune status or vaccination status is not known or not sure, then the HCP is given the first dose of a measles containing vaccine (MR or MMR), excluded from work for 5–21 days and a second dose of the vaccine is repeated after 28 days. In those HCPs where a definite history of receiving a single dose of a measles containing vaccine is available, she/he should be given the second dose and allowed to continue to work. Data suggests that giving the measles containing vaccine within 72 hours of exposure will prevent or modify the disease.

22. What about the risk of mumps in HCPs?

The CDC does not consider HCPs to be at increased risk of mumps. HCP-related transmission of mumps continues to be reported as infrequent probably as 40% of the exposed remain asymptomatic. A single dose of the mumps vaccine induces an immunogenicity of around 80-85% and this increases to nearly 79-95% with the second dose. So in the West, all HCPs are assumed to be vaccinated and immune to mumps.

23. What about the status of immunity against mumps of HCPs in India?

Since mumps vaccine has never been a part of the universal immunization program (UIP) in India and also not included in the recent MR campaign, it is difficult to comment on the immune status of the community or the HCPs against mumps in India.

24. How do we manage HCPs who have been exposed to a mumps patient?

If the HCP has not been vaccinated with a mumps containing vaccine or the immune status is not known, then she/he should receive the first dose of the vaccine (which would be MMR in India), excluded from duty from day 12 of the first exposure through day 25 of the last exposure. If the HCP had ever received a dose of a mumps containing vaccine, then she/he should be given a repeat dose of MMR and allowed to continue to work.

25. Will the MMR vaccine harm the HCP if she/he is already incubating the mumps virus?

No, the MMR vaccine will not result in any exacerbation of the symptoms.

26. Are HCPs in India immune to rubella?

Since the rubella vaccine has never been a part of the UIP, and was only added recently as a part of the MR campaign in 2018, it is assumed that most of the population is not immune to rubella.

27. What is the role for rubella vaccination in HCPs in India?

All HCPs must get a dose of the rubella or the MMR vaccine prior to or immediately after employment. Being highly immunogenic, a single dose of the vaccine can give protective antibodies of > 99%. There is no role of postexposure rubella vaccination.

DIPHTHERIA, PERTUSSIS AND TETANUS

28. Should HCPs receive protection against DPT?

All HCPs are at increased risk of acquiring pertussis and diphtheria from the patients, as well as transmitting them to other patients. The WHO recommends that all HCPs should receive a dose of Tdap as a priority, and should continue to receive protection against diphtheria every 10 years. So, the first vaccine to be given is Tdap followed by Td every 10 years.

29. What should be the schedule followed in HCPs exposed to a diphtheria case?

Following exposure, the HCP must receive a dose of Tdap (if not received before) followed by Td every 10 years. If the HCP has already received Tdap in the past, the booster or postexposure vaccination is to be done with Td. The same schedule is also recommended for protection against tetanus.

VARICELLA

30. Is varicella of concern in HCPs?

Varicella is highly contagious with very high secondary attack rates, which can reach up to 90% in susceptible contacts. Adults who have not received the two-dose series of the varicella vaccine remain highly susceptible to get varicella infection, and that too a severe form of the disease. In addition to this, nosocomial varicella is known to occur because of spread from HCPs. A single HCP can infect >30 patients and >30 employees from a single exposure.

31. What is the recommendation for varicella vaccine in HCPs?

The WHO and CDC both recommend that all potentially susceptible HCPs (i.e., those who were unvaccinated or with no history of natural varicella infection), should receive two doses of the varicella vaccine 4–8 weeks apart.

MENINGOCOCCAL VACCINE

32. Is the meningococcal vaccine recommended for all HCPs?

The meningococcal vaccine is recommended in those HCPs who fulfill the following criteria:
- If they have asplenia or persistent complement deficiency
- If they are HIV positive
- If they travel to a country where the meningococcal disease is hyperendemic, or to a place where there is an epidemic
- Clinical microbiologists and researchers who are routinely exposed to samples which may harbor Meningococcus.

33. What are the most prevalent serotypes of *Neisseria meningitidis*?

The most prevalent serotypes worldwide are A, C, W, Y. Serotype B and C are prevalent in the USA, New Zealand, Australia and some parts of Europe. In India, the most prevalent serotype is A and C, with occasional reports of B.

34. What are the recommendations for the meningococcal vaccine?

All HCPs who fall in the high-risk category as described in Q32 should get 2 doses of the conjugate quadrivalent ACWY Meningococcus vaccine 8 weeks apart, with a repeat dose every 5 years.

TYPHOID

35. Do HCPs need to be vaccinated with the typhoid vaccine?

The CDC and WHO recommend that microbiologists and other HCPs who work closely with *Salmonella typhi* and professional food handlers should be vaccinated against the disease.

36. Which typhoid vaccine should be used?

The WHO has currently approved a single dose of the Vi polysaccharide conjugate vaccine in all countries endemic for typhoid.

POLIO

37. Should HCPs receive the polio vaccine?

As per WHO, all HCPs should have completed a full course of the primary vaccination against polio. It is expected that all HCPs in India are fully vaccinated against polio due to its inclusion in the UIP.

38. What should be done in those HCPs who may not have received the polio vaccine at all or is not sure of the status of polio vaccination?

Vaccination of adults is not recommended in India. The CDC recommends a three-dose series of inactivated polio vaccine (IPV) at 0, 4, 8 weeks followed by a booster at 6–12 months.

CATCH-UP/TRAVEL VACCINES FOR HEALTHCARE PROFESSIONALS

39. Is the Japanese encephalitis (JE) vaccine indicated in all HCPs?

Currently, only HCPs at high risk in JE endemic areas or those involved in vector control, or are traveling to a JE endemic area to be vaccinated against the JE virus.

40. Which JE vaccine is to be recommended in HCPs?

The inactivated Vero cell derived vaccine (SA-14-14-2 strain) currently available in India with the brand name of JEEV-™, is to be used in a two dose schedule 4 weeks apart at a dose of 0.5 mL containing 6 µg of the antigen. As per the latest CDC recommendations (MMWR Recomm Rep. 2019), subjects in the age group of 18–65 years, can receive two doses of 0.5 mL of IXIARO™ vaccine (or JEEV™ in India) at the interval of 7 days also. For all age groups, the 2-dose series should be completed at least 1 week before potential exposure to JE virus.

A second inactivated Vero cell culture derived Kolar strain vaccine is also available for use in children in India. Studies recommending its efficacy and dosing in adults is awaited.

41. Is there a need for a booster dose of the JE vaccine?

Those HCPs who have received their primary immunization more than a year back, may be given a booster dose if there is an ongoing epidemic or a re-exposure risk to JE.

RABIES

42. Do HCPs need to be immunized against rabies?

Those HCPs who provide care to the rabies patients are the highest risk and should receive a pre-exposure prophylaxis with the antirabies vaccine with 2 doses intramuscular (IM) or intradermal (ID) at two sites on day 0 and day 7.

43. What should be done in those HCPs who are at continual or frequent risk of exposure to rabies?

In these HCPs, a regular serological assessment for vaccine-induced neutralizing antibodies (VNA) and if the VNA is <0.5 IU/mL, a one site ID or IM booster is to be administered. If it is not possible to get a VNA done, then a one-site ID or IM booster is to be given after proper risk assessment.

44. Do HCPs require to be vaccinated against yellow fever?

Healthcare professionals are not at increased risk of yellow fever infection and hence only travelers to yellow fever endemic zones are recommended to take a single dose of the vaccine.

45. How can we improve vaccine uptake of HCPs?

Since many HCPs including doctors still do not take most of the recommended vaccines, a regular teaching of the need for these vaccines in HCPs, and a national level policy from the government for mandatory vaccination of HCPs is the need of the hour.

SUGGESTED READING

1. ACIP, CDC. Immunization of Health-Care Personnel, Recommendations of the Advisory Committee on Immunization Practices (ACIP). MMWR. 2011;60(7): 1-45.
2. Grohskopf LA, Alyanak E, Broder KR, Blanton LH, Fry AM, Jernigan DB, Atmar RL. Prevention and control of seasonal influenza with vaccines: recommendations of the Advisory Committee on Immunization Practices- United States 2020-21 influenza season. MMWR. 2020;69(8):1-24.
3. Haiduven-Griffiths D, Fecko H. Varicella in hospital personnel: a challenge for the infection control practitioner. Am J Infect Control. 1987;15:207-11.
4. Health Ministry to immunize healthcare workers with Hepatitis- B vaccine. New Delhi: Press Information Bureau, Government of India, Ministry of Health and Family Welfare; 2018.
5. Healthcare Professional Vaccination Recommendations. Immunization Action Coalition, Saint Paul, Minnesota. 2017.
6. Hills SL, Walter EB, Atmar RL, Fischer M. Japanese encephalitis vaccine: Recommendations of the Advisory Committee on Immunization Practices. MMWR Recomm Rep. 2019;68(2):1-33.
7. Seasonal influenza: Guidelines for vaccination with influenza vaccine. New Delhi: Ministry of Health & Family Welfare, Directorate General of Health Services (National Centre for Disease Control, Government of India); 2017.
8. Seasonal influenza: Guidelines for vaccination with influenza vaccine. New Delhi: Ministry of Health & Family Welfare, Directorate General of Health Services (National Centre for Disease Control, Government of India); 2018.
9. WHO. Summary of WHO position papers: Immunization of healthcare workers. Geneva: WHO; 2018.
10. World Health Organization. Vaccines and vaccination against yellow fever: WHO position paper. Wkly Epidemiol Rec. 2013;88;265-84.
11. World Health Organization. Japanese encephalitis vaccines: WHO position paper. Wkly Epidemiol Rec. 2015;90:69-88.
12. World Health Organization. Diphtheria vaccine: WHO position paper. Wkly Epidemiol Rec. 2017;92:417-436.
13. World Health Organization. Typhoid vaccines: WHO position paper. Wkly Epidemiol Rec. 2018;93:153-72.
14. World Health Organization. Rabies vaccines: WHO position paper. Wkly Epidemiol Rec. 2018;93:201-20.

ANNEXURES

Annexure 1: National Immunization Schedule 2020

Annexure 2: Indian Academy of Pediatrics—Advisory Committee on Vaccines and Immunization Practices Recommended Immunization Schedule 2019

ANNEXURE 1

National Immunization Schedule 2020

NATIONAL IMMUNIZATION SCHEDULE

Age	Vaccines given
Birth	Bacillus Calmette-Guérin (BCG), oral polio vaccine (OPV)-0 dose, and hepatitis B birth dose
6 weeks	OPV-1, pentavalent-1, rotavirus vaccine (RVV)-1***, fractional dose of inactivated polio vaccine (fIPV)-1, and pneumococcal conjugate vaccine (PCV)-1***
10 weeks	OPV-2, pentavalent-2, and RVV-2***
14 weeks	OPV-3, pentavalent-3, fIPV-2, RVV-3***, and PCV-2***
9–12 months	Measles and rubella (MR)-1, Japanese encephalitis (JE)-1*, and PCV booster***
16–24 months	MR-2, JE-2*, diphtheria, pertussis, and tetanus (DPT) booster-1, and OPV booster
5–6 years	DPT booster-2
10 years	Tetanus toxoid (TT)/tetanus and adult diphtheria (Td)
16 years	TT/Td
Pregnant mother	TT/Td-1, -2 or TT/Td booster**

*JE in 231 endemic districts.
**One dose if previously vaccinated within 3 years.
***Rotavirus vaccine and PCV in selected states/districts as per details below:

- *Rotavirus*: Andhra Pradesh, Assam, Haryana, Himachal Pradesh, Jharkhand, Madhya Pradesh, Odisha, Rajasthan, Tamil Nadu, Tripura, and Uttar Pradesh.
- *Pneumococcal conjugate vaccine*: Bihar, Himachal Pradesh, Madhya Pradesh, Uttar Pradesh (12 districts), and Rajasthan (9 districts).

NATIONAL IMMUNIZATION SCHEDULE FOR INFANTS, CHILDREN, AND PREGNANT WOMEN (VACCINE-WISE)

Vaccine	When to give	Dose	Route	Site
For pregnant women				
Tetanus toxoid (TT)/tetanus and adult diphtheria (Td)-1	Early in pregnancy	0.5 mL	Intramuscular	Upper arm
TT/Td-2	4 weeks after TT-1	0.5 mL	Intramuscular	Upper arm

Contd...

Contd...

Vaccine	When to give	Dose	Route	Site
TT/Td booster	If received two TT doses in a pregnancy within the last 3 years*	0.5 mL	Intramuscular	Upper arm
For infants				
Bacillus Calmette-Guérin (BCG)	At birth or as early as possible till 1 year of age	0.1 mL (0.05 mL until 1 month of age)	Intradermal (ID)	Left upper arm
Hepatitis B— birth dose	At birth or as early as possible within 24 hours	0.5 mL	Intramuscular	Anterolateral side of mid-thigh
Oral polio vaccine (OPV)-0	At birth or as early as possible within the first 15 days	Two drops	Oral	Oral
OPV-1, -2, and -3	At 6 weeks, 10 weeks, and 14 weeks (OPV can be given till 5 years of age)	Two drops	Oral	Oral
Pentavalent 1, 2, and 3	At 6 weeks, 10 weeks, and 14 weeks (can be given till 1 year of age)	0.5 mL	Intramuscular	Anterolateral side of mid-thigh
Pneumococcal conjugate vaccine (PCV)^	Two primary doses at 6 and 14 weeks followed by booster dose at 9–12 months	0.5 mL	Intramuscular	Anterolateral side of mid-thigh
Rotavirus vaccine (RVV)^	At 6 weeks, 10 weeks, and 14 weeks (can be given till 1 year of age)	3 mL	Oral	Oral
Inactivated polio vaccine (IPV)	Two fractional doses at 6 and 14 weeks of age	0.1 mL ID	ID two fractional doses	ID: Right upper arm
Measles and rubella (MR)^ first dose	9 completed months to 12 months (measles can be given till 5 years of age)	0.5 mL	Subcutaneous	Right upper arm
Japanese encephalitis (JE)-1**	9 completed months to 12 months	0.5 mL	Subcutaneous	Left upper arm
Vitamin A (first dose)	At 9 completed months with measles and rubella	1 mL (1 lac IU)	Oral	Oral

Contd...

Contd...

Vaccine	When to give	Dose	Route	Site
For children				
Diphtheria, pertussis, and tetanus (DPT) booster-1	16–24 months	0.5 mL	Intramuscular	Anterolateral side of mid-thigh
MR second dose	16–24 months	0.5 mL	Subcutaneous	Right upper arm
OPV booster	16–24 months	Two drops	Oral	Oral
JE-2	16–24 months	0.5 mL	Subcutaneous	Left upper arm
Vitamin A*** (second to ninth doses)	16–18 months. Then one dose every 6 months up to the age of 5 years	2 mL (2 lac IU)	Oral	Oral
DPT booster-2	5–6 years	0.5 mL	Intramuscular	Upper arm
TT/Td	10 years and 16 years	0.5 mL	Intramuscular	Upper arm

*One dose if previously vaccinated within 3 years.
**JE vaccine is introduced in selected endemic districts after the campaign.
***The second to ninth doses of vitamin A can be administered to children 1–5-year-old during biannual rounds, in collaboration with Integrated Child Development Scheme (ICDS).
^Rotavirus vaccine and PCV in selected states/districts as per details below:

- *Rotavirus*: Andhra Pradesh, Assam, Haryana, Himachal Pradesh, Jharkhand, Madhya Pradesh, Odisha, Rajasthan, Tamil Nadu, Tripura, and Uttar Pradesh.
- *Pneumococcal conjugate vaccine*: Bihar, Himachal Pradesh, Madhya Pradesh, Uttar Pradesh (12 districts), and Rajasthan (9 districts).

ANNEXURE 2

Indian Academy of Pediatrics—Advisory Committee on Vaccines and Immunization Practices Recommended Immunization Schedule 2019

INDIAN ACADEMY OF PEDIATRICS IMMUNIZATION SCHEDULE 2018–2019 (TABULAR FORM)

The Indian Academy of Pediatrics (IAP) recommended vaccines for routine use are as follows:

Age (completed weeks/months/years)	Vaccines	Comments
Birth	BCG OPV-0 Hepatitis B1	• Administer these vaccines to all newborns within 7 days. Hepatitis B vaccine preferably within 24 hours
6 weeks	DTwP-1/ DTaP-1 IPV-1* Hepatitis B2 Hib-1 Rota-1 PCV-1	*DTP:* • Both DTwP and DTaP or their combinations can be used in primary series • Immunogenicity and longevity of immune response is better with DTwP • DTaP/DTwP combination vaccines may be offered as an alternative in view of nonavailability of standalone IPV preparations in the private sector. DTaP combination vaccines may be offered in view of parental anxiety of increased reactogenicity with DTwP. *Polio:* • No child should leave the facility without polio immunization (IPV* or OPV). • Continue birth dose OPV and OPV on SIAs • Ideally IPV should replace OPV completely as early as possible • Three doses of IM IPV in primary series is the best option • Two doses of IM IPV instead of three doses for primary series if started at 8 weeks, with an interval of at least 8 weeks between two doses • In case IPV is not available or feasible, the child should be offered bOPV (three doses). In such cases, two fractional doses of IPV at a Government facility or at least one dose of an IM IPV either standalone or as a combination at least at 14 weeks of age.

Contd...

Contd...

Age (completed weeks/months/years)	Vaccines	Comments
		Rotavirus: • Two doses of RV-1 or three doses of RV-5 and RV-116E and BRV-PV • RV-1 can be given at 6 and 10 weeks. *Pneumococcal conjugate vaccines:* • *Minimum age:* 6 weeks • Both PCV-10 and PCV-13 are licensed for children from 6 weeks to 5 years of age (although the exact labeling details may differ by country) • Additionally, PCV-13 is licensed for the prevention of pneumococcal diseases in adults >50 years of age • *Primary schedule (for both PCV-10 and PCV-13):* Three primary doses at 6, 10, and 14 weeks with a booster at age 12 through 15 months.
10 weeks	DTwP-2/ DTaP-2 Hepatitis B3 IPV-2 Hib-2 Rotavirus-2 PCV-2	• Only two doses of RV-1 are recommended • If RV-1 is chosen, the second dose should be given at 10 weeks.
14 weeks	DTwP-3/ DTaP-3 Hepatitis B4** IPV-3 Hib-3 Rotavirus-3 PCV-3	• If any dose in series was RV-5 or RV-116E or BRV-PV, a total of three doses of RV vaccine should be administered • **Fourth dose of hepatitis B permissible for combination vaccines only.
6 months	Influenza vaccine (flu vaccine)	*Influenza vaccine:* • Inactivated influenza vaccine (IIV) is recommended for routine immunization of children having 6 months to 59 months of age • Children 6 months to 59 months are grouped as "high risk" and should be offered routine influenza vaccine. • Beyond 5 years of age, only high-risk group as listed below • Both TIIV and QIIV are licensed in India • QIIV is preferred if available • *Minimum age:* 6 months for trivalent/quadrivalent IIV • *First time vaccination:* – 6 months to below 9 years: Two doses 1 month apart; 9 years and above: Single dose • Annual revaccination with single dose 2–4 weeks before flu season.

Contd...

Contd...

Age (completed weeks/months/years)	Vaccines	Comments
6 months onward	Typhoid conjugate vaccine (TCV)	Single dose of any of the licensed TCV can be administered Can be administered with MMR vaccine if started at 9 months Sufficient data on safety and immunogenicity available for 25 µg TCV
9 months	MMR-1/MR	Currently available data is insufficient for making any recommendation for 5 µg TCV. *MMR/MR*: • Standalone measles will no more be available • Measles-containing vaccine (MMR/MR) ideally should not be administered after completing 9 months of age • The second dose must follow in second year of life • MR is not available in private sector as on date. If available, it should be offered instead of MMR • Additional dose during MR campaign for children 9 months to 15 years, irrespective of previous vaccination status.
12 months	Hepatitis A1 Japanese encephalitis (JE) vaccine (for endemic areas)	*Hepatitis A*: • Single dose for live-attenuated H2 strain hepatitis A vaccine • Two doses for all inactivated hepatitis A vaccines are recommended. *Japanese encephalitis vaccine*: • Any of the licensed JE vaccine can be administered • Two doses to be given 1 month apart • Live attenuated SA-14-14-2 is not available in private market.
15 months	MMR-2 Varicella-1 PCV booster	*MMR*: • The second dose must follow in second year of life • However, it can be given at any time 4–8 weeks after the first dose. *Varicella*: • The risk of breakthrough varicella is lower if given 15 months onward • MMRV as a combination is more reactogenic at 15–18 months.
16–18 months	DTwP-B1/ DTaP-B1 IPV-B1*** Hib-B1	• The first booster (fourth dose) may be administered as early as age 12 months, provided at least 6 months after the third dose • Both DTwP and DTaP as combination vaccine can be offered • No child should leave the facility without booster dose of IPV (standalone or combination) or bOPV vaccination.
18 months	Hepatitis A2	*Hepatitis A*: • Second dose for inactivated vaccines only

Contd...

Contd...

Age (completed weeks/months/years)	Vaccines	Comments
4–6 years	DTwP-B2/ DTaP-B2 MMRV or MMR-3 + Varicella-2	• Tdap is not recommended here *Varicella*: A total of two doses of varicella vaccine should be administered • The second dose of varicella vaccine should be given at 4–6 years of age or at 3 months after the first dose • MMRV can be used without increased risk of adverse reactions at this age • MMR third dose is recommended at 4–6 years of age.
9–12 years	Tdap/Td HPV	*Tdap*: Recommended age is 10 years • Tdap is preferred to Td followed by Td every 10 years • Minimum age for Tdap is 7 years. *HPV*: • Only two doses of either of the two HPV vaccines for girls aged 9–14 years • For girls 15 years and older and immunocompromised individuals three doses are recommended • For two-dose schedule, the minimum interval between doses should be 6 months • For three-dose schedule, the doses can be administered at 0, 1 or 2 (depending on brand), and 6 months

*In case IPV is not available or feasible, the child should be offered bOPV (three doses). In such cases, two fractional doses of IPV can be provided at a Government facility.

**Fourth dose of hepatitis B permissible for combination vaccines only.

***bOPV, if IPV booster (standalone or combination) is not feasible.

(BCG: Bacillus Calmette-Guérin; DTaP: diphtheria, tetanus, and acellular pertussis; DTwP: diphtheria, tetanus, and whole-cell pertussis; Hib: Haemophilus influenzae type b; HPV: human papillomavirus; IPV: inactivated polio vaccine; MMRV: measles, mumps, rubella, and varicella; OPV: oral polio vaccine; PCV: pneumococcal conjugate vaccine; Td: tetanus and adult diphtheria; Tdap: tetanus, diphtheria, and acellular pertussis)

INDIAN ACADEMY OF PEDIATRICS RECOMMENDED VACCINES UNDER SPECIAL CIRCUMSTANCES

- Influenza vaccine
- Meningococcal vaccine
- Japanese encephalitis vaccine
- Cholera vaccine
- Rabies vaccine
- Yellow fever vaccine
- 23-valent pneumococcal polysaccharide vaccine (PPSV-23).

Rabies Vaccine

- Four-dose schedule of anti-rabies vaccine is recommended for post-exposure prophylaxis

- Rabies monoclonal antibody is as effective as rabies immunoglobulin and is a cost-effective option.

Japanese Encephalitis Vaccine
- Only for individuals living in endemic areas
- For travelers to JE-endemic areas provided their expected stay is for a minimum period of 4 weeks
- Any of the licensed JE vaccine can be administered
- Live-attenuated SA-14-14-2 is not available in private market.

Meningococcal Vaccines
Any of the licensed vaccine can be administered.
- *9 months through 23 months*: Two doses at least 3 months apart
- *2 years through 55 years*: Single dose.

Cholera Vaccine
- *Minimum age*: 1 year (killed whole-cell *Vibrio cholerae*)
- Not recommended for routine use in healthy individuals; recommended only for the vaccination of persons residing in high-endemic areas and traveling to areas where risk of transmission is very high
- Two doses 2 weeks apart for >1-year-old child.

Yellow Fever Vaccine
Refer to topic on Travelers Vaccination.

High-risk category of children:
- Congenital or acquired immunodeficiency [including human immunodeficiency virus (HIV) infection]
- Chronic cardiac, pulmonary (including asthma if treated with prolonged high-dose oral corticosteroids), hematologic, renal (including nephrotic syndrome), liver disease, and diabetes mellitus
- Children on long-term steroids, salicylates, immunosuppressive, or radiation therapy
- Diabetes mellitus, cerebrospinal fluid leak, cochlear implant, and malignancies
- Children with functional/anatomic asplenia/hyposplenia
- During disease outbreaks
- Laboratory personnel and healthcare workers
- Travelers
- Children having pets in home
- Children perceived with higher threat of being bitten by dogs such as hostellers, risk of stray dog menace while going outdoor
- Influenza vaccination annually is recommended yearly for high-risk children from 5 years of age onward.

INDIAN ACADEMY OF PEDIATRICS—ADVISORY COMMITTEE ON VACCINES AND IMMUNIZATION PRACTICES IMMUNIZATION SCHEDULE

	Birth	6 weeks	10 weeks	14 weeks	6 months	9 months	12 months	13 months	15 months	16–18 months	2–3 years	4–6 years	9–14 years	15–18 years
BCG	BCG													
Hepatitis B	HB1	HB2	HB3	HB*2										
Polio	OPV-0	IPV**-1	IPV**-3	IPV**-3						IPV**-81				
DTwP/DTaP		DTP-1	DTP-3	DTP-1						DTP-81		DTP-82		
Hib		Hib-1	Hib-2	Hib-3						Hib-81				
Pneumococcal		PCV-1	PCV-2	PCV-3					PCV-81				PCV	
Rotavirus		Rota-1	Rota-2	Rota-3****										
MMR						MMR-1			MMR-2			MMR-2/MMR		
Varicella									Varicella-1			Varicella-2		
Hepatitis A							HepA1			HepA2*****				
Typhoid					TCV#									
Influenza							Influenza (yearly)							
Meningococcal						MCV-1	MCV-2				MCV			
JE							JE-1	JE-2						
Tdap													Tdap	Td
HPV##													HPV-1, and -2	HPV-1, -2, and -3
Cholera									Cholera 1 and 2					

	Range of recommended age for all children
	Range of recommended age for high-risk children/area
	Range of recommended age for catch-up immunization
	Not recommended

Contd...

Contd...

*Fourth dose of hepatitis B permissible for combination vaccines only
** In case IPV is not available or feasible, the child should be offered bOPV (3 doses). In such cases, give two fractional doses of IPV at 6 weeks and 14 weeks
***b-OPV, if IPV booster (standalone or combination) not feasible
****Third dose not required for RV1. Catch-up up to 1 year of age in UIP schedule
*****Live attenuated hepatitis A vaccine: single dose only
******Begin influenza vaccination after 6 months of age, about 2–4 weeks before season; give 2 doses at the interval of 4 weeks during first year and then single dose yearly till 5 years of age
#TCV = Typhoid conjugate vaccine, ## HPV = human papilloma virus
Meningococcal vaccine (MCV): 9 months through 23 months; 2 doses, at least 3 months apart; 2 years through 55 years; single dose only
Japanese encephalitis (JE): For individuals living an endemic areas and for travelers to JE endemic areas provided their expected stay is for a minimum period of 4 weeks
HPV: 2 doses at 6 months interval 9–14 years age; 3 doses (at 0, 1–2) and 6 months) 15 years or older and immunocompromised
Cholera vaccine: Two doses 2 weeks apart for > 1 year old; for individuals living in high endemic areas and travelling to areas where risk of transmission is very high
(BCG: Bacillus Calmette–Guérin; DTaP: diphtheria, tetanus, acellular pertussis vaccine; DTwP: diphtheria, tetanus, whole cell pertussis; Hib: Haemophilus influenzae type b; HPV: human papillomavirus; IPV: Inactivated poliovirus vaccine; MMR: measles-mumps-rubella; OPVO: oral poliovirus vaccine at birth; PCV: pneumococcal conjugate vaccine; Td: tetanus, reduced dose diphtheria toxoid; Tdap: tetanus, reduced dose diphtheria and acellular pertussis vaccine)

Source: Balasubramanian S, Shah A, Pemde HK, et al. Indian Academy of Pediatrics (IAP) Advisory Committee on Vaccines and Immunization Practices (ACVIP) Recommended immunization Schedule (2018-19) and Update on immunization for children aged 0 through 18 years. Indian Pediatr.2018;55(12):1066-74

Index

Page numbers followed by *b* refer to box, *f* refer to figure, *fc* refer to flowchart, and *t* refer to table.

A

Abscess 97
Acellular pertussis 43, 84, 246, 253
   vaccine 228, 230, 238*t*, 242
Acquired immunodeficiency 370
   syndrome 35, 191, 329, 364, 366, 476, 477
Activation-associated protein-1 664
Active bacterial core surveillance 373
Acute encephalitis syndrome 64, 67, 410, 411*f*
Acute flaccid
   myelitis 219
   paralysis 64-67, 69, 71, 218, 219
Adaptive immune system 23
Adaptive immunity 4*t*
Adenocarcinoma in situ 451
Adhesin-based vaccine 591
Adjuvant 656
   functions of 656
   limitations of 666
   vaccines, newer 656
Adolescent immunization 47, 677
Adolescent travellers, vaccines for 688*t*
Adolescent vaccination 677
Adult polio vaccination 212
Adverse drug reactions 95
Adverse effects following immunization 527
Adverse event following immunization 40, 93, 94*t*
   types of 94
Advisory Committee on Immunization Practices 316, 317, 421, 456, 476, 522, 686
Advisory Committee on Vaccines 78
   and Immunization Practices 45, 318, 376, 438, 477
Aedes aegypti 525, 620
Aerosol infection 390
Agammaglobulinemia 298
Alanine aminotransferase 600
Allergic disorders, vaccines against 635
Alleviate pain 48

Alpha-synuclein 650
Alzheimer's disease 643, 650
Ambiguous vaccine-derived poliovirus 203
American Academy of Pediatrics 329, 542
Amino acids 7
Anaphylaxis 453
Anesthesia, superficial 48
Angiotensin-converting enzyme 2 560
Animal exposure, management of 391*t*
Animal rabies
   signs of 402
   transmit 389
Antibody 607
   affinity 7
   containing products 55, 86, 326
   dose of 87*t*
   titers, correlation of 19*f*
   vaccine-induced neutralizing 719
Anti-cyclic citrullinated peptide 651
Antigen
   presenting cells 5, 631, 647, 649, 657
   specific cells 11
   specific immune effectors 11
   tumor
      associated 634, 648
      specific 634
   vaccine, liver-stage 513
Anti-inflammatory response 234
Anti-rabies
   vaccination 392
   vaccine 152, 393, 394, 399
   types of 394
Antiretroviral therapy 191
Anti-tetanus prophylaxis 392
Antitubercular therapy 181
Anti-Vaccination Society 169
Anxiety-related reaction 97
Apical membrane antigen-1 vaccines 513
Arthus reaction 240, 249
Aseptic meningitis 275*t*
Aspiration 50
Asplenia, functional 86

736 Index

Asthma 521
Atypical measles 259
Autoimmune diseases 650
Autopsy, conduction 99
Auxiliary nurse midwives 95
Avian influenza 464
Avidity 7
    index 351
AYUSH doctor 155

B

B cells 5
B lymphocyte 24
    primary 77
Bacillus calmette-guérin 12, 26, 43, 46, 59, 60, 82, 105, 111-113, 161, 162, 178, 183-186, 189, 190, 192, 194, 565, 687, 692, 724, 730
    adenitis, management of 182b
    immunization 193
    role of 563
    scar 180f
    status of 177
    strains 194
    vaccination 180, 181f, 193, 196, 564t
    vaccine 16, 41, 177, 178, 190-192, 194, 195, 197, 262, 549
        characteristics of 177
        effects of 184
Bacterial colonization 11
Bacterial meningitis 68
Basic reproductive number 31
Basic transmission cycle 406
Bat-infested caves 390
B-cell lymphoma 643
Bell's palsy 219
Bioterrorism 215
Bivalent oral poliovirus vaccine 43, 200
Bleeding disorders 90
Blindness 259
Blood
    stage vaccine 513
    test 296
B-mannosylceramide 662
Bone marrow plasma cells 471
Booster doses 20
Bordetella 236
    pertussis 224, 232, 236, 661
Bovine spongiform encephalopathy 134

C

Calicivirus 589, 590
    infections 589
Calmette-guérin and rubella 51

Campaign vaccination 429
Campylobacter jejuni 588-590
Cancer immune therapeutics 634
Candidate Shigella vaccines 593
Candidate vaccine, subunit 593
Capsular polysaccharide 483
Catch up immunization 91, 679, 683
    schedule 46t
Catch-up vaccination 266, 679
Cell culture rabies vaccines 394
Cell culture-derived
    influenza vaccines, advantages of 468
    vaccines 468
Cell-based flu vaccine production 468
Cell-mediated immunity 3, 319, 662
    role of 449
Cellular immune responses 657
Cellular immunity 657
Centers for Disease Control and Prevention 99, 318, 453, 590
Central Drugs Standard Control Organization 129
Cerebrospinal fluid 219
    leaks 487
Cervarix 452t
Cervical cancer 446, 448
    burden of 447
    cause of 446
Cervical intraepithelial neoplasia 2 448
Chickenpox 327
    vaccine 319, 684
Chikungunya virus 525, 617, 617f, 619, 619f, 620, 620f, 621, 622
    biology of 617
    development, vaccines for 624
    fever
        diagnosis of 621
        treatment for 622
    infection 620, 622, 624
    phylogenetic 618
        tree of 618f
    prevention of 623
    role of 623
    vaccine 617, 622, 624
        status of 624
Child and adolescent immunization schedule 79f
Childhood diarrhea 588b
Childhood vaccination schedule 269
Childhood vaccines 262, 399
Chimeric gene 639
Chimeric universal influenza vaccine 470
Chimeric vaccine 426, 639, 640
    development of 426f
Chimpanzee adenovirus 602

Chinese vaccines, efficacy of 420
Cholera 491, 492, 679, 692, 703
　　epidemic 492
　　protective immunity in 493
　　toxin 491, 493
　　vaccine 491, 494, 696, 730, 731
　　　　role of 496
Chronic diseases 89
Clostridium perfringens 588
Cochlear implants 89
Cocooning 708
Cold chain 104, 105
　　and vaccine storage 104
　　breach 115
　　components of 105
Cold spots 109
Cold-sensitive vaccines 110
Combination vaccines 519, 520, 520t
　　advantages of 520
Common mucosal immune system 664
Complex regional pain syndrome 453
Congenital rubella syndrome 64, 162, 268, 678
Conjugate vaccines 10
Consumed milk 399
Contact immunity 32, 34
Control pertussis resurgence 247t
Cord antibodies levels 240f
Coronavirus 173, 556, 632, 643
　　vaccine 563
COVID 19 25, 36, 189, 556, 557, 559, 560, 563, 564t, 566, 691, 711
　　epidemic 121
　　infection 37, 122
　　pandemic 167
　　vaccines 556
COVID laboratory results, interpretation of 558t
Crohn's disease 650
Cryptosporidium parvum 589
Culex
　　mosquitoes 407
　　tritaeniorhynchus 405
Current immunization schedule 159
Cytokines 3
Cytomegalovirus 574, 577, 578, 703
　　candidate vaccines 578b
　　infection 574, 575
　　prevention of 581
　　vaccination 575
　　　　targets for 576b
　　vaccine 574, 576, 578t, 579, 580
　　　　development 577
Cytosine phosphate guanine 578
Cytotoxic T lymphocyte cell 8, 578, 609

D

Danger signals 5
Deadly disease 533
Dendritic cell 5, 6f, 24f, 651, 657
Dengue 498, 499, 499f, 678
　　cases, distribution of 499f
　　disease, burden of 498
　　fever 640
　　vaccine 498, 501, 503, 505, 507, 683
　　　　development of 502
　　virus 498, 506, 525, 641
　　　　immunity against 501
Dengvaxia 504
　　vaccine 504b
　　　　contraindications of 504
Deoxyribonucleic acid 11, 25, 185-187, 281, 285, 287, 446, 468, 502, 561, 609, 629, 630, 630f, 631, 633, 635, 639
　　vaccine 513, 572, 605, 613, 629, 630
　　　　action of 631f
Dermonecrotic toxin 248
Diabetes mellitus
　　insulin-dependent 185
　　type 1 521, 651
Diarrhea 589
　　acute 588
Diarrheal disease 588, 589f
　　vaccines 588
Diarrheal episodes 589
Dimethyldioctadecylammonium 662
Diphtheria 35, 50, 54, 66, 69-71, 717
　　acellular pertussis, and tetanus vaccine 151
　　and tetanus 105, 111-113
　　　　toxoids 50, 59
　　pertussis tetanus 84
　　tetanus vaccine 59, 60
　　toxoid 12, 43, 253, 340
　　vaccine 34, 45
Diphtheria, pertussis 69
　　and tetanus 52, 69, 105, 111-113, 151, 153, 418, 519, 692, 717
　　　　vaccine 178, 442
　　measles, mumps 34
Diphtheria, tetanus acellular, and pertussis 112
Diphtheria, tetanus and pertussis 60, 110
　　vaccines 22, 224
Diphtheria, tetanus toxoids
　　and pertussis 112
　　vaccines 249
Diphtheria, tetanus, and acellular pertussis 43, 46, 359, 519, 730
　　vaccine 227, 248, 687

Diphtheria, tetanus, and pertussis 43, 227, 254, 267, 515
   vaccine, doses of 226f
Diphtheria, tetanus, and whole cell pertussis 43, 46, 519, 522, 687, 730
Disease estimation 29
Disease surveillance 62
District Immunization Officer 98
Dog bite 393
   management of 707
Dog transmit rabies 398
Domestic refrigerator, types of 108

E

Ebola 35, 532
   disease 533
      kinds of 532
      hemorrhagic fever 532
      vaccines 532
   virus 532, 534
      disease 532, 533
Echovirus 9 219
Encapsulated bacteria 11
Encephalitis 259, 268, 390
Endgame strategy 213
Engerix-b 289
Entamoeba 118
Enterotoxigenic escherichia coli 591
Enteroviral vaccines 582
Enterovirus 582
   vaccination for 582
Enterovirus A71
   infections, complications of 582
   vaccine, development of 584
Environmental mycobacteria 194
Environmental surveillance 74
Enzyme immunoassay 603
Enzyme-linked immunosorbent assay 533
   technique 377
Epitope suppression 342
Equine rabies immunoglobulin 392
Equipment cleaners, types of 285
Escherichia coli 432, 458, 494, 589, 591, 597, 661, 665
Ethics Committee, responsibilities of 132
European Medicines Agency 515
Expanded Program on Immunization 12, 339, 414

F

Facial paralysis 219
Families vaccine hesitant 169
Febrile seizures
   risk of 279, 384, 385, 515
   simple 68

Fever, low-grade 169
Fine-needle aspiration cytology 181
Flu 462
   causes of 462
   danger signs of 464
   vaccine 128, 465, 467b, 469, 478, 705, 716, 728
      egg-based 468
Fluorescent-antibody-to-membrane-antigen 313
Food and drug administration 453, 468, 559
Furious rabies 390

G

Gardasil 452t
General vaccination 1
Genetic Engineering Approval Committee 134
Genetic vaccines 629
Genital warts 451
Geometric mean titer 306, 317, 450
Germinal centers 6
Giardia lamblia 118, 589
Glatiramer acetate 650
Glaxosmithkline 305, 436
   tuberculosis vaccine 190
Glutamic acid dehydrogenase 651
Glycoconjugate vaccines 11
Glycoprotein B vaccine 579
Good clinical practice guidelines 132
Good manufacturing practice 417
Granulocyte-macrophage colony-stimulating factor 649
Guillain-Barré syndrome 249, 453, 466, 485, 590

H

H1N1 304
H3N2 475
Haemophilus B conjugate 358
Haemophilus influenzae 10, 63, 64, 67, 89, 110, 158, 204, 228, 298, 343, 357, 371, 692
Haemophilus influenzae type B 8, 12, 43, 46, 59, 60, 84, 112, 356, 359-361, 374, 519, 687, 730
   disease 356, 357
   glycoconjugates 12
   infection 357
   meningitis 361
   vaccination 360
   vaccine 356, 356f, 357, 357t, 358-361
Hand-foot-mouth disease 582, 583f
   signs of 582
   symptoms of 582
Hansenula polymorpha 458

Healthcare professionals, vaccines for 711
  travel 719
Heat sensitive 111
Heat shock proteins 661
Helicobacter pylori 659
Hemagglutinin 462
Hematopoietic stem cell transplant 85
Hemolytic uremic syndrome 591
Heparan sulfate proteoglycans 449
Hepatitis 59
  A2 729
  birth dose 162
  D 286
  vaccine 308
    inactivated 308
  virus 304
Hepatitis A 12, 43, 302, 309, 519, 679, 692, 702, 703
  infection 304, 307, 695
  prevention of 89
  vaccination 309
  vaccine 82, 84, 161, 295, 302, 305, 307, 308, 681, 695
    inactivated 308
    live 306
    live attenuated 305
    side effects of 307
  virus 302-304
    infection 308
    vaccines 305*t*
Hepatitis B 12, 15, 16, 22, 43, 68, 76, 105, 111-113, 152, 161, 165, 281, 285, 294, 498, 519, 679, 702, 703, 711, 724
  acute 284, 285
  birth dose 301
  carriers 309
  core 287
    antibody 287
    antigen 287
  during pregnancy 707
  E-antigen 282, 285-287
  immune globulin 713
  immunoglobulin 286, 299
    role of 298
  infectivity of 711
  laboratory nomenclature 287*t*
  panel results 286
  prevention of 89
  schedule for 294
  signs of 284
  surface 287, 299
    antibody 287, 713
    antigen 285, 287, 294, 297, 299, 713
  symptoms of 284
  testing 286, 287*t*, 294
  vaccination 179, 301
    adverse effects of 291
  vaccine 56, 84, 281, 286, 289, 290, 291, 295, 297, 298, 300, 308, 681, 712
    against 45
    dose of 292
    efficacy of 290
    monovalent 293
    single antigen 296
    types of 288
  virus 8, 97, 281-285, 285*t*, 287, 298, 299, 299*t*, 601, 659, 707
    core protein 584
    infection 282, 286, 296, 300, 308
    infection, chronic 284, 286
    infection, transmission of 282
    maternal 288
    prevalence of 281
    role of 298
Hepatitis C 599
  infection 599
  vaccine 599, 600
    development 601
  virus 97, 609, 657
    infection 600, 652
    infection, epidemiology of 599
Hepatitis E 703
  chronic 594
  infection, prevalence of 594
  vaccines 594
  virus 594
    combination vaccine of 597
    components of 595
    infection 594
Herd immunity 32, 35
Herd protection 33, 34
Herpes simplex virus 26, 188, 657, 703
Herpes zoster 318, 320
Heterologous immune 27
Hip dysplasia 54
Histocompatibility complex, major 5, 633, 643
Hodgkin disease 370
Human coronavirus 563
Human cytomegalovirus 578
Human enterovirus 582
Human immunodeficiency virus 35, 97, 190, 191, 201, 206, 262, 329, 366, 380, 441, 454, 477, 489, 553, 559, 568, 568*f*, 569, 601, 605, 643, 657
  biology of 568
  infection 291, 316, 361, 370, 504, 653
  vaccine 568, 569
    development of 570
Human interleukin, recombinant 578
Human leukocyte antigen 5, 607, 609

Human papillomavirus 14, 43, 84, 161, 446-450, 519, 576, 585, 652, 659, 678, 687, 692, 702, 704, 730
  diseases 454
  infection 448
  vaccination 455
    during pregnancy 704
    protection after 459
  vaccine 446, 450t, 453, 454, 456, 457-459, 507, 679
Human rabies immunoglobulin 392
Human-to-human transmission 406
Humoral immunity 657
Hyperimmunoglobulins 54
Hyperventilation 97
Hypocalcemic seizures 252
Hypoglycaemia, severe 185

I

Ibuprofen 22
Ice-lined refrigerator 111, 112
Ideal adjuvant, features of 657
Idiopathic thrombocytopenic purpura 326
Immune globulin 310
Immune memory 23
Immune response
  primary 18
  secondary 18
Immune system 4, 6, 23
  maturation of 350
Immunity
  active 120
  evidence of 319
  nonspecific 4
  specific 4
  types of 119
  vaccine-induced 233, 449
Immunization 60, 81
  adverse effect of 75
  after pregnancy 702t
  anxiety-related reaction 94
  before pregnancy 702t
  before travel 691
  maternal 237, 700
  practices 264
  primary 161, 254, 423
  program 105
  purpose of 39
  record 156
  regular 155
  schedule 39, 42, 162
Immunized child 161
Immunizing pregnant women 90
Immunocompromised children 298
Immunocompromised conditions, types of 77

Immunodeficiency, severe combined 441
Immunogenicity 291, 417
  data, long-term 351t
Immunoglobulin
  A 12, 18
  G 12, 18, 273, 316, 335, 558, 559
  M 18, 287, 482, 558, 559
Immunosuppressive agents, categories of 81
Inactivated vaccine, trivalent 377, 466
Inconsolable crying 250
Indian Academy of Pediatrics 153, 267, 306, 395, 471, 486, 727, 732
Indian Council of Medical Research 145, 566
Infant antibodies 700f
Infant pertussis
  immunization 242
  vaccination 243
Infection
  bite by rabid dog, risk of 403
  chronic 303
  control 120
Infection and prevention of disease, prevention of 550
Infectious disease 31, 35, 35t, 36t, 118, 119, 121, 122
  control and eradication of 118
  incidence of 121
Influence vaccine hesitancy 168
Influenza 12, 35, 462, 679, 714
  A 466, 715
    viruses 474, 475
  B 464, 474, 715
    victoria lineage 466
  complications of 463
  intranasal 12
  surveillance 464
  symptoms of 463
  vaccination 472, 479
  varicella and zoster infection 78
  virosomes 305
  virus 462, 463, 463f, 469
    types of 462
Influenza vaccine 128, 377, 462, 467, 471, 473, 476, 477, 680, 715, 728, 730
  coverage of 471
  inactivated 468, 472, 475, 477
  live attenuated 59, 466, 468, 702, 707
  production 468fc
  recombinant 476
  trivalent 705
  types of 466
Injectable polio 156
Innate and adaptive immunity 3, 4f
Innate cells 24
Innate immunity 4t, 183
Integrated Disease Surveillance Program 63, 100

Integrated vector management, role of 623
Interferon-gamma 8, 347, 635
Intravenous immunoglobulin 54, 327, 328
Invasive bacterial infections surveillance 356
Invasive cervical carcinoma 448
Invasive pneumococcal disease 363, 370, 373, 380
Ipsilateral inguinal lymphadenopathy 192
Isothermic cold boxes 114

J

Japanese B encephalitis 688
Japanese encephalitis 67, 68, 99, 158, 405, 408, 409, 410f, 411f, 498, 679, 692, 703, 724
   disease 405
   epidemiology of 408, 409
   risk of 408f, 430
   transmitted 405
   virus 405, 406, 639
      genotypes of 427
      transmission, rethinking 407f
Japanese encephalitis vaccine 158, 414, 414b, 415t, 420, 429, 430, 431b, 681, 696, 697, 697b, 719, 729-731
   cost-effective 430
   current status of 414
   dose of 165, 719
   inactivated 428b
   live attenuated 414
   new generation of 431
   recombinant 432
   types of 430b
   use of 428b
Jeryl-Lynn strain 275

K

Kidney diseases, chronic 89
Killed oral vaccine 591

L

Lapsed immunization 91
Latent tuberculosis infection 549
Leishmaniasis 642
Leningrad-3 strain 275
Leukemia 328
Leukocyte migration inhibition test 179
Linked-epitope suppression 236
Lipoidal biocarriers 572
Live viral vaccine 42f, 529
   measles vaccine 261
Liver disease, chronic 89, 309
Low birth weight
   babies 209
   infants 293

Lower respiratory infection, acute 541
Lymph node 181
   activation 13
Lymphocytic choriomeningitis virus 578
Lymphoid tissue, mucosa-associated 662
Lymphoreticular tissue, nasopharyngeal-associated 664
L-zagreb strain 275

M

Macrophages 3
Malaria 509
   control and prevention 510
   Elimination Program 509
   elimination, technical strategy for 509
   Policy Advisory Committee 515
   transmission 512
Malaria vaccine 509, 510
   development 511, 512
   explored for 512b
   Implementation Programme 517
   initiative 511
   timeline of 511t
   types of 512
Master cell bank 134
Maternal antibody 11, 16, 42f
   concentrations 246
   influence 16, 41
Measles 12, 35, 111
   hepatitis, and varicella 11
   modified 259
   risk for 716
   vaccines against 45
   virus, strains of 261
Measles and rubella 66, 69, 71, 72fc, 724
   elimination 68
   initiative 268
   surveillance project 73fc
   vaccination program 263
   vaccine 152, 274
Measles vaccination 262
   adverse reactions of 261
   contraindications of 261
   regular 260
   schedule of 261
Measles vaccine 162, 259-261, 263
   role of 263
Measles, mumps and rubella 55, 111, 152, 261, 264, 266, 269, 271-274, 276-278, 315, 683, 716, 730
   and varicella 317, 519, 521, 730
      vaccines 279
   dose of 274, 269, 271
   third dose 269
   vaccination 272

vaccine 43, 46, 59, 60, 266, 267, 270t, 271, 273, 274, 276-278, 683, 693, 702
    doses of 272, 276
Membrane vesicles 352, 483, 593, 642
Memory B cell 15, 236, 449
    hallmarks of 19
Menacwy vaccines 489
Meningitis 268
Meningococcal conjugate 12
    vaccine 481, 482, 576, 692
Meningococcal disease 642, 703
Meningococcal polysaccharide vaccine 482
Meningococcal recombinant protein vaccines 481
Meningococcal serogroup B vaccines 489
Meningococcal vaccination 487
Meningococcal vaccine 11, 481, 487, 488, 680, 688, 694, 718, 730, 731
Meningococci, types of 481
Meningococcus 693
Meningoencephalitis 219
Merozoite surface protein-1 vaccines 513
Messenger ribonucleic acid 468, 561, 631, 632
    vaccines 561
        types of 561
Metered-dose inhaler 330
Micro-ribonucleic acid 187
Middle ear infection 259
Middle east respiratory syndrome 632
    coronavirus 643
Miliary tuberculosis 177
Ministry of Health and Family Welfare 145
Monocytes 3, 13
    epigenetic reprogramming of 187f
Moraxella catarrhalis 371
Mouse brain 414
Mucosal adjuvants 664
Mucosal immunity 213, 572
Multiepitope fusion vaccine 591
Multiple sclerosis 453, 650
Multiple vaccines, administration of 56b
Multivalent combination vaccines 336
Mumps 12, 35, 37, 269, 678
    containing vaccine 268f
    infection 273
    measles rubella 82
    vaccine 275t, 683
    virus 717
Muramyl dipeptide 665
Mutants matter 285
Mutational antigens 634
Mycobacterium
    avium 194
    bovis 196
    intracellulare 194
    marinum 194

tuberculosis 11, 25, 549
    infection 183

N

Nasal mucosa 3
Nasopharyngeal swabs 558
National Drug Regulatory Authority 101
National Immunization Program 164, 229, 373, 385, 436
National Immunization Schedule 44t, 158, 161, 163, 206, 723
National Immunization Technical Advisory Group 145
National Institute for Communicable Diseases 399
National Institute of Virology 67
National Institutes of Health 444
National Technical Advisory Group on Immunization 147, 149
National Vector Borne Disease Control Programme 410, 509
Neisseria meningitidis 10, 89, 642, 718
Neoantigens 648
Neomycin 48
Neonatal immune responses 16
Neonatal sepsis, severe 184
Nephrotic syndrome 330, 370
Nerve tissue vaccine 393
Neuraminidase 462
Neutrophils 3
New pertussis vaccines 247
New vaccine, approval of 136
Noninvasive pneumococcal disease 374
Nonlive vaccines 6
Nonsterile injection, causes of 97b
Nonsteroidal anti-inflammatory drugs 621
Nontuberculous mycobacteria 194
Norovirus 35, 590
Norwalk virus 589
Novel antigen candidate vaccines 593
Novel oral polio vaccine type 2 220
Nucleic acid vaccines 560
Nucleocapsid protein 559

O

Onchocerca volvulus 664
Optimal immunization schedules 39
Oral cholera vaccine 495, 688
Oral polio vaccine 16, 82, 156, 178, 182, 199, 200, 201, 207-217, 418, 439, 521, 724, 730
    cessation 215
    contraindications of 201
    doses of 8, 208, 211
    monovalent 200
    side effects of 201

stockpiles 221
trivalent 199
types of 199
Oral poliovirus vaccine 46, 60, 105, 112, 113
Oral rehydration solution 442
Oral sex 284
Orally administered vaccines 49
Orchitis 268
Organ transplants 390
Orthomyxoviridae virus 462
Otitis media 371
    acute 363, 371

P

Pancreatitis 268
Paracetamol 22
Paralytic poliomyelitis, vaccine-associated 201, 202, 210
Paralytic rabies 390
Parasitic infection 195
Paratope 7
Paratyphoid fevers 334*f*
Parenteral vaccines, administration of 49
Parkinson's disease 650
Passive neonatal immunity 703
Passively acquired immunity 119
Pathogen-associated molecular patterns 8
Pediatric dengue vaccines, development of 502
Penta vaccine, dose of 97
Pentamer protein complex 577
Pentameric complex 578
Pentameric vaccines, soluble 579
Pentavalent vaccine 162
Pentaxim 228
Peptide vaccines 602, 651
Pertussis 35, 66, 69-71, 239
    booster 54
    disease 234
    epidemiology of 224
    resurgence 246
    samples 71
    toxin 248
    toxoid 253
    vaccination 230, 249
    vaccine 227, 237, 238*t*, 247, 251*t*
        against 45
        doses of 252
        live attenuated 248
Pet dog, vaccinated 398
Peyer's patches 664
Phagocytic function disorders, primary 77
Pichia pastoris 458
Pivotal trials 423
Placental transfer, percentage of 703*f*
Plasma cells, long-lived 19

Plasmodium falciparum 513
    circumsporozoite protein 512
    bacteria vaccines 513
Pneumococcal conjugates 12
    vaccine 20, 43, 158, 243, 363, 367, 370, 371, 373-377, 379, 380, 383*f*, 385, 693, 705, 724, 725, 730
    against pneumonia 372
Pneumococcal disease 364
    high risk for 380*t*
Pneumococcal pneumonia and mortality, burden of 365
Pneumococcal polysaccharide vaccine 20, 367, 378, 679, 681, 730
Pneumococcal vaccine 84, 158, 680
    candidates 386
Pneumococcus 693
    serotypes of 366
Pneumonia 259, 364*f*
    episodes, severe 365*f*
    rotavirus, measles, mumps and rubella 692
Polio 11, 35, 692, 718
    campaign 212
    eliminated 163
    free status 212
    global eradication of 214
    immunization 206, 207, 209, 218
    like syndrome 219
    outbreak simulation exercise 219
    sabin 12
    salk 12
    transition 220
    vaccination 206, 209
        schedule 207*t*
        status of 718
    vaccine 41, 102, 199, 204-206, 216, 399, 697
        against 45
        inactivated 34, 43, 84, 97, 112, 153, 161, 199, 203, 205, 207-213, 692, 724, 730
        sabin inactivated 216, 217
        schedule 207
        vaccination 206
Poliomyelitis 199
    clinical spectrum of 199*t*
Poliovirus 76
    vaccine
        derived 65, 202, 203, 210
        inactivated 46, 519, 522, 687
Polymerase chain reaction 558
    real-time 67
Polyradiculitis 268
Polyribosylribitol phosphate-outer membrane protein 358
Polysaccharide 12, 339

conjugate vaccines 592
vaccine 10, 14, 335
   unconjugated 481, 482
Population for vaccination 120
Positive rubella titer 272
Postexposure prophylaxis 271, 299*t*, 307, 309, 310, 396, 397*t*, 707
Postexposure vaccination 712
Postpolio eradication strategy 214
Postural orthostatic tachycardia syndrome 453
Post-vaccination
   blood test 284
   serologic testing 714*fc*
Pre-erythrocytic vaccine 512
Pre-exposure prophylaxis 394, 688
   against rabies 396
Pre-exposure vaccination, schedule of 395
Pregnant woman traveler 694
Preservatives, roles of 48
Pretransplant 85
Primary complement deficiency 77
Prophylactic B cell combined vaccines 602
Prophylactic paracetamol 23
Prophylactic T cell combined vaccines 602
Prophylactic vaccine 608*t*
   candidates 608
Prostatic acid phosphatase 649
Protein
   polysaccharide conjugate vaccine 339, 339*t*
   subunit 571
   vaccines 483
Pseudomonas aeruginosa 340
Psoriasis 650
Pulmonary tuberculosis 177, 183, 549
Pulse
   Immunization Program 218
   oral polio vaccine 218
   polio immunization 218
Purified chick embryo cell vaccine 394
Purified formalin inactivated vaccine 615
Purified protein derivative 179
Purified vero cell rabies vaccine 394

Q

Quadrivalent conjugate 702
Quadrivalent influenza vaccine 466
Quarantine 120

R

Rabies 12, 679, 692, 719
   higher risk for 391
   immunoglobulin 392, 393
   monoclonal antibodies 392
   period of 390

postexposure treatment 398
tissue culture vaccines 399
transmission of 389
types of 390
vaccinated against 695
vaccination 400
   prophylaxis of 394
   route of 401
vaccine 389, 401, 402, 688, 730
virus 390
Randomized controlled trial 454, 565
Rapid fluorescent focus inhibition test 399
Recombinant vaccines, live 572
Refrigerator, purpose-built 106*f*
Renal failure, chronic 370
Resistant pathogens, surveillance of 367
Respiratory infections, acute 464
Respiratory syncytial virus 26, 188, 541, 560, 703
   burden of 541
   infection, risk factors of 541
   vaccine 541, 543
      snapshot of 544*t*
      strategies 542
Retinoblastoma 634
Rheumatic diseases, chronic 89
Rheumatoid arthritis 650
Ribonucleic acid 302, 462, 463, 502, 558, 559, 599, 629
   vaccine, modified 615
Roseola 259
Rotavirus 12, 43, 436, 588, 725
   disease 434, 435
   gastroenteritis 435
      severe 435, 438*t*
   infection 434
   serotypes 441
   vaccination 441, 442, 444
      guidelines for 443
   vaccine 41, 158, 434, 435, 437, 438*t*, 439-441, 443, 724
      adverse effects of 440
      doses of 438
      preterm babies receive 439
Rubella 12, 35, 111, 259
   titer, negative 272
   vaccination
      certificate 684
      role for 717
   vaccine 278, 684
Rubini strain 275

S

Saccharomyces cerevisiae 288, 514
Safe injection practices 48

Safe vaccine storage 109
Salmonella
   enterica 337
     minnesota 661, 665
     typhi 8, 10, 34, 120, 718
       strain 336
     typhimurium 607
Scar formation 180, 182
Sclerosing panencephalitis, subacute 262
Seasonal flu vaccines 474f
Seizures 259
Sentinel and population-based surveillance 65f
Sentinel surveillance 64
Serious side effects 485
Seroconversion rates 349
Serum
   immunoglobulin 54
   specimen testing protocol 73fc
Severe acute respiratory syndrome 121, 691
   coronavirus 2 26, 35, 188, 558, 559, 632
Sexual transmission 282
Sexually transmitted diseases 447
Shigella
   flexneri 184
   infection 592
   sonnei 592
Shigellosis 592
Sick child 58
Sickle cell disease 86, 379
Smallpox 35
Solid organ transplant 85, 576
Spirit test 400
Staphylococcus aureus 588, 665
Stem cell harvest 85
Strengthen polio 215
Streptococcus
   group B 703
   pneumoniae 10, 78, 363, 372
Streptomycin sulfate 48
Superfluous antigen, administration of 522
Swachh Bharat Abhiyan 335
Synthetic flu vaccines 468
Synthetic influenza vaccines 469
Synthetic peptide vaccines 584

T

T cell 607
   dependent 10
     antigens 14
   independent immune 10
   receptor 5
   response, vaccine with 601
T lymphocyte 24
   activation pathway 9f
   defects 77

Tetanus 11
   immune globulin 255
   neonatal 66, 69, 71
   protein 359
   single-antigen 255
   vaccine 45, 152
Tetanus and diphtheria 43, 46, 163, 519, 679, 730
   and acellular pertussis, dose of 256
   and pertussis 576
   vaccine 679, 706f
Tetanus, diphtheria and acellular pertussis 519, 678, 679, 692, 730
   products 254
   vaccination 249
   vaccine 237, 245, 256, 692
Tetanus toxoid 54, 60, 102, 105, 111-113, 152, 253, 340, 723
   vaccine 706f
Tetravalent dengue vaccines, live attenuated 503f
T-helper cell type 233
Therapeutic cancer vaccines 647-650
Therapeutic vaccination 553, 616
Therapeutic vaccine 459, 608t, 647, 651
   current status of 650
   pipeline 2019 653t
   status of 651
Thimerosal causes autism 278
Thrombospondin-related adhesive protein 512
   vaccine 513
Tick-borne
   encephalitis 432, 703
   fever 640
Tissue culture vaccine 394, 397
Toll-like receptors 8
Towne vaccine 577
Towne-toledo chimera vaccines 577
Toxic shock syndrome 262
Tracheal cytotoxin 248
Trained immunity 185
Trained innate immunity 25f, 186f, 187f
Transcriptase-polymerase chain reaction, reverse 466, 526, 557, 559
Transverse myelitis 268
Tuberculosis 12, 66, 70, 162, 549, 657
   disease 550
   incidence, estimate of 29f
   protection against 184
   types of 177
   vaccine 190, 551
     newer 549
Tumor
   antigens 647
   necrosis factor 26, 188
     alpha 347

Twinrix™ vaccine 308*t*
Typhoid 80, 333, 679, 718
   conjugate 12
      vaccine 335, 339, 341*t*, 342*t*, 729
   fever 334*f*, 335, 349, 692
      status of 333
   immunity 347
   vaccine 333, 335*f*, 353*b*, 682, 695, 718
      inactivated 84
      types of 335, 336*t*

U

United Nations International Children's Emergency Fund 146
United States Food and Drug Administration 523
Universal flu vaccine 469, 470
Universal immunization 301
Universal Immunization Program 148, 151, 158, 224, 268, 412, 436, 438, 443, 471, 716
Universal influenza vaccine 469, 470, 470*b*
Upper respiratory tract infection 58, 498

V

Vaccinating Healthcare professionals with flu vaccine, advantages of 714
Vaccination 75, 82, 101
   contraindications to 486
   dose and route of 527
   epidemiology in 28
   in adolescents 552
   in adults 552
   in infants 552
   in special situations 75
   instructions for 48
   issues of 81
   practice of 48
   program 30
   role of gender-neutral 451
   routine 429, 679
   schedule 39, 156, 398
      of routine 53*b*, 289
Vaccine 84, 91, 131*f*, 170*b*, 595, 723, 727
   administration of 44
   adverse effects of 596
   all-in-one 22
   approval 137*t*
      permission of 134
   attenuated 8, 577
   available 481
   brands 91
   candidates 505
   carriers 115

   characteristics 22
   clinical development of 125
   communication, reframing of 171
   confidence 102
   conjugate 359
   contents in 527
   current status of 597
   delivery, methods of 536
   derived polio viruses 163
   development of 124, 126, 127*f*, 129, 129*t*, 571
      roadmap of 124*t*
   doses of 14, 41, 56*b*
      and schedule of 595
   efficacy 30, 452*t*
      estimates 419*t*
   egg-based 467
   egg-derived 468
   failure 290
      causes of 314
   formation of 596
   handling of 58
   hesitancy 103, 167, 169-172
      communication 171*b*
      spectrum 168*f*
      types of 167
   immunity 102, 234
   immunogenicity 30
      role in 8
   immunology of 3, 4
   in pipeline 496, 535, 539
   inactivated 8
   induced immunity, correlates of 12*t*
   interchangeably 455
   licensing of 124
   lightsensitive 111
   like particles 470
   live 8, 13, 15, 82*t*, 327, 704
      attenuated 585, 591, 592
   manufacturing 129
   maternal 700
   newer generations of 507
   non-live 83*t*
   performance of 6
   poxvirus-based 432
   preventable disease 17, 62, 90, 154, 161, 267
   product-related reaction 94
   protection of 596
   quality defect-related reaction 94
   reaction, type of 97
   refrigerator 110
   responses, effectors of 11
   safe 101, 709
   safety testing of 126*f*

schedules 158
sensitivities 112*t*
side effects of 313
simultaneous 519
single-antigen 296
storage 58, 107, 108
    domestic refrigerator for 107*f*
    equipment 105
subunit 560
third-generation 629
transmission-blocking 514
types of 304, 401, 437, 526, 584
    combination 519
    inactivated 304
use to store 108
vaccination schedule for nonlive 17
vectored 579
vial monitor 273
    stage of 201
with humoral immune response 602
Vaccine-derived poliovirus
    circulating 203
    types of 203
Vaccine-preventable disease 67, 69*t*
    surveillance 62
        types of 64
Vaccinia ankara virus, modified 653
Vaccinia virus
    herpes, and influenza 184
    modified 652
Varicella 54, 80, 111, 273, 327, 329, 679, 717
    breakthrough 313, 315
    immunization 326
    vaccination 318, 325
    vaccine 312, 316, 320, 321*t*, 325-330, 683, 717
        contagiousness of 329
        content of 312
        efficacy of 313
Varicella zoster 63
    immune globulin 327, 328
    virus 312
Venous thromboembolism 453
Verbal autopsy 99
Vertical transmission 282
Vibrio cholera 491, 588
    types of 492
VI-CPS vaccines, limitations of 338*b*
Viral infections 35
Viral pandemics 25
Virosomes 665

Virus
    like particles 12, 502, 572, 584, 609, 665
    vaccine, replication-defective 579
    vectors 665
Vitamin A 165, 725
Vomiting 97
Vomits dose 439
Vulvar intraepithelial neoplasia 451

W

West Nile
    fever 640
    viruses 432
Whole virus vaccines 560
Whole-cell cholera vaccine 494
Whole-cell pertussis 50, 84
    vaccine 230, 238*t*
Whole-limb swelling 240
Whooping cough 101
Wild polio 211
    eradication of 214
    transmission 213
    virus 203, 215
Wild virus 577
Working cell bank 134
World Health Organization 78, 549, 594, 711
Wound
    management, part of 255
    suturing of 401

Y

Yellow fever 525, 525*f*, 526, 679, 688, 692, 703
    symptoms of 526
    vaccinated against 719
    vaccination 530
    vaccine for 525, 526, 730, 731
    virus 525
Young age immunization 15, 17

Z

Zika 35
    fever 611
Zika virus 525, 611, 613
    infection 611, 612*f*, 613, 697
        epidemiology of 611
    live attenuated 615
    structure of 612, 612*f*
    vaccine 611, 614*t*
        developing 616

Other Best-selling Books

IAP TEXTBOOK OF VACCINES

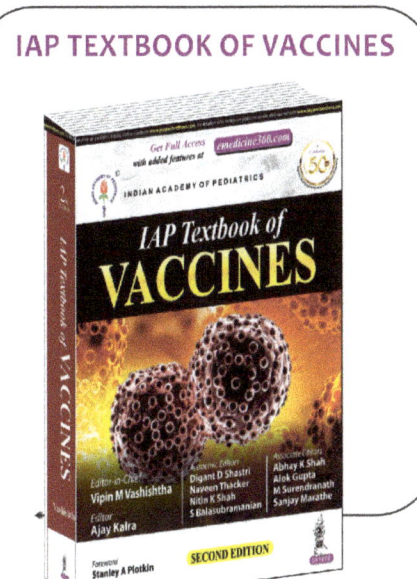

Vipin M Vashishtha, *et al.*

Two Colour | Soft Cover | 2/e, 2020
8.5" x 11" | 900 Pages | 9789352709892

- A comprehensive textbook on vaccines and immunization practices from Indian Academy of Pediatrics
- Around 80 state-of-the-art chapters on basic and advanced vaccinology
- Authored by more than 80 national and international experts of repute
- Five sections covering comprehensively all the facets of contemporary vaccinology from general aspects of vaccination to vaccines in development and new vaccine strategies
- Provides in-depth information to the professionals working in the field of vaccination in India and neighboring south central and south eastern Asian countries
- Special emphasis to disease epidemiology and vaccine needs of India and neighboring countries
- A reference material for international health agencies, vaccine developers, national immunization program managers, vaccine-funding agencies, etc.
- Special foreword by legendary, Dr Stanley A Plotkin, the father of modern vaccinology.

CASE BASED REVIEWS IN PEDIATRIC INFECTIOUS DISEASES

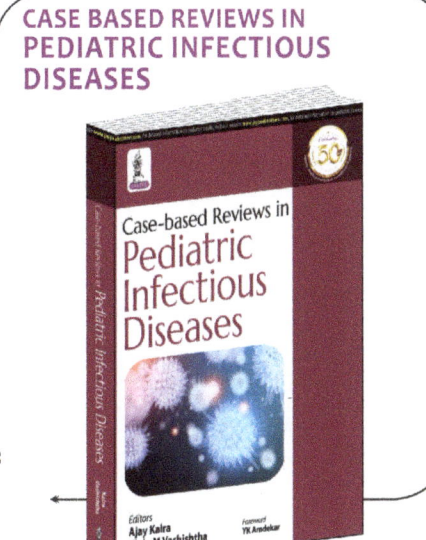

Ajay Kalra, *et al.*

Two Colour | Soft Cover | 1/e, 2021
6.75" x 9.5" | 238 Pages | 9789352706730

- Comprehensive coverage of all aspects of pediatric infectious diseases in a crisp and to-the-point format
- The book has been divided into 24 chapters on various infectious diseases
- Every chapter begins with a case and followed by how-to-do-it right approach for managing the patient
- Each chapter is supported by a take home message that summarizes the discussion
- Written by experts with extensive research and clinical experience
- The book is a valuable resource for pediatricians, physicians and postgraduate students.

JAYPEE
The Health Sciences Publisher

Please visit our website
www.jaypeebrothers.com or Scan the QR Code

www.ingramcontent.com/pod-product-compliance
Ingram Content Group UK Ltd.
Pitfield, Milton Keynes, MK11 3LW, UK
UKHW051433250425
457755UK00002BA/3